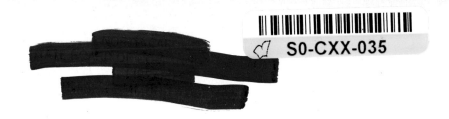
Mental Health and Illness

A Textbook for Students
of
Health Sciences

Mental Health and Illness

A Textbook for Students
of
Health Sciences

Editors

Robert Kosky
BSc, MD, FRANZCP

Hadi Salimi Eshkevari
MD, DPM, MRCPsych

Vaughan Carr
MD, FRCP(C), FRANZCP

Butterworth-Heinemann

Sydney Oxford Boston Guildford London Munich
New Delhi Singapore Tokyo Toronto Wellington
1991

National Library of Australia
Cataloguing-in-Publication entry

Kosky, Robert J.
    Mental health and illness.

    Includes index.
    ISBN 0 409 30139 6.

    1. Mental health. 2. Psychiatry. I. Salimi Eshkevari,
    Hadi. II. Carr, Vaughan. III. Title.

616.89

Typeset in Times Roman and Optima by Midland Typesetters, Maryborough, Victoria

Printed in Australia by Macarthur Press

Acknowledgments

We would like to thank our distinguished contributors for their invaluable efforts in writing the chapters in this textbook.

We are indebted to Mr John Coxhill, Manager, Butterworth-Heinemann, and Ms Eve Ross, Publishing Manager, Manuscripts, and other staff.

Our special thanks go to Mrs Avril Easton, book editor, without whose impetus and skilful sub-editing this work could not have been finished so quickly.

We would like to thank Mrs Barbara Wood, secretary, for her sterling effort in typing manuscripts. Finally, we thank other secretaries and staff for their enthusiastic help.

10 January 1991   *R Kosky*
H Salimi Eshkevari
V Carr

Contents

		Page
Acknowledgments		*v*
Preface		*xiii*
Contributors		*xv*

Part 1
History

| 1 | A Brief History of Mental Health Services in Australia and New Zealand
R Pargiter | 3 |

Part 2
Normal Development

2	The Developing Child *H Salimi Eshkevari*	15
3	Pregnancy, Birth and Parenthood *J Condon*	40
4	Adolescent Development *J Jureidini*	49
5	Middle and Later Life *F Hughes and S Ticehurst*	57
6	Neglect and Abuse of Children *P Hazell*	62
7	Death, Disharmony and Divorce *C Tennant*	67
8	Fostering and Adoption *R Kosky and H Salimi Eskhevari*	73

Part 3
Disorders of Development

| 9 | Mental Retardation
H Moloney | 81 |

10   Pervasive Developmental Disorders
     H Salimi Eshkevari   88

11   Learning Disabilities
     H Salimi Eshkevari   93

12   Encopresis
     R Kosky   98

13   Nocturnal Enuresis
     J Bollard   101

14   Personality Disorders
     J Grigor   106

Part 4
Assessment and Classification

15   Interviewing 1: Children
     G Carter   115

16   Interviewing 2: Adults
     R Goldney   121

17   Classification: General
     G Mellsop   129

18   Classification: Childhood and Adolescence
     J Rey   132

19   Biological Investigations
     J Kulkarni, D Copolov and N Keks   136

20   Neurological Investigations
     R Burns   143

21   Brain Imaging in Psychiatry
     E Gordon and D Copolov   146

22   Psychological Testing
     A Gannoni   152

Part 5
Psychiatric Syndromes

23   Disruptive Behaviour in Children and Adolescents
     J Rey and D Blyth   161

24   Attention Deficit Hyperactivity Disorder
     F Levy   167

25   Developmental Aspects of Emotional Disorder in Children and Adolescents
     R Kosky   171

26 School Refusal
    S Ward   180

27 Anxiety Disorders
    L Evans and F Judd   184

28 Affective (Mood) Disorders
    P Joyce   190

29 Suicidal Behaviour
    R Goldney   199

30 Obsessive Compulsive Disorders 1: Children
    F Levy   208

31 Obsessive Compulsive Disorders 2: Adults
    N McConaghy   210

32 Psychoses in Adolescence
    R Kosky and B Waters   214

33 Schizophrenia
    V Carr   220

34 Pain: Psychiatric Aspects
    I Pilowsky   231

35 Post-traumatic Stress Disorder
    A McFarlane   236

36 Eating Disorders
    A Hall   241

37 Obesity
    A Hall   247

38 Problems of Psycho-sexual Development and Function
    B Boman   250

39 The Psychiatry of Late Life
    S Ticehurst   256

40 Dementia
    S Ticehurst   266

41 Delirium
    S Ticehurst   272

42 Alcohol Dependence and Related Problems
    R Pols   276

43 Other Substances Abuse
    R Pols   287

Part 6
Community

44   Community Psychiatry
     G Smith and M Harries   297

45   Aboriginal Mental Health
     E Hunter   305

46   Remote Australia
     H Connell   313

47   Multicultural Psychiatry: General Considerations
     G Boranga   320

48   Emergencies
     A Davis   328

49   Forensic Psychiatry
     J Grigor   335

50   Mental Health Acts
     J Durham   345

Part 7
Contemporary Issues

51   A Feminist Perspective
     L Achimovich   361

52   Immunology and Mental Illness
     D Silove   365

53   AIDS 1: In Children and Adolescents
     B Waters and J Ziegler   370

54   AIDS 2: In Adults
     F Judd and B Biggs   377

55   A Parent's Loss: The Sudden Infant Death Syndrome
     S Beal   383

Part 8
Treatment

56   Medication 1: In Children and Adolescents
     B Waters   389

57   Medication 2: In Adults
     T Stedman and H Whiteford   395

58   Psychotherapy
     V Carr   400

59 Family Therapy 1: General Considerations
    P Hazell   408

60 Family Therapy 2: Clincial Aspects
    C Quadrio   412

61 Behaviour Therapy
    A Gannoni   419

62 Hypnosis
    F Judd and G Burrows   423

63 Nursing for Mental Health
    M Clinton   427

64 Social Work
    R Bland   433

65 Occupational Therapy
    A Passmore   438

66 Speech Therapy 1: Children
    K Robinson, S Hogben and K Eddy   447

67 Speech Therapy 2: Adults
    J Hooper   452

68 Prevention
    R Kosky   460

Part 9
Research

69 Epidemiology 1: Child and Adolescent Disorders
    M Sawyer and P Baghurst   471

70 Epidemiology 2: Adult Disorders
    P Joyce and M Oakley-Browne   476

71 Statistical Inference in Psychiatry
    W Hall and K Bird   480

Index   491

Authors' note

There is no accepted genderless pronoun in English. Therefore, throughout the text we have used 'he' and 'his' where either the masculine or feminine pronoun would be appropriate. This is not an expression of prejudice but a convention to facilitate a simple writing style. Where, however, the masculine pronoun would be inappropriate, the feminine pronoun has been used.

Preface

There have been many exciting developments in the field of mental health in Australia and New Zealand over recent years. What was the exclusive province of medical practitioners and asylum attendants at the beginning of the century slowly broadened to include, first, the nursing profession and then the discipline of psychology. Since the Second World War the field has opened up more dramatically, particularly in the last 25 years or so to incorporate contributions from several professions, such as social work, occupational therapy and speech pathology. There has also been a concomitant increase in the involvement of volunteers and members of various self-help and support groups. As mental health and illness have become areas of interest and concern to an ever widening range of people, so the clinical task of understanding and treating mental illness is now, more than ever, a multi-disciplinary activity. The aim of this book is to try to bring together contemporary knowledge in psychiatry for people with diverse training backgrounds and skills, particularly those likely to participate in the multi-disciplinary management of people with mental illness.

For many students of the health sciences, recent developments in psychiatry can be disorienting, particularly as there are many valid, but sometimes apparently contradictory, pathways to the understanding of mental health and illness. While the collision of ideas and the different perspectives generated by the various disciplines in the field is exciting, and also very promising for future advances at the cutting edge of psychiatry, students new to the subject can become unsure about the nature and basis of clinical practice.

For these reasons, in preparing this book a number of distinguished researchers and clinicians from Australia and New Zealand were asked to provide an account of their current areas of interest and expertise. Mostly, these have come from the disciplines of psychiatry and psychology so there is a bias towards representation of these points of view. However, many of the contributors would regard themselves primarily as clinicians or scientists, able to take a broad view, acknowledging that much recent knowledge informing clinical practice comes from many sources. Ideas and knowledge have been derived from the traditional sciences and mathematics, physiology and psychology. As well, there have been major contributions from such fields as sociology, law, cybernetics, philosophy and so on. The convergence of these lines of knowledge, at the level of the individual clinical encounter or in the interaction between public health administration and the community, entails the integration of these various contributions and their transformation into useful practice to reduce suffering from mental illnesses and to improve mental health.

Not only has the provision of mental health services become an interdisciplinary activity but developments at the research front have increasingly involved collaboration between investigators from different disciplines as well. With the 'team' approach in both clinical practice and research activities, it is even more urgent that integration of the disparate sources of knowledge occur and that an appreciation of their complementarity develops. It is hoped that this book will provide an elementary framework for viewing the field of psychiatry and enable those who work in various disciplines to see more clearly where and how they may make useful contributions.

The book has nine parts and it will be seen at once that these divisions are quite artificial and merely provide one method for the organisation of thinking about mental health and illness. The material in the parts overlap to some degree, as does the material in the individual chapters. For example, treatments will be found both in the part dealing with treatment as well as in the chapters dealing with specific syndromes. Perhaps it is best to look on the parts as each providing a view of the issues of mental health and illness taken from a different perspective, rather like illuminating the same room through different windows. Indeed, this metaphor is also very useful when looking at the contributions to mental health and illness that are made by the various disciplines. Each may be valid in its own right but the illumination of the room provided by one window is limited and needs to be complemented by illumination through other windows.

This is a book for students in nursing, social work, medicine, psychology, occupational therapy, speech pathology, physiotherapy, and other disciplines in schools of health science who will need to know about mental health and who, later, may work with those who suffer from mental illness. We also hope that it will be a useful book for health care administrators, lawyers, pastoral care and other hospital and welfare workers who come into contact with mental health issues and the mentally ill. It is not a text for psychiatrists or trainees in psychiatry. Its contents are a condensation of a fraction of the total knowledge and thinking in contemporary psychiatry. However, in asking our contributors to define their clinical knowledge for students in the disciplines listed above, we hope to have made some of the most useful material accessible to those who will work in mental health-related professions in the future.

August 1990

R Kosky
H Salimi Eshkevari
V Carr

Contributors

Achimovich L	MB BS, FRANZCP Private Practice in Psychiatry, Fremantle, Western Australia, Australia
Baghurst P	PhD Principal Research Scientist, Division of Human Nutrition, CSIRO; Visiting Research Fellow, Department of Psychiatry, University of Adelaide, South Australia, Australia
Beal S	MD Consultant Paediatrician, Adelaide Children's Hospital, South Australia, Australia
Biggs B A	MB BS, FRACP, MRCP Consultant Physician, Fairfield Infectious Diseases Hospital, Melbourne, Victoria, Australia
Bird K D	PhD Senior Lecturer, School of Psychology, University of New South Wales, Australia
Bland R	PhD Lecturer, Department of Social Work, University of Queensland, Australia
Blyth D	B Soc Studies Social Worker, Rivendell Child, Adolescent and Family Services, Royal Prince Alfred Hospital, Sydney, Australia
Bollard J	PhD Clinical Psychologist, Department of Psychiatry, Adelaide Children's Hospital, South Australia, Australia
Boman B	MB BS, PhD, FRANZCP Senior Consultant Psychiatrist, Department of Psychiatry, Repatriation Hospital, Concord, New South Wales, Australia
Boranga G F	MD, FRANZCP Superintendent Psychiatrist, Multicultural Psychiatric Centre, Health Department of Western Australia
Burns R	MB BS, FRACP, FRCP Senior Director of Neurology and Associate Professor of Medicine, Flinders Medical Centre, South Australia, Australia
Burrows G	AO, BSc, MD, DPM, FRANZCP, FRC Psych Professor of Psychiatry, University of Melbourne, Victoria, Australia
Carr V	MD, FRCP(C), FRANZCP Professor of Psychiatry, University of Newcastle, New South Wales, Australia
Carter G	MB BS, FRANZCP Director of Child Psychiatric Services, Division of Mental Health Services, Hunter Area, New South Wales, Australia; Clinical Lecturer, Discipline of Psychiatry, University of Newcastle; Director, Newcastle and Central Coast Post-Graduate Psychiatry Training Association
Clinton M	PhD, BA, RGN, RPN Professor of Nursing and Head, School of Nursing, Queensland University of Technology, Australia

Condon J	MB BS, FRANZCP Senior Consultant Psychiatrist, Repatriation General Hospital, Dow Park, South Australia; and Senior Lecturer, Department of Psychiatry, Flinders University of South Australia, Australia
Connell H	AM, BSC, FRANZCP, FRCPsych Associate Professor in Child Psychiatry, University of Queensland; Director of Postgraduate Studies, Division of Youth Welfare and Guidance, Health Department, Queensland, Australia
Copolov D	MB BS, DPM, PhD, FRANZCP Director, The Mental Health Research Institute of Victoria, Australia
Davis A T	MB BS, FRANZCP Senior Consultant in Psychiatry, Royal Adelaide Hospital, South Australia, Australia
Durham J	MB BS, FRANZCP Director of Psychiatry, St Vincent's Hospital, Sydney, Australia
Eddy K	B App Sc (Sp Path) Speech Pathologist, Division of Child and Adolescent Mental Health Services, Adelaide Children's Hospital, South Australia, Australia
Evans L	MB ChB, FRANZCP, FRCPsych, DPM Associate Professor, University of Queensland, Australia; Head, Anxiety Disorder Clinic, New Farm Clinic, Brisbane, Australia
Gannoni A	BA, M Psych Chief Clinical Psychologist, Department of Psychiatry, Adelaide Children's Hospital, South Australia, Australia
Goldney R	MD, FRANZCP, FRC Psych Clinical Associate Professor, Department of Psychiatry, Flinders University of South Australia; and Senior Visiting Psychiatrist, Glenside Hospital, South Australia, Australia
Gordon E	MB BCh, PhD Senior Lecturer, University of Sydney Cognitive Neuroscience Unit, Westmead Hospital, New South Wales, Australia
Grigor J	MB ChB, FRANZCP, FRCPsych, DPM, Dip Crim Director, Forensic Psychiatry, Health Department, Victoria, Australia
Hall A	MB ChB, FRACP, FRANZCP Associate Professor, Wellington School of Medicine, University of Otago, New Zealand
Hall W	PhD Associate Professor and Deputy Director, National Drug & Alcohol Research Centre, University of New South Wales, Australia
Harries M	BA, M Soc Admin Lecturer, School of Social Work and Social Administration, University of Western Australia, Australia
Hazell P	B Med Sc, MB ChB Lecturer in Psychiatry, University of Newcastle, New South Wales, Australia
Hogben S	B App Sc (Sp Path) Speech Pathologist, Division of Child & Adolescent Mental Health Service, Adelaide Children's Hospital, South Australia, Australia
Hooper J	B App Sc (Sp Path) Chief Speech Pathologist, Queen Elizabeth Hospital, South Australia, Australia
Hughes F	BA MSc Head, Discipline of Psychology, Division of Mental Health Service, Hunter Area Health Service, New South Wales, Australia
Hunter E	MD, MPH, MA, FRANZCP Research Fellow, New South Wales Institute of Psychiatry; and National Drug and Alcohol Research Centre, Sydney, Australia

Joyce P R MB ChB, PhD, FRANZCP Professor, University Department of Psychological Medicine, Christchurch School of Medicine, Christchurch, New Zealand

Judd F K MD, FRANZCP Clinical Associate Professor, University of Melbourne, Department of Psychiatry, Austin Hospital, Victoria, Australia

Jureidini J MB BS, FRANZCP Director, Adolescent Psychiatric Services, Adelaide Children's Hospital; Clinical Lecturer in Psychiatry, University of Adelaide, South Australia, Australia

Keks N MB BS, MPM, FRANZCP Senior Lecturer, Monash University, Department of Psychological Medicine; and Associate Investigator, Mental Health Research Institute, of Victoria, Melbourne, Australia

Kosky R BSc, MD, FRANZCP Professor of Child Psychiatry, University of Adelaide, South Australia, Australia

Kulkarni J MB BS, MPM, FRANZCP Consultant Psychiatrist, Royal Park Psychiatric Hospital, Melbourne; and Associate Investigator, Mental Health Research Institute of Victoria, Australia

Levy F MD, FRANZCP Senior Staff Paediatric Psychiatrist, Avoca Clinic, Department of Child and Adolescent Psychiatry, Prince of Wales Hospital, Sydney, New South Wales, Australia

Molony H MB BCh, DPM, DPH, FRANZCP Consultant Psychiatrist, Department of Developmental Disability, Prince of Wales Hospital, Sydney, New South Wales, Australia

McConaghy N DSc, MD, FRANZCP Associate Professor, University of New South Wales, New South Wales, Australia

McFarlane A MD, FRANZCP Professor of Rehabilitation Psychiatry, University of Adelaide, South Australia, Australia

Mellsop G MD, FRANZCP Professor of Psychological Medicine, Wellington School of Medicine, University of Otago, Wellington, New Zealand

Oakley-Browne M A BSc, MB ChB, FRANZCP Senior Lecturer, Department of Psychological Medicine, Christchurch School of Medicine, Christchurch University, New Zealand

Pargiter R MB BS, FRANZCP Consultant Psychiatrist, Royal Hobart Hospital, Tasmania, Australia; Formerly Archivist, Royal Australian and New Zealand College of Psychiatrists

Passmore A E Grad Dip Hlth Sci, B App Sc, OT Lecturer in Psychosocial Processes, School of Occupational Therapy, Curtin University of Technology, Western Australia, Australia

Pilowsky I MD, DPM, FRACP, FRANZCP, FRC Psych, FASSA Professor and Head, Department of Psychiatry, University of Adelaide, South Australia, Australia

Pols R MB BS, FRANZCP Director, National Centre for Education, Training and Research in Addictions, Flinders University of South Australia, Australia

Quadrio C MB BS, FRANZCP Senior Lecturer, School of Psychiatry, University of New South Wales, Prince of Wales Hospital, New South Wales, Australia

Rey J MB BS, PhD, FRANZCP Director, Rivendell Child, Adolescent and Family Services, Royal Prince Alfred Hospital, New South Wales, Australia

Robinson K   B App Sc (Sp Path) Chief Speech Pathologist, Division of Child and Adolescent Mental Health Services, Adelaide Children's Hospital, South Australia, Australia

Salimi Eshkevari H   MD, DPM, MRCPsych Senior Consultant Psychiatrist, Adelaide Children's Hospital, South Australia, Australia

Sawyer M   MB BS, FRCP(C), FRANZCP Director, Evaluation Unit, Department of Psychiatry, Adelaide Children's Hospital, South Australia, Australia

Silove D   MB ChB, FRANZCP Professor of Psychiatry, University of New South Wales, Australia

Smith G P   MB BS, MRANZCP Principal Policy Consultant, Psychiatric Services, Health Department of Western Australia, Australia

Stedman T J   MB BS, FRANZCP Senior Psychiatrist, Clinical Studies Unit, Wolston Park Hospital; and Hon Senior Lecturer, Department of Psychiatry, University of Queensland, Australia

Tennant C   MPH, MD, FRANZCP, MRCPsych Professor and Head of Department, Sydney University Department of Psychiatry, Royal North Shore Hospital, Sydney, New South Wales, Australia

Ticehurst S   MB BS, FRANZCP Director, Psychogeriatric Service, Division of Mental Health Services, Hunter Area Health Services, New South Wales; and Clinical Lecturer in Psychiatry, University of Newcastle, New South Wales, Australia

Ward S   MB BS, FRANZCP Visiting Psychiatrist, Department of Psychiatry, Adelaide Children's Hospital, South Australia, Australia

Waters B   MD, FRCP(C), FRANZCP, Dip Psych Professor of Child and Adolescent Psychiatry, University of New South Wales, New South Wales, Australia

Whiteford H   MB BS, FRANZCP Director of Psychiatric Services, Queensland Department of Health, Brisbane, Australia

Ziegler J B   MB BS, FRACP Head, Paediatric AIDS Unit, Prince of Wales Childrens' Hospital, Randwick, New South Wales; and Senior Lecturer in Paediatrics, University of New South Wales, Australia

Part 1
History

Chapter 1

A Brief History of Mental Health Services in Australia and New Zealand

R Pargiter

The development of mental health services in Australia is unique. No other modern nation had its origins as a penal colony in an isolated remote and, for Europeans, inhospitable country. The land had already been occupied by people with a culture many thousands of years old. They had some five hundred different clans and tribes with their own ancient systems of managing the sick. It can be said that what we now know as psychiatry was practised in Australia long before its European colonisation in 1788. The intermingling of sickness and its management with basic cultural beliefs characteristic of the aboriginal societies was in contrast to European mechanistic concepts of cause and effect. The European colonists failed to appreciate that the aboriginals' mental and physical health depended on their relationship with their environment and was governed by their sophisticated and complex systems of beliefs.

Not only did the Europeans bring to Australia alcohol and sickness, but they had their fair share of mental illness among both the convicts and their keepers. This quickly became apparent in the fledgling colonies where harsh conditions fostered the development of both physical and mental diseases, accelerated by the early common currency of alcohol.

Mental health services

The first Australian hospitals were nothing but tents and huts and there was little segregation of the physically ill from the mentally sick. It was a matter of chance whether or not the insane were housed in gaols or hospitals and often there was not much difference between the two.

Governor Phillip, founder of the New South Wales colony, had been instructed to provide for lunatics in the same way as they were provided for under the 'Great Seal of Great Britain'. However, in England at the end of the eighteenth century, public inquiries had revealed that the conditions of the men, women and children confined to mad houses in England were uniformly appalling. Moreover, they were the object of exploitation and public derision. In one year, late in the eighteenth century, the foremost mad house in London, Bethlem, had 96,000 public visitors, each of whom paid one penny to witness the inmates 'at play'. The King himself had not been spared brutalising treatments when, in 1790, he became temporarily insane.

Many people, professional, religious and philanthropically-minded lay persons, sought a new way of dealing with the insane. In 1806, D D Davis, a physician to the Sheffield General Infirmary, United Kingdom, translated Pinel's 'Treatise on Insanity' into English and this book, outlining a treatment of non-restraint, validation of the human qualities of the insane and rational treatments, became available to the British medical profession. At the same time, the work of the Quaker family Tuke at their Retreat for their insane brethren at York became widely publicised. Many visitors to the Retreat marvelled at the apparently free atmosphere and the dignity and humanity of the staff. Patients would be invited to meals with the staff and restraint was rarely used. The idea of a retreat or an asylum for the insane where they could be both treated with dignity and subjected to corrective rational treatment (the moral treatment) rapidly spread throughout Britain.

These developments influenced the first attempts in the New South Wales colony to create a mental health service. While at first the mentally ill were housed in gaols or sheds, early colonial governors sought to develop asylums for various disadvantaged groups of people—orphans, the destitute and the mentally incapacitated. The first asylum for the insane was opened at Castle Hill in Sydney in 1811. The first important superintendent of a lunatic asylum in Sydney was Digby. He was a lay person who, with his wife, had come from England where he was well versed in the principles of the Tuke's Retreat. He attempted to establish the Tarban Creek Asylum along the lines of the Retreat and, although dogged by financial insecurity, was judged to be relatively successful in maintaining a reasonable establishment with a minimum of restraint.

Around 1848, however, anonymous articles began to appear in the Sydney newspapers accusing Digby and his wife of poor management of Tarban Creek. About this time in Britain, the asylum movement had come under the control of the medical profession who were anxious to try to establish a scientific basis for mental illness. The real argument against Digby and his wife seemed to be that because of their lack of medical qualifications and scientific training they were unable to classify the conditions they dealt with or describe their natural history. After an inquiry Digby was dismissed and Campbell, a medical graduate from Edinburgh, was appointed as superintendent. He began to keep meticulous clinical notes which are still available today. Digby became the senior warden. This arrangement established the medical and 'nursing' systems for the asylums and was copied everywhere throughout the colonies.

The rapid development of asylums by way of increase in number and size, characteristic of the British mental health scene between 1850 and 1920, was reflected also in the Dominions. In some ways it was made more intense in the Australian colonies because of the explosive population growth largely due to development of the agricultural industry and the discovery of gold. The populations of Victoria and New South Wales trebled in a single decade between 1850 and 1860. The strain on all community services was intense.

The asylum systems became so complex and scandals so numerous that in most colonies Commissions were established to oversee the operations of the asylum services. In 1881 in New South Wales 2.84 per thousand of the population were resident in asylums. The Commissions were eventually replaced by bureaucracies headed by a medical practitioner variably entitled Director or Inspector General of the Insane, many of whom were bravely outspoken and introduced many necessary reforms. Federation of the Commonwealth in 1901 had little effect on the various mental health services since under the new Constitution health remained a State responsibility.

The impact of two world wars on psychiatry was immense. The establishment of the Repatriation Commission during the First World War (now Department of Veteran Affairs) and its mental hospitals in 1915 provided the first nationally unified system of mental hospitals. The psychiatric morbidity of war was acknowledged by governments and specialised hospitals, outpatient and inpatient units grew up to manage war trauma and for many years provided the best psychiatric services available in Australia.

The Australasian Association of Psychiatrists was founded in 1946 and the first report on psychiatric services nationwide was circulated by this Association in 1950. Although this report concentrated largely on the poor physical state and the obvious overcrowding of State mental hospitals it also addressed the needs of psychogeriatric, child psychiatric and intellectually handicapped services.

In 1950, Cunningham Dax, chairman of the Mental Hygiene Authority of Victoria, showed the then Prime Minister of Australia, Robert Menzies, the appalling conditions at the Kew Cottages for intellectually handicapped people. As a result, the Federal Minister of

Health commissioned Stoller and Arscott to report on 'Mental Health Facilities and Needs of Australia'. Their report was published in 1955. It is a comprehensive report which left no doubt as to the poor state of mental health services throughout Australia. Their final remarks commented on the gross overcrowding. This was virtually the only matter on which the Commonwealth Government took action by providing grants to the States to extend, rebuild and replace the worst of their mental hospitals. Ironically, within a few years, the psychopharmacological revolution and more active rehabilitation approach led to the gradual reduction of patients resident in mental hospitals, many of which then became redundant. Other recommendations in the Stoller Report concerned the needs to provide community services, improve standards, expand professional staff, and the need for research.

While the Commonwealth Government under Menzies took responsibility for the state of higher education in Australia and financed the development of universities, no real support was provided to the States for health matters. In particular, under the voluntary health insurance scheme then operating, the chronically mentally ill were severely disadvantaged, since insurance was not usually available to them. This meant a significant burden of caring for these people was placed on the State mental health systems. The mainstay of that care has continued to be the State asylums up to the present time. The disadvantaged position of the chronically mentally ill has continued under the national health insurance schemes—the various Medicare systems have led to the anomalous situation where mentally ill people treated in general hospitals have health insurance status and those treated in the State mental hospitals do not. In 1988, Eisen and Wolfenden were asked to prepare a national mental health services policy for consideration by the Australian Minister for Health. Their report points to considerable deficiencies in both Commonwealth and State mental health services despite an estimated total expenditure of $2745.5m. Their report and recommendation will be made available for wide consultation with various interested parties.

Australian States and New Zealand

For 130 years following the colonisation of New South Wales, the history of mental health services in that State was virtually that of the lunatic asylum, always starved of funds and subject to scandal. Initially the control of the asylums and the care of the inmates were in lay hands but this situation gave rise to many bitter conflicts. By 1849 medical administration became the rule. Many of the medical administrators were significant figures. Far sighted and brave Norton Manning, the New South Wales Inspector General of the Insane from 1878 to 1898, was held in high public esteem and this helped break down the barriers between the community and asylum. He instituted many reforms, carried out research, established statistical baselines, set up outpatient clinics and endeavoured to make psychiatry into a medical science with an academic basis.

The second colony to be founded, Tasmania, developed on similar lines to New South Wales with the same problems of lack of funds, no segregation of criminals from the insane, and the lingering legacy of convict transportation which eventually centred around Port Arthur. The ill, the infirm and the invalids were scattered about the colony. Accommodation for the insane in 1806 was in tents and huts. By 1811 they were being lodged in houses and in the newly built colonial hospital. In 1823 a start was made on a 'barracks for invalids' some 37 kilometres up the River Derwent from the capital Hobart. It did not take its first insane patient until 1829 and remained a mixed institution before becoming exclusively a mental hospital in 1848. It went through the customary vicissitudes but better management was attained by the appointment of public spirited commissioners, one of whom was the renowned Roman Catholic Bishop Willson who stood up for the rights of the mentally ill and their humane management. Slowly the hospital developed into the Lachlan Park Hospital and the Royal Derwent Hospital.

Until 1839 Victoria was under the jurisdiction of New South Wales. In 1848 the first of the many lunatic asylums in Victoria was opened at Yarra Bend. As each of the colonies developed so did their asylums with their location often dictated by economic forces. In Victoria in the late nineteenth century this was the Gold Rush. Asylums were built on the gold fields at Ararat and Beechworth where they remain today. Victoria had its great administrators, Beattie Smith, Ernest Jones and Springthorpe, the first becoming, like Norton Manning, one of the first private alienists (psychiatrists). He advocated psychiatric nurse training and the use of female nurses on male wards. Jones was influenced by eugenics and advocated segregation of the intellectually handicapped.

South Australia was established as a free colony without the problems of mentally ill convicts; nevertheless, there were in South Australia many difficulties similar to those in the 'penal' colonies. The colonial authorities attempted to remedy these in a unique manner for Australia at that time—by privatisation. A private mental hospital was established in 1841 with a government contract to accommodate the insane. It failed financially so the insane were again lodged in gaols and in two rented houses, until the completion of the Parkside Hospital (later renamed Glenside Hospital) in 1870. Enfield Receiving House, which could take voluntary patients, was opened in 1922.

Queensland started as a penal outpost of New South Wales and remained under its jurisdiction until 1859. Initially the mentally ill were housed in gaols, general hospitals or sent to New South Wales. Woogaroo Lunatic Asylum (later to become the Goodna Hospital) was opened in 1864. It was dogged throughout by scandal, maladiminstration and overcrowding which culminated in a Royal Commission in 1915. It was not until 1918 that early treatment facilities were available at the Brisbane General Hospital.

Early psychiatry in Western Australia is notable in that the first recorded insane patient was a medical practitioner who was confined in a wrecked ship. From 1831 both prisoners and lunatics were lodged in the Round House—a fort. The impetus to build an asylum arose from the increased prevalence of mental illness following the introduction of the convict system in 1850. The large Fremantle asylum took its first patient in 1857. There-

after the pattern of development of mental health services followed that of other States but was delayed by a slower economic development. The replacement for the Fremantle Asylum, Claremont, was not opened until 1903. The Perth Public Hospital was the first general hospital in Australia to open a ward for psychiatric patients in 1908 but this was, unfortunately, replaced by the Heathcote Reception House in 1929.

The development of mental health services in New Zealand should have differed from that of the Australian colonies because it did not start as a penal colony and always had a central system of government. Unfortunately, the pattern of early development is distressingly familiar with inappropriate housing and detention of the mentally ill in gaols and chronicles of scandal, overcrowding and financial stringency in asylums. Ironically, New Zealand was a pioneer nation in social welfare. In 1844 a pauper lunatic asylum was attached to the Wellington gaol. In 1851 there was a public appeal to build a lunatic asylum in Auckland. This opened in 1853, followed by another in Wellington in 1854. Not to be outdone Christchurch and Dunedin opened their asylums in 1863. There was a second asylum opened in Auckland in 1867. The Seacliff Mental Hospital outside Dunedin was opened in 1878. This rapid growth of asylums to some extent reflects that of the population itself which rose from approximately one hundred thousand in 1861 to seven hundred and seventy thousand in 1901.

Early treatment methods

The colonists brought with them all the problems of the old world and some of their solutions. The practices characteristic of Eighteenth Century Bedlam (the Bethlem Royal Hospital, United Kingdom) of restraint, purging, bleeding, emesis and blistering were partly derived from the ancient theory of Galen's Humoral pathology which was known to the early colonists. However, the first superintendent of the early Tarban Creek Asylum in New South Wales, Mr Digby, had worked with the Tuke family in the Quaker Asylum at York. He introduced principles of non-restraint and ideas of dignity and rational order which were associated with the moral treatments introduced by Pinel in France and the Tukes in England. His influence was, however, limited.

After 1850 the treatments of restraint were modified and supplemented by hydrotherapy (alternating hot and cold baths or showers), primitive forms of electrotherapy and, most significantly, synthesised drugs such as the bromides, chloral hydrate and paraldehyde. Individual psychotherapy had little place in overall asylum management.

Alongside these more humane developments, were others, less constructive, which resulted from the beginnings of modern pathology. Together with misinterpretations of Darwinism, some of these early biological ideas led to the opinion, widely held, that insane persons represented instances of mental degeneracy, an evolutionary line destined for extinction, and that mental illness itself was a manifestation of some yet to be identified underlying brain disease which was irreversible. Naturally, such theories led to therapeutic nihilism. To some extent these views were fostered by what was then known about generalised paralysis of the insane (GPI) with its inexorable progress of mental and physical dissolution leading to death. Yet, ironically, it was from experiments in the management of this disease, together with the growth of the psychoanalytic movement, which led to the modern therapeutic revolution.

The discovery that GPI was due to tertiary neurosyphilis led to the first truly rational physical treatment for a syndrome characterised by mental phenomena, viz malarial therapy. The deliberate and risky innoculation of malarial parasites into patients with GPI to produce fever was used in Victoria and New Zealand in 1924 and New South Wales in 1926. The fever temporarily arrested the disease progress. This treatment was rendered obsolete with the introduction of penicillin. The pursuit of physical treatments for mental illness led to deep insulin coma treatment for schizophrenia. This was introduced into Victoria and New Zealand in 1938. Electro convulsive therapy was used in Australia and New Zealand in the early 1940s and, of the original physical treatments, it is the only one

which has remained in common use.

Pre-frontal leucotomy for mental illness was performed in New Zealand in 1942 and Victoria in 1943. Victoria and New South Wales both developed specialised psycho-surgery units but the number of operations done over the last two decades has dwindled to a mere trickle.

The introduction of these rationally based physical treatments raised the morale of nurses and doctors treating the mentally ill. Theirs became a more respectable vocation and it began to attract those who saw in the speciality a major modern challenge. John Cade introduced *lithium* treatment for mania in Australia in 1949. Rather belatedly this became the standard prophylactic treatment of manic depressive psychosis. Cade's discovery antedated the second major development in psychopharmacology by three years when Delay, Deniker and Harl in 1952 reported on the first truly antipsychotic drug, chlorpromazine. Since its introduction there has been a flood of psychotropic drugs available for use in therapy. Their advent was probably the single greatest factor affecting the contemporary management of the severely mentally ill. Along with the antidepressant drugs which quickly followed the antipsychotics, the population of mental hospitals was at lease halved. These drugs provided rapid control of the acute symptoms and enabled more active rehabilitation, and allowed the development of a community based psychiatry.

The profession of psychiatry

In a large country with great problems in communications, professional development was isolated and largely derivative. In the United States and the United Kingdom in the mid nineteenth century there developed associations of superintendents of asylums. In the United States there was the influential American Psychiatric Association and in the United Kingdom the Royal Medico-Psychological Association (now the Royal College of Psychiatrists). In Australia, each of the colonies established a medical society which became branches of the British Medical Association (BMA). In the 1960s the

7

Australian Medical Association was formed. Several of the old BMA branches had sections of Psychological Medicine and Neurology. Many were very innovative. In 1911, the secretary of the New South Wales Section invited Freud, Jung and Havelock Ellis to read papers at the Australasian Medical Congress in Sydney. All sent papers which were read at the meeting.

In 1946, Maudsley of Melbourne, Bostock of Brisbane and Dawson of Sydney founded the bi-national Australian and New Zealand respresentative body of psychiatrists. The Australasian Association of Psychiatrists had a founding membership of 67. In 1989, its successor, the Royal Australian and New Zealand College of Psychiatrists (RANZCP), had 1700 members. In 1962 the Australian Association of Psychiatrists had established its own bi-national standard of psychiatric specialisation, the Diploma of Psychological Medicine (DPM). Later, this was replaced by the examination for Fellowship of the RANZCP.

Australia exported many fine psychiatrists, such as Sir Aubrey Lewis, Professor of Psychiatry at London University. The first Australian Chair in Psychiatry was founded at the University of Sydney in 1923, the foundation Professor being Sir John Macpherson. He was followed by Dawson. In 1940 John Bostock was appointed Research Professor of Medical Psychology at the University of Queensland. There are now 22 full time professors of psychiatry in Australia and New Zealand of whom four are professors of child psychiatry—a welcome, if belated, recognition of the crucial significance of this sub-speciality. In New Zealand there has been a similar development starting at the medical school in Dunedin extending to the other cities of both islands, Christchurch, Wellington and Auckland.

Until recently, most of the management of the mentally ill has been in the public sector. The first alienist in private practice was probably Fishbourne of Melbourne. In 1881, with his daughters, he set up the first day school for the intellectually handicapped.

With the development of various health insurance schemes, private psychiatry has become an important segment in the psychi-atric services, more so in Australia than New Zealand. Its development probably began with units for the treatment of alcoholism, some of which later became private psychiatric hospitals. Perhaps the most prestigious is Ashburn Hall, Dunedin, founded in 1882. There is now a network of private psychiatric hospitals throughout New Zealand and Australia which provide valuable services, carry out research and have standards recognised by accreditation from the appropriate Australian Councils on Healthcare Standards.

The first psychotherapist professing to be such was the Reverend Frazer, a renegade Presbyterian minister, who eventually resigned from his church. Whilst practising psychotherapy, he studied medicine in Sydney and graduated in 1909. The high prevalence of psychiatric disorders in soldiers following the First World War led to the recognition of the value of psychotherapy for certain neurotic conditions. Although some practitioners were influenced by Freud, psychoanalysis did not officially reach Australia until 1931, when Winn started to practise in Sydney. Its further establishment was aided by the flight of many intellectuals from pre-war Germany and its European neighbours. Institutes of Psychoanalysis were founded in Melbourne in 1941 and in Sydney in 1951. Through their training programs, they were a great influence in ensuring that the central tenets of psychoanalytic doctrine were understood by psychiatrists and other mental health professionals.

Psychiatric nursing

The first psychiatric nurses were merely the more able and perhaps artful convicts who were put in charge of their fellows. As the mental hospital systems developed, they were replaced by wardsmen and attendants whose quality was often the subject of complaint. It was not an attractive nor popular occupation in those days.

In Europe reforms in general nursing were underway prior to 1850. They were accelerated and strongly influenced by Florence Nightingale and her highly publicised experiences in the Crimean War. Subsequently, she led an unrelenting pursuit for better hospital conditions with the emphasis on a professional approach to nursing. These changes affected the whole Brisith Empire and what happened in general hospitals eventually flowed through to mental hospitals. In Australia the process was slow because of the size of the country and parochial attitudes which survived Federation. Nevertheless matrons, usually from the Nightingale School of Nursing or the Edinburgh Royal Infirmary, were imported in the latter part of the nineteenth century and in 1887 the systematic training of psychiatric nurses began at Gladesville Hospital in Sydney.

The most significant single event which hastened professionalisation of nursing was the statutory requirement for registration. In each of the States of Australia and New Zealand there were established Nursing Registration Boards between 1912 (Queensland) and 1933 (Australian Capital Territory) which ensured that standards were met and maintained. In due course these reforms flowed from general to psychiatric nursing until the establishment of training courses and eventually schools of psychiatric nursing.

General hospital and community psychiatric services

Intermediate between the asylum and community psychiatry, was the development of general hospital psychiatric units and outpatient clinics. The enormous gulf existing between the community and the mentally ill was emphasised in Australia and New Zealand by the geographical and social isolation of communities. In these circumstances general hospitals were often the first facility contacted by the mentally ill and in the early days they were often the reluctant providers of accommodation. This lynch pin position was gradually enhanced by the establishment of comprehensive psychiatric services without which no large general hospital is now considered complete. Close links were then developed between psychiatrists and other specialists in the general hospitals—an important step towards the ideal of considering any patient and their illness as a whole person. Outpatient clinics were

established in Victoria in 1911 and other States soon followed.

In New Zealand, by 1925, there were outpatient clinics and observation wards in many general hospitals.

As far back as 1841 there was provision in New South Wales for voluntary admission to mental hospitals. Other States were slow to adopt similar provisions but eventually did so. This allowed the shift from focus on the management in the mental hospital towards treatment and management in the community. The move towards community psychiatry has been encouraged by various studies such as the recent Richmond Report in New South Wales. This movement has greatly enhanced the role of psychiatric nurses, occupational therapists, social workers and clinical psychologists. In the more traditional hierarchical systems of the mental hospitals their roles were more clearly delineated. With the concept of multi-disciplinary teams working in the community these roles and their associated responsibilities are more flexible.

Community psychiatry, particularly in the United States and Italy, has come under criticism for having de-institutionalised patients without providing sufficient resources in the community. There is some concern Australia may make this mistake although the protagonists of community psychiatry point out that the problems in community psychiatry are usually due to the traditional underfunding of psychiatric services in general.

Allied health professionals

The contribution of psychology to the development of mental health services in Australia and New Zealand has been slow and tentative. The discipline of psychology in many instances derived from academic philosophy and it was not until the late nineteenth century that psychology was established in a clinical setting. The major path of the introduction of psychology into mental health services was through assessment of the intellectually handicapped. Psychometry was used by Berry at the Melbourne Children's Hospital in 1921 and by Porteus in 1930. The latter was the first Australian to have his name attached to a psychological test (Porteus

Maze). He was the first headmaster of a 'special' school for the intellecutally handicapped in Melbourne.

The other major influence on the development of clinical psychology was the psychoanalytic theories of Freud and Jung, and the clinical application of behavioural psychology as elaborated by Watson and Skinner. Many psychologists trained as psychoanalysts and many more of recent years have made therapeutic contributions through behaviour therapy. Through their interest and training in child development together with their expertise in psychometrics, psychologists have been active in the field of child psychiatry, from whence the basic model of the multidisciplinary team has spread to all areas of psychiatry. The academic background of the psychologist's training emphasises the scientific method so it is hardly surprising that one of the major contributions of psychology to psychiatry has been in research partnerships between psychiatrists and psychologists.

The social work profession has a history of its own with diverse roots in charitable and benevolent organisations and hospital almoners. While mental hospitals were largely custodial and community psychiatry fragmentary there was little development. With the psychodynamic, psychosocial and psychobiological revolutions of the last 70 years, social work has developed into an essential element of the complementary care and management of the psychiatric patient whether in hospital or in the community. Social work has become important at all levels of diagnostic assessment, therapy (especially with families), rehabilitation and as the 'broker' between the patient and the component agencies in their social network.

In Australia and New Zealand, unlike the United Kingdom, most social workers receive a generic training rather than becoming specialised psychiatric social workers. There were five training bodies in social work spread over New South Wales, Victoria and South Australia by the outbreak of the second World War. Despite that, in 1941 there were only 95 social workers in the whole of Australia. The output was increased when University courses were established in the early 1940s

and they became increasingly linked with outpatient clinics, mental hospitals and community psychiatric services. Schools of Social Work are now present in all Australian States and New Zealand providing a diversity of academic backgrounds with various levels of qualification from degree courses to shorter more specialist certificate and diploma courses.

The concepts underlying occupational therapy have an ancient origin, for its value was appreciated by the earliest medical writers of Greece and Rome. In the late eighteenth and early nineteenth centuries the powerful pragmatic work ethic, expressed as the aphorism that the devil finds work for idle hands, led to the employment of the mentally ill. A great deal of early 'occupational therapy' was in reality imposed domestic work which enabled asylums to run more cheaply. The appointment of craftsmen and tradesmen to instruct patients slowly grew and with it the realisation that there was something more to it than keeping people usefully occupied. The valuable benefits of socialisation became obvious.

Although there are frequent references to occupational therapy in asylums, such as mat and carpet making in the Lachlan Park Hospital in Tasmania in 1856, occupational therapy as a discipline was slow to develop beyond its traditional image. Stoller in 1955 reported a dearth of occupational therapists and facilities. The first occupational therapy school was established by Docker in Sydney in 1942 which was followed by a smaller Melbourne establishment which was active in the early 1950s. The first occupational therapist in Western Australia was appointed in 1949. Since then courses have been developed in occupational therapy and the subject has become most diverse with skills for assessment, testing, measuring psychosocial effects and counselling as well as the traditional craft skills.

Self help groups are a relatively recent feature of Australian and New Zealand mental health and their potential is as yet a largely untapped resource. In each State of Australia, and in New Zealand, there are active mental health associations. More specialised groups have been formed such as ARAFMI

(Association for the Relatives and Friends of the Mentally Ill), the Schizophrenic Fellowship, Huntington's Disease Associations, OCD (Obsessive Compulsive Disorder) Foundation, Alcoholics Anonymous (AA) with its auxiliaries, friends and after care associations.

Conclusion

The history of Australasian psychiatry shows that developments have been largely modelled on those in Western Europe and the United Kingdom in particular. In the early periods mental health problems associated with convicts and the soldier establishment were dealt with largely in general medical settings often in primitive conditions. By the late nineteenth century the Asylum movement had swept across New Zealand and Australia, and asylums were especially prominent features of the landscape in many cities and country towns, particularly in the gold fields. Asylums, later mental hospitals, were a focus for public mental illness care for the next 100 years, although psychiatric care in general hospitals continued and academic departments developed during this century. The last 20 years have seen major developments in mental health care with major contributions from many disciplines and sciences. This has enabled a recent re-appraisal of mental health services in Australia and New Zealand.

Further Reading

Bostock J, *The Dawn of Australian Psychiatry*, Australasian Medical Publishing Co Ltd, Sydney, 1968.
Cawte J, 'Aboriginal Medicine' in *Ways of Healing* (ed Joske R and Segan W), Penguin, Australia, 1987.
Eisen P and Wolfenden K, *A National Mental Health Services Policy: A Report of a Consultancy*, Commonwealth Government, 1988.
Lewis M, *Managing Madness: Psychiatry and Society in Australia 1788–1980*, Australian Government Publishing Service, Canberra, 1988.
Stoller A and Arscott W, *Mental Health Facilities and Needs of Australia*, Australian Government Publishing Service, Canberra, 1955.

Part 2
Normal Development

Chapter 2

The Developing Child

H Salimi Eshkevari

The mental development of children consists of a series of progressive qualitative and quantitative changes following one from the other in an order which is the same for every child. It depends on central nervous system intactness and its maturation. A child is never ready to develop until his central nervous system is ready. However, development is affected by many factors such as those present before and during gestation and birth, individual characteristics, genes, culture, family atmosphere and interactions, social factors and other elements. In this section, we are only concerned with those aspects of development which are related to thought, behaviour, affect and interpersonal relationships.

Factors influencing development

Preconception, gestation and birth

Parents' childhood experiences and the attitude towards them of their own parents affect their interaction with their own children. Also, the parents' personality, the type and style of their family life and their security in the past and present are important in dealing with their children. For instance, if they were physically abused during childhood they may abuse their own children. Other factors like social class, parents' age at pregnancy, the time of the pregnancy after marriage, the duration between two consecutive pregnancies and order of birth of the child play some role in parents' behaviour towards their children. Maternal health and nutrition during pregnancy, smoking, physical illnesses, drugs and birth difficulties may cause abnormal

development in the child. A prolonged delivery and/or drugs used during delivery may cause the child to cry and wake frequently after birth. Poor economical conditions have adverse effects on the infant's development. Boys are more sensitive than girls to maternal malnutrition.

Genes and constitution

The development of each individual is determined, in part, by their genes. Constitutional characteristics of an infant are the result of genetic factors associated with the environment of the intra-uterine life. Genetic potentialities become manifest whenever the combination of genetic predisposition and external factors reaches a critical level for occurrence. Genetic factors are evident in traits such as the smiling response and some fear reactions in infancy. However, when children are born, they are not only under the influence of genetic factors, but also the intra-uterine factors.

Temperamental differences

Temperament means the style of behaviour, that is, how an individual reacts to his environment and affects it. Gesell, the American paediatrician, was one of the first workers to investigate temperament. He found 15 behavioural traits which were present in the first year of life and were still present at five years of age. Thomas and colleagues, in a longitudinal study in New York, found nine categories of behavioural styles. These included activity level or energy output, rhythmicity of biological functions such as the sleep–wake cycle, hunger/satiety, intensity of emotional reaction, distractibility and attention span, quality of mood, threshold of sensory responsiveness and approach or withdrawal to new situations. Children in the first few months of life differ markedly in these features, a conclusion supported by other investigators. However, activity level and adaptability were more stable than the other factors over an eight year age span.

Children are not passive individuals but affect others with their temperament. It is therefore necessary for parents to be sensitive to their child's temperamental characteristics. Individual differences in response forms the basis for identifying temperamental differences between children. The age of the child, his maturation from conception to birth, genetic factors and the sex of the child all influence such difference. There are slight differences between boys and girls at early infancy, but these are greater later in life, due to economic, psychosocial factors and the secretion of different hormones.

Stability of temperament

Stability is evident in some, but not all temperamental traits. The most stable traits are rhythmicity, activity and adaptability. The least stable traits are approach or withdrawal, persistence and distractibility. Activity, emotionality and sociability are relatively consistent from three to seven years of age. Social inhibition occurs early and is stable up to the age of two years or more.

Personality and temperament

The relation between early temperament and later personality is not clear, but activity, sociability and emotionality show a close relationship with similar later characteristics. Early high levels of activity predict extraversion in adolescence.

Response to stress

Children differ in their response to stressful situations and use different strategies to cope with or reduce the anxiety provoked by the stressor. These differences partly depend on previous experiences and partly on their temperament. Thus, children with high activity

level reduce the adverse effects of institutional care by interacting more with others as well as themselves. However, they often, later, cause conflict with peers and teachers at school. Birth of another child in the family may cause disorders of sleep pattern, toileting and clinging behaviour in those children who show extremes in their intensity of emotional response.

Difficult temperaments

Children with audio-visual problems are more difficult to manage than normal children. Children with neurological impairments often show low activity, low persistence and short attention span, but do not necessarily exhibit difficult temperament. There is significant association between children with low birth weight and later difficult temperament. The range of temperament in children with mental retardation or brain damage is not usually especially different from normal children.

Psychiatric disorders are more common in children with difficult temperaments. The rate of accidents is also higher among children with difficult temperaments. Children with difficult temperaments can be the scapegoat of parents with marital problems.

Experience and environment

Active children participate in more activities compared with passive and withdrawn children. Physical disabilities, mental retardation and educational handicaps restrict the nature and range of experience and the ability to master new situations. Educational segregation hinders adjustment to the same experiences that other children encounter.

Ability and disability

Individual differences in some skills and abilities are related to normal or abnormal outcomes. Thus, children with mental retardation or reading disability have a higher rate of psychiatric disorders than those who do not have such problems. On the other hand, some skills like athletic prowess or superior IQ have social significance for the rapid development of competence.

Child rearing practices and family functions

Feeding

From the psychosocial point of view, the important factor in feeding is not whether the milk comes from breast or bottle, but it is the attention given to the baby during feeding, talking and cuddling which will affect development.

Overprotection and constraint

The most facilitating psychological environment for children is provided by parents who are warm, nurturent and supportive, but provide adequate and realistic expectations. Insecure and apprehensive children usually have controlling parents who are less nurturent and tend to frighten or threaten them. Such children's parents show more marital discord than control groups. Parents of impulsive–aggressive children are poorly controlling, less demanding and less organised. It is the way that parents apply control to children that causes anxiety. The level of control over children's leisure time has no relationship with emotional disorders.

Parents of neurotic children are not more protective than other children, but parents of school phobic children tend to foster their child's dependency on them. They have a high level of contact with their children and give prolonged infantile care. They prevent the child's independence, guard them, fight their battles and encourage them to come to them in times of stress. However, these children also have some characteristics that make their parents behave in such a way. Thus, it was found that mothers of school refusers were often afraid of losing the child during pregnancy, had difficulty in falling pregnant, gave birth to the child a long time after marriage owing to infertility, had a history of abortion or death of another child or had severe complications in pregnancy. Many school refusing children had life threatening illnesses or chronic illnesses and multiple operations. Many of the mothers lacked love and warmth during their own childhood and desperately wanted to give something to their children that they had lacked. The fathers also had problems. They tended to be passive and inattentive to family life. The parents' social life was limited and they had sexual disharmony.

Overprotection on the part of some mothers might be compensating for feelings of hostility towards, and rejection of the child. Emotional disorders in parents can result in unrealistic expectations of the child.

Overprotection can result in predisposition to emotional disorders and depression in later life. Excessive anxiety in parents can be associated with a high level of constraint of children. Severe constraint interferes with the development of social competence and autonomy in children. Social incompetence and low self-esteem in turn make an individual less able to cope and deal with stresses.

Discipline and aggression

The parents' methods of discipline affect children's reactions. Intermediate levels of severity of discipline, namely neither lax nor strict, work best for the development of children's behaviour. Authoritarian parents tend to make rules that must be obeyed by their children without discussion. But this approach does not foster the development of a conscience in children. On the contrary, it leads to a child's low self-esteem, misery and social withdrawal.

Indulgent–permissive parents do not adequately control their children, neither do they set limits for them. Instead, they accept their children's demands without questions. This approach leads to lack of self-reliance in the child and poor impulse control, often with aggressive outbursts. Sometimes, such lack of impulse control and aggression leads to intolerance in their parents who then, inconsistently punish their children.

Parenting that is indifferent, uninvolved and neglecting, leads to aggression, low self-esteem, poor self-control and problems of interpersonal relationships in the children. In families of aggressive children there is a lack of parental supervision and a lack of discipline to monitor children's behaviour. Such parents, therefore, cannot improve their children's behaviour. Such parents have no clear rules or expectations of their children. Children with conduct disorders know that their parents cannot set limits for their behaviour. These parents do not react to their child's abnormal behaviour, as they are disorganised themselves. They avoid confrontation on key issues and lack a systematic approach. They often give commands to their children, but their commands are inconsistent. They are often irritable and nag and shout, and punish their children more than other parents. Their coercive actions make the children more aggressive. They do not follow a disciplinary plan and cannot give praise for good behaviour or consistent punishment for bad behaviour. Their reactions are more reflection of their mood than their children's behaviour. However, it must be noted that aggressive behaviour is found in normal young children and may be precipitated by hunger, fatigue and boredom. Aggression may be expressed physically or verbally.

Physical aggressive behaviour may take the form of grabbing objects from others, destruction of toys, beating others with fists, kicking or rigid resistance on being dressed. Some children may grind their teeth or beat themselves when they can not release their aggressive feeling on others.

Verbal aggression is expressed in temper tantrums, rebellion, screaming and shouting, swearing, coughing, arguing, negativism and disobedience. Although disobedience is common between one and three years of age (the 'terrible twos') it generally decreases with increasing age.

Temper tantrums are manifested by sudden outbursts of anger, which are usually associated with screaming and shouting, stamping feet on the floor, and occasionally with destruction of objects belonging to self or others.

These aggressive behaviours occur more frequently in boys than girls in all cultures.

Persistent or severe aggression is often a sign of insecurity and is thought to be a form of attention seeking behaviour. Some young children show aggressive behaviour when separated from parents. Sibling jealously is also a common reason of aggression in children. Other reasons for aggressive behaviour are imitation, particularly of aggressive parents, and culturally determined behaviour. Frustration also leads to aggression, since it arouses feelings of anger.

Parents can cause intense frustration in their children by being overly critical, carping or rejecting at times of need or providing little emotional warmth and support. Inconsistent behaviour by parents also causes frustration in their children. Expressions of aggression do not generally appear to diminish the level of arousal. It is not known whether or not competitive sports reduce or increase aggression in children but high levels of competition in a child's life lead to conflicts with others which may in turn cause aggressive behaviour. Aggressive sports tend to increase aggressive behaviour in participants.

Aggressive responses to a child's aggressive behaviour only increases aggression by providing the reward of parental attention. Also, anger or aggression in parents towards children may function as a reward to the children as they see their parents lose self control. Parental behaviour can be a model for children.

The effect of punishment for aggression is, therefore, inconsistent and not very effective. Punishment is only effective if the child can find another way of coping with his frustration. Punitive parents do not generally praise their child's *appropriate* behaviour and are often cold and rejecting towards their children, and it is this poor interaction which leads to even more aggressive behaviour on the part of the child.

Discussion about the reasons for the child's frustration may reduce the child's aggressive feelings. Children's perception of frustration can be altered by sympathetic attitudes and positive approaches. Participation by parents and children in co-operative activities leads to reduction of conflict and hostility, particularly if they develop a common goal and make decisions collectively.

Watching aggressive films increases the expression of aggression in children, particularly if children watch these kinds of films constantly. On the other hand, aggressive or maladjusted children, particularly boys, tend to choose to watch aggressive movies more often than other children. However, television seems to have a minor role in causing aggressive behaviour in children. Aggressive behaviour seen on TV has an effect in leading to the *expression* of aggression in normal young children, and especially in those children who are feeling frustrated and have psychosocial problems. Prolonged exposure to aggressive films also reduces inhibitions against aggression and increases acceptance of aggression as a means of solving problems, dealing with frustrations and as a permitted and normal response in human interactions.

Aggression as a symptom is common in psychiatric disorders. Among children reported to child psychiatric services, between 10 and 50 per cent have disorders of conduct and in one survey of a child psychiatric clinic, fighting, bullying and aggression was reported as a symptom in 11 per cent of 0–5 years olds, 23 per cent of 6–11 year olds and 30 per cent of 12–15 year olds. Some depressed children may show aggressive behaviour as part of the symptom of irritability. Occasionally, children with schizophrenia may be impulsively aggressive. Aggression is commonly found in children with early childhood autism, and less frequently in mentally retarded children. Irritability may be seen during or after a physical illness in young children, and in temporal lobe epilepsy, aggressive behaviour may be seen during epileptic attacks.

To improve children's behaviour, it is useful to attract their attention and then orient them to a desired direction. Then parents should ask them to do a particular job. Children should not be asked, suddenly, to change their activities and requests should be parallel with ongoing activities. Reasoning does not, necessarily, make children accept requests. It is useful to emphasise the effect of their actions and behaviours on peers. However, warm and affectionate expression and emphasis on reparation, play an important role on developing reasonable behaviour.

Family size

Large family size may affect slightly the child's intellectual functioning and development, depending on the social class. Children from large families may get less adequate care during infancy, less encouragement in schooling than other children, fewer financial and material resources, less verbal skills, less intensive interaction and less communication

from parents. The poor education and socioeconomical conditions of most people who have a large family size contributes to these factors. Nutrition, which plays a very important role in the development of the child in early infancy, may also be inadequate in poorer families. Children of large families may show a higher rate of conduct disorders than other families; this may be due to overcrowding and social disadvantage.

Ordinal position

Order of birth has only minor effects on a child's development when other factors such as sex, temperament of the child and family relationships are considered. Last born children are more at risk for educational failure, but first borns are slightly more at risk for emotional disorders than last borns. Parents treat first born children differently, talk and play more with them, but also they can be more anxious and restrictive with them.

Sociocultural factors

Childrens' experiences outside the family atmosphere are important in their development. School, social, economic and political changes influence childrens' behaviour. Cultural values affect child rearing practices. School is influential in promoting normal development, but delinquency, absenteeism and under-achievement can also be learnt. As well as its educational role, school must be considered as a social organisation which promotes social relationships and values in which the composition of the student body, the efficiency of classroom management and the relationships between child–teacher and other staff are operating factors.

Social class

Social class has strong associations with a child's educational achievement. The reasons for this association relate to the collective experiences that a child gains from the life style and social value of his family. Among social class factors, the education of parents is the most important factor, not their occupation.

Children from higher social classes tend to ask more questions than those in lower socio-economic families and they get clearer and more complete answers from their parents. Children from lower class families spend less time reading books and have less opportunity for social and leisure activities to broaden the range of their experiences.

Ethnic groups

Younger children are usually willing to migrate but older children are not necessarily so. In migrating, children lose friends and close relatives and may miss them for months or even years afterwards. They have to face the stresses of a different environment, a different language and life style. Finding friends might be a problem for them, particularly due to poor ability to communicate. Their educational achievements and attainment can be below average for a few years, but most of them overcome these problems when they become competent in the language. The colour of their skin may be a factor in being teased by peers at school and/or making friendships with others.

Parents usually want to keep their own culture, including their religion, but children like to take on the new country's culture. Adolescents may have conflict with their parents on some cultural issues. However, there is a suggestion that adolescents and young children can cope fairly well with the new culture. 'Culture shock' is rare in children and is more due to family discord and the parents' poor adaptation to new culture. The presence of psychological problems is more due to adverse experiences such as poor living conditions, poor economy due to unemployment or social discrimination in housing, job and poor language. In a survey of consecutive referrals to a child psychiatric service in Perth, Western Australia, children whose parents were from overseas were not over-presented among the referred cases.

Theories of development

Three of the more well-known theories of psychological development are: social learning theory, psychoanalytic theory and Piagetran theory of cognitive development. As social learning is described later in chapters 58 and 61, only the second and third theories are discussed here.

Psychoanalytic theories of development

Psychoanalytic theories consider that all mental functions are meaningful and are motivated, and that the ultimate motivating forces are instinctual drives which possess energy and propel the behaviour. The most important drive is sexuality which has a biological root. The existence of a drive related to self-preservation is also accepted.

Sigmund Freud (1856–1939), an Austrian neurologist, was the proponent of psychoanalysis. He proposed a topographic system of the mind, namely unconscious, preconscious, and conscious parts. He called the mental mechanism governing functioning of the unconscious 'primary process'. This operates on the principle of pleasure. Those of the conscious, he described as 'secondary process' and they operate to adjust function to reality. He later put forth another theory of the mind's structure which consisted of an id, ego, and a superego. Freud emphasised development and he proposed several sequential stages of psychosexual development: oral, anal, phallic, latent, and genital, which correspond to the infant, the toddler, the three to five year old, the school aged child and the late adolescent, respectively.

Anna Freud, his daughter, also a psychoanalyst, accepted this phasic theory of psychosexual development, but she emphasised ego development, including mechanisms of defence against anxiety, and cognitive development. Erik Erikson , a psychoanalyst, attempted to integrate social and cultural factors in development.

Oral phase (first year)

The central feature of the oral phase is said to be primary narcissism. Before the baby can invest his environment with psychic energy, expect gratification from it, or develop confidence or trust, the baby must first experience comfort. Without body comfort the infant is not able to develop stable expectations, gratification, or hope. A healthy outcome results when the child experiences the world as nurturing, reliable and trustworthy. This leads to the capacity for satisfying personal relationships. When comfort is not adequately satisfied, impaired capacity for intimacy, or 'mistrust' (Erikson, 1963), will develop.

The baby's nursing activities are his way of 'working for a living', and conquering the difficulty presented by them is his first experience of mastery. Some consider that the oral phase contributes to character formation, and this is the foundation and background for the work of psychoanalysts of different emphasis. Some psychoanalysts believe that the period of the very first weeks after birth is an undifferentiated phase and that the baby is in a state of lack of consciousness about the self, all feeling being centred on the baby's own body and action.

In this phase, mouthing and sucking are the dominant behaviours of the infant, and the mouth is the main source of sensual pleasure. However, the development of attachment to the care giver which is the most important feature of the first year of life does not primarily depend on sucking and feeding and the infant spends much time on play activities of a non-oral kind.

Anal phase (1 to 2 or 3 years)

Traditional psychoanalytic theory emphasises toilet training in the second year of life, the so-called anal phase, because psychoanalysts thought that in this stage, the child's sexuality focuses around defaecation. Others consider that there are many more important developments in the second year of life. During the second year, attachment to the care giver, for example, mother, becomes more intense, the child tries to explore the world, develop language and speech, and the ability to play progresses rapidly. Motor activity and cognitive ability expand. Negativism, self-assertion, and self-reliance develop in parallel with these aspects of development.

Many investigators have failed to find significant association between the timing or severity of toilet training and the so-called 'anal' personality traits which are seen in obsessional people.

Freud considered that in the second year,

the child was dominated by an instinctual drive which included sadism, and a wish to control the mother. He also considered that the child–parent relationship was the prototype of all significant relationships in later adult life, and the experience of each stage of sexual development determined the future personality of the child. However, Freud's belief is not widely accepted these days.

Erikson viewed the second year of life as the stage of autonomy. The child should be able to control himself. In the second year, the child becomes more self confident and enjoys acquiring control over bladder, bowel and body. Failure to achieve these objectives leads to 'shame and doubt'. Erikson, in contrast to S Freud, did not relate anal activity to sexual pleasure in this phase.

Mahler invented the term 'psychological symbiosis', to describe a phase which exists between the infant and mother immediately after birth. According to her, an 'autistic' state develops in the infant during the first week of life, during which the infant is disorientated (and hallucinated). Then 'separation and individuation' begins to develop in the infant between 4-9 months. Later, between 16-25 months, internalisation of the parents' values and rules occurs.

Phallic phase (3 to 5 years)

In this phase, interest is directed towards the genital area and is expressed in the child's talk, play and actions between age three to five. Children identify with their parents but more with the same-sexed parent. Identification, in which imitation is to some extent involved, occurs for the sake of power and needs satisfaction. Thus, a boy identifies himself with his father, wants to be his mother's companion and feels hostile to his father, since he is his (the child's) rival—the 'oedipus complex'. This hostility causes anxiety in the boy that his father may castrate him—the so-called 'castration anxiety'. The same phenomenon happens in girls when they identify themselves with their mothers and wish to replace them with their fathers. Psychoanalysts believe that girls feel inferior due to the lack of a penis and develop an 'electra complex'. However, there is still controversy about this matter. Castration anxiety and oedipus complex occur in some, but not all children, and their importance in development is doubtful. Hostility of the child to the same-sexed parent depends on the family pattern of relationships and family situations and conditions. In any case, most children are able to solve the conflict of hostility by the end of this phase.

At this stage, children know their own and other children's sex from physical characteristics, appearance and clothes. They relate more with the same sex but to a lesser extent with the opposite sex in group activities. Sexual play and/or exploration are not uncommon in this phase. Children may like to see and/or touch friends', siblings' and parents' genitals. Family romance, namely a fantasy of having another family, are apparent in many children.

Erikson referred to 'initiative vs guilt' in this phase. Children can perform many acts and feel guilty if they are not able to do them. Children think they should obey parents' demands, otherwise they may get angry with them, or even that they (the parents) may destroy them. Consequently children's negativism diminishes and they becomes more compliant, cooperative and obedient. Children's obedience is usually due to fear of and love and respect for their parents, and their concept of 'goodness' depends on obedience of parents' commands accordingly.

Development of a conscience is established, and defence mechanisms are formed to reduce anxiety and guilt.

Attachment behaviour, which existed intensely in the previous phase, diminishes at three to four years of age. There is a rapid growth of language, symbols, imitation and play. Also, cognition and socialisation develop enormously.

Latency period (5 to 11–12 years)

Freud believed that children do not think much about sexuality in this period, but other workers doubt the existence of sexual latency, and consider that children are interested in the same and the opposite sex. Masturbation is performed by both sexes but is more common in boys than girls.

Erikson referred to 'industry' vs 'inferiority' for this stage. The child is capable of learning enormously and is very productive during this period of life. Thus, the child gets satisfaction from performing many actions and consequent recognition from others.

Children learn to read, write, solve mathematical problems and can do many other cognitive tasks to increase their abilities and knowledge. They also form ideas about their capacities and limitations, work out patterns of social behaviour, are active or passive, leader or follower. Standards of social behaviour become more refined and the child's growth of personality continues up to adulthood. However, although children take interest in and are curious about their immediate environment and also the universe, they cannot comprehend in the earlier years of this period the explanation given to them by adults. For example, the child asks his parents about the 'origin of man'; and 'how he was born'; 'who was the first teacher'; 'how earth or other stars were formed and work'. If a child is incompetent in learning and productivity for any reasons such as physical or mental disability, he will feel inferior with poor self-esteem. The latter is a central issue at this stage. Cognitive ability progresses in a suitable environment, and language becomes sufficiently improved for verbal communication in this period. Play gradually takes the form of games with rules and is more orientated towards social and physical activities from the age of six to seven years onwards. Attachment to parents becomes less intense but social relationships with peers tend to develop steadily and progressively.

Morally, children's conscience progresses in the direction of accepting adults' ideals and demands but they also apply and use their own judgement. It is in the next stage, namely 'formal operation' from 11 to 12 years onwards, that children gradually use their own judgements. Defence mechanisms continue to be present during this period and later in life.

Defence mechanisms

Defence mechanisms have been defined as unconscious intrapsychic processes which are protective of a person's emotional stability and are used to relieve anxiety arising from conflict between one's drives or impulses and the prohibitions against their expression.

Defence mechanisms exist in children, adolescents and adults. The most common are:

1. Identification. In this process an individual patterns himself on another, usually an important and respected person and incorporates characteristics of that person into himself. It is extremely common for children to identify themselves with their parents (for example, a child wears his mother's shoes and says 'I am mum'). Later they identify also with other relatives, friends, and then with their teachers. In adolescence, this defence mechanism takes place in relation to pop stars and heroes. Still later in life it occurs with other important people, depending on the individual's interests and values, for example, a medical student may identify with a Nobel prize winning physician.

2. Intellectualisation involves using logic, reasoning and abstract thinking to avoid confrontation with an unacceptable impulse or desire.

3. Denial. In this process some aspect of external reality is disavowed. For example, a child denies having been punished by his parents in order to maintain his self-esteem.

4. Displacement is a process whereby the individual redirects feelings about a person or situation towards another person or situation.

5. Dissociation which is the separation or splitting between certain mental processes and activities so that the normal integration of consciousness is lost. It exists in dissociative disorders and in fugue states.

6. Introjection involves the internalisation of various characteristics of a loved person and so establishes psychological closeness to or a sense of, the constant presence of, that person. One of its functions is to reduce anxiety in the face of losing the loved person. Hence, an individual may feel that their beloved is present even if they are not there or are dead. In addition, fear of destructive impulses or aggression from others can be introjected and thereby seemingly place the aggression under one's own control. The aggression is thus no longer felt as coming from outside, but from within. The person does

not then feel threatened but strong. For instance, a child says, 'I am a lion' in play if frightened, or wanting to be strong, because the lion is strong.

7. Isolation involves separation or splitting of an idea or memory from its accompanying feeling. Unacceptable ideas are rendered free from their unpleasant or disturbing emotional tone. For example, a person recalling a particularly frightening recent experience may do so without any feeling or display of emotion.

8. Projection is said to occur when unacceptable inner mental contents, feelings and behaviour are attributed to others, rather than the self. Projection exists in paranoid states in adults.

9. Rationalisation involves justification of behaviours by the application of reassuring or superficially plausible explanations which are actually convincing fallacies.

10. Reaction formation involves expression of unacceptable impulses in antithetical form. In persistent conflict, reaction formation can become a character trait on a permanent basis such as in obsessional character. For example, somebody with a desire to steal money from others may instead become a strong defender of law and order.

11. Regression entails a partial or total return to earlier behavioural patterns of psychosocial development, such as when a ten year old child talks like a baby. This process may occur in response to external stress such as illness or disaster.

12. Repression is the unawareness of or failure to remember unacceptable memories.

13. Somatisation is the transformation of some psychic phenomena into physical symptoms. For example, a child worried about going to school (or to work in the case of adults) may complain of a headache or abdominal pain.

14. Sublimation involves gratification of an impulse where the aim or object is retained, but the content is changed from a socially unacceptable one to a socially acceptable one, for example, aggressive feelings channelled into competitiveness in sports or games.

15. Undoing involves behaving in a way that symbolically makes amends for or negates unacceptable impulses. It is a form of magical expiatory behaviour, repetitive in nature, which is observed in an obsessive–compulsive disorder.

The use of defence mechanisms is normal in all ages, provided that they are not excessive and do not dominate a person's character. Some, such as projection, isolation, regression, somatisation and undoing are only found rarely in normal development.

Piaget's concepts of cognitive development

Intelligence has been defined as 'the ability of the organism to adjust itself to a new situation', or 'the sum total of all those thought processes which consist of mental adaptation' or 'the degree of availability of one's experiences for the solution of one's present problems and the anticipation of one's future needs'.

Jean Piaget (Swiss psychologist, 1896–1980) held the view that intelligence was only one aspect of general biological adaptation to the environment and intellectual adaptation was a progressive integration of innate reflex mechanisms modified by experience. He believed that mental activities and the growth of intelligence could be seen as a progressive transformation of motor patterns into thought patterns. The differentiation of nervous reflex structures[1] and their functions lead to mental operations[2], by which a person can conceive objects, time and place, causality and logical relationships, which are the basis of scientific thought. He considered that intellectual functioning consisted of two factors: organisation and adaptation. Adaptation is subdivided into two inter-related components: assimilation and accommodation. Adaptation refers to those organism-environment exchanges in which assimilation and accommodation are in equilibrium, neither one predominating. These provide the crucial links between biology and intelligence.

Piaget considered that intelligent activity was always an active, organising process of assimilating new knowledge to old and of accommodating old to new. This process begins with the interaction of individual and environment.

Piaget divided the course of cognitive development into four major periods: the sensorimotor, pre-operational, concrete operations and formal operations.

Sensorimotor period

1. From birth to one month. Activity consists of nervous motor reflex responses to the environment.

2. From 1–4 months. During this period, the infant co-ordinates his reflex activities and responses, such as hand and eye movement to reach out to touch or grasp an object, or co-ordination of eye–head muscles to search for the origin of a sound etc. First, simple habits such as finger sucking develop. There is no intention on the part of the child to develop these habits, but his reflex activities in meeting with the environment lead to new results, for example, when he moves his hand in front of his eyes, he notices the existence of his hand. The hand becomes a new stimulus for him which causes a response, namely, to move it again in order to see it. Piaget called this type of repetitive activity 'primary circular reaction', in which the infant uses his own body.

3. From 4–8 months. During this period, the infant actively acts on the environment to cause some change in it and he sees the result of his action, for example, he shakes a rattle to hear the noise and then repeats the action. Piaget calls these sorts of activities 'secondary circular reactions'. In this stage, the relationship between objects and actions is established. Although initially there is no intention for action, later, the infant acts intentionally.

4. From 8–12 months. During this stage, the co-ordination of secondary schemas[3] and their applications to new situations occur. The infant co-ordinates two or more independent behaviours. The infant also establishes the

1 Structures are the organisational properties of intelligence, which are created through functioning and are inferable from the behavioural contents whose nature they determine.
2 An operation is an interiorised action. It is a symbolic act which is a part of an established conceptual organisation.

3 The schema is the organised overt behavioural content, a plan of action and a strategy.

idea that objects have 'permanence', even when out of their visual field, so that a child will set aside an obstacle in order to obtain another object behind it.

5. From 12–18 months. In this stage the child manifests unexpected behaviour patterns and tries experiments (trial and error) in order to find out in what respect the object or event is new, and also discovers fluctuations in the results. He distinguishes object from act, explores distant space, constructs his representation of movement, letting go or throwing objects in order to pick them up, watches the body in motion, looks at an object for a long time when it has fallen and solves problems which demand new and unfamiliar means. An example of trial and error is when a child has a key holder, tries to insert the keys one by one in the key hole, turns to unlock and continues until he finds the right key. This type of activity is called 'tertiary circular reaction'.

6. From 18–24 months. In this stage, there is invention of new means through mental combinations, which includes the spontaneous re-organisation of earlier schemata. These are accommodated to the new situation through assimilation. They are the first crude representations of reality and the combination of these internally helps deduce new solutions. For example, the child puts a book under his feet to become taller to get an object out of reach.

Pre-operational period

This consists of two substages: pre-conceptual and intuitive.

1. Pre-conceptual substages

The pre-conceptual stage develops from about one and a half or two to three or four years. Thinking is action orientated and concrete. Children have difficulty in establishing true concepts and recognising stable identities in the midst of contextual changes. Children do represent reality, but their representations are closer to overt actions and their cognitive functions are based on mental experimentations. They involve themselves in a limited point of view and ignore the rest. For example, a child may concentrate on the length of an object, but not on the width, or may look at only one side, right or left, when crossing a street while cars are moving in two different directions. The latter example may apply up to the age of six to seven years.

Children lack awareness of their own mental operation and because of this lack of 'introspection' have difficulty in entering into any one else's point of view and fail to take into account others' informational requirements.

Children cannot play the role of the other person but only their own role ('egocentrism') and cannot coordinate with others: this is evident in their talk, play, action and relationships. A child cannot differentiate between his action and the action of objects, for example, if he throws a ball, he doesn't know whether it is he who moves the ball, or the ball moves itself.

The child judges events from their appearance. For example, a ball seems 'different' when it is under a table from the same ball when lying on the floor.

Children believe that everybody thinks like them. Their thoughts and reasonings are self-referential. A child believes that others can understand him without his feelings and thoughts being expressed by him. For instance, when a child is hungry, he does not necessarily ask for food, because the child thinks that his parents are aware of his hungry feeling. The child's thoughts and reasons are based on the 'idea of proximity', for example when a child walks with his father and falls, he may think his father was the cause of the fall, since the child's father was near him. During this period symbols develop and the child uses language and play.

2. Intuitive substage

Intuitive thoughts develop between about three to four and seven years. In this period, the child's thoughts are reasonably goal directed, but are still impressionable and unsystematised. However, the child can now use symbols and therefore words and language.

Children use words in their mind and can express thoughts in words, which is in contrast to the previous substage when they could only express them in actions. For example, the child in the previous substage would kiss his parents to express his love and affection, but at this substage he says 'I love you'. Also, the child talks to himself (egocentric speech). The child believes that the 'word' has the power to cause actions. For example, if his parents call him 'fat', the child may think that the word 'fat' makes him 'fat'.

Classification or grouping of objects begins to develop according to similarity and differences such as shape, colour or size, but logical connections are limited. Children call all kinds of birds 'birdy' or call all creeping creatures 'snake'.

Children can tell their right and/or left hand but have no true conception of 'right' or 'left'. Rank and relativity have no meaning to them except on two opposite poles, such as 'good' or 'bad' and nothing in between.

The child orients only on one aspect of objects, either quantity or quality (appearance) but not on two or more aspects, the so-called 'one dimensional thinking'. However, 'two dimensional' thinking begins to develop at the end of this substage at around age six years. For example, children think of 'length' and 'width' at the same time. They begin to draw a house with both frontal and lateral views at the end of this substage, whereas previously they could draw only a square with a triangle over it as the symbol of a house. Also, they start to look at the right and left when crossing a street (usually after the age of six years).

At the beginning of this substage, the child thinks that any active object (such as a car when its engine is on) is alive, but at the final period of this stage, he thinks that any object that moves (for example, an animal) or has energy (for example, sun or a heater) is alive. Dolls are still alive, have ideas and feelings for the child. That is why he talks and plays with them and expects them to react to him.

In this period, language, play and other congitive functions develop enormously and he is able to form concepts in language and gradually to construct more complex thoughts.

Concrete operations period

This stage of development starts from seven years of age and ends at 11–12 years. The child's intelligence is now based on the perception of objects and events. A child can focus on two or more dimensions of a problem simultaneously and process them mentally. He can focus on changes, rather than states. For example, if we pour water from a transparent, thin but tall glass, into a transparent, wide but short glass, he now knows that the amount or volume of water hasn't changed, although the level of water in two glasses is not equal. Hence, the principle of 'conservation of quantity' has been developed. He knows that some changes have happened and that water in a thin glass has higher height, but its diameter is less than the other glass. So the principle of 'compensation' has been established. Also, he takes notice of two dimensions, namely, both height and width at the same time.

At the early period of this stage, children have not yet developed the true concept of 'weight' and numerical relations. Although they know their times table by rote memory, they do not know what these calculations signify.

However, children gradually develop the concept of 'number'. For instance, if we show a child two rows of 'five' objects sitting together in horizontal lines with different spaces between them, for example:

· · · · ·

· · · · ·

he knows that the number of objects in each row is equal at the beginning of this period, whereas he used to say that the longer row contained more objects than the shorter one.

The child at seven to eight years can deal with logical classes and things and with logical relationships, that is, sets of rules for classes and relationships. Serialisation, namely arrangement of objects according to their length, colour or size, develops. The principle of 'invariance' is established after the age of eight years. The child knows that an object with the same amount (weight) or *quantity* can be transformed in different shapes. For example, a piece of plasticine in the shape of a sausage can be altered to a ball-like shape without its quantity being changed—'conservation of the quantity'. At the age of 9–11 years, the child accepts the principle of 'reversibility', for example, a piece of

26

plasticine in the shape of a ball can be altered into the shape of a snake and vice versa, without its quantity being changed.

Relativity and rank of objects, quantity and quality are established. For example, the child uses 'darker', 'longer', 'larger' and later 'darkest' etc. At 12 years the child can understand the meaning of decimals, fractions and proportions. The child knows the concept of 'age', 'old', 'older' or 'younger' and doesn't judge people's age according to 'height' or 'body size' as he used to do in previous stages. He knows that the origin of dreams is in himself and does not relate them to external events.

After this period, the child enters another (the last) stage of cognitive development, namely, 'formal operations', which is discussed in chapter 4 'Adolescent Development'.

Social behaviour

Social behaviour starts in the first year of life. Within a few months the baby seeks contact with other human beings. Infants' *gazing* is the indicator of this feature and the basis of their sociability. Further development is heralded by the *smile. Emotional attachment* to one or both parents develops and the infant tries to relate to other humans, besides their attachment figures, in this period.

The first sign that the infant is becoming socialised appears at the age of 9–10 months when the baby accepts the parental command, which is usually 'no' or 'don't'. An early sign of social achievement in the infant is the ability to let mother out of sight without anxiety and rage, because her presence has become an inner certainty to him and he is able to predict her continued care.

The second year of life sees a clearer emergence of *peer interactions*. Successful toilet training is also considered a sign of *socialisation*, since it indicates an acceptance of the parental rules for this behaviour.

From the third year onwards, the child's interaction with peers increases markedly and this is observed in group play. Children up to puberty prefer making friendships with children of the same sex. However, gradually, they mix equally with both sexes. It is sometime after puberty that they tend to have relationships with the opposite sex and occasionally sexual intercourse occurs between them. However, these friendships do not usually last very long and changes of relationship are common during adolescence.

The formation of the 'gang' of the same sex begins at puberty or even earlier and the co-operative activities, such as playing sports, going to movies, libraries etc, are performed as a group.

Independence from parents gradually begins and the child enjoys the company of friends more than that of his parents.

A sense of *morality* develops early (gradually from the age of two years) in the child. This includes differentiating wrong from right, a sense of self-criticism, a sense of guilt and fear of punishment. The child accepts his parental values and their standards up to the age of 6–7 years old, after which time he uses his own values to a greater extent (see psychoanalytic theories of development).

Smiling

Spontaneous smiling occurs a few hours after birth during alert inactivity, drowsiness, irregular sleep and during the rapid eye movement phase of sleep. It is also expressed after feeding. Spontaneous smiling is a neurmuscular reflex and is mediated through brain stem mechanisms.

Social smiling is a function of cerebral maturity. It involves a period of social exposure during which the infant relates to the Gestalt of two other eyes and a mouth seen in a face, often the mother's. Some consider that this reaction is an innate species specific pattern and that it is not a learned conditioned response as proposed by other investigators. Piaget considers that the social smile is an emotional recognition behaviour and primarily a reaction to a familiar image. He places it in the second stage of the sensorimotor period. Smiling appears gradually from the mouthing of a four week old baby to clear smiling when six weeks old.

The baby vocalises one to two weeks after the social smile appears. The early appearance of social smiling is a strong indicator of superior intelligence and its delay after eight weeks may be sign of mental retardation, autism, severe deprivation or congenital muscular paralysis.

Babies smile most easily at a moving smiling human face. Sounds elicit smiles in wakefulness, but a human face is more effective in eliciting smiles than a bell.

Before 20 weeks of age, social smiling becomes selective to familiar and unfamiliar faces. Differential smiling appears at 6–7 months, by which time the infant only smiles at those to whom he is attached.

Attachment

Theories of attachment between members of higher order species were proposed by Bowlby and Harlow, simultaneously and independently. Attachment behaviour in humans is any form of behaviour that results in a person attaining or retaining proximity to some other differentiated and preferred individual. In children it includes crying and calling to elicit care, following and clinging to mother (or caregiver) and also protesting behaviour should a child be left alone or with strangers. Attachment behaviour decreases in frequency and intensity with increasing age, but attachments continue throughout life. There is a 'sensitive' period that appears to be optimal for the formation of a strong affection and maternal *bond* and this is soon after birth. About the age of seven months, the child develops an attachment to a specific person. However, there is a great variation in different children. Attachment behaviour also depends on previous experiences the child has had with attachment figures.

Bowlby considered that there was an innate basis for an infant to be attached, especially to a parenting figure and that this primary attachment differs in kind from attachment to other figures. Attachment theory is different from Freud's theory of psychosocial development, as it is not based on physical care and feeding. Rather, it depends on playing with the infant, giving him a lot of attention, showing sensitivity to the infant's signals and bringing comfort in distress.

Attachment is different from *bonding*. Bonding is a selective positive attachment which persists over time, even during a period of no contact with the bonded person. Bonding enables the child to feel secure and to explore in strange situations. Very severe clinging and following behaviour results from an insecure, neglectful or anxious relationship between the infant and his mother.

Separation distress, fear of strangers and secure-base behaviour are seen as the prime indicators of positive attachment to a parent. The onset of negative reactions to strangers at about 8 months of age indicate that the mother has taken on a new meaning for the infant.

Acute distress reaction on separation

Acute distress appears following separation of emotionally attached infants from the mother-figure. Many, but not all, young children show an immediate reaction of acute distress with panic, crying and angry screaming (the phase of protest). This is followed by misery, apathy, unhappiness, eating and sleeping disorders, thumb sucking and rocking (the phase of despair). Finally, there may be a phase in which the child becomes apparently contented and loses interest in his parents (the phase of detachment).

This acute distress reaction does not always involve all the stages of protest, despair and detachment. When parents return to the child he may ignore them at first or turn away and seem to reject them but later cling and follow them everywhere. The presence of familiar possessions during separation, the companionship of another familiar child, or parenting from a skilled and familiar foster parent can decrease the intensity and persistence of the acute distress reaction.

Rutter, in a review of studies, found that the following factors had adverse influences on separated children:

1. age between six months and four years;
2. male sex;
3. poor previous relationship between the child and parent;
4. on-going parental discord;
5. a strange environment;
6. an unhappy experience of separation;
7. lack of, or low stimulation after separation.

Temperamental characteristics in terms of poor relationships with others, uncommunicativeness and aggressiveness were apparent in separated children who had these features.

Play

Definition

Play has been defined in various ways by different authors. It involves the fragmentation, exaggeration or re-arrangement of goal oriented behaviour. However, some writers believe that it is non-goal directed behaviour, non-serious and free from the constraints laid down by adults. It is self initiated, undertaken for intrinsic satisfaction and may or may not be constrained by rules. Piaget, considered that play helped to assimilate experienced events by their repetition in fantasy and that this may also help to bear mental pain. He considered too, that it helped resolve conflicts present in real life or in the mental life of the child. Other writers have emphasised that the child may be exploring feelings, lessening fears, increasing excitement or trying to understand a puzzling event by its graphic representation. Sometimes play may be directed towards seeking confirmation of a hazy memory or altering an event to make it more pleasant.

Some authorities have emphasised that play is a useful tool for developing a sense of achievement and with helping to practise developing new skills, particularly intellectual skills and those relating to the co-ordination of hands and eyes. Others have emphasised that play is aimed towards mastering anxiety or ideas and impulses that lead to anxiety if they are not in control. Freud wrote that 'play is determined by the child's wishes, mainly a single wish, to be big and grown up and for achieving this, he imitates adults' life'. Psychoanalysts since Freud have emphasised that play can be considered in the same way as daydreams in adults. Erikson considered that play, like language, serves an intrapsychic function as well as enabling interpersonal interactions. In this role, play is a way of communicating inner events and, of course, this can be useful for the clinician.

Culture and play

The type of culture in which the child grows up can affect the quantity and quality of play. In children from lower socio-economic groups in Western culture, there tends to be a reduction or delay in symbolic play among them. Also, there is a difference in the emphasis in which these groups of people encourage their children to play outside or to play with their peers or to settle their disputes without reference to adults. In certain cultures play may also be developed with religious motives.

Sex

There is some evidence that girls act out relatively fewer roles, mainly domestic, and those in more detail than boys. Boys' play tends to be more gross body activity, such as running, jumping and wrestling, than girls' play. Young girls are more active in doll related activities, particularly in the care of dolls—such as brushing and combing the dolls' hair. However, these differences are not apparent before the age of 21 months but, after that, marked differences in play material and imaginative themes are evident. To what extent this is determined by culture has still to be clearly understood. It is apparent that symbolic play does not develop spontaneously in all its forms and that its nature is highly determined by interactions with adults who may determine the choice of play materials and suggest the themes of the play. Sex role stereotypes carried by the culture may be passed on to the child at an early age in terms of play activity.

Type of play

It is apparent that there are many types of play. Some are passive, such as looking at pictures or listening to stories; others involve make believe or illusion; others involve games of construction or games with rules, and in early childhood there is simply a functional play which may involve rattles or hitting noisy, mobile, colourful toys in the pram.

Piaget has divided games into four types which are: (a) practice play, (b) intermediate, (c) symbolic, and (d) games with rules.

Practice play

Practice play is a primitive form of play at the sensorimotor level. The act is repeated by the child for the sake of the pleasure it gives. Practice play at the sensorimotor level involves the physical knowledge of objects, such as whether they are soft, hard, pliable etc as well as a mathematical knowledge of the spatial organisation of sets of objects. The functional use of objects is not apparent until about nine months of age and this announces the onset of the capacity to develop ideas for specific situations. Thus, at four months, the child simply bangs rattles. At 11 months the child can use different objects for different purposes. At 12 months, children can feed with utensils, for example, drink from a cup or feed themselves with a spoon. Playing with dolls appears at this early stage but objects are still more often used for non-specific purposes.

Exploratory behaviour, such as looking at things, fingering them and turning toys around reaches its peak at 12 months and declines after about 18 months but never stops entirely. Some workers report that manipulation with toys, such as throwing, banging and waving, declines within 15 months and should stop at 18 months. Certainly, after this time, parents identify this behaviour as being 'destructive'.

Spatial play indicates the presence of spatial concepts and also the ability to compare and relate schemata. Spatial play includes stacking and grouping of objects and bringing together two objects for use in play. The child, at this point, may show increased interest in contents and containers, such as repeatedly putting objects in and out of a box. The peak age for container play is around 15 months. Stacking play, which occurs also at about 15 months, requires that objects are put on top of each other and this means that the child must understand the relationship between objects and is aware of vertical dimensions. Grouping, in which objects are clustered or lined up together, occurs at between 18 and 21 months, and is the expression of early categorisation.

Symbolic play

There are many terms used to describe this type of play. It is make believe, imaginative, socio-dramatic, thematic, creative, fiction and pretend play. The main functions of symbolic play appear to be the fulfilment of wishes and resolution of inner conflicts and the adaptation of a reality to the inner world. Imitation plays

some role in symbolic play and sometimes exact imitation of reality occurs in the play itself.

Symbolic play begins between 18 and 24 months and declines after the age of seven years. It indicates a development of mental images and symbols and thus the transition from the sensorimotor stage to a symbolic period of thought. The onset of language reflects the expression of this change and is itself expressed in symbolic play. Piaget states that de-centralisation marks the beginning of true symbolic play and this is apparent when the child's play activities are transferred from his own body onto the object's. True symbolic play appears between 19 and 26 months, during which time children handle many objects in an adult-like fashion, know their physical properties and can combine toys in a drama play.

During the third and fourth years of life, the child likes to hold or carry a favourite object, which is usually a soft object such as a cuddly toy, a teddy bear or a blanket. This most often occurs at bed time and the object is rubbed against the face or the lips while playing with it with one hand and sucking the thumb of the other hand. The smell of the object is very important in this play to the extent that the child objects to the play material being washed. Winnicot called such objects *transitional objects* and believed that they serve a link with the mother when she wasn't present. One of the features of this transitional object is that it cannot easily be replaced by anything else and the child will strongly resist any attempts to change the behaviour.

Making up stories in symbolic imagination is typical of this type of play. In these stories many of them send wishes which are combined and not necessarily rationally connected. The stories may be often difficult for others to follow with their strange mixture of fact and fantasy.

The occurrence in play of asking people questions seems to be due to the fun of asking without much interest in the answer and appears to be a sort of mental exercise. However, this form of play may also be due to the child's curiosity and interest in learning and practising words, communicating with others and obtaining reassurance of his knowledge base.

Games with rules

Games with rules develop after the age of about six years but particularly when children go to school. They seem to reach their height during the years before early adolescence. They include many activities, beginning with skipping games and hopping games, many of which have been handed down from generation to generation of children. Often there are rhymes to go with these games, some of which like 'London Bridge is Falling Down', and 'Eeny Meeny Miny Mo' are ancient. Some authorities have claimed that the skipping rhyme 'Ring o ring o roses,

> A pocket full of posies,
> A tishoo, a tishoo,
> All fall down'

goes back to the time of the Great Plague, and its words are a reference to the plague deaths.

Children at this age may also make up games and make up their own rules. Many of these become fashionable for a while and then fall into disuse. Chasing and hiding games are particularly played in the ages between seven and ten. Children after the age of ten also become interested in more formal games which include soccer, cricket and other sporting activities as well as more purely intellectual games such as chess and cards. There are many, many forms of these games which are also then carried on into adulthood.

Play therapy

Play, including drawing, has been used regularly by clinicians in child therapy, particularly with young children since they are often unable to verbalise their problems in a direct fashion. It also seems easier for children to express their thoughts, feelings and worries in actions during play. Clinicians can recognise children's reactions, aggressions or sympathy and the family relations by observing children's playing. Play can also be used for assessment of the mental development of the child. For instance if a child fails to show any sign of symbolic play at the age of two years, then mental retardation might be expected.

Drawing

Drawing or graphic image[4] is at first an intermediate stage between play and mental image and it rarely appears before the age of two or two and half years. Drawing is like symbolic play in its functional pleasure and like the mental image in its effort to imitate the real. The first form of drawing is a pure exercise play; then the child recognises forms in aimless scribbling. Later, modelling from memory develops and this is imitative and imagery drawing.

Drawing in any phase is related to space and reflects the child's intellectual development. On this basis, the Goodenough (1926) test has been developed. Drawing represents affective contents too. It not only depends on brain maturation, but also on perceptual and cognitive experiences and the capacity to understand and form *symbols*. There are a series of stages of drawing, involving first, placement, then shapes and designs and finally, pictures. These stages are universal and are as follows:

1. Sensorimotor scribbling. These are the traces of the vertical and horizontal extensions of the arms bending at the elbow and the scribbles are like curved forms and arcs. The child pays little or no attention to the boundaries of the page. There is also no focused attention to the drawing.

2. On the way to an awareness of form, which occurs between sixteen to twenty months of age, children pay attention to form, placement, line quality and intentionality. They recognise the page as a space and draw in the centre of the page and acknowledge its boundaries. There is a predominance of circular forms and two-dimensional circles, which is possibly due to similarity to the human face. Some children draw only one form and move on, but others draw one form on the other one. Children see the causality in their own activities.

3. Children draw new types of lines and sometimes several types on the same page. They can draw circular and oval lines, dots,

---

4 Image is an internalised or deferred imitation which is rooted in motor activity, or an internalised action, a covert but active accommodation.

continuous lines, but may stop and start again. Directionality of lines becomes apparent.

4. Another stage appears at the age of two or after two years. There are loops, angled figures, straight line segments, dots and their combinations in this stage. The child draws greater and smaller sizes of forms. Representation of a space within a space develops. Children draw the internal parts of an object (transparency) which is an indicator of ability to draw the face and body. The representation of people is apparent. Different ideas come to the child's mind at the same time which represent the ambivalent feeling about the same object. They talk about what they draw, and name the figures. They first draw, and then name it. They draw letters, or ask others to write for them, or write their names on the paper, which shows the pride of children on their own identity. Awareness and utilisation of colours develops and more than one colour may be used on the same page (at the age of four years).

It is believed that vertical lines precede horizontal ones. After these lines, loops, zig-zags and wavy or jerky trailing appear. It has been found that up to the age of four years, children's drawings represent squares, quad-rangles, circles and oval-like enclosed curves and that they cannot draw straight lines and angles in proper shape but draw them as curves. Horizontal lines and crosses are drawn as open curves.

The course of drawings are as follows (see also Figures 1 to 8):

May scribble by imitation, back and forth
at . . . . 12 months (m)
Strokewises and then scribbles at . . . . 15 m
Scribbles spontaneously at . . . . 18 m
Imitates vertical and circular strokes at . . . . 2 years
Imitates vertical and horizontal strokes
at . . . . 2½ years
Holds crayon in fingers as adults at . . . . . 2½ years
Names what he has drawn on request, copies a circle without demonstration and a horizontal line, cannot copy a cross from a model, but can do it by imitation, names the incomplete man
at . . . . 3 years
Can draw a plus (+) at . . . . 3½ years
Draws a square, copies diagonal lines (\ /)
at . . . . 4 years
Draws a man with six parts at . . . . 4½ years

Draws a triangle, a cross (X), a man with all facial details, a house at . . . . 5 years

Draws a with long horizontal diameter, or a square (or triangle) and a circle which contact each other in one point. Draws a person with trunk, fingers, ears, nostrils and feet at . . . . 6 years

Copies a , draws a person (includes clothing), trunk length greater than width, arms and legs in two dimensions. Copies at . . . . . 7 years

Copies , draws a person (with neck, fingers, waistline and complete clothing) at . . . . . . 8 years

Draws a person who shows an 'action', eg running, sitting, etc, at . . . . 9 years

Use of drawing in clinical practice

Drawing, like play, has been used by therapists for children and sometimes for adolescents (see 'Play', earlier). Drawing represents intelligence, visuo-motor (fine motor) ability and neuromuscular integrity. It is below average in mentally retarded children and/or in children with brain damage and neuromuscular disorders.

Drawing of any child, even when scribbling, should not have any signs of shaking, trembling or wavy lines, otherwise neuromuscular disorders would be suspected. Drawing also is related to hand writing in school children, in that poor drawers show poor hand writing.

Dreams

Dreams are a succession of vivid, discrete, yet integrated, hallucinated images. There is a relationship between sleep with rapid eye movements (REM sleep) and dreaming. Although REM sleep is present from birth, the presence of dreaming from birth has not yet been demonstrated.

However, dreams begin very early in the life of children. Most investigators accept that they can not tell exactly when dreaming

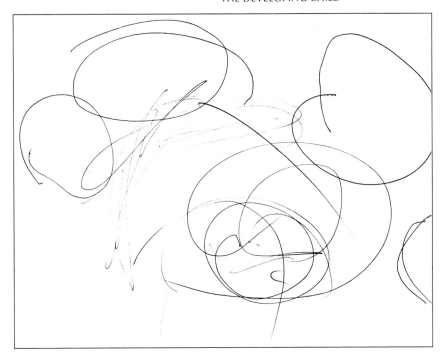

Figure 2. *Circles at 3 years (51% photoreproduction).*

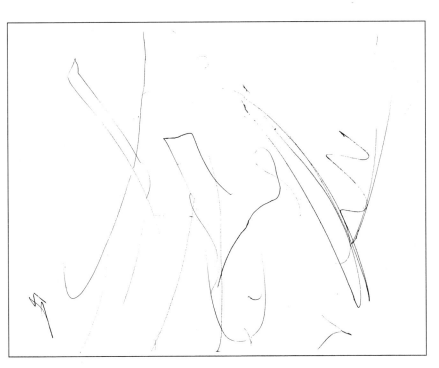

Figure 1. *The first scribbling at 11 months by Ertimiss (51% photoreproduction).*

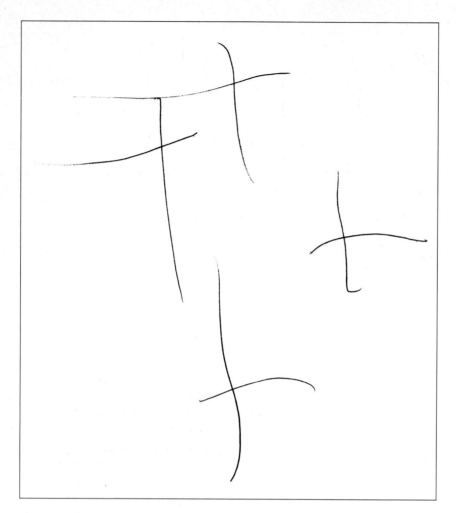

Figure 3. *Pluses at 3½ years.*

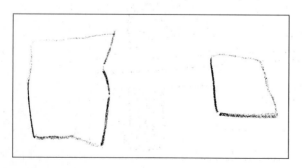

Figure 4. *Squares at 4 years.*

34

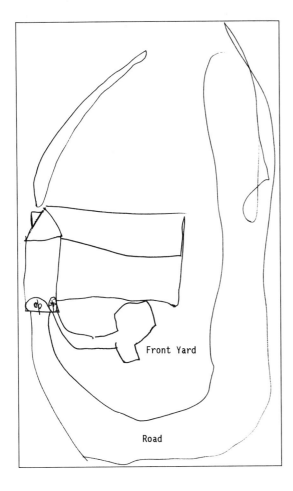

Front Yard

Road

Figure 5 (left). *A house at 6 years (63% photoreproduction).*

Figure 6 (below). *A car at 13 years (65 % photoreproduction).*

Figure 7 and **Figure 8**. *Colour drawings by 6 year old and 7 year old appear overleaf.*

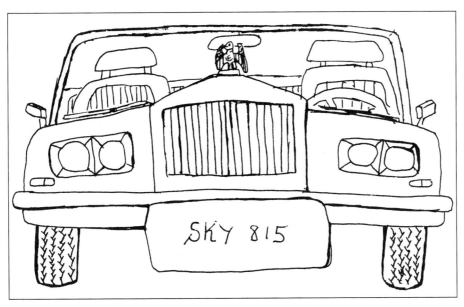

SKY 815

begins, but consider that they start at the same time as language and speech develop. The author considers that dreams can begin with the establishment of memory traces, or the establishment of stable internal representations of people and that the earliest age that children talk in their sleep is about 15 months. Piaget found that the earliest age of dreams was 21 months, when his children talked in their sleep and told him about their dreams. He believed that at a very early age children think that their dreams originate from outside themselves, and when they talk about them later, they arrange them in their own way, and make them into story with the element of play. He also stated that dreams, may, at the beginning, be very disconnected, but gradually take a more total form and may reflect happy feelings, anger, anxiety, fear, sadness, wish fulfilment or sometimes a physical stimulus. The content of dreams depends on the child's cognitive development, and also on the sex of the child. At the age of seven years, the child knows that the dream arises from inside himself, and he does not relate them to external factors as he used to do before this age.

Dream content of young children is often about parents. Two year old children may dream about being bitten, or being chased by animals. At the age of 5-6 years, they have dreams of ghosts and other imaginary creatures. The significance of dreams has been variously interpreted. Some consider they are meaningless and are reflections of the brain's random activity.

Freud believed that dreams were the guardian of sleep, and represented a wish fulfilment which was achieved through the hallucinated images. The wish may express pleasant or unpleasant desires. Jung saw dreams as messages expressed in a primitive language, compensating for the deficiencies in the dreamer's conscious life, and informing him of what he should do to achieve balance and wholeness in life. In Jung's view, dreams were an essential counterbalance to a rational conscious existence.

Adler's view was that dreams were concise reflections of the subject's present attitudes and anxieties. Piaget believed that dreams were a continuation of play.

Sleep and its disorders

Sleep is defined as a periodic state of rest in which there is diminution of consciousness and activity and from which arousal easily occurs.

The newborn infant sleeps an average of 16.5 hours per day, the three week old infant 14.5 hours per day, the six month old infant 14 hours per day and the 12 month old infant 12 hours per day. The time spent in sleep gradually decreases to 11 hours by six years of age. Up to the age of three months, the child sleeps three to four times in a 24 hour cycle and at the age of one year, he sleeps two to three times per day. During the first four weeks, most babies awaken twice for feeding in the night, and this may last up to the age of 10 weeks. The sleep-wake cycle of neonates is approximately three to four hours.

The amount of sleep taken by a child depends on age, sex, personality, intelligence, psychological atmosphere, and the physical health of the child. Boys are more restless than girls in sleep. An active child sleeps less than the placid one. There are individual difference in the quantity and quality of sleep from birth. A more intelligent child sleeps less than a less intelligent child. Parental presence helps sleep.

Some children may lie awake for a long time in the evening, talking or playing until they fall asleep. Toddlers may fuss on awakening in the morning when they are 2-3 years old.

Most children develop a ritual before going to sleep; this seems to be a protective device to make safer the withdrawal from reality into the world of sleep. Rituals may develop from nine months onwards. It may take the form of rocking, head banging, head rolling, thumb sucking etc.

The best indicator of adequate sleep is the child's lack of tiredness in the day time. Also, a happy mood and the lack of fussing or nagging in the day are other indicators that the child is getting adequate sleep.

Sleep disorders

Sleep disorders are common in children and adolescents, but they are not necessarily

36

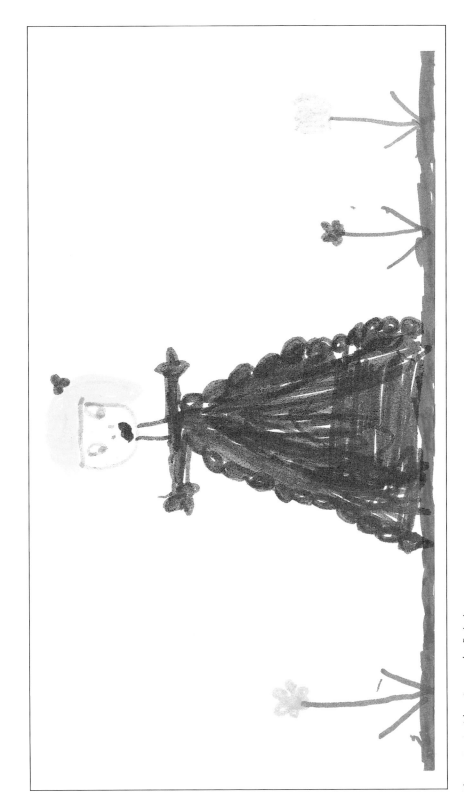

Figure 7. *A girl at 6 years by Ertimiss.*

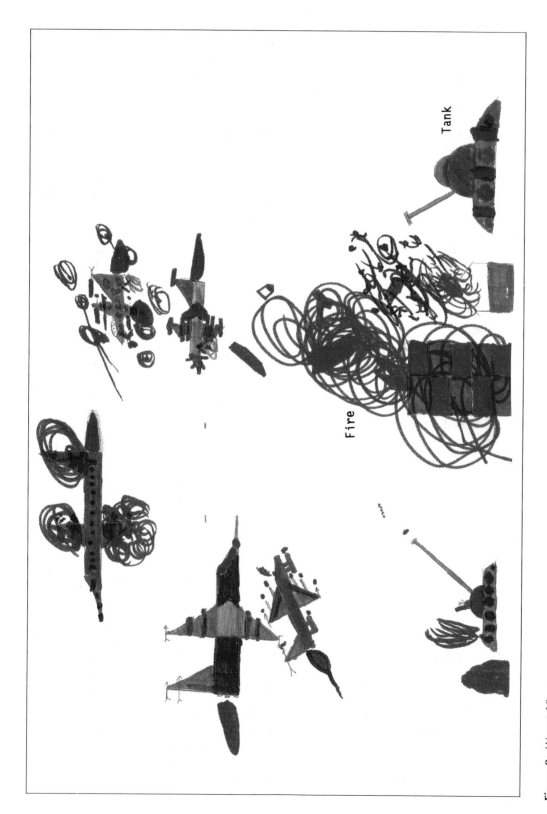

Figure 8. *War at 10 years.*

associated with psychiatric disorders. However, severe and prolonged disorders of sleep are usually associated with psychiatric disorders. Poor sleep causes restlessness, poor concentration and impaired memory, irritability, temper tantrums and fatigue during the day time.

There are different kinds of sleep disorders which are as follows:

1. Restlessness

Restless sleep occurs in some children, during which they move frequently (toss and turn). It reaches its peak at the age of 11 years. Some children show jerking movements in a group of muscles during sleep. A general jerk (in all muscles) at the beginning of sleep and/or waking is considered normal.

Restless sleep is usually associated with restlessness during the day. It may be due to overactivity, overstimulation or overexcitation during the day.

2. Insomnia

Sleep disorder may take the form of insufficient amount of sleep overall, inability to sleep which may occur at the beginning, middle or terminal period of sleep, or a combination of these.

Physical reasons of insomnia include most physical illnesses, particularly those associated with pain, fever, asthma, severe and frequent coughing. Some drugs such as central adrenergic blocking agents, bronchodilators, steroids, amphetamines or other psycho-stimulants, such as methylphenidate, usually cause insomnia.

Insomnia is associated with *most psychiatric disorders*. Disturbance of sleep as a single symptom is usually due to excessive tiredness, separation anxiety, particularly in young children, and fears, especially fear of the dark, burglars and ghosts. Also children may fear dying, being attacked or may worry about parental disharmony. Some children wake up and sit for a short time during sleep and show rocking movements or may bang their heads. Hyperactive children go to sleep late but wake up early in the mornings.

3. Hypersomnia

Occasionally, children sleep longer than expected usually in response to stress. Environmental or emotional understimulation may cause lack of interest in the environment, and consequently they may sleep during the day time, or longer at night. Sometimes, in *depressive disorders* in adolescence, the patient may sleep during the day or longer hours at night. Schizophrenic adolescents may wake up late in the morning, usually at lunch time, but they go to sleep very late at night.

In narcolepsy 'sleep attacks' may occur at any time even during the day, and anywhere. In these attacks, sleep is irresistible for the patient. Some antihypertensive drugs, and marijuana (cannabis) cause hypersomnia. After elimination of amphetamine in abusers, hypersomnia occurs. Occasionally, the reason for hypersomnia is Kleine Levin Syndrome, and in rare conditions, hypersomnia may be due to cerebral tumor.

4. Nightmares

Nightmares or 'incubus' or 'dream anxiety disorder' manifest during sleep with a sudden cry which is associated with anxiety symptoms, namely: sweating, dilated pupils, difficulty in breathing and palor. This is due to a frightening dream which awakens the child. Young children usually cry. Then, the child sleeps again but remembers his dream in the morning when he gets up. Fifteen per cent of 21 month old children have been recorded as having frightening dreams, but the frequency of anxiety dreams is at a peak between the age of eight to ten years. Nightmares occur during rapid eye movement (REM) sleep.

The cause of nightmares is not quite clear, but it is believed to be a disorder of arousal mechanism. Anxiety due to any reasons such as separation from parents, being attacked by a burglar, threat to self-esteem, hearing frightening stories, watching terrifying movies and so on, may cause nightmares. Extreme tiredness and a change of bedroom are also contributory factors in some cases.

5. Night terror

'Night terror' or 'sleep terror disorder', or 'pavor nocturnus' occurs during stages three and four of sleep, during non rapid eye movements (NREM). It is manifested by extreme motor activities and autonomic system arousal. After a short period of psychomotor over activity, the child sits up in his bed with open eyes. He is pale, confused, perspires profusely, shows rapid pulse and respiration, and piloerection. The child can't be awakened during the attack of night terror. He has no recall of events on the following morning. It lasts for up to 15 minutes, and then the child sleeps again.

Night terrors occurs in 1-4 per cent of children between 3-8 years of age and do not happen after puberty. The cause is not quite clear, but some investigators think that it is due to a disorder of arousal mechanism. It happens more when the child has extreme fatigue, is under stress or with a raised temperature. Night terror needs to be considered more seriously than nightmares as it can be of considerable concern to parents and may, if persistent, interfere with the whole family function by reducing the sleep of anxious parents.

Night terrors need to be differentiated from nightmares. The latter can be recalled by the child on awakening but this is not so with night terrors where there is no dream content to remember.

6. Sleep walking disorders (somnambulism)

Somnambulism occurs in one to six per cent of children at some time during childhood and adolescence, most frequently between the ages of 6 and 12 years. It usually ceases around the age of 20 years but it may begin for the first time in later adulthood with recurrent episodes. A child with somnambulism gets out of his bed and walks with blank staring face around the house, sometimes going outside, or he may sit and show semipurposeful motor activities such as picking at a blanket. It is sometimes associated with crying or talking. The child's awareness of his external world is disturbed, and usually he can not recall the activity on awakening, although he may recall some part of it. The child is *not* careful or safe during the episode of somnambulism. He can not be awakened unless with intense stimulation. Sleepwalking lasts from a few minutes to around 30 minutes.

The aetiology of sleepwalking disorder in children is not completely known but it may be a disorder of arousal mechanism. Stress, fatigue and raised body temperature contribute to its development. It is more frequent in first degree relatives of sufferers than in the general population. Night terror is more common in children with sleepwalking disorders; so there might be an aetiological link between these two phenomena.

Sleepwalking must be differentiated from psychomotor epilepsy. The latter is associated with the attacks during waking (but occasionally during sleep) and with EEG abnormalities.

7. Sleep talking

Sleep talking is very common in children. The child's talk may be clear, or unintelligible, or a combination of both. The content of speech of the child is a reflection of his thoughts, feelings and daily activities. Sleep talking is found in normal children but is also common in children with fever or severe anxiety.

Treatment of sleep disorders

Infants may need the presence of their parents in their room before falling asleep. Some young children and infants sleep easily if parents hold them in their arms and move them rhythmically. For pre-school children, lying in bed beside the child, telling a story, or reading a book, cuddling and giving affection are helpful. Other factors such as bathing, having milk or a light meal before bedtime make sleep easier. Some children can sleep with their most favourite toy and they should be allowed to take it to bed with them. Other children like to play until they fall asleep. Some children prefer to sleep with the light on, since they are frightened of the dark. It is helpful for the child to go to bed at a regular time every evening.

When sleep disorder is one of the associated symptoms of psychiatric disorders, the latter should always be managed primarily. Very occasionally, a few children may need medication since their insomnia is severe and persistent (see chapters 56, 57).

Further Reading

Biber B, *Children and Drawing*, Bark Street College of Education Publication, New York, 1962.
Bowlby J, 'The Nature of the Child's Tie to his Mother', *International Journal of Psychoanalysis*, Vol 33, 1958, pp 350–73.
Bowlby J, 'Separation Anxiety', *International Journal of Psychoanalysis*, Vol 41, 1960, pp 89–113.
Bowlby J, *Attachment and Loss*, Basic Books, New York, 1969.
Bowlby J, 'The Making and Breaking of Affectional Bonds, I, Aetiology and Psychopathology in the Light of Attachment Theory', *British Journal of Psychiatry*, Vol 130, 1977, pp 201–10.
Broughton R J, 'Sleep Disorders; Disorder of Arousal', *Science*, Vol 59, 1968.
Carey W B, 'A Simplified Method for Measuring Infant Temperament', *Journal of Paediatrics*, Vol 77, 1970, pp 188–94.
Ellingsson R, 'Autogenesis of Sleep in the Human', in *Experimental Study of Human Sleep*, Elsevier, Amsterdam, 1975, pp 129–46.
Emde R N, McCartney R D and Harmon R J, 'Neonatal Smiling in REM States, IV, Premature Study', *Child Development*, Vol 42, 1971, pp 1657–61.
Erikson E H, *Childhood and Society*, 2nd edn, Norton, New York, 1963.
Fenichel C, *The Psychoanalytic Theory of Neurosis*, W W Norton and Co, New York, 1945.
Flavell Y H, *The Developmental Psychology of Jean Piaget*, Ian Nostrand, Princeton, 1963.
Freud A, *The Ego and Mechanisms of Defence*, International Universities Press, New York, 1964.
Freud A, *Normality and Pathology in Childhood*, Penguin, Harmonsworth, 1966.
Freud S, *'The Interpretation of Dreams'*, Standard Edition, Vols 4 and 5, 1900.
Freud S, *'Narcissism'*, Standard Edition, Vol 14, pp 73–102, Hogarth Press, London, 1914.
Freud S, *The Ego and Id*, Standard Edition, Vol 19, 1923.
Freud S, *Three Contributions to the Theory of Sex*, Modern Library, New York, 1938.
Gesell A, 'The Ontogenesis of Infant Behaviour', *Manual of Child Psychology*, (ed Carmichael L), 1946.
Gesell A and Amatruda, *Developmental Diagnosis*, Hoeber, New York, 1947.
Goddard H H, 'A Suggested Definition of Intelligence', *American Journal of Mental Deficiency*, Vol 50, 1934, pp 245–50.
Harlow H F, 'The Nature of Love', *American Psychologist*, Vol 13, 1958, pp 637–85.
Illingworth R S, *The Normal Child, Some Problems of the Early Years and their Treatment*, 9th edn, Churchill Livingston, Edinburg, 1987.
Kellog R, *The Psychology of Children and Art*, CRM-Random House, San Diego, 1967.
MacFarlane Y W, Allen L and Honzik M P, *'A Developmental Study of the Behaviour Problems of Normal Children between 21 Months and 14 Years'*, University of California Press, Berkeley, 1954.
Mahler M S, Pine F and Bergman S, *The Psychological Birth of Human Infants*, Basic Books, New York, 1975.
Milstein J M, 'Sleep Disturbances', in *The Practice of Paediatric Neurology*, Vol 1, Molsey, Saint Louis.
Nutherg J J, *The Anatomy of Sleep*, Roche Laboratories, Chapter 3, 1966.
Piaget J, *The Psychology of Intelligence*, Routledge and Kagan Paul, London, 1950.
Piaget J, *Play, Dreams and Imitation in Childhood*, 3rd edn, Routlege and Kagan Paul, London, 1972.
Piaget J, *The Origin of Intelligence*, Harmonsworth, Penguin, 1977.
Roche Laboratories, *Roche Laboratories*, Nutley, New Jersey, 1966.
Rutter M, 'Maternal Deprivation, 1972–1978: New Findings, New Concepts, New Appoaches', *Child Development*, Vol 50, 1979, pp 283–305.
Rutter M and Hersov L, *Child and Adolescent Psychiatry: Modern Approaches*, 2nd ed, Blackwell Scientific Publication, Oxford, 1985.
Salimi Eshkevari H, *Development in the First Three Years of Life: A Cultural Perspective*, Kitchener Press, Adelaide, 1988.
Schaffer H R, 'Early Social Behaviour and the Study of Reciprocity', *Bulletin of the British Psychological Society*, Vol 27, 1974, pp 209–16.
Stern L W, 'The Psychological Methods of Testing Intelligence', *Educational Psychology Monograph*, No 13 (translated by Whipple G M), 1914.
Thomas A and Chess S, *Temperament and Development*, Breuner-Mazel, New York, 1977.
Tizard B and Harvey D, *Biology of Play*, SIMP, London, 1977.
Winnicot D W, *Play and Reality*, Tavistock, London, 1971.

Chapter 3

Pregnancy, Birth and Parenthood

J T Condon

This section presents a theoretical framework which is helpful for understanding the psychological experiences of normal men and women in relation to child bearing, together with the psychological tasks which both members of a couple usually face during pregnancy. It also addresses a number of situations which could be viewed as crises and which may potentially disrupt the transition to parenthood. These include infertility, miscarriage, perinatal bereavement and postnatal depression.

One unifying framework which is particularly useful for understanding the psychology of pregnancy is that of attachment and loss. Attachment is usually defined as an 'emotional tie' and, in its broadest sense, may be a tie to another person, a foetus, a fantasy (such as having a particularly desired type of childbirth) or an aspect of the self (such as 'career woman'). The breaking of an attachment bond occurs when an object of attachment is lost, and this is normally followed by a grief reaction in the course of which the individual emotionally comes to terms with (resolves) the loss. The occurrence of this type of desirable outcome may be influenced by a variety of biological, psychological and social factors. Crucial among these is the nature of the original attachment as illustrated by the statement of a young woman bereaved by stillbirth: 'it's extraordinarily difficult to say goodbye to someone you have never properly said hello to'.

The psychology of normal pregnancy

The desire for children

In our society, the desire in both men and women to have a child is determined by many factors. Whether a human maternal (or paternal) instinct is of importance is controversial. Certainly there is evidence that human adults exhibit responses to infants which may well be genetically preprogrammed. Thus, for humans 'instinct' may be more relevant in this regard than a specific biological drive to achieve parental status.

Of greater relevance to the development of an urge to procreate in our species is probably the experience of being cared for and nurtured oneself. Certainly, in the play of young children of both sexes, a recurring theme is the co-existence of a wish to 'care for' as well as to 'be cared for'. Most authorities believe that identification with the same-sex parent is probably a crucial milestone in the formation of 'fatherliness' and 'motherliness'. For example, the young pre-school age girl will often utilise her own mother as a model in nurturing (or punishing) her dolls in play. This process of building up a mental picture of what constitutes 'a mother' continues throughout childhood, adolescence and early adulthood. The concept of mother which eventually results, is influenced by the woman's perceptions of her own mother, other female role models and a variety of factors including social stereotypes. As elaborated below, the final representation may not necessarily be free of conflict or well integrated. Thus, it seems probable that humans are psychologically primed for parenthood.

A variety of other influences may impinge upon this psychological substrate, and individuals may vary greatly in their degree of conscious awareness of these. Examples would include social expectation, the belief (often erroneous) that having children will strengthen the marital relationship or, the seeking of a kind of immortality by surviving through one's children. In addition, some men and women may feel a need to validate their masculinity or femininity in this way or experience the hope that a child will fill an emotional void arising from previous unresolved losses or underlying depression.

If an individual has had a traumatic psychological development, this can alter the motivation for child bearing in ways which are quite difficult to predict. Some such women and men experience an overwhelming compulsion to have a child, possibly seeking to provide for their own children the nurturance and affection which they themselves were deprived of during their own childhood. Others may find the prospect of parenthood exceedingly threatening either for fear of rejection by (or of) the child or, because 'sharing' the partner with a third party is excessively anxiety provoking. Finally, it seems probable that most parents experience mixed feelings (ambivalence) to some extent towards parenthood due to an awareness of both the potential advantages and disadvantages in assuming the parental role. However, in some individuals the issue becomes so conflicted that they become paralysed by their ambivalence. Unfortunately the latter dilemma is often solved by leaving conception 'to chance' or by having an 'accident on purpose' rather than via discussion, counselling or psychotherapy.

It should be apparent that motivation to have a child is complex and to dichotomise pregnancy into 'planned' versus 'unplanned' is rather simplistic. Such terms define extreme ends of a continuum and in between are many pregnancies which are neither planned nor unplanned. For example, one frequently encounters pregnancies which have resulted from contraceptive failure which, on further exploration, seems far from accidental.

Losses and threats for prospective parents

For both men and women, the transition to parenthood inevitably involves both losses and threats. The former may cause depression while the latter tend to cause anxiety. Losses

for the woman may include career, freedom, physical well-being or figure. Threats for both sexes may include physical injury to the woman at delivery, the possibility that the child will be born deformed or dead, doubts about the ability to cope with the parental role. Many men fear that their partner's involvement with the child may result in her becoming less close to them. One aspect of the transition to parenthood which is difficult for many individuals arises from the fact that parenthood inevitably confronts them with their status as adults rather than as children. It places them on a developmental level equivalent to their own parents and thus they must relinquish their status as 'child'. This is a psychological task which unfortunately is far from straightforward for many women and men. In clinical practice, it is very striking how frequently psychological problems in families with young children have their origins in one or both parents remaining, in a developmental sense, a child who then looks to the real child to nurture them.

The developmental crisis of pregnancy

Research on the psychology of pregnancy strongly supports the notion that it is time of crisis for both expectant parents. There is virtually no research support for the idealised view of pregnancy as a time of enhanced physical well-being and psychological contentment for either parent. The potential difficulty of the psychological tasks inherent in the transition to parenthood should not be underestimated. A considerable body of research suggests that approximately 20 per cent of parents of both sexes are overwhelmed by them and have a negative outcome of the crisis. Thus, they fail to regain pre-pregnancy levels of psychological adaptation and functioning.

Successful negotiation of the psychological tasks of pregnancy strongly favours (but does not guarantee) a healthy postnatal adaptation. The tasks can be conceptualised as involving the development or restructuring of four crucial relationships.

First, each parent normally develops an emotional 'attachment' to the unborn baby. The word 'attachment' is often used somewhat loosely in the literature. In the present context it is defined as a collection of (interconnected) desires or needs. These include: to want to interact with the foetus in fantasy and reality and derive pleasure therefrom; to want to 'get to know' what the foetus is like; to want to protect and safeguard the foetus and meet its needs (even at the expense of one's own) and to want to avoid separation from or loss of the foetus. Such desires and needs may often (but not always) find expression in corresponding 'attachment behaviours'.

As shown in Figure 1, the first experience of foetal movement is an important milestone in the development of this attachment for both parents as is the experience of visualising the foetus at ultrasound. Both experiences render the foetal existence more 'real' and create a sense of 'separateness' from the mother. Figure 1 also shows that, in the third trimester, the attitude towards the foetus is quite different from the attitude towards the 'pregnancy state' per se; disenchantment with the latter is very common but quite compatible with strong attachment to the foetus.

A desire to protect is intrinsic to any attachment and is an important motivation for abstaining from nicotine or alcohol during pregnancy. Protective behaviour is also evidenced by maternal care with diet and compliance with antenatal care. Somewhat ironically, attachment is low in the first trimester when the foetus is, of course, most vulnerable to failure of maternal protective behaviours.

As gestation progresses, the foetus is experienced in increasingly human terms and comes to be conceptualised as a 'real little person'. Most parents have imaginary monologues with their foetus and derive pleasure from these kinds of behaviours and interactions. Finally, with the increase in attachment there is an increased fear of loss and hence fears concerning stillbirth or deformity are ubiquitous in both parents in the third trimester.

A variety of pathological developments can occur in the parent-foetus relationship. For example, the existence of the foetus may be denied; the relationship may be intensely ambivalent; hostility towards the partner may be displaced on to 'his' or 'her' baby, or exces-

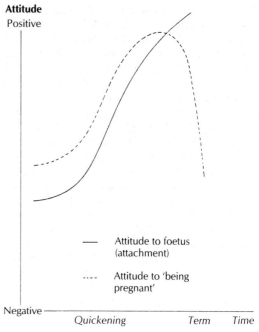

Figure 1. *Schematic representation of changes in male and female expectant parents' attitudes towards the unborn child and the pregnancy state (Reproduced from Condon J T,* Journal of Psychosomatic Obstetrics & Gynaecology, *Vol 4, 1985, pp 271-84).*

sive fears of loss may preclude the development of attachment. In clinical practice, one may encounter young women who present requesting termination of pregnancy in their mid trimester, following the experience of foetal movement. The existence of the unwanted pregnancy has been completely denied until the experience of movement renders such denial no longer possible. Termination at this late stage of pregnancy is usually refused and the resultant hostility may find expression as foetal abuse or neglect.

The second task involves a re-working of the relationship between the expectant parent and their own same-sex parent which often includes a re-evaluation of the quality of parenting they themselves received. If their own same-sex parent is seen as 'good' the task is one of identification, and the parent feels content to follow in their own parent's footsteps and feels confident, if they do so, that their child will be well cared for. If however, the same-sex parent is experienced as 'bad' or inadequate, the task is considerably more difficult. The individual must then struggle against identification with that parent and seek an alternative parent figure or model with whom to identify. Expectant parents often feel a need for more interaction with their own parents (or parental models) especially in late pregnancy and this is one outer manifestation of this inner restructuring.

The third relationship requiring restructuring is that with the partner. Often for the first time each parent now begins to evaluate his partner, not only as a partner, but as a future parent. In addition, there arises the requirement to 'share' the partner with another. Individual men and women differ greatly in their ability to share without feeling excessively deprived or excessively jealous. Men in particular often experience difficulties in resolving the transition from a dyadic to a triadic relationship.

The fourth 'relationship' which must often be reworked is that between the parent and his self-concept. The ability to grieve the abovementioned losses is central to this restructuring. Adolescent expectant parents are particularly vulnerable in this regard as they are often being asked to relinquish what they have never tasted, let alone lived to the full. The older pregnant woman who, for example, has derived enjoyment and satisfaction from a career may experience its loss as painful yet resolution will usually be less conflictual.

The foregoing description of the tasks of pregnancy is both oversimplified and over-generalised. Although these four tasks have been described separately, they are intimately interdependent. For example, the quality of parent-foetus attachment has been shown to be strongly determined by the quality of the marital relationship and, to a lesser extent, by the perception of their own same-sex parent. Moreover, considerable individual variation can occur without necessarily any implication of pathology or 'abnormality'.

Birth

During pregnancy, both parents normally develop a set of expectations about what the baby will be like, in terms of appearance, gender and temperament. Thus, childbirth, from a psychological perspective, is a confrontation of fantasy and reality. If there is a reasonable degree of congruity between the 'fantasy baby' of pregnancy and the real baby, then feelings which have developed towards the foetus can be transferred relatively smoothly to the neonate. If not, the later may be experienced as the 'wrong baby' for these feelings and the parent may have to begin the relationship de novo. For example, if an already much-loved and wanted boy turns out to be a girl, the parent faces two tasks. First, an attachment bond has been broken and the loss of the wished-for or expected boy must be grieved. This is a necessary prerequisite for completion of the second task, viz the formation of a new attachment to the girl.

Many problems of early parent-infant bonding have their origins in failure to grieve. If a baby is lost through stillbirth or cot death, some parents may embark immediately upon a further pregnancy to 'replace' the infant whose loss is never fully grieved. This would seem a hazardous course from a psychological viewpoint and, following the birth of the new baby, parents are suddenly confronted with the fact that the new baby is different from (and therefore cannot replace) the baby who has died. Resentment and early bonding difficulties often occur under these circumstances.

In our society, many women have an intense emotional investment in having a particular type of childbirth experience. Failure to achieve this goal may result in shame, guilt or an intense feeling of failure and these may predispose to postnatal depression or early bonding difficulties. Unfortunately, *some* types of childbirth education classes tend to foster expectations which many women are ultimately unable to fulfil.

Recent research has demonstrated that 40 per cent of primiparous women and 25 per cent of multiparous women feel indifferent or negative in their early encounters with their baby. Many such women feel obliged to feign 'love at first sight' and experience substantial guilt and shame at its absence. Most women develop strong attachment in the subsequent weeks. Delivery variables (especially intensity of pain) may play a role in determining the first impression, as may incongruity between the fantasy baby and real baby. Incongruity is usually much greater for the less experienced primiparous women, hence their higher incidence of negative or indifferent feelings.

Bonding during the 'critical period'

In many animal species, it has been demonstrated that there is a period of time immediately following the birth during which contact between the mother and newborn is essential for the mother to bond. This is the so-called 'critical period' for bonding and if mother and newborn are separated after birth during this period, the mother will reject her offspring when reunited with it.

In a series of experiments during the 1970s, Klaus and Kennell claimed to have demonstrated that women who did not have skin-to-skin contact with their neonates in the hours following birth suffered impaired bonding which failed to normalise even after several years.

Klaus and Kennell's work provided a major impetus for more humane changes in labour ward routines and many other reforms such as postnatal rooming-in. Unfortunately, women who could not have such contact were sometimes led to believe that they would never feel 'fully attached' to their babies.

The methodology of Klaus and Kennell's studies has been repeatedly reviewed by a variety of authorities and found to have quite severe short-comings. In addition, the majority of studies attempting to replicate their findings have failed to do so. Even much of the early animal work has also subsequently been shown to be of dubious validity.

At the present time, the critical period theory is best regarded as unproven. One could legitimately argue that the psychological events occurring over the nine months of pregnancy are considerably more important than those of the first one or two hours following delivery. The available evidence supports the notion that men and women deprived of early contact quite rapidly bond to their infant once contact is resumed. Thus, parents deprived of contact during the first

few weeks of the baby's life do not differ in their relationship with the six month old infant as compared to parents who have had contact throughout.

Accidental crises in human reproduction

The transition to parenthood is itself a crisis of a developmental type. However, a variety of unforeseen events can arise in the context of human reproduction which are best considered as accidental crises. The framework of attachment and loss is helpful in understanding the psychological implications of such events.

Infertility and the new reproductive technology

Comprehensive reviews of the psychological impact of infertility have been published and brief mention will be made here of only three aspects. First, there is the loss of the anticipated child. Second, there is the loss inherent in the failure of the individual's reproductive system which, for many individuals, represents a severe blow to self-esteem and identity. Thus, the individual may feel incomplete or defective. Third, for the partner, there is the loss of a 'fertile partner' and potential resentment and hostility may arise as a result of feelings of being 'cheated out of' the opportunity to have children.

In our society, infertility is treated as a medical matter and, by implication, a disease. Like any disease it can arouse primitive feelings of guilt or be experienced as punishment for past transgressions, especially of a sexual nature. Thus, the diagnosis of infertility is a psychological crisis for both members of the couple.

The new reproductive technologies have offered hope to many infertile couples. At the same time, they have raised formidable moral, ethical and legal issues. The latter have sometimes eclipsed psychological issues. From the psychological viewpoint, the new fertility interventions can be divided into two categories, namely those in which the foetus resides in the uterus of the woman who is to be its mother and those in which it does not (mother surrogacy).

There is no empirical evidence that a child's genetic origins substantially influence antenatal or postnatal attachment. Thus, if a pregnancy is created in the future mother by donor insemination, in vitro fertilisation (IVF) or gamete intrafallopian transfer, then the psychological tasks which require negotiation during pregnancy do not differ substantially from those described above for pregnancies conceived by conventional means. Such foetuses and infants are usually very much 'wanted' and antenatal attachment in both parents is exceptionally strong even before quickening. Such parents rapidly come to identify the foetus as their own and their intellectual knowledge of its genetic origins seems to make less impact than the emotional experiences engendered by the physical presence of the child in the uterus. Those few parents who do experience difficulties in bonding in their IVF infants would probably have had the same difficulties in an ordinary pregnancy, since the origins lie in their own personality development or in marital disharmony (the latter may, of course, have been exacerbated by the fertility problem).

Both clinical and research observations suggest that participation in IVF or similar programs is extremely stressful. Success rates are low (variously quoted at 5–25 per cent on each cycle) and the protracted and intrusive nature of testing and treatment can severely undermine closeness in the marital relationship including its sexual aspects. Each successive failure can further erode the self-esteem of both members of the couple and engender increasing hostility. Psychological stress can, in turn, have a detrimental impact on the likelihood of success by influencing gonadotrophin releasing hormones; by affecting (via catecholamines) utero-tubal functioning; by interfering with the immunological mechanisms which prevent rejection of the embryo at implantation or by predisposing to excessive alcohol or drug use detrimental to the foetus.

A major psychological difficulty with such programs involves the decision regarding when to stop trying. Both animals and humans may have considerable difficulty abandoning

any activity which is associated with a random chance of reward, especially if that reward is emotionally charged. IVF and related processes make each step of the reproductive process visible to the couple who thus, see themselves approaching their goal. Positive indication may be construed as signs that success is imminent and many couples seem to believe that their chances improve with the number of times they try, rather than seeing each attempt as an independent chance event.

A sense of finality of loss is a necessary prerequisite for resolution of the grief associated with that loss. Repeated attempts at IVF and other programs may provide, for some couples, a rationalisation for avoiding the pain of grief. Thus, as long as there is the possibility of yet another attempt or yet another program, the loss of fertility goes unmourned.

Surrogacy, as a solution to infertility, is of two types. In *altruistic* surrogacy, there is no financial payment made to the surrogate mother. In contrast, in *commercial* surrogacy the pregnant woman receives a fee for carrying the child. From a psychological view point, both types of surrogacy carry significant risks for *all* concerned. First, the commissioning couple must constantly deal with the anxiety surrounding the possibility that the surrogate may renege on the contract. Second, the surrogate must endeavour to inhibit her attachment to the foetus. If she fails, the grief at relinquishment may be very intense and greatly conflicted by guilt (especially, in commercial surrogacy where she has given up the child for money). If she succeeds in attaining detachment, she may also fail to protect the foetus since such protection derives much of its impetus from attachment. Third, the foetus, as well as being potentially less protected, may as a child experience difficulty coming to terms with its unusual origins. For example, to have been relinquished for adoption carries a rather different meaning than to have been 'sold' as in the case of commercial surrogacy. Finally, the finding that a very substantial percentage of surrogate mothers have previously had either a termination of pregnancy or relinquished a baby for adoption suggests that such women may be attempting to resolve a psychological problem or conflict in what is potentially a very maladaptive way.

The crisis of miscarriage

Fifteen per cent of confirmed pregnancies miscarry. Most of these occur before the experience of foetal movement, and lie on the low attachment segment of the curve shown in Figure 1. Most women experience a definite but transient grief reaction and major psychological sequelae appear to be rare.

Recurrent miscarriage or habitual abortion (defined as three or more consecutive miscarriages) is however, of much greater significance. The psychological impact is similar to other forms of infertility as discussed above. There is a good deal of evidence from both animal and human studies that psychological stress is an important aetiological factor in miscarriage, the likely mechanisms being as outlined above. If each loss is dealt with by immediately embarking upon yet another pregnancy (rather than resolution by grief), the intense anxiety experienced during the new pregnancy, which will usually peak at the 'gestational anniversary' of the loss, may well cause stress-induced physiological changes likely to cause miscarriage of yet another foetus. On each successive pregnancy the cycle may be repeated with ever increasing anxiety levels and accompanying physiological disturbance.

The crisis of perinatal bereavement

Approximately one per cent of babies are stillborn and a further one per cent die in the first few hours of life. In the last decade, there has been a profound improvement in the psychological management of stillbirth, intrauterine death and other perinatal bereavements. Previously, the dead baby was removed as rapidly as possible in the mistaken belief that if the parents avoided visual or tactile contact they would not 'attach' and thereby their grief and sense of loss would be diminished. What was unrecognised was the fact that most parents have already developed a very significant emotional attachment to the unborn baby during pregnancy and hence a grief reaction is inevitable.

A number of negative consequences ensued from this approach. First, the parents had no accurate awareness of what was lost and many either had horrific fantasies or came to doubt that a baby ever existed at all. Second, the parents' sense of loss and experience of grief was invalidated by staff and relatives, the latter, often taking the view that, because the parents had not seen the child, their sense of loss should be fairly negligible. Third, a great deal of hostility was engendered in these parents by remarks such as 'it's not like losing a child, you didn't even see it', and also by the feeling that their baby had been taken away from them by staff. Finally, heavy sedation was often administered to these women which not only impeded the initiation of the grief process but impaired recollection of the events surrounding the loss.

Fortunately, most major hospitals now recognise the psychological significance of perinatal bereavement and parents are given an opportunity to see and hold the dead baby if they wish. Likewise, their expression of grief is accepted and validated. As a result, the very high incidence of serious adverse psychological sequelae in women bereaved by stillbirth (quoted in most older studies as 25–30 per cent) is now considerably reduced. Nevertheless, adverse reactions are not uncommon, especially when the attachment to the foetus was highly ambivalent or where there had been a previous elective termination of pregnancy.

Postnatal depressive states

Approximately 50 per cent of women experience a transient period of incipient or actual tearfulness around the third day postpartum. This is referred to as the 'three day blues' and is of little clinical significance. Despite intensive hormonal and biochemical studies, no biological explanation of the phenomenon has been generally accepted. Likewise, the search for psychological correlates has been unsuccessful.

Approximately 10 per cent of women experience a mild to moderate depression which lasts up to one to three months postnatally. The aetiology is again uncertain. Hormonal factors may predispose, however, there is a clinical impression that many of these women have been overwhelmed by the transition to parenthood and have not been able to resolve the losses involved. Treatment is usually supportive psychotherapy with a grief work component. In some cases, especially if neurovegetative changes are apparent, antidepressant medication is indicated in addition to the above.

Approximately one in five hundred women experience severe psychiatric illness in the puerperium known as postpartum psychosis. Approximately three-quarters of these illnesses are depressive in nature and most of the remainder are manic. There is controversy as to whether the phenomenology of these illnesses differs from that of their non-puerperal counterparts, however, the physical treatments are identical. Management must, in addition, ensure the physical safety of both mother and baby, minimise the disruption to bonding and, if the mother is breast feeding, ensure that drugs such as lithium and benzodiazepines are not used.

Conclusion

Both research and clinical practice in psychosomatic obstetrics have tended to lack a sound theoretical framework for integrating the biological, psychological and social determinants of the transition to parenthood. Utilising the framework of attachment and loss, this chapter has attempted to address the psychological tasks inherent in this transition and explore the effect of various crises which may arise. One advantage of this approach lies in its ability to encompass both aetiological determinants and psychotherapeutic strategies.

George Vaillant has, in one short paper, arguably conveyed more about the true nature of attachment and loss than most other writers of more weighty volumes. Two quotations from his paper will serve to close this chapter:

Contrary to folklore and psychiatric myth, separation from and loss of those we love do not cause psychopathyology. Rather, failure to internalise those whom we have loved—or never having loved at all—causes psychopathology.

Grief work is remembering, not forgetting; it is a process of internalising, not extruding. Attachment, if properly treated, provides a strength forever.

References

Bibring G L, Dwyer T F, Huntington D S, and Valenstein A F, 'A Study of the Psychological Processes in Pregnancy and the Earliest Mother–Child Relationship', *Psychoanalytic Study of the Child*, Vol 16, 1961, pp 9–72.
Condon J T, 'The Parental-Foetal Relationship: A Comparison of Male and Female Expectant Parents', *Journal of Psychosomatic Obstetrics & Gynaecology*, Vol 4, 1985, pp 271–84.
Condon J T, 'Management of Established Pathological Grief Reacton after Stillbirth', *American Journal of Psychiatry*, Vol 143, 1986, pp 987–92.
Condon J T and Dunn D J, 'Nature and Determinants of Parent-To-Infant Attachment in the Early Postnatal Period', *Journal of American Academy of Child & Adolescent Psychiatry*, Vol 27, 1988, pp 293–9.
Kennell J H and Klaus M H, *Maternal-Infant Bonding*, Mosby, St Louis, 1976.
Reading A E, 'Psychological and Social Aspects of the New Reproductive Technologies', in Von Hall E V and Everaerd W, *The Free Woman*, Panthenon, Lancs, 1989.
Robson K M and Kumar R, 'Delayed Onset of Maternal Affection after Childbirth', *British Journal of Psychiatry*, Vol 136, 1980, pp 347–53.
Vaillant G E, 'Loss as a Metaphor for Attachment', *American Journal of Psychoanalysis*, Vol 45, 1985, pp 59–67.

Further Reading

Brockington I F and Kumar R, *Motherhood and Mental Illness 2: Causes and Consequences*, Wright, London, 1988.

Brockington I F and Kumar R, *Motherhood and Mental Illness.* Academic Press, London, 1982.

Grossman F K, Eichler L S and Winickoff S A, *Pregnancy, Birth and Parenthood*, Jassy-Bass, Washington, 1976.

Pines D,'Pregnancy and Motherhood: Interaction between Fantasy and Reality', *British Journal of Medical Psychology*, Vol 45, 1972, pp 333-43.

Sluckin W, Herbert M and Sluckin A, *Maternal Bonding.* Basil Blackwell, Oxford, 1983.

Chapter 4

Adolescent Development

J Jureidini

Adolescence is defined by the *Collins English Dictionary* as 'the period in human development that occurs between the beginning of puberty and adulthood'. The usual criteria which define adulthood are largely culturally and socially determined. The biological markers of puberty are distinct but, in practice, additional variables are used in defining the onset of adolescence, so that an Australian prepubertal 14 year old would be considered adolescent. Adolescence is therefore not clearly circumscribed, and has many biological, psychological and social continuities with childhood and adulthood. For epidemiological purposes, the World Health Organisation classifies as adolescent those individuals between 10 and 19 years of age.

Some clinicians find it useful to divide adolescence into an *early* phase where physical and cognitive changes predominate; a *middle* phase characterised by increased emphasis on peer relationships and the emergence of an adolescent subculture; and a *late* phase in which decisions about the future and the development of intimate relationships figure most strongly.

This section adopts a different but complementary approach, by dividing development into physical, cognitive, emotional and socio-cultural streams. The emphasis here is on psychological development but with recognition of the dynamic interaction with biological development and the individual's socio-cultural context. It is always important to consider the interaction between the different streams. If development in one area is significantly advanced or delayed in comparison to others, there can sometimes be problems.

The mentally handicapped teenager's cognitive disability may result in those around him ignoring changes in his physical and emotional needs as adulthood approaches. Conversely the physically and cognitively advanced adolescent may be treated as an adult with neglect of his persisting needs as a child.

Similarly, demands from one developmental stream may conflict with the needs for another. For a student, academic needs may be best served by repeating a year while emotional and social needs may suffer if he is not promoted.

Physical development

The onset of puberty is defined as the appearance of discernible secondary sexual characteristics. The first changes in boys are increase in the size of testicles and penis. In girls it is the appearance of breast buds. These changes are the direct result of the pubertal activation of the hypothalamic–pituitary gonadotropin–gondal apparatus (gonadarche). About two years earlier there will have been an increase in adrenal androgen secretion (adrenarche). It is the adrenal hormone which is responsible for axillary and pubic hair development. The brain also undergoes some further maturation during puberty, mainly an increase in myelination in cortical association areas.

The normal range for the onset of puberty is from 9 to 13 years in girls and 10 to 14 years in boys. Girls complete secondary sexual development in a mean of 4 years (range 1.5 to 6 years); boys in a mean of 3.5 years (range

49

of 2 to 4.5 years). First ejaculation (semarche) and first menstruation (menarche) usually occur in the first two years after the onset of puberty. Percentile charts are available that allow the stage of puberty to be determined. Plotting the child's sexual development on these charts can reassure adolescents and their families that development is proceeding normally.

The physical changes of puberty have complex effects on emotional development. Delayed puberty is more often a normal variation than a pathological condition, but in males it may have a negative effect on the development of age–appropriate social skills.

Androgens, especially testosterone (produced primarily by the testes but also in both sexes by the adrenals) can increase physical activity and aggressiveness. A change in these characteristics may occur in a young person prior to the appearance of overt signs of puberty and can be the precipitant for psychiatric presentation in the prepubertal period. Puberty brings about a great increase in strength so that aggression in the form of temper tantrums which might be relatively easily controlled in small children can become dangerous in adolescents.

Chronic diseases can be more difficult to manage during adolescence, because of the effects of growth, alterations in metabolism (including drug metabolism) and changes in psychological attitudes towards illness and its potentially restrictive effect on lifestyle. Epilepsy can manifest itself for the first time or become unstable during puberty. There are also changes in anticonvulsant pharmacology so that an increase in drug half-life can result in toxicity.

Pubertal growth and the associated changes in the hormonal environment probably result in changes in insulin requirements for young people with diabetes. More importantly the young person increasingly wants control over his own body and life, and is intolerant of those aspects of illness which make him feel different from his peers. As a result compliance frequently deteriorates just at the time when diabetic control can be most difficult. The psychological adjustment to chronic disability in the teenage years is complicated by the growth retardation and delayed puberty that occur in conditions like chronic renal failure.

Cognitive development

Characteristically early adolescence brings a rapid development in cognitive abilities. Piaget describes a qualitative shift whereby the individual is not only able to think about concrete things (concrete operations), but also about thoughts, reasons and ideas (formal operations). An analogy can be drawn to the relationship between arithmetic manipulation of actual numbers, and algebraic manipulation of concepts. These qualitative changes are accompanied by an improvement in the power and efficiency of existing cognitive skills. The results can include a new ability to understand jokes and proverbs; an increase in the ability to see things from the other's point of view; an ability to conceptualise ideals and a realisation that actual events or people fall short of such ideals, and a recognition that ambiguity is more common than absolute right or wrong.

Young people do not always feel comfortable with these new skills. For example, they may become overwhelmed by the difficulty of making sense of a world where nothing is absolute or perfect. In attempting to lessen anxiety a young person might adopt an extreme position which denies that there are other sides to an argument. Such attempts to master an increasingly uncertain world provide a partial explanation for the capacity of adolescents to elicit extreme reactions from adults. A negative reaction from an authority figure can feel preferable to living with uncertainty.

The capacity for formal operations is not universal amongst adults. It is dependent on practice and experience as well as intelligence, and once achieved it can be lost through disuse. Adult cognitive competence is, therefore, not simply defined by the presence or absence of formal operational thought but rather by the development of a repertoire of cognitive skills that equip the individual to function as an adult in the society.

The acquisition of new cognitive skills is facilitated by play. Play is used here in the sense of playing around with ideas or experimenting, rather than playing at formal games. Adolescence brings an increase in appetite for experimentation, including risk taking. Many factors will contribute to an individual taking a risk, including desire for acceptance by peers, the mimicking of adult models, attempts to overcome fear, and the presence of self-destructive or suicidal feelings. Risk taking is also an important way of experimenting with the limits of one's power and influence and with the limits that are set by parents and other authority figures.

Teenagers make a variety of more or less adaptive attempts to cope with the physical, cognitive, emotional and social changes that confront them. Some of their attempts seem maladaptive and ill-directed, and 'acting out' is said to be characteristic of adolescence, although it occurs throughout development. 'Acting out' occurs when individuals who are unable to express feelings through words or tears, translate them into action.

A 16 year old boy was being teased by his peers about the residual deformity of his cleft lip. He could not directly express his distress and anger at this teasing but behaved cruelly towards his non-disabled younger brother.

The non-compliance of ill adolescents to their treatments sometimes represents an 'acting out' of their anger and unhappiness at being ill.

Emotional development

Adolescence is the time when the physical and cognitive changes of puberty are conceptualised as threatening our sense of continuity, in what Erikson has called the 'identity crisis'. Moves towards independence are accompanied by increasing doubts about whether we can think or function independently. Over several years successful mastery of these threats leads to identity formation: that is, in spite of major changes in roles, relationships, beliefs, etc, we have a sense of continuity and remain capable of making decisions and functioning with at least some degree of independence from external constraints.

The concepts of identity crisis and identity formation are useful but can be misleading. The term 'crisis' suggests that adolescence must be a time of dramatic conflict and distress: 'storm and stress'. In fact it has been shown that many young people pass successfully through adolescence without such manifestations. More importantly, it is very dangerous to dismiss distress in adolescence as 'just adolescent turmoil'. Too often clinicians accept superficial explanations for an adolescent suicide attempt (for example, 'I didn't want to do the exam'). Suicidal behaviour should prompt an exploration for deeper disturbance which will often reveal a significantly depressed young person and/or major family discord.

There is an implication that identity formation starts only with puberty and must be completed by the end of the teenage years. On the contrary, children probably begin to grapple with their separateness and sense of constancy from earliest infancy and most of us have times of uncertainty about these issues well into adult life. For any individual, the timing will be influenced by family, social and cultural factors.

In discussions about identity formation, the achievement of a capacity for separateness is often emphasised at the expense of the capacity for relatedness. These qualities may seem to be alternatives but greater separateness makes possible a higher quality of relatedness and vice versa. Together they constitute the overriding goals of emotional development. The process of identity formation can be considered as a number of more concrete tasks which are grouped according to their emphasis of separateness or relatedness.

Growth in the capacity for separateness

Separation, the process of moving away emotionally from the parents, is complemented by *individuation*—the attainment of the qualities required to be able to stand alone. Separation–individuation implies a capacity to function separately rather than actual physical separation from the parents. In many cultures the child never moves away from the physical presence and influence of the parent but still achieves individuation. Separation–individuation is not something which begins in adolescence. Its basis is in the earliest parent/infant relationships which builds on experiences like weaning and going to school. For most teenagers, cognitive and physical changes and new social expectations make the process more intense.

Relinquishing the old pattern of the parent/child relationship is likely to be a painful loss for both parties. Childhood has usually been a time when parents have taken the responsibility for decision making and the child's safety. The child in turn has accepted the parental mores and usually believes 'my Mum and Dad know best'. Now the child begins to see the parents more realistically and recognise their inadequacies. To become truly independent, individuals must develop the capacity to tolerate not only their own disillusionment, but also the parents' disapproval and disappointment in them. Siblings are often important supports in this task.

Many children who are deprived and/or abused are prematurely forced to be independent. They lack the cognitive and emotional maturity necessary to successfully negotiate separation–individuation and their overall development is threatened, even if they make a superficial adjustment.

An 11 year old girl, the eldest child of a single alcoholic mother, was a competent housekeeper and caregiver for her two younger siblings. Although she functioned precociously in this role she was under-achieving at school and had no satisfactory peer relationships.

Development of a relatively stable self-image is central to establishing a capacity for separateness. Self-image refers to our own concept of how we look, feel and behave and develop from earliest infancy. For example, many disabled children are acutely aware of their difference from other children by the age of three or four. Puberty is a time of preoccupation with one's own origin (especially for those who are adopted or belong to an ethnic or cultural minority) and self-image. There is intensive self-examination and comparison with others, and young people tend to be harsh on themselves in such comparisons. Their discomfort is intensified by the broader socio-cultural idealisation of the beautiful, thin, confident and sexual adolescent.

Sexuality is an integral part of self-image. Gender identity is stabilised in the first two to four years of life and sexuality is probably most strongly influenced by biological and social factors that have already exerted their influence before puberty. Hormonal changes, the onset of reproductive capability and social pressures interact to confront adolescents with their sexuality. A positive identification with the same-sex parent is a great asset in meeting this challenge. Young people often become preoccupied with their inadequacies and genuinely frightened by what they regard as abnormalities (for example, temporary breast development in pubertal boys is not uncommon, but can cause severe anxiety). In spite of adequate sex education, teenagers can become guilty or anxious about masturbation, especially if it is prohibited by culture or religion. They may even mistakenly believe that they are doing themselves physical damage through masturbation.

Teenagers are frequently threatened by the thought of heterosexual relationships. Sexually-orientated play among peers of both sexes is common in our culture. Precocious sexuality may suggest that the child has been exposed to inappropriate sexual activity, which has prematurely aroused sexual interest and promoted inappropriate sexual behaviour; or that anger towards the parents is being expressed by challenging their sexual values. Teenagers often do not enjoy their first sexual experiences, and they may be a source of guilt and anxiety.

Chronically ill and disabled youngsters may be preoccupied with the effects of their illness on their sexuality and reproductive capabilities, but reluctant to voice their concerns. Health workers must therefore ensure that these teenagers have opportunities for adequate and appropriate counselling.

Self responsibility allows the individual to rely less on others to regulate behaviour and feelings. Social influences always have a powerful effect on behaviour, but people are more independent if they have a set of internal rules to guide them which are not overly harsh or inflexible. As described above, the need for internal controls over behaviour and emotions is increased by the gains in strength and effectiveness and possibly increased lability of mood which are a consequence of puberty. A young person who lacks these internal controls risks destructive conflict which may impair development and invite society to exert external controls.

There are also dangers with over-control, although over-controlled individuals attract less attention from mental health professionals. Teenagers who are fearful of their feelings, and the fantasised consequences of them, or who have harsh and forbidding internal rules, can become emotionally and behaviourally restricted. Consequently they are less able to experiment playfully. Instead of evolving an identity for themselves they often fulfil a role based on their perception of what others expect of them, sometimes called 'identity foreclosure', or 'false self' in Winnicot's terms. This state of superficially good adjustment with quiet compliance, 'pseudomaturity', tends to be associated with a constricted emotional repertoire and lack of expressiveness. Such individuals often lack satisfying interpersonal relationships and are vulnerable when placed under stress. Because they create little fuss, their dysfunction is frequently missed.

Role of the parents

As young people undergo the changes of the separation–individuation process, the parents have complex complementary tasks. For example, as adolescents take more responsibility for their personal life and decision making, they may adopt a stance at odds with the parents' beliefs or values. In response, the parents must balance the risks on the one hand of trying to impose their own ideal on their children and, on the other hand, of giving way over personal beliefs or principles. For example, how should a father behave if his strong political beliefs lead him to conclude that his son's behaviour is socially irresponsible?

Sometimes parents become envious of their children's youth and opportunities. They may respond by imposing unreasonable restrictions or by channelling their children into activities which vicariously satisfy the parents but may not take sufficient account of the adolescent's wants and needs. Although it is important for the parents to relinquish some responsibility over their adolescent's personal life, they should retain their right to be in charge of family life; that is, to set reasonable rules and requirements for behaviour within the home. Other authorities, such as teachers, should do the same within their own territories. Adolescents become uncertain about their powers and limits as they grow physically, cognitively and emotionally, and they need clear limits within which to experiment. The art of parenting is to provide limits that are narrow enough to ensure that the adolescent is, and feels, relatively safe but broad enough to allow experimentation. Adolescents learn best when behaviour progresses to its natural conclusions and consequences rather than being interrupted by rules or limits. Parents, teachers and other adults who deal with young people need to be authoritative without being authoritarian; that is, neither to shirk taking authority when it is appropriate nor to take authority just for the sake of it.

All of these tasks may be more difficult for ill and disabled young people and their families. Although individuation is a psychic rather than a physical process, a dependence on help for physical care may inhibit the achievement of emotional independence. Disabled people are often frustrated in their attempts to establish their individuality.

A young man with cerebral palsy was busy with his tertiary studies. Nevertheless it was important for him to make time to maintain his own flat, rather than have his parents do it for him.

Health professionals will be placed in the role of parental figures in dealing with ill and disabled adolescents, who will often select an aspect of their handicap or treatment as a focus for a struggle over independence. The health worker may be drawn into a struggle as he defends what is believed to be optimal care. Like parents, professionals become involved in a complex process of negotiation, yielding and, at times, authoritative insistence. The aim should be for the adolescent to take appropriate responsibility for his own health.

Growth in the capacity for relatedness

Increasing separateness needs to be complemented by finding a place in the world—*a social context*. Prior to adolescence the family has been the dominant context, although school and peers will have become increasingly important. With the teenage years, the peer group and idealised outsiders often replace the family as the primary influence. At the same time, cognitive development brings an increasing ability to see things from more than one point of view as well as more effective, if erratic, powers of reasoning. The adolescent often questions the family's *values* for the first time. This may lead to some confusion and, in the absence of other values can lead to the adoption of what has been called a negative identity—'I don't know what I am, but I know what I'm not'. The stereotype is of an intellectual questioning of parental and societal standards but this can be misleading. Challenging of parental and societal values need not be an intellectual process. Many adolescents behave in a way which challenges their parents and society without verbalising or perhaps even being aware of their dissent. Nor is major rebellion against parental values universal. Some young people can comfortably adopt the ideals of their culture and family without foreclosure.

The *adolescent sub-culture* is characteristic of the middle years of adolescence. Young people identify with a group or adopt a role prescribed by that group, gaining access to ready-made identities. Such groups are accepting of the individual provided they adhere to rules which are both stated and unstated. Their rules provide guidance and structure, but because they are different from the rules of adult society, they allow different forms of experimentation. There are destructive gangs and altruistic clubs but more often groups display aspects of both. Within one or more groups, the adolescent can try a variety of roles, ideally retaining and integrating those aspects which are prositive for them, and rejecting the rest.

The *capacity for peer relations* is both a test of and a resource in adolescent development. An important quality of early adolescent friendships is the mirroring function. Adolescents use friends to find out about themselves, both through talking about each other and through vicariously experimenting with roles that one or more members of the group may adopt.

One teenager in a group may try out an illicit drug and bring the experience back to the group, allowing them to decide their own attitudes towards that drug.

Vicarious experimenting can have positive effects with only one rather than all the adolescents exposed to risk; on the other hand, the group may influence one member to take a risk that no individual would have taken of their own accord.

A group of teenagers had been preoccupied for some time with suicidal fantasies, often daring each other to act and entering into suicide acts that never eventuated. Eventually one of the more vulnerable individuals did commit suicide.

With increasing age, there is a tendency for peer groups to progress from single to mixed gender, with the beginning of heterosexual relationships. For some time, however, the primary relationships are to the group and often to the same sex peers. It is only in late adolescence that the couple becomes the primary unit.

The achievement of *intimate reciprocal relationships* and establishing realistic *expectations for the future* are the two markers of relatedness that signal a readiness to take adult responsibility. The intimate relationships of adulthood develop out of the friendships and infatuations of adolescence. One important change is the greater acceptance within an adult intimate relationship of how the partner is in reality. There is less pressure on each partner to meet some ideal and a lessening of the lability that is characteristic of adolescent relationships. In a truly intimate relationship, there will be a mutually satisfying balance of giving and taking.

Future expectations in our culture are most clearly manifest in choices about career and family structure and this can be a source of considerable anxiety. The amount of choice and control over the future varies according to the circumstances. Whether we begin from a position of privilege or deprivation, maturity involves the relinquishing of unrealistic and idealised goals in favour of potentially achievable, but challenging expectations about future life. Within the family, the increasing relatedness of adolescence leads to a re-negotiation of the relationship between parent and child towards predominantly adult to adult. Remember that the achievement of independence is quite compatible with still allowing oneself to be looked after by one's parents or to turn to them for advice. For the ill and disabled, some dependency is usually inevitable and it is the capacity to appropriately establish independence at some times or in some areas that is important.

Social and cultural context

The most important part of the environment for the growing teenager is the *family* (or its substitutes). The importance of the family lies in the complementary role of parents and siblings in the emotional development of the adolescent, and examples have already been given. Note that at least 25 per cent of adolescents do not grow up with both parents in nuclear families and the potential effects of this experience must be taken into account when talking about 'normal' adolescence.

The other major influence on teenagers is the *school*. There is good evidence that some schools produce less delinquency, less behaviour disturbance, less absenteeism and higher levels of educational attainments than other schools serving demographically equivalent populations. The important variables are not the school size or the physical facilities, but the characteristics of the student population and the teachers—the school culture. At-risk children do better where there is a high proportion of other children without major problems, an accepting environment without isolation from peers and opportunities to take responsibility. Successful schools have teachers who provide good models of behaviour for children, respect their students, and have appropriately high expectations of

them. The teachers offer well planned classroom management techniques, good discipline with sparing use of punishment and a pleasant working environment and are willing to give attention to individual worries or problems. The successful school supports teachers with an organisational structure which encourages staff to work together and provides leadership and decision making at the senior level. Those most at risk in the school system include those from migrants or minority groups; the physically, intellectually or learning impaired; those whose parents have low educational achievements; and those who come from deprived backgrounds. Although these are risk factors in many other aspects of life, a child with strengths within the educational system is often able to overcome major adversity in other areas.

We have seen how the growing adolescent needs to adjust to internal and external changes. In the process, he will be pressured to fill a role in society, which will vary according to the nature of the society and the status of the individual. Adult society overtly and covertly encourages young people to experiment with alcohol, weight reduction, promiscuity and other risk factors. Adolescents may experiment with behaviours which the broader society then may or may not adopt. For instance, in the democracy movement in China in 1989, it was the students who openly protested most and took the greatest casualties. The immediate response of the leaders was to reject the values expressed by the students and to increase conservatism and social controls. Conversely, in Australia, adolescents played a major part in the Vietnam Moratorium that led the country in a change of attitude towards that war.

Adolescents are over-represented amongst the unemployed and research has demonstrated that Australian unemployed young people have much higher levels of psychiatric and other dysfunction, raising the possibility of a causal relationship. Other physical or cultural factors which lead the society to define an adolescent as 'different', such as disability or ethnic origin, also place additional pressures on young people. In particular the tasks of establishing self-image, relating to a peer group and finding a place in the peer subculture can be more difficult in the face of such feelings of difference.

Different cultures place different demands on their adolescents. It is generally accepted that adolescence is prolonged in Australia, compared with smaller scale societies. It is sometimes further assumed that in such small scale societies (for example, traditional aboriginal culture in its undisturbed state), the transition from childhood to adulthood is made easy by formal Rites of Passage and the availability of clearly determined adult roles; however there are stresses and conflicts associated with achieving adult status in all cultures.

Further Reading

Blos P, *The Adolescent Passage,* International Universities Press, New York, 1979.

Erikson E H, *Identity: Youth and Crisis,* W W Norton, New York, 1968.

Evans J, *Adolescent and Pre-adolescent Psychiatry,* Academic Press Inc, London, 1982.

Laufer M, *Adolescent Disturbance and Breakdown,* Penguin Books, 1975.

Offer D, *The Psychological World of the Teenager: A Study of Normal Adolescent Boys,* Basic Books, New York, 1973.

Rutter M, Maughan B, Mortimor E and Ouston J, *15,000 Hours: Secondary Schools and their Effects on Children,* Open Books, London, 1979.

Steinberg D, *Clinical Psychiatry of Adolescence: Clinical Work from a Social and Developmental Perspective,* John Wiley and Sons, Chichester, 1983.

Chapter 5

Middle and Later Life

F Hughes and S Ticehurst

Midlife generally includes the years from 35 to 65 and old age from 65 years onwards. It is only in comparatively recent times that living to a relatively advanced age has become common. One hundred years ago only 27 per cent of males and 35 per cent of females survived to age 70 years. In 1982, 63 per cent of their generation for males and 79 per cent for females were at least 70 years old. Research into middle and old age has grown with the increasing numbers of elderly people in the community. However, the greater interest in people in these age groups is not just a product of the increasing numbers of older people. Our increasing awareness of middle and old age is also related to the rapid pace of social change itself. Successive generations (or cohorts) grow up in different social environments. To some extent each learns differently, develops different norms and, very significantly, develops different expectations about the course and pace of individual lives. These features then become characteristics which differentiate one generation from the next.

It is important to distinguish cohort effects, or differences in socialisation and life experience, from age effects when comparing generations. For example, the assignment of life priorities and the development of schedules for achieving them are very much affected by social conditions experienced during life. Some of the generation which lived through the economic depression of the 1930s developed a distrust of banks while the children of that generation placed great importance on owning a home.

The increasing rate of social change in this century has accentuated the diversity between and within generations. It used to be thought that the developmental tasks of getting married, having children, establishing a career and reaching career plateaux could be timetabled or scheduled in a fairly uniform way. For example, in a series of studies conducted in the late 1950s, Bernice Neugarten and her associates asked, among other questions 'What is the best age for a man (or woman) to marry?'. Most respondents thought somewhere between 20 and 25 years of age. Similarly, it was agreed that a man should be settled in a career by age 26 and hold his top job by 40. There is thus a type of mental map which people used to judge their progress in life. While it is probably true that people still attempt to plan or map out their lives, it is unlikely that such maps are as uniform in detail as they used to be. For today's generation of young people a question such as 'What is the best age for a person to marry?' would probably elicit a response to the effect that it depends on the person.

In middle and old age the problems by uncertainties about social norms become apparent. Feelings of vulnerability seem to prompt many people to question the direction of their lives. The popularity of books which describe in a prescriptive fashion the stages of adult life can be attributed to the needs of many of today's middle aged people to understand themselves and to find satisfactory purposes for their lives.

Systematic study of midlife and old age is a relatively recent phenomenon. The traditional view of developmental theorists was that personality was shaped early in life and remained fixed thereafter. It was thought that intellect reached its peak in adolescence and was followed by gradual deterioration. This view was based on a belief that psychological functioning paralleled physical functioning. As a physical unit, the body becomes less efficient with advancing age. This process is genetically determined and has death as its end point. There is a great deal of individual variation. Further, there are differences between organ systems with each system reaching optimal function at a different age and declining at a different rate. For instance, visual acuity reaches a peak in early adolescence and declines thereafter. It took a long time to realise that psychological and physiological functioning were not parallel.

A person's awareness of and adjustment to their body changes in midlife does have great psychological significance. Some people react to the first signs of physical decline (for example, the first set of spectacles) with anxiety and panic. Others seem to regard the deterioration as an inevitable part of ageing over which they have little control. The important point is that while physiological deterioration does not necessarily imply psychological stagnation, psychosocial development in midlife occurs against a background of biological ageing.

Stages and themes

The psychoanalyst, Erikson divided the life span into eight developmental stages. Each stage is characterised as a conflict between opposite poles of a central theme.

The seventh stage of life in this scheme is late adulthood (middle age) which represents a conflict between generativity and stagnation. The person becomes concerned with issues of productivity and the value of his life's work. For many middle-aged people, self-esteem derives from successful work performance. If this is challenged or threatened, for example, by failing to gain promotion, then the person may question the effort put into the work. Some people begin to wonder whether there is any prospect of their being useful to anyone and, indeed, whether their lives are worthwhile. This reaction has a strong depressive component

and is perhaps found more frequently among middle-aged people who lose their jobs or experience a sudden decline in health (for example, a stroke). For others, feelings that they are not appreciated may come to dominate them. In this type of reaction, feelings of self doubt are mixed with bitterness. Escapist fantasies in which the person gives up his job and adopts a radically different lifestyle, usually free of significant responsibility, may be prominent.

According to Erikson, the outcome of the late adult stage may be positive or negative. A positive outcome involves a renewed commitment to a productive life. The recognition that self-esteem does not depend exclusively on successful work performance, and the identification of goals still to be achieved in life are fundamental to a positive resolution of this stage. A frequent and important component of being 'generative' in later life is the passing of expertise or skills to the next generation. A negative outcome means a withdrawal of energy from productive activity and profound feelings of futility.

In the scheme advanced by Erikson, old age is the final period of life and the developmental issue is here summarised as ego integrity versus despair. With increasing age, people become aware that the end of their life is near. According to Erikson, such an awareness is a threat to ego integrity. The elderly person looks back on his life to appraise whether there has been any meaning or pattern to it. They may be aware of deterioration in physical or psychological functions. The person is also conscious of the fact that remaining life is short; there is not enough time to do much that will be significant or to make up for lost opportunities. Successful resolution of this stage involves the person coming to see that life has been worthwhile. Although there may be tasks left incomplete, the person feels satisfied to live each day as it comes. A negative outcome or failure to resolve the issues involved in this stage leaves the person with a sense of despair. The person may withdraw from life, almost as if he were giving up. An alternative negative reaction sometimes seen is denial of the ageing process.

Erikson's ideas have stimulated theoretical and empirical studies. The concept of life review, which is implicit in his description of the last stage, ego integrity versus despair, has been elaborated extensively. Life review usually refers to the spontaneous intrusion into consciousness of memories of past events, particularly those events which are associated with unresolved emotional conflicts. When these memories are considered carefully, emotional conflicts in them can be resolved. Life reviews have been put forward as a therapeutic tool which can be used to facilitate adjustment to middle and old age. They seem useful if the failure to adjust is the product of unresolved emotional conflict. Another use of a life review is as a technique for affirming the value of people whose sense of self integrity is threatened because of degenerative disease, especially dementia. The rationale here is that by reminding people of past successes we are saying to them that they were once valuable.

There are two major problems with the stages and themes approach developed by Erikson and others. The first has to do with the proposition that stages follow a fixed sequence. Erikson advocated that successful resolution of one stage is a necessary condition for advancement to the next stage. However, in reality the lives of most adults do not conform to such precise staging. An issue such as the value of one's work is usually con- sidered many times between early middle age and the years after retirement. Further, individual differences are more pronounced with increasing age and it becomes more difficult to impose a conceptual schema which applies to every person.

The second problem with the themes and stages approach is that the themes described are usually abstracted from personal accounts which are themselves summaries of experiences. The problem is that while such abstraction is useful for descriptive purposes, it can be misleading when used as a basis for predicting behaviour. As an example, consider the 'empty nest' syndrome which was put forward by people who had been influenced by Erikson's stage of generativity versus stagnation as it applied to adulthood. Basically, this predicts that women whose children leave home become depressed, and that they are of no further value. It is a simple

and elegant concept. However, it occurs in only a few cases. Surveys indicate that many women are more distressed by adult children who do not leave home than they are by those who do!

Developmental sequences

More recently, the approach to the changes in midlife and old age has been based more on findings from empirical research. Several studies have followed-up adult subjects longitudinally through two or more decades. These studies and cross-sectional research yield a picture of normal development in later life which is different from commonly held views.

It is widely thought that intellectual performance declines in midlife and that intellectual deterioration is one of the major characteristics of old age. The Seattle longitudinal study which was conducted over 28 years by Schaie and his colleagues separated the effects of belonging to a particular generation from the effects of ageing. People born early in the century generally received less education than people born later. Unless a study is carefully designed, this type of generational effect is confused with the effects of ageing. Schaie found that the effects of belonging to a particular gen- eration were very significant. Performance on tests of verbal meaning, spatial perception and reasoning improved with every generation from birth year 1896 onwards. On the other hand, word fluency declined with each generation since 1889.

The major finding of the Seattle study was that, apart from a decline in speed-related intellectual operations in the sixth decade, the intellectual performance of most people remained reasonably constant into the eighth decade of life. This finding was consistent with those of other longitudinal studies. Of the other studies, the Duke University study is particularly interesting because of the effort made to discover variables which correlated with intellectual decline when it did occur. Best correlations were achieved with cardio- vascular abnormalities, electroencephalo- graphic slow waves and levels of immuno- globulin in the blood. These findings led the

Duke researchers to conclude that intellectual deterioration in old age was associated with compromised functioning of body systems. In other words, while people remained physically healthy they could reasonably expect to maintain their intellectual functioning into advanced old age. Intellectual deterioration seems to be unusual and sometimes is the product of potentially correctable pathology.

Vaillant followed a group of men for 35 years after they had graduated from college in the early 1940s. He was interested in how people used defence mechanisms to adapt to the demands of life. He proposed that defence mechanisms belonged to one of four groups, with each group being progressively more adaptive (see chapter 2). These were (i) primitive (for example, denial); (ii) immature (for example, projection, hypochondriasis, acting out); (iii) neurotic (for example, intellectualisation, displacement, dissociation); (iv) mature (for example, altruism, humour, sublimation). Vaillant classified the subjects according to the highest level of adaptive functioning they exhibited. He found that many had not progressed past defences he considered immature. Less than a third showed mature defence mechanisms. He concluded that while there is development and enrichment of personality throughout the adult lifespan for some people, for others there is very little change after early adulthood.

Vaillant found that health status was correlated with the emotional defences used by a person. Most of the subjects whose highest level of coping was still immature either died or developed a chronic, incapacitating physical condition by the age of 55. Mature copers were significantly better than immature copers when measured by physical health indices, work satisfaction, marital stability, friendship patterns and social activity levels.

It is tempting to postulate that there is, in midlife and old age, a strong positive correlation between good health, stability of intellectual functions, use of mature defences and social adjustment. However, such an hypothesis would grossly oversimplify the potential variations in individual functioning. There are some tasks on which the performance of older people is inferior to that of people in late adolescence or early adulthood. Elderly people are slower in processing visual information. They also do not perform as well as younger people in complex auditory vigilance tasks. It is probable that this difference reflects an age related decline in short term memory. Increasing age is also associated with comparative difficulty in learning new relationships and in situations where there are many distractions.

However, there are tasks where people in midlife and old age do better than younger subjects. Older people respond more creatively to social judgement tasks involving ambiguous situations (for example, will a woman who has indicated that she will leave her drunken husband, do so?). They analyse information on human interaction in a more complex way and are more sophisticated in interpreting non-verbal communicative cues. Older people are slower but more creative on some psychological tasks. It is interesting that older people become quicker on such tasks but only by giving common responses (that is, by becoming less creative). The apparent slowness of older people may, therefore, be an indication of more complex cognitive processing. In the area of memory, for example, older people do not find it easy to recall detail, but instead, put effort into extracting and memorising the meaning of material.

There are other tasks where older and younger perform differently and there is disagreement about the interpretation of such differences. These tasks usually involve logical analysis and one view is that older people think more concretely than younger people and are unable to separate their real world knowledge from the process of logical analysis. This interpretation has been criticised because it judges the performance of people in midlife and old age by standards and tasks which are appropriate for adolescents. The alternative view is that older people find formal approaches to problem solving and logical analysis to be unsatisfactory precisely because such approaches fail to take account of the real world. This can be seen as an advantage because it enables older people to make decisions on the basis of probable outcomes. Older people seem aware that despite predictive certainty, formal logic does not adequately capture the complexity of everyday life.

Contextual factors

Across the population of middle-aged and old people marked variations exist in measures of intellectual and personality functions. This variation in part may be due to differences in situations and lifestyles. Intelligence, at least as measured by standardised tests, seems to be responsive to environmental conditions. Performance on tests of visuospatial perception, memory and response speed can also be modified by training. Performance on cognitive tests therefore probably varies with the amount and type of intellectual stimulation a person has experienced in his life. Moreover, cognitive deterioration in midlife or old age, when it does occur, is not necessarily irreversible. Elderly people can and do learn. It is not uncommon for a person in their sixties or seventies to undertake a course of tertiary study and succeed.

Experiences such as unemployment, divorce, severe illness and hospitalisation may, for some people, mark a transition from one developmental stage to the next. Feelings of anxiety or of not being in control of one's life can be associated with periods of life transition. While there is evidence that such experiences may be stressful for many people, the evidence that they are associated with a systematic reorganisation of personality is only slim.

Conclusion

The study of development in midlife and old age is comparatively new. Despite this, significant progress has been made in defining norms and in clarifying the dimensions of personal development. The field is now moving beyond describing simple chronological changes. The most interesting questions being considered by current researchers concern the mechanisms which initiate and maintain development in adulthood.

Why is it that some people in midlife and old age have managed to free themselves from rigid emotional defences adopted in adolescence? Why is it that some people in midlife and old age develop quite complex cognitive processes, especially to do with their reasoning about themselves and other people? Why is that some of these people also display an integration of affect and thought? Why is that some people do not show any of these developments? Attempts to answer these questions make the study of midlife and old age one of the most interesting and important areas of present day psychology.

Further Reading

Birren J E and Schaie K W, *Handbook of the Psychology of Aging*, Van Nostrand Reinhold Co, New York, 1985.

Erikson E H, *Childhood and Society*, Triad/Paladin, Frogmore, St Albans, Hertfordshire, 1977.

Levinson D J, Darrow C N, Klein E B, Levinson M H and McKie B, *The Seasons of a Man's Life*, Ballantine, New York, 1978.

Schaie K W, *Longitudinal Studies of Adult Psychological Development*, Guildford, New York, 1983.

Vaillant G E, *Adaptation to Life*, Little Brown, 1977.

Chapter 6

Neglect and Abuse of Children

P Hazell

The neglect or abuse of children arouses concern and strong emotional reactions from the community. To some extent this may be a reaction against the previous lack of regard for the rights of children prevalent in Western Society until this century. Children were being used as cheap labour well into the nineteenth century in England. In the United States, in 1872, the 'Society for the Prevention of Cruelty to Animals' had to intervene to protect an abused child because there was no statutory basis to protect children. This led to the establishment of the 'Society for the Prevention of Cruelty to Children' in New York in 1875, and in England in 1883, and the development of child protection laws. Failure to thrive as a result of psychosocial deprivation was described early this century. Child abuse, or the 'battered child' syndrome, was not generally recognised by health professionals until the 1960s. The acknowledgement of the existence of child sexual abuse has been a phenomenon of the 1980s.

Neglect

The best documented form of child neglect is the so-called 'nonorganic failure to thrive syndrome'. This syndrome is defined as a failure to grow and develop normally, in the absence of any physical disorder that could account for the abnormality. Neglect also includes an inadequacy of parents or guardians to meet the nutritional, medical, educational, and social needs of a child, for example, failure to obtain medical assessment and treatment for an ill child. Frequent changes of caregivers may also lead to neglect. Failure to thrive is most commonly seen in

infants under the age of two years. Such infants often demonstrate an associated persistent failure to initiate or respond to social interaction. Older children may be overfriendly with strangers. Children with this form of neglect improve after the institution of adequate care in hospital.

The prevalence of nonorganic failure to thrive within the community is unknown, but psychosocial causes are thought to account for approximately one third of all cases of failure to thrive. 'Deprivation dwarfism' is a result of neglect occurring in older children where the prominent feature is short stature rather than malnutrition. The mechanism appears to be a decreased activity of growth hormone, and it has been proposed that this may be due to malnutrition.

In the past an important cause of failure to thrive was the lack of consistent and adequate parenting due to continuous institutional care. Contemporary cases are more likely to be caused by impaired parent/infant attachments. Studies examining parental factors leading to impaired attachment have identified three types of vulnerable parents: (i) those who are capable but temporarily overwhelmed due to the presence of stressors or mental illness (ii) those who are emotionally immature and themselves deprived (iii) those who reject the baby. Infant attributes that contribute to poor attachment include poor responsiveness and difficult feeding. These attributes may result from temperament or underlying organic pathology. There is debate whether the primary deficit leading to failure to thrive is lack of affection or lack of nutrition.

Management includes the adequate feeding

of the child and the assessment of: (i) the child's health (ii) the mother's physical and emotional health (iii) the mother's social circumstances (iv) the quality of the interaction between infant and mother. Less severe cases of failure to thrive often respond to counselling of the parents about feeding and infant care as well as the provision of social support. These parents and their infants are successfully followed up by mothercraft or family care units. More severe cases may require psychiatric treatment for the mother or father.

Studies of the long term outcome of infants with nonorganic failure to thrive show that with adequate nutrition and parenting, growth and intellectual development can improve, but generally they are below the height, weight and intelligence quotient (IQ) that might otherwise have been expected. In addition, they are at greater risk for emotional and behavioural problems. One reason for this may be a result of impaired brain development due to malnutrition. Another could be a consequence of prolonged social disadvantage. A common feature in children with a history of nonorganic failure to thrive is a continued impairment in their attachments to others in later life. Often, they show behaviour that invites rejection from others. Children who do not have stable and permanent caregivers often move from one temporary care situation to another. Each time there is a brief 'honeymoon' phase in which the caregiver feels that they can form some bond with the child, usually followed by a series of problems leading to the removal of the child.

Physical abuse

The physically abused child has been defined as 'any child who receives non-accidental physical injury (or injuries) as a result of acts (or omissions) on the part of his parents or guardians'. Sometimes it is difficult to determine what is abuse and what may be considered within the normal spectrum of discipline. Physical abuse must be suspected when a child presents with injuries that are inconsistent with the story provided by parents, or where the history is implausible

(for example, a two year old child walked into a door handle injuring his eye socket) or where the injuries themselves are suspicious (for example, cigarette burns, scalding to the buttocks). Injuries can include haemorrhage into the brain or eye from shaking, head injuries, broken bones, burns, genital injuries, poisoning and parents causing simulated illness in the child.

Australasian studies have found a prevalence of child abuse of approximately 2.6 per 10,000 children, but these figures are thought to be an underestimate. Physical abuse of children is reported more commonly from lower socio-economic groups although no social class is free of it. It is commonly associated with a parental history of neglect and abuse. Child abuse is also associated with parental psychiatric illness, particularly post partum depression and alcohol and drug abuse. Some researchers have identified a range of factors associated with child abuse which include social isolation of the family (for example, having an unlisted telephone number), distorted parental perceptions of the child including unrealistic expectations, fear of spoiling, emphasising punishment as a positive value, and having an impaired ability to empathise with the child. Child characteristics associated with abuse include temperamental and physical factors leading to an unresponsive baby.

Abused children with injuries may present to hospital for treatment. Recognition of child abuse therefore will depend on the vigilance of emergency and primary care staff. A thorough and well documented history and examination is essential, preferably with photographs to illustrate the nature and site of injuries. It is generally recommended that a senior physician be involved in the management of the case. Child protection issues are most important at the point of diagnosis and will be discussed below under the heading 'Prevention'. The child should be regularly examined for further injuries. Treatment ideally should involve engagement of both parents. Unfortunately this is not always possible. It is often deemed too great a risk for the child to remain at home and removal of the child from the family, temporarily or in the long term, is necessary.

Treatment of the abusing parent begins with encouraging the parent to accept responsibility for their behaviour towards the child. Some parents, for example, will say that they could stop hitting their child if the child would only behave better. The response from the therapist is that a parent must not harm a child, regardless of the child's behaviour. Parents are given counselling on alternative strategies for dealing with difficult behaviour in their child. Treatment of a parent's alcohol and drug abuse often has a positive influence on parenting behaviour. In addition, the parent may require assistance with other social problems such as finance and housing.

The abused child may require treatment for post traumatic symptoms such as persistent nightmares and anxieties. More commonly the child may require treatment for behavioural or emotional problems that have arisen due to the social circumstances which have also contributed to the abuse. Head injured children may have special difficulties due to intellectual impairment. Essential to the successful management of child abuse cases is adequate liaison between health, welfare and legal professionals.

Some abused children show long term intellectual impairment and emotional and behavioural disturbance. A concern is that some of these children will become abusing parents.

Child sexual abuse

Child sexual abuse is the involvement of children in sexual activities which they cannot fully comprehend, to which they cannot give informed consent, and which violate the law. Child sexual abuse includes incest, extra-familial sexual abuse, child pornography and child prostitution. As with physical abuse it is often difficult to draw the boundary between behaviour in a family that may be considered normal and that which is pathological. Sexual abuse is generally considered to include a range of behaviours from exposure and genital fondling through to rape with violence and sadistic sexual activity. Intrafamilial abuse is often persistent and may involve a number of children in a family. Many children do not report their experience, or only report their experience when they are much older. Sadly, the partner of an abusing parent may often fail to recognise the presence of abuse, or deny it and may only report abuse when there are other issues such as disputes over child custody.

In recent years there has been increased public awareness of sexual abuse but it is still likely that child sexual abuse is under-diagnosed. Current estimates suggest up to 20 per cent of girls and 10 per cent of boys less than 16 years of age have experienced some form of inappropriate sexual contact although in less than one per cent does this involve genital contact.

Penalties for sexual abuse of children are severe, hence there is a lot at stake in the accurate diagnosis of child sexual abuse. While clinical experience indicates that a warm, accepting and non threatening approach is the most appropriate and therapeutic for the child, it may have insufficient rigour to meet the needs of a legal assessment. This has led to a cumbersome division between assessment for therapy and assessment for court hearings, and can lead to prolonged and unnecessary investigation of children which may of itself be stressful to them.

Recognition of sexually abused children often lies with professionals other than doctors such as teachers, kindergarten staff and welfare workers. Sexually abused children may present with medical complications including genital or anal trauma, sexually transmitted disease, pregnancy, persistent vaginal discharge and urinary tract infections. Infection with HIV virus is now a matter of concern. Behaviours which overtly emphasise sexual activities, especially if they seem inappropriate to the child's age, are a possible indication of child sexual abuse. These include preoccupation with sexual matters, inappropriate sex play, seductiveness, sexual aggression, excessive masturbation and inappropriate sexual knowledge. Many sexually abused children show emotional and behavioural disturbances which are also found in other children under stress, for example, nightmares, anxiety, depression and suicidal ideation.

Assessment of a child who has been sexually

abused should be undertaken by a professional who is skilled with children, competent in regard to child emotional and behavioural problems, and one who is sensitive to the needs of the child. As with children suspected of being physically abused, a thorough medical examination is essential.

Adults who sexually abuse children are often members of the child's family or are well known to the family. Betrayal of trust therefore plays an important part in the phenomenology of child sexual abuse. This may lead to problems for the child in developing trusting relationships with other people.

The adverse consequences of child sexual abuse are thought to derive as much from the conditions that permit abuse to occur and to be sustained as from the sexual acts themselves. Since child sexual abuse is illegal and socially abhorrent, the child is usually forced to maintain it as a secret (often under threat from the abuser). Discovery can itself be traumatic, since the child may be disbelieved, blamed and even rejected.

Treatment focuses on the child and the family. Individual therapy for the child may consist of support through the notification and investigation process, providing a supportive relationship in which it is possible for the victim to express his feelings of anger and guilt, and promoting a healthy development beyond the abuse experience. Where there has been extrafamilial abuse, the family may need to be supported in coping with the experience and dealing with feelings of guilt often associated with their perceived failure to protect the child from the abuser. With intrafamilial abuse, the abusing parent or family member can be engaged in family therapy and come to acknowledge their responsibility for their actions. This is not always possible, so that the focus of management may be primarily directed to protection of the child. It is not always recognised that the non abusing parent may require considerable individual support during the notification and investigation process, as well as the child victim.

Depressed mood is common amongst children who have been sexually abused. Some children are more severely affected and may make suicide attempts, run away from home or display behaviours imitative of the offence. Older children may become promiscuous, and there is possibly a link between the experience of sexual abuse in childhood and prostitution. The whole family may be affected by the abuse and its legal consequences, sometimes leading to a severe disruption in family life. Adult adjustment following the experience of childhood sexual abuse is determined by the nature of the abuse (especially whether it was violent), the family circumstances which permitted the abuse to occur, and the sensitivity with which the abuse experience was handled by the family and professionals. Enduring psychological harm is uncommon amongst adults who have been exposed to mild sexual abuse experiences in childhood (for example, exhibitionism or fondling). Those exposed to more severe sexual abuse, especially if accompanied by violence or threats of violence, may experience sexual maladjustment, general unhappiness and marital discord, even in the absence of psychiatric illness.

Prevention

Ideally, the neglect and abuse of children should be prevented. Considerable emphasis has been given by some to the importance of successful early attachments by the mother to the infant as a protective factor against subsequent neglect or abuse. Work in this area has led to a significant improvement in perinatal practice, including the emphasis on early warm contact between the parents and the infant. There is a danger that the significance of this early period may be overvalued. Recent research indicates that parents begin to form meaningful attachments to their baby long before its birth. The most hopeful preventive interventions are based on the identification of mothers and infants at risk during the antenatal period. Those parents most at risk may have only sporadic contact with health professionals and often avoid follow-up. Interventions generally consist of parental support and counselling, with the provision for statutory investigation and even removal of the child if the parents are not compliant, or if there is evidence of abuse.

At this time there has been no systematic study into the efficacy of these interventions. It is important to note that it is unrealistic to expect that all child abuse will be eradicated, regardless of the effort spent on the early detection of risk. Some professionals approach child abuse with a sense of personal failure, or a need to blame other professionals or agencies with inadequacy.

The primary prevention of child sexual abuse is an equally difficult area. While the ideal is an alteration in the attitudes of some adults to children and their developing sexuality, the most usual preventive intervention has been teaching 'protective behaviours' to children. In the classroom or in small group settings children are taught to recognise appropriate and inappropriate behaviours towards them, how to rebuff sexual overtures that are made to them and how to enlist the assistance of other adults if they perceive themselves to be at risk. Such classroom programs are controversial and await adequate evaluation.

Secondary prevention involves the early recognition and action against abuse and neglect, which is usually referred to as 'child protection'. Child protection involves the rapid assessment of the child and family where abuse has occurred, or where there is considerable suspicion. Appropriate action is then taken based on the assessment. In approximately 10 per cent of notified cases this action involves the removal of the child from the family, either to hospital or to foster care. Welfare legislation makes provisions for temporary custody orders while further

assessment can be made. In intrafamilial child sexual abuse the preferred option is for the alleged perpetrator to leave the family voluntarily. Where this does not occur, the child and often other siblings at risk may be removed to temporary care. Assessment of the need for therapy of the child and family forms part of secondary prevention. Not all children who are abused require psychiatric intervention, but indications include persistent emotional or behavioural disturbance, for example, depression or suicidal behaviour, or an expressed desire on the part of a child for further support.

Tertiary prevention refers to steps taken to prevent a future occurrence of abuse. This may include family intervention and monitoring, and teaching the child protective behaviour. Some children find it hard to escape the tag of having been previously abused. It is important to assist the child in adjusting to abuse but it is also important to recognise when discussing the past is not helpful, and when it is better to allow the child to get on with planning for the future.

Child abuse and neglect is an important concern for health professionals because of the immediate and long term consequences to the emotional and physical development of the child. Systematic research is still required to determine the most effective ways of predicting risk and of intervening when abuse has occurred. The major challenge facing health professionals is to prevent the transmission of abusive behaviour from one generation to the next.

Further Reading

Finkelhor D, *Sexually Victimised Children*, Free Press, New York, 1979.
Kosky, R, 'Incest: What Do We Really Know About It?' *Australian and New Zealand Journal of Psychiatry*, Vol 21, 1987, pp 430-40.
Muir R C, Monaghan S M, Gilmore R J, Clarkson J E, Crooks T J and Egan T G, 'Predicting Child Abuse and Neglect in New Zealand', *Australian and New Zealand Journal of Psychiatry*, Vol 23, 1989, pp 255-60.
Oates K, *Child Abuse. A Community Concern*. Butterworths, London, 1982.
Oates K, *Child Abuse and Neglect. What Happens Eventually?* Butterworths, Sydney, 1985.
Rutter M, 'Maternal Deprivation, 1972-1978: New Findings, New Concepts, New Approaches', *Child Development*, Vol 50, 1979, pp 283-305.

Chapter 7

Death, Disharmony and Divorce

C Tennant

For some considerable time the long term effects of parent loss in childhood have intrigued mental health workers. Early preoccupations were with the psychological significance of the traumatic loss itself and, perhaps understandably, with depression being the long term likely outcome. Later workers broadened this argument further by concluding that childhood loss per se, be it separation from or death of a parent, was not the critical factor. They argued that such loss may subsequently lead to a range of adverse social and psychological experiences which could prove more damaging than the parental loss itself. This cascade-like effect could then culminate in psychological illness in later life. In effect, loss would be regarded in this framework as the precipitant for a range of other noxious experiences.

One of the major problems in 'parent loss' research has been the very wide-ranging use of the term 'loss'. Greater specification is necessary. In particular, death and separation should be distinguished. Only 5–8 per cent of children experience parental death compared to 30–40 per cent of children who face 'loss' of a parent through divorce. Unfortunately, the non-specific term 'loss' continues to be used by some researchers, which may lead to inappropriate conclusions and contribute to inconsistency in published findings.

Death of a parent

There may be a range of severe behavioural and emotional reactions in the immediate aftermath of parental death. However, generally there is a negligible long term psychopathological effect. When the data is available to distinguish different types of loss, parent-child separations are usually associated with psychological problems later in life, but parental deaths are not. The research findings in this area do not always agree however. Some studies show no significant relationship between early separations and depression in patient samples or normal populations. In those studies where 'loss' did seem to predict depression, the effect can largely be attributed to prolonged separations from parents, and this is most often due to divorce.

Concerning the effects of other types of childhood separation experience on later adult psychological function, in one community study, prolonged separations due to marital problems and parental illness were associated with increased risk of psychiatric disorder.

While the research evidence seems to suggest that, as a group, children who suffer the death of a parent do not suffer serious psychological problems in the longer term, in clinical circumstances longer term problems may be observed. In individual cases, long term effects could be expected when the surviving parent cannot cope with the death of a spouse or when the long term parenting abilities are affected by the loss. Similarly, if there is gross social disruption, such as severe and prolonged economic hardship, then there may be adverse effects in later life. It would appear that such consequence are not the norm, and families usually cope adequately in the long term, despite the immediate devastating effects of the death.

Family disharmony and divorce

In the 1970s, over 30 per cent of children in the Western world, including Australia and New Zealand, experienced parental divorce. Estimates from the United States of America indicate that, of children born in the early 1980s, some 45 per cent will experience parental divorce, 35 per cent a subsequent parental remarriage and 20 per cent a second divorce.

Whether or not the increase in the Australian divorce rate since 1975 has resulted in improved awareness of and catering for the children's needs, has not been studied. Despite the fact of divorce becoming increasingly 'normative', most of the child's experiences surrounding it are not. They include practical problems: there may be a decline in family income, children may move to a new house and school, lose friends, their mothers may commence work, a new parental partner may appear and there may be a change in the pattern of contact with other relatives and friends. Continuing parental conflict and loss of contact with the non-custodial parent, usually the father, are not uncommon. Other important consequences include parental emotional distress, loss of confidence, feelings of incompetence and thus the possibility of impoverished parenting, especially in the early aftermath of the parents' separation. These factors may be reinforced by disruption in the parent's social support network. Before reviewing the evidence about the effects of separation due to family discord, one needs to be aware of factors which confound most of the studies and may lead to erroneous conclusions in some instances.

The first issue to consider is the various definitions of 'divorce'. Sometimes divorce may simply be an official acknowledgment of a change in marital status which appears in the mail. In other cases, it may be a process including the parents' relationship from the time they met to after they are divorced and embracing all the psychological, social, economic, educational and other effects which that may have on a child. For most children, 'divorce' is a complex ongoing process. No studies have been able to address the full complexity of this process. Two other important factors to consider are parental mental illness and the long term quality of parenting.

Parental mental illnesses, especially affective disorders, antisocial personality and alcohol abuse may be one important cause of marital disharmony and divorce. Parental psychopathology can also have a deleterious effect on the child's social and emotional environment. Poor parenting causes psychological morbidity in children. To complicate this effect is the genetic transmission of the disorders to the children. Both genetic and environmental factors may thus contribute to the effects of childhood separations and contribute to subsequent psychopathology. It is important that studies on the effects of parental separation take into consideration the complicating effects of parental emotional disorders. This has not always been done, especially where subjects have volunteered to be involved or where welfare agency cases are used.

It is also crucial to consider the effects of the quality of parenting prior to separation. The relative importance of predivorce parent–child relationships is highlighted in a study in which the quality of pre-separation parenting predicted the later development of depression in adulthood but post-separation parenting did not.

The relationship between divorce and a child's personality development is far from simple. There are a number of possibilities. Firstly, childhood personality factors preceding divorce may play a role in the development of later disorders. Secondly, it is possible that such problems or a child's psychopathology generally may strain the parents' marriage and contribute to their divorce, a causal relationship not in the direction generally proposed by most researchers. Finally, there is also the likelihood that divorce and its sequelae have some influence on later personality development in children.

In two longitudinal follow-up studies, emotional disturbance in children immediately following parental divorce was initially substantial, but diminished over the next two years. Problems were most marked in boys, with aggressive behaviours being prominent.

Most separations were from fathers, and parenting problems were greatest for mothers in dealing with their sons. In another longitudinal study there was, interestingly, considerable overlap in parental disharmony in divorced and in intact families. Parental disharmony predicted the child's emotional disturbance whereas divorce per se did not.

In an uncontrolled follow-up study, one third of children were judged to be depressed at the fifth year of follow-up. At 10 years post divorce, when most were young adults, some 30 per cent had engaged in moderately serious illegal activities and many had shown educational or occupational decline from their earlier middle class family status. However, in a six year follow-up study, which controlled for social class, economic factors, other life events and marital discord, it was also demonstrated that divorce per se did not predict the child's subsequent emotional problems.

In summary, despite the plethora of studies appearing to show parental 'loss' in childhood causes adult psychiatric illness, especially depression, the evidence is somewhat fragile. When one distinguishes for instance between parental death and separation, there is no good evidence to suggest that parent death has any significant impact on adult depressive disorders. With parent–child separations, only those occurring in relation to family discord appear to have any long term impact and even this data is brittle.

Factors modifying effects on children

1. Parenting

Parenting problems following any childhood loss would appear to be the most important potential mediator of the effects of divorce. The available evidence, while confirming the importance of poor parenting as a risk factor for depression generally, does not specifically address its role as a mediating factor between childhood separations and adult problems. In one study of children who had experienced a loss, the relationship with the custodial parent and the stability of home life following the loss were important factors for the development of depression in later life.

However, other studies have not confirmed these findings.

Longitudinal studies of divorce have also assessed post divorce parenting and tried to measure its effects. All describe an early deterioration in quality of parenting in the first year and this predicted disturbed behaviours in the child. Positive parent–child relationships lessened the adverse emotional effects in children. These behaviour problems in the child were worsened by ongoing spouse conflict. It should be stressed that relationships between parenting problems and disturbed behaviours in the children are reciprocal and this reciprocity is greatest in mother–son interactions. Despite early difficulties, parenting generally improves over time and may eventually be better than that occurring before divorce.

Considerable overlap is found in the quality of parenting in divorced and intact families. Parenting factors are generally better predictors of children's psychological outcome than whether the family is divorced or intact.

Is it better for children to remain in intact but stressed families or to face parental separation and its consequences? The evidence suggests that when divorce leads to a significant reduction in parental conflict then the outcome for children is likely to improve. Continuing spouse conflict is an important mediating factor. If family discord is continuous, then separation is likely ultimately to benefit the children.

2. Parents' post divorce contact

Another mediating variable is that of the degree of continuing contact with the father, since fathers are more usually the non-custodian parent. There is some evidence that the father's absence in the first five years has some effect on educational attainment, particularly on mathematical abilities and that these are more marked in boys. For girls, father's absence may have more effect around puberty. A central factor is the quality of continuing contact with the non-custodial parent. Continuing contact can be beneficial if there is lack of conflict between the parents. Contact with mother is important also and has some bearing on the issue of whether mothers should work full time. Improved maternal parenting is noted when finances improve and mothers work but there is a short-term adverse effect on children if mothers work in the immediate aftermath of separation.

Of course, many children are reared in single parent families. There is some evidence to suggest that these children show less satisfactory social and academic development than children raised in two parent families. These effects are more marked in single parent families resulting from divorce than those resulting from widowhood. However, such families are likely to have considerable financial hardships. When this influence is accounted for, the effect of single parenthood alone is not great. There is no substantial difference between mother-headed and father-headed families.

3. Remarriage

On the surface, remarriage should provide significant benefits in that it restores a dual caregiver family and economically the family benefits from the presence of the extra income of the step-parent. In addition, one might assume somewhat less social stigma in this situation. These factors must however be balanced against the negative effects which can include adverse changes in the child's relationship with both the custodial and non-custodial parent and, because of custody issues, increased friction between the natural parents. Furthermore, the merging of two families of children can significantly disturb the relationship within the new marriage.

Several studies show no difference between the adjustment of children with no fathers at home and those with step-fathers. A few have reported better adjustment. However most studies, both in the United States and United Kingdom, show adverse effects on the children. One showed increased bed-wetting in children in remarried families. Anti-social behaviours, low self-esteem and 'psycho-somatic' symptoms have also been reported. In prospective studies, which provide stronger evidence, the findings are also generally adverse. In one cohort there was a worse outcome for children in remarried families and in this same sample some 50 per cent of the remarried females had split up again after three years. In another study wives failed to cope with their former husband's re-marriage and had increased feelings of depression, anxiety and anger. Children's contact with their father usually decreased with his remarriage, especially for his daughters. Problems in the family were greatest between step-father and step-sons which were worse if remarriage occurred when the children were older rather than younger. Problems for sons were identifiable at both two and six year follow-up but there were no adverse effects on daughters. In general, from the child's viewpoint, remarriage of the parents can be problematic.

4. Institutionalisation

Children separated from both parents, and institutionalised as well, appear to have a poor psychosocial outcome. Whether or not these adverse effects are due to the institutionali-sation and subsequent experiences, or factors preceding it, is unclear. Nonetheless, girls reared in institutions show considerable levels of personality disorder, marital discord and separations, and poor parenting skills in adult life. However, their psychosocial adjustment may owe more to ongoing social problems than to the childrearing they experienced. The 'effect' of institutionalisation may also be related to the social circumstances experienced by the child apart from those provided by the institution, emphasising the importance of the social and family environment prior to institutionalisation. Adverse effects of emotionally or socially deprived backgrounds fortunately seem remediable; for example by a subsequent supportive marital relationship.

5. Social relationships

The school environment has some influence on behaviour problems; less disturbance is found when there are clear standards and the environment is predictable.

6. Economic factors

The maintenance of two households clearly leads to economic restrictions and this is especially true of households headed by women. Lower income can have a negative effect on the children by way of poorer housing, fewer holidays, and the mother being forced to work so that she is more often absent from the house.

Adult life

1. Attitudes to marriage and premarital pregnancy

Young adults ten years after parents divorce remain apprehensive about repeating their parents' differences. Women especially are anxious about close interpersonal relations. This is more marked if divorce had occurred later in childhood rather than earlier. Children of divorce, when grown up, often express powerful personal commitments to marriage and fidelity within it. However, in some empirical studies marital instability in one generation seems to predict similar instability in the next.

2. Marriage and its quality

In contrast to common belief, the experience of parental death appears to have no adverse impact on subsequent marriage. In fact, parental death in childhood can be associated with later marital closeness, a greater desire to have children and with lower rates of marital separation and divorce.

Unlike childhood experiences of divorce, childhood bereavement does not seem to affect the potential to become an effective parent.

3. Vulnerability to other life stressors

It has been argued that early childhood experiences such as parental death and separation render children more vulnerable to subsequent life stressors apart from marriage and parenting. This could occur because they perceive subsequent events as being more stressful, but this has not been confirmed. Secondly, it could occur because they actually experience more acute life events. However, there is no evidence of a relation between parental loss and the number of acute life events experienced in later life.

Summary

Parental loss through separation and death has preoccupied psychiatry for many years and has been widely accepted as a significant risk factor for adult psychopathology. However, there is little evidence that parental death is a significant risk factor for later depression. There is however some evidence that separations, especially those occurring in the context of family or parental discord, may contribute to later personal difficulties. In no study has loss or separation been shown to be a risk factor for later psychiatric disorder when the effects of subsequent experiences of parenting are controlled. In other words, optimal parenting following loss or separation can offset the possible psychologically harmful effects of such loss or separation. Parental separation may even be beneficial when it terminates earlier family turmoil.

The evidence would appear to show that if family breakdown occurs and does not seriously affect the quality of parenting in the longer term, then long term psychopathology in the children is unlikely. Parent–child separations occurring in the context of marital disharmony are often indicators of poor earlier parenting as well as impoverished parenting post divorce.

The evidence is increasing that poor parenting of children has short, intermediate and long term consequences. However, its effects are mediated through a diversity of personal, interpersonal and social factors. These factors, not necessarily the loss event itself, need to be addressed clinically.

Further Reading

Hess R D and Camara K A, 'Post Divorce Family Relationships as Mediating Factors in the Consequences of Divorce for Children', *Journal of Social Issues*, Vol 35, 1979, pp 79-96.

Hetherington E M, Cox M, and Cox R, 'Effects of Divorce on Parents and Children', in *Nontraditional Families: Parenting and Child Development*, (ed Lamb M E), Lawrence Eribaum Association, Hillsdale, N J, 1982, Ch 9.

Rutter M, 'Maternal Deprivation, 1972–1978: New Findings, New Concepts, New Approaches', *Child Development*, Vol 50, 1979, pp 283–305.

Tennant C, Bebbington P and Hurry J, 'Parental Death in Childhood and Risk of Adult Depressive Disorders', *Psychological Medicine*, Vol 10, 1980, pp 289–99.

Wallerstein J S and Kelly J B, *Surviving the Break Up: How Children and Parents Cope with Divorce*, Blackwell Scientific Publications Ltd, London, 1980.

Wallerstein J S, 'Children of Divorce: Preliminary Report of a Ten Year Follow-up of Older Children and Adolescents', *Journal of the American Academy of Child Psychiatry*, Vol 24, 1985, pp 545–53.

Chapter 8

Fostering and Adoption

R Kosky and H Salimi Eshkevari

Health and welfare professionals are commonly involved in the adoption and fostering of children. There are many questions for professionals working in this area.

All children need affection and care during their development. In the past, many illegitimate children, orphans and neglected children (foundlings) were reared in institutions. While some institutions were of high quality and provided continuous good care, others were poor and the children in them lacked adequate care and food, received little stimulation and were often worked as drudges. In other cases, foundling children were removed from their environments and under such schemes as those of Barnado and Fairbridge, many thousands of children, some only three or four years old, were shipped from the United Kingdom to Canada, Australia and South Africa. While some prospered, many were cruelly exploited. These schemes ceased during the 1960s.

The reports of children who had inadequate, institutional care indicated that they had a tendency to suffer from emotional disorders especially depression or to become antisocial later in life. At school, such children tended to be disruptive, overactive, inattentive and to have poor social skills.

Women reared in institutions tend to have poor parenting skills themselves (although this is not the case for about one in three), so alas, a pattern of inadequate parenting can be repeated.

Previously in Australia and New Zealand, adoption was often a private arrangement between people usually arranged by a family doctor. Fostering was usually a matter for the Department of Child Welfare, but in many cases was a fairly flexible arrangement. Bernard Smith, a distinguished Australian art critic, has written affectionately of his foster childhood in Sydney during the 1920s and 1930s. His foster parents, who fostered many other children, were pleased to allow him access to his mother and the government inspectors behaved in a benign paternalistic fashion. For others, the arrangements were not always so good. Some foster parents were more interested in the payment they received than the care they gave. Some of the children were difficult, and multiple placements were not uncommon for fostered children. A considerable degree of exploitation may have occurred. This was especially true for aboriginal children. Many were forcibly taken from their parents by government officials and placed in institutions or fostered to white people. In the latter case, many children, especially the girls, were trained to provide domestic service. It is impossible now to know the extent of the exploitation of the children involved, but the practice, which continued in West Australia into the 1960s, has left a bitter legacy among the aboriginal people.

Against this background of concern about the effects of institutionalisation and exploitation, much greater attempts have been made to develop and monitor adequate adoption and fostering arrangements in recent years.

Fostering

The present practice is for fairly strict control of fostering situations, and many welfare departments provide training and support for foster parents.

Fostering may be *short term*, for a few days

or weeks while a crisis is resolved. This is an often difficult task for foster parents, as the fostered child may be very upset and disturbed. In these circumstances, foster parents may need support from mental health and welfare professionals.

More *long term* foster placements are provided for children who cannot live at home. In these cases, the foster parents develop close relationships with the child. These relationships may have a powerful stabilising influence on a disturbed child's mental state. The foster parents can provide the child with consistent limit-setting on behaviour, so that the child can develop some internal control. In these cases, foster parents can be decidedly therapeutic. The fostered child may also use the foster parents as models. However, in most cases, the foster parents' role is temporary and reunion with the natural family is the goal. Sometimes considerable therapeutic work is necessary with the natural family before this can be achieved.

Medium length fostering is also used in some places in Australia as an alternative to custody for children who are in trouble with the law. Such foster placements need to be closely supervised and the foster parents carefully selected for their experience and capacity to exert control over the child in a non-punitive fashion. Also, the effects on the foster parents' own children need to be considered before placing a delinquent child with the family.

Long term foster home placements until the child is 18 years old can occur when the natural family relations are irreversibly broken down. Natural parents' access in these cases must be carefully considered. The overall policy should be to help the foster parents wherever possible. As the child grows, it is important to be honest with him and flexible in trying to meet his needs for information about his natural parents and allowing him access to them if this is suitable.

Despite the best support, a considerable proportion of foster placements break down (up to 50 per cent). Breakdowns should not be taken lightly as it can induce guilt, sadness and anger on both sides. Breakdowns are more likely for mentally retarded and emotionally disturbed children. They are more likely when the foster parents have financial problems and inadequate room in the house. Furthermore, foster parents can develop marital problems and the parents can separate during the course of the fostering with additional problems for the child.

Adoption

Adoption is a permanent arrangement and the adoptive parents take legal responsibility for the child. Between one and two per cent of Australian children from birth to 15 years are adoptees. The aim is to give the child a permanent home where the relationships will be emotionally, not less than legally, stable and the same as if the child was born into the family.

Attempts are made by adoption agencies to screen adoptive parents and to provide a physical and intellectual match between adoptee and adopting parents. It is unclear whether these practices affect a better adopting arrangement. Many willing parents feel angry if they are judged unfit to adopt. Given that there is a long wait for adoption in Australia, many parents find it more satisfying to adopt a child from a deprived situation in another country.

In the past, infants were often kept for several months, even years, in institutions awaiting adoption. In these circumstances affection was often minimal and care was more mechanical. Today, it is recognised that such a practice is harmful and is likely to severely impair the child's later chances of developing attachments to adopting parents.

Adopted children are usually healthy, but care needs to be taken to inform adopting parents of any impairment or hereditary condition that may be present, so that they can take these into consideration and be prepared for the associated difficulties as the child grows.

Studies comparing the development of adopted children to those raised in other circumstances show that adopted children in general do better on most measures of intellectual, emotional and social development than do children reared in institutions and children who are fostered. Studies comparing adopted children to children raised by natural parents give variable conclusions, but overall it can be said that adopted children do no better and no worse than children reared by biological parents. There is just as much variation in outcome. There are, in any case, significant methodological problems in such outcome studies.

Nevertheless, adopting parents and adoptees face several problems unique to their situation and not shared by children raised by biological parents.

While follow up studies have generally indicated that the risks concerning the subsequent development of adopted children are in no way greater than the risks for children in the general population, this is so provided that the adoptive homes are of good standard and well prepared for the task of rearing a non-biological child.

A 15 year follow up on Swedish children registered for adoption showed that the prospects for adopted children were 'very good, irrespective of their social and genetic background'. On the other hand, the study indicated a considerable risk for maladjustment and school failure among adopted children who, due to the indecision of their mothers or of the social agencies, were first placed and reared in foster homes. No association was found in this study between registered criminality and alcohol abuse among the biological fathers and the adjustment of children in non-biological homes, although a connection was found between these characteristics in the biological mother and later difficulties with the child reared in an adoptive home. This may indicate a genetic link between mothers and their children in adoptive and foster homes or it may indicate subtle damage to the foetus due to alcohol, smoking or poor nourishment during pregnancy.

Special problems

It is generally considered that adoption placements are best made at an early age, indeed, as early as possible. However, if the care of the infant and child during the period before adoption has been adequate, there appears to be no reason why the adoption cannot be successful. One American study of children who were adopted between the ages of 5 and 12 years, following the need for care because of abuse and neglect by the natural parents showed that, even in these cases, the outcome was good for most children. Only where the child had already demonstrated behavioural problems, had experienced multiple foster placements or still possessed a strong attachment to the natural mother, was the outcome unfavourable.

However, children adopted at a later age are more likely to have been medically unwell and to have suffered neglect and abuse. Adopting parents need to know about this and to expect potential emotional and behavioural problems and to have adequate access to skilled professional help if problems arise.

Adopted children are referred to child psychiatric services more commonly than would be expected. For instance, in West Australia, six per cent of children referred for psychiatric assessment were adoptees, while the best estimate of the base rate of adoptees of 0–15 years olds in the general population was 1.8 per cent.

There may be several reasons for this high referral rate. In the first place, adoptees in West Australia may be at greater risk than the general population for emotional and behavioural disorders, which may reflect procedural practices in that State. In particular, it may reflect the prevalence of the practice of private arrangements for adoption and possibly a high incidence of cross cultural adoptions. Several of the referrals were of aboriginal children who were adopted by white parents. In these cases, the adoptee had entered adolescence and faced significant issues about cultural identity and a desire to find natural parents. An alternative explanation for the higher than expected referral rate may be that adoptive parents are more sensitive to emotional problems in their children, or more ready to seek help from health professionals, than other parents.

Some aboriginal boys who have been adopted by white people are very concerned about the extent to which they should claim their aboriginal heritage. Most have maintained contact with family members of the original aboriginal extended family. In a few cases they had done this unbeknown to the adoptive parents, and were secretly contacted by aboriginal relatives. Decisions about learning the tribal lore, its history and the learning of the language are of particular importance to these boys and their adoptive and natural families at about age 12 years, since this is the traditional time of initiation in tribal ceremonies. It is also an age when all young people must begin to make decisions about their future. Cross cultural adoptees and adoptive parents may need special help and advice during the child's adolescence.

In Australia, particularly among rural families and also in aboriginal families, it has not been uncommon for children to be adopted by aunts and uncles or grandparents. In some cases, tension can occur when this is kept 'secret' or when natural parents seek to reclaim their children. Sometimes, the adoption is kept from the adoptee, although it is readily known among the extended family. In one case, the adopting parents who were an aunt and uncle, planned to reveal the child's adoption when he was 14 years old. However, he had known about it since he was 6 years old because a cousin had told him.

There has also been a trend in recent years to extend adoption services to include more children with special needs for adoption. Among these children are those with the intellectual and physical handicaps, although usually it has been difficult to obtain adoption for these children. However, with better social support services for adoptive parents, it has been possible to assess parents to care for such children.

Relinquishing parents

It has been estimated that over 2000 women in Australia will relinquish a baby for adoption in a single year. Several studies have shown that such women are at high risk for psychological disability. These women are generally young, single, unprepared for parenthood, unable to provide financially for a baby, or are unsupported socially, or have been raped.

Relinquishing mothers tend to have higher levels of anxiety and depression than others. Many report intense anger subsequent to relinquishment. Most report that they received little support from family or friends and professionals. Some use alcohol and sedatives to help them cope with the feelings of relinquishment. A proportion consider they are overprotective towards their subsequent children.

It is possible that these findings represent a measure of psychological morbidity which was present in these women prior to relinquishing their children, or the study designs are not sufficient to establish a casual link. However, most of the women perceive that their grief is a result of relinquishing their baby.

One striking finding is that anger, sadness and guilt about the relinquishment remains for a considerable number of years after the event. Some report intensification of feelings, especially anger. Overall, it can be said that a considerable proportion of relinquishing mothers suffer grief reactions which do not reduce with the passage of time, which manifest predominantly as depression and psychosomatic illness. Some of these women benefit from counselling and support from self help groups such as the Australian Relinquishing Mothers' Society. For more severe profound symptoms, psychiatric help may be necessary.

It has been suggested that relinquishing mothers should have the right to obtain information about the wellbeing and progress of their children. This may be sufficient to enable these women to endure their grief. New adoption laws being developed in several States have taken a more enlightened approach to the needs of the relinquishing mothers.

It has been suggested that relinquishing mothers be allowed to breastfeed their child during the first month. This may help to reduce guilt because the mother feels she is giving the infant the best help before he leaves her. On the other hand, too close contact can be cruel. In the hope of preventing suffering, it is sometimes arranged that the relinquishing mother does not see her child at all. This does not seem to be a helpful practice and may lead to long term resentment and guilt.

Adoptive parents

Most adopting parents come from the middle socio-economic stratum which is generally a result of the selective criteria of adoption agencies. Most tend to be older than natural parents due to adoption policies and also because of the period of childlessness and decision making. Some studies have suggested that adoptive parents had poorer physical health than natural parents, which may be a reflection of their older age and the circumstances of infertility. Couples who are marginally eligible for adoptive status because of age, health and who have a desire to move quickly are more likely to accept children with special needs.

One of the purposes of adoption is to enable married couples to fulfil their desire for parenthood. There have been few follow up studies of this aspect of adoption, but there is some suggestion that in the majority of cases, this is achieved. In general, it is considered that a successful outcome is more likely if the adopting parents are happily married, cheerful, emotionally stable and with a good social network. Adoptive parents who have proved successful with one child are likely to successfully build a large family with further adoptions.

Special circumstances

It is rare that mental illness in the natural parents is a barrier to adopting the child. In most cases of neurotic conditions, the genetic component is negligible. A strong family history of depressive psychosis, schizophrenia or epilepsy should signal a risk for later developments in the child, but again, the environmental aspects of these conditions are strong and such a family history is in itself no barrier to adoption. It is imperative though, that clear cut hereditary degenerative conditions, such as Huntington's disease, if known, should be clearly notified to potential adopters.

The position regarding adoption of children whose parents are mentally retarded is a complex one. Many of their children prove to be of normal intelligence and there are cases of children of exceptional intellect who were natural children of mentally defective parents. However, it may be that a period of trial fostering by the prospective adoptive parents can provide a valuable guide to the child's developmental potential and to any likely problems.

Examination of the child to discover any mental, neurological and sense organs defect can be an important means of determining if the child will have any special needs for adoption and if the prospective parents are likely to require any special help and consideration.

Temporary adjustment problems

Sometimes adopting parents are not adequately prepared. After a long wait, during which they have made their individual adjustments in life without a child, they suddenly find their request for adoption is granted. Having a baby requires a considerable amount of time and effort. Unpreparedness, anxiety and sometimes lack of support may lead to a temporary loss of confidence. Mostly, this can be dealt with by sympathetic guidance from a family doctor.

Telling the child

In the past, adoption was often kept from the child, and some people discovered their adoptive status quite late in life when, inevitably, it produced a considerable shock. The more recent practice is for the matter to be dealt with more naturally. In response to a child's question about his origins, adoptive parents can answer truthfully without expecting that the child will reject them. Children assimilate the knowledge within the context of love and acceptance by the adoptive parents. However, they do so at an appropriate developmental age level, so adoptive parents can expect to have to repeat the answer at several times throughout the child's life.

It is a mistake to expect the child to be active in this process. A question about 'where I come from' should not be answered by a child being told that there are papers in a drawer which the child can look at any time. If papers are to be shown to the child, it should be with the adoptive parents alongside, so the child feels the context of acceptance.

Adolescents may wish to find their natural parents. This can be a dilemma for the adoptive parents but by and large, no harm will come from helping the young person if this is what they wish. Moreover, often, when help is offered, many youngsters quietly forget about it. Government adoption agencies are normally most helpful. However, some adolescents can experience considerable conflict of loyalties in these matters. We have found that such children can benefit from short term psychotherapeutic help.

Rejection of the adopted child by the adopting parents can occur, likewise the child can reject the adopting parents. These situations normally lead to marked behaviour problems in the child and the sooner the situation is recognised the better, as the situation can lead to tension and possibly violence.

Conclusion

Many studies have shown that adopted children develop as well as those reared in natural homes. Fostered children usually come from situations where their natural family has disintegrated or is in turmoil. The results of fostering are variable, but on the whole, it is considered preferable to institutional care. However, while the latter is currently held in low regard among many health and welfare professionals, some children do flourish in good quality institutions.

Adopted, fostered and institutionally raised children do have special needs and unique circumstances which must be taken into consideration by health professionals.

Further Reading

Condon J T, 'Psychological Disability in Women who Relinquish a Baby for Adoption', *Medical Journal of Australia*, Vol 144, 1986, pp 117–19 (and editorial comment p 113).

Hersov L, 'Adoption' in *Child Psychiatry, Modern Approaches*, (ed Rutter M and Hersov L), Blackwell Scientific Publication, Oxford, 1985.

Kosky R, McAlpine I, Silbun S and Richmond J, 'A Survey of Child Psychiatry Outpatients', *Australia and New Zealand Journal of Psychiatry*, Vol 19, 1985, pp 158–66.

Part 3
Disorders of Development

Chapter 9

Mental Retardation

H Moloney

Mental retardation, a term used in classification systems such as ICD-9 and DSM-III-R in preference to intellectual handicap, mental subnormality, or developmental disability, refers to a condition in which a person's intellectual functioning has not developed fully or has been impaired because of damage, disease, malformation or maldevelopment of the central nervous system. It occurs before the end of the early developmental period, taken arbitrarily as the age of 18 years. Persons with mental retardation are slow in passing the normal developmental milestones of childhood and adolescence, and have difficulty in learning at an average rate. Mental retardation refers to a person's *level* of intellectual functioning and is not the same as mental illness, which refers to a *disturbance* of a person's normal mental state, regardless of their level of intelligence.

The revised version of DSM-III, in seeking to differentiate between mental retardation and mental illness or other psychiatric disorders, has categorised mental retardation as a developmental disorder, that is, usually first evident in infancy, childhood or adolescence, on AXIS II of its multiaxial system. It refers to people with significantly sub-average general intellectual functioning (an Intelligence Quotient (IQ) of 70 or below) and concurrent deficits or impairments in adaptive functioning that is, the person's effectiveness in meeting the standards expected for his age and cultural group in social skills, communication, daily living skills, personal independence and self-sufficiency.

There are over 100 conditions or diseases which can cause mental retardation, so the group is quite heterogeneous. Four degrees of severity are recognised, namely mild (IQ 50-55 to approximately 70), moderate (IQ 35-40 to 50-55), severe (IQ 20-25 to 35-40) and profound (below 20 or 25). Borderline intellectual function (IQ range 71-84) is not considered to warrant a diagnosis of mental retardation.

There are 25 to 30 persons with mild mental retardation in every 1000 of the population compared with 3 to 4 per 1000 with moderate, severe or profound handicap.

Psychiatric disorders in mentally retarded people

It has long been recognised that people with mental retardation of all levels are more vulnerable than others to the development of virtually all psychiatric disorders. For the most part, particularly in the mildly retarded, they are recognisable, and can be treated by the same techniques as used in the normal population.

The moderate to severely mentally retarded (IQ below 50) have more brain abnormalities and thus they have greater deficits in language and communication, more marked motor, sensory and perceptual problems and higher rates of epilepsy. They show more disorganised, less predictable and less easily classified groups of symptoms, often referred to as 'severe behaviour disorders' or 'challenging behaviours'. These include outbursts of hyperactivity and restlessness, impulsivity, episodes of aggression and destruction, repetitive rituals (known as stereotypies), self-stimulating mannerisms (hand flapping, body rocking), self-injurious behaviours (head banging, eye gouging, face slapping) which can result in serious self-injury or mutilation, pica (eating rubbish or inedible material) and disorganised psychotic or autistic behaviours.

The most reliable surveys of prevalence carried out on community samples show that psychiatric disorders occur in up to 50 per cent of people with mental retardation. Surveys of institutionalised populations examine a biased sample because residential care is most frequently sought for retarded people who have behavioural problems. Institutionalisation itself may create, or prolong, certain forms of behavioural disturbance. Most community surveys show that schizophrenia, manic-depressive psychoses, neurotic and conduct disorders and adjustment reactions occur more frequently among mentally retarded persons than in the general population.

Clinical features

The limitations implicit in mental retardation affect the way psychiatric disorders manifest themselves. In mentally retarded people with significant brain abnormalities causing changes in perception, discrimination, attention, concentration and the ability to abstract, conceptualise and verbalise, the expression of emotional or behaviour disorders or mental illness is modified accordingly. The mentally retarded person's usual patterns of behaviour, their individual personality, level of intelligence, language and communication, their memory and what they have been taught, all need to be taken into account when attempting a psychiatric assessment.

The standard mental state examination may not be appropriate and may need modification. Ascertaining whether a mentally retarded person is oriented in time, place and person may be dependent on whether that person has been taught or is capable of reading the time, knowing the day and date or being aware of the months of the year. Modified interview techniques, with more concrete illustrations or pictorial representations which accord with the retarded person's verbal ability and level of comprehension, are more useful.

Diagnosis is normally dependent on the patient's subjective account. The mentally retarded person is often unable to discuss his problems clearly. The extent of a mentally retarded person's degree of insight or reality testing may be difficult to judge. Some clinicians argue that schizophrenia cannot therefore be reliably diagnosed in severely or profoundly retarded people. Maladaptive behaviours such as aggression, irritability or self-injury may be the first manifestations of a psychiatric disorder, regardless of the underlying psychiatric diagnosis.

Because of the lack of a good personal history, observations and information from family, friends and care givers are necessary to obtain a clearer picture.

A longitudinal personal and developmental history of the intellectually handicapped person should be obtained. Complete assessment necessitates obtaining details of pre-, peri- and post-natal periods, milestones of development, significant life events, coping styles and previous personality type and behaviour. It is important to look broadly in the environment for stress factors. Developmental regression with loss of previously acquired skills and a return to an earlier stage of development may be seen in the face of significant emotional stresses.

Too much reliance on verbal presentation should be avoided. The clinician will need to be empathetic to the non-verbal messages which are implicit in the patient's expressions, gestures, posture, responsiveness, feeling tone and levels of activity.

Early and more subtle changes in behaviour, which are the first signs of emotional disturbance, may be obvious only to those who know the person well. This is especially important in the case of mood disorders such as depression which are not uncommon and often underdiagnosed in the mentally retarded. Depressive illnesses have been diagnosed even in profoundly retarded persons and they have responded to treatment.

Retarded people may be dependent and anxious to please the interviewer so that direct questioning is more likely to elicit a response they think is preferred. Open-ended enquiries or the presentation of alternatives is a better approach to eliciting information. Longer and repeated interviews may be needed in order to gain trust and confidence, establish rapport and overcome initial anxiety as well as to build up a broad picture of the person and his circumstances.

Play-therapy techniques with the use of toys and play materials or other assessment tools are appropriate for intellectually handicapped children. It is essential to establish a non-threatening atmosphere in which free expression of feelings and ideas is encouraged.

When judging whether any particular piece of behaviour in an intellectually handicapped person is abnormal, it is important to be aware of their functional or mental age as opposed to their chronological age. For example, an intellectually handicapped child may continue to hold conversations with imaginary friends long past the age when these are given up by normal peers.

The full range of social, biological, psychological and cultural factors should be taken into account in making a psychiatric diagnosis. A thorough examination of family interaction patterns and recent environmental changes as well as intra-psychic phenomena must be carried out. Interdisciplinary assessment with allied health professionals such as social workers, psychologists and therapists may be useful. The schematic diagram below illustrates one method of approach to the consideration of the clinical features and presentation of psychiatric disorders in the mentally retarded person.

A multi axial diagnostic classification such as DSM-III-R where the mental disorder or psychiatric illness is coded on AXIS I, the level of intellectual functioning on AXIS II, physical disorders and conditions on AXIS III and on AXIS IV and V the severity of psychosocial stressors and global assessment of functioning, mirrors this biopsychosocial approach to assessment very well.

Causes of mental illness in mentally retarded people

Psychiatric disorder in mentally retarded persons is multi-determined. The development of personality, emotions and self-concept and factors which contribute to the normal adjustment of the non-disturbed mentally retarded

person have been studied only rarely. Often there seems to be denial of the mentally retarded person's capacity for experiencing or expressing emotions. Clinicians often focus on the person's intellect and tend to ignore other phenomena. Despite this the determination of possible aetiological factors in individual cases is often easier than expected.

The parent's reactions to having a child with a disability, how these reactions were handled from the start and what supportive services were available are directly relevant. Distorted patterns of child-rearing which vary from over-protectiveness and over-anxious handling to parental guilt, anxiety, withdrawal, depression, denial of the fact of handicap, projection of blame on to others and rejection of the child or even physical or emotional abuse, are frequently encountered and can form the basis for the development of disturbed behaviour. Rejection by peers or adults, constant experiences of failure and the loss of close emotional attachments, play an important part in causing emotional disturbance. These factors can produce a cycle of disturbed behaviour leading to further rejection and undesirable behaviour, 'unattractive' personality characteristics and deepening emotional disturbance.

Marital discord and family instability, economic and social deprivation may adversely affect the vulnerable slow learning and slow developing child. The reactions of siblings are often complex. They may feel neglected because of the needs of the handicapped child and they may experience anger and guilt. Temperament can affect the adaptability of retarded children to different circumstances. Early placement in poor quality institutional care with lack of stimulation and rigid, insensitive regimes with no individual child care may give rise to early emotional disturbance. Nevertheless, a good institution may be better than a bad parental home and not all retarded children in care become disturbed. The range of social experience may be more limited but sometimes the structured environment and relationships with like peers can provide positive experiences for intellectually disabled people.

The social learning experiences of a handicapped child can also determine the presence of maladaptive behaviour. The badly behaving retarded child is often inappropriately reward by focus on the disruptive behaviour. Learning theory has provided information about the development of maladaptive behaviours in the retarded. Many treatments based on the rules of behaviour modification have been extremely effective, particularly with more severely retarded or autistic people.

Language and communication impairments are increasingly recognised as the basis for many disturbed behaviours in mentally retarded children. Feelings of frustration and helplessness as a result of not being able to get one's message across manifest as angry outbursts, aggression and destructive behaviour or as social withdrawal and acts of self-abuse. These reactions can be modified if effective communication is established.

The social, personal and emotional immaturity associated with delayed development results in behaviour more appropriate to a younger age. The seeking out of companions who are chronologically younger but mentally equivalent can be misinterpreted. The pressures of sexual drives at puberty are often difficult for an intellectually handicapped adolescent, particularly when associated with social rejection or lack of opportunities for sexual expression or sublimation.

Cerebral damage is present in many moderately and severely mentally retarded persons and is often associated with behaviour disorders and epilepsy. Brain dysfunction probably increases any child's susceptibility to psychiatric disorder. Neurosurgical removal of scars or damaged cerebral tissue may strikingly improve behaviour, as well as reduce the number of seizures. Children who have had brain diseases such as encephalitis or meningitis frequently show hyperactivity, poor frustration tolerance and outbursts of irritable behaviour afterwards. Brain damage can affect the behaviour of retarded children because of its location, its extent, or the developmental stage at which it occurs.

The presence of pain and discomfort due to an underlying medical illness, or the side effects of drugs (for example, motor restlessness from psychotropic drugs) may precipitate

disturbed behaviour, particularly in people without speech. Visual, hearing and language impairments predispose to the development of self-injury in mentally handicapped people.

The usual genetic predispositions to the development of schizophrenia or manic-depressive psychosis are thought to operate in intellectually disabled persons so a family history of mental illness should always be sought.

Syndromes in mentally retarded people

Autism

Mental retardation is sometimes associated with early childhood autism (see chapter 10).

Attention-deficit disorder

Hyperkinesis can be associated with attention deficits, learning problems, behaviour disorders, emotional lability, impulsivity, aggressiveness and destructiveness (see chapter 24). It is frequently seen in association with mild mental retardation in children. Occurring mainly in males, it can be a major problem in families with poor socio-economic circumstances. Interventions which combine environmental change, respite care, behaviour management and medication can break the 'vicious spiral' of problems created at home and school in which the overactivity causes anger and intolerance in carers which leads to more anxiety in the child and thus, to increased motor activity.

Organic mental disorders

Dementia is becoming more common as intellectually handicapped people are living longer. The brains of almost all people with Down's Syndrome over the age of 40 show the characteristic neuropathological changes of Alzheimer's disease. Clinical dementia does not occur in all cases despite the brain abnormalities. Dementia shows up initially as increasing withdrawal, apathy and loss of interest in previous occupations, with personality and mood changes. Later manifestations include progressive disorientation, loss of social and cognitive skills and eventual incontinence, seizures and increasing paralysis.

The early stages of dementia are particularly difficult to detect in severely and profoundly retarded institutionalised persons unless serial records of cognitive and adaptive functioning have been made. Repeated neurological investigations are used to confirm the presence of brain atrophy. Hypothyroidism (also common in Down's Syndrome) and depression must be excluded as differential diagnosis.

Schizophrenia

Mildly retarded people who develop schizophrenia usually present with personality change, withdrawal, apathy, loss of interest and delusional ideas with auditory and visual halluncinations (see chapters 32 and 33). Some respond very well to treatment with psychotropic drugs (Chlorpromazine, Thioridazine, Haloperidol). Generally, schizophrenia is associated with a poor prognosis in the mentally retarded. Neurological side-effects from psychotropic drugs are common. In severely and profoundly retarded persons where behaviour changes suggest the diagnosis, a trial of drugs can be made provided frequent monitoring is also instituted.

Affective disorders

Mood disorders (depression and mania) occur in mentally retarded people at more than twice the rate of the general population. Mentally retarded people may not complain of mood changes or feelings of sadness, so reliance must be placed on their appearance, or accounts from people who know them well. When depressed, they look unhappy, have decreased motor activity, weight loss, anorexia and disturbed sleep. When manic, retarded people become elated, overactive and aggressive. Observation of changes in behaviour occurring cyclically may suggest a diagnosis of manic-depressive illness. Precipitating factors include bereavement, losses, childbirth and viral illnesses. There may be suicide attempts. The usual drug treatments tend to be effective. They should be combined with supportive management of

the patient and family and any necessary therapeutic environmental changes (see chapters 25, 56 and 57).

Anxiety disorders

It is often hard to distinguish anxiety disorders from many of the other apparently abnormal behaviours of mentally retarded people. For example, ritualistic behaviours are common. These are not necessarily the results of distressing anxiety but can be a source of pleasure and are sought out rather than resisted. Nevertheless, mentally retarded people may become distressed, and attention to pain, surroundings and difficulties along with helpful support are required when this occurs. Drug treatments are not usually recommended for anxiety as drug dependence can develop with anxiolytic drugs (see chapters 26, 56 and 57).

Personality disorders

Antisocial and socially deviant traits can sometimes be recognised in mentally retarded people. These traits may lead them to activities which result in gaol sentences. Antisocial or delinquent acts in mild and borderline retarded males can bring them to the attention of the police but the legal system is sometimes reluctant to prosecute and instead, may prefer residential or hospital treatment. Management is often very difficult. Education, behaviour modification and counselling programs are most commonly recommended (see chapter 14).

Conduct disorders

These are frequent at all ages among the mentally retarded and may be related to environmental factors such as family conflict, school problems or difficulties with staff in residences or workshops. They are usually amenable to intervention but some families and staff find it very difficult to change their ways of reacting to a particular handicapped person (see chapter 23). In such cases, separation from the family may be the only effective solution for the emotional problems of adolescent and young adult people with mental retardation. Acute crises often clear up with a change of day activity or allowing the person more independence. Suitable group home placements need to be made more freely available for these patients. The stereotyped, repetitive, self-stimulating or self-injurious behaviours of the more severely retarded, the aetiology of which is multi-factorial, require a different approach. Specialised behavioural techniques are the most effective.

Treating mental illness in mentally retarded people

Most mentally retarded people can be treated in main stream psychiatric services, others in their place of residence. It is important to stress that the approach to the treatment of mental illness in mentally retarded people must be open-minded, flexible and pluralistic with a preparedness to use a variety of techniques and to involve other disciplines. Individual solutions will need to be formulated for each situation. The drug treatment of mental illness in the intellectually handicapped is well established but needs special safeguards because of the tendency to develop side-effects and an unfortunate history of excessive and unwarranted use in institutions.

Psychotropic drugs should not be used to control behaviour problems which are the result of situational factors like boredom, understimulating environments and inappropriate care or lack of educational or activity programs. When carefully monitored and used as *part* of a management plan, medication can be helpful in certain circumstances, such as disorganised, agitated, noisy, destructive and aggressive episodes. Regular monitoring and review is essential. Individual, group and family therapies have their uses, particularly with the mild and moderately retarded and with families of young handicapped children. Community support services and adequate respite care facilities are important. Community nurses, social workers and psychologists provide support through home visiting and designing and implementing home-based behaviour management programs.

The application of early intervention (therapy and special education) programs as soon as disability is discovered has an important role in the prevention of many behavioural problems. The limitation of premature institutionalisation prevents the personality and intellectual damage resulting from early parental separation and deprivation however, some problems may require management in special treatment units. Most mildly retarded persons can be accommodated within the general psychiatric services. Behavioural methods, used by specially trained personnel, form the main treatment of behaviour problems for more retarded people who are in institutions. Details of appropriate behaviour therapy techniques can be found in more specialised texts. A hierarchy of procedures ranging from reinforcement methods whereby adaptable skills are developed through to aversive conditioning are described. A model which utilises the least restrictive and least intrusive method is preferred.

The provision of adequate social, vocational, leisure and recreational activities in a supportive environment is essential. For some mentally retarded people long term residential placement is still necessary. Recent moves away from hospital care into the community under the philosophies of 'deinstitutionalisation', means that remaining residential units are small, specialised and community-based.

The diagnosis, assessment, treatment and management of psychiatric and behaviour disorders in mentally handicapped children and adults remains the primary role of the psychiatrist working with this special group of people. The members of the multidisciplinary support team will increasingly utilise the psychiatrist as consultant as more mentally retarded people live in the community.

Sexuality and the retarded

The sexual development of mentally retarded young people is often a major issue for parents, teachers and care givers. One common fear is that the youngster will be unable to understand or control the sexual feelings which arise during puberty. In fact, mentally retarded people are rarely a danger to the community. Rapists and those committing aggressive sexual crimes are more often of normal intelligence. Psychiatrists and other clinical personnel are often called on for advice during the adolescence of a retarded person, particularly where issues of contraception or sterilisation are involved. Emphasis is now increasingly being placed on educational programs. A proportion of adolescent retarded girls may be at risk, because they indiscriminately seek affection from others or, because they misinterpret sexual advances as affection. Sexual abuse and incest can occur with this group. Men and women who cannot understand issues of safe sex, also may be at risk for AIDS (see chapters 53 and 54). Public masturbation or exhibitionism in males can sometimes be a problem where the person is unaware of the public consequences. Instruction may be needed to promote the expression of sexual drives in an appropriate manner and setting.

Questions of the rights of mentally retarded persons to sexual and emotional relationships, marriage and childbearing are issues of current concern, often creating heated debate.

Many situations can be resolved by common sense and humanitarianism. The right of a mentally retarded person to have children has to be balanced against the right of children to adequate parenting. It is now legally mandatory in most States of Australia to obtain informed consent for all operative procedures including those for sterilisation. This requires empathic enquiry and patient explanation. Hysterectomy or tubal ligation as forms of permanent contraception and termination of pregnancy are problematic issues. For totally dependent women, who are incapable of self care during menstruation, removal of the uterus may improve the quality of their life substantially, and may need careful consideration. Mildly retarded men and women can be trained to use ordinary contraceptive measures. Each case must be judged on its merits, there should be careful consideration of all options and consultation with relevant professionals, family, patient advocates and properly constituted authorities.

Further Reading

Mayou R, 'Mental Retardation' in *Oxford Textbook of Psychiatry*, (ed Gelder M, Gath D and Mayou R), Oxford Medical Publications, Oxford, UK, 1983, pp 686-713.

Oliver R, *Mental Handicap*, Current Reviews in Psychiatry, 1, (ed Paykel E S and Morgan G), Churchill Livingstone, Edinburgh, London, Melbourne and New York, 1985.

Reid A H, 'Psychiatry and Mental Handicap' in *Mental Handicap: A Multidisciplinary Approach* (ed Craft M, Bicknell J and Hollins S), Bailliere Tindall, London, 1985, pp 317-32.

Szymanski L S, 'Psychiatric Diagnosis of Retarded Persons' in *Emotional Disorders of Mentally Retarded Persons: Assessment, Treatment and Consultation*, (ed Szymanski L S and Tanguay P E), University Park Press, Baltimore, 1989, pp 61-81.

Chapter 10

Pervasive Developmental Disorders

H Salimi Eshkevari

Autistic disorder is the only disorder of pervasive developmental disorders (PDD) which has been mentioned in DSM-III-R. However, there are other similar disorders which are called *'PDD, not otherwise specified'*. These disorders are similar to autism in some features, but they differ from it in a number of ways.

Autism

The syndrome of autism, or early infantile autism, was first described by Kanner (1943). It is rare in children, affecting 4–5 per 10,000 live births. It afflicts boys more than girls in the proportion of 3–4:1 (although girls tend to be more severely affected). It is found in all social classes and cultures, but there is a tendency to occur more in higher and upper middle classes.

Criteria for diagnosis

Autism is diagnosed by the following criteria:
1. Disorders of social behaviour (see Table 1).
2. Disorders of language and speech (see Table 2).
3. Obsessive–compulsive phenomena (see Table 3).
4. Other symptoms (see Table 4).
Age of onset is before 2½ years (at most 3 years).

Table 1. Social behaviour

Gaze avoidance (evades looking at other people)

No attachment behaviour (including anticipatory response, delay in recognition of parents)

No responsiveness to people (eg no smiling or saying hello when meets a familiar person, does not say goodbye on leaving, does not shake hands)

No play with peers (constructive and/or imaginative)

Ignores the presence of other human beings

Lacks response to other people's emotion or distress

No social/emotional reciprocity

Rarely initiates interactive conversation and/or play with others

Rarely seeks others for comfort or affection, or offers affection

Disturbed affect, (eg giggling, crying or screaming without any apparent reason)

Absence of emotional response, no facial expression in response to familiar people

Self absorption

Table 2. Disturbance in language and speech

Abnormal vocalisation

Very poor understanding of language (comprehension)

Deviation and delay in speech, echolalia, perseveration of speech, abnormal production of speech, eg literalness, using 'he' for 'I'

Abnormality of speech tone, rhythm, rate, pitch, stress and intonation

Deficit in using gesture or understanding other people's gesture, lack of imitation (except in speech)

Does not respond when called by name

Table 3. Obsessive-compulsive phenomena

Repetitive behaviour such as hand flapping, whirling, spinning object, teeth grinding, posturing, rocking, protrusion of the tongue, head turning to the right and left, etc

Resistance to change (or morbid sameness)

Morbid attachment to unusual objects, such as a branch of a tree, washing powder, a thread, plate, bead, etc

Morbid preoccupation (eg talking about the same subject over and over)

Table 4. Other symptoms of autism

Abnormal fear (eg fear of harmless objects or, no fear of danger)

Destructiveness, aggression to self or other (eg biting, head banging, poking eyes)

Eating peculiarities, (eg refusing having certain foods, drinking a large volume of water)

Mouthing objects, throwing objects, smelling or sniffing objects

Abnormal reaction to sensory stimuli (eg looking at or avoiding sunshine, hypo or hypersensitivity to sounds, stiffening or hypotonicity on holding, poor sense of pain, peculiarities in eating (sense of taste), smelling objects instead of touching)

Associated features

At least 50 per cent of children with autism are mentally retarded, so it is important to consider their symptoms according to their mental age, and not their chronological age. For example, a normal two year old child can speak simple sentences. Obviously, a two year old mentally retarded child is not able to talk like a normal two year old child, but his lack of speech does not necessarily indicate autism.

Autism is associated with epilepsy. Mentally retarded children develop epilepsy earlier than autistic children with normal intelligence.

Depression may develop in some cases in adolescence as a response to their distressing condition. Very few autisitc children develop schizophrenia during adolescence or later in life. Attention deficit-hyperactivity disorder is a common feature in autistic children which occurs intermittently or continously.

Aetiology

The main deficit in autism is language and cognitive disorders. In one study, it was found that about a quarter of the relatives of autistic children suffered from mild degrees of cognitive disabilities. Autistic children can not interpret external stimuli properly, or can not perceive environmental factors appropriately. Consequently, they can not process information in their central nervous system. In other words, they have deficits in coding and decoding of information.

It is believed that the cause of the language and cognitive disorder in autism is a combination of predisposing genetic factors and an insult to the brain in prenatal life or at birth. Twin studies show a higher rate of autism in identical twins than dizygotic twins. In a study of a series of 21 same-sexed pairs, one of whom was an autistic child, there was a 36 per cent concordance in monozygotic (identical) pairs and 0 (zero) per cent concordance in dizygotic (non-identical) pairs. Autism also occurs slightly more often in siblings of children with autism than in the general population.

Impairment of brain development by a variety of diseases may be associated with autism. These include maternal rubella, tuberous sclerosis, encephalitis, infantile spasms, untreated phenylketonuria (PKU), fragile X syndrome, severe cyanosis, cerebral lipoidosis and neurofibromatosis. However, organic brain dysfunction per se is not the necessary cause of autism, since there are many organic factors which cause brain damage but do not result in autism. For instance, cerebral palsy is associated with brain damage and gross motor abnormalities but not autism. In most cases of autism no gross cerebral abnormality of structure or histology is demonstrated. Also, autistic children are usually physically normal. aetiology of autism, but they can affect the course of this syndrome. Parents may show abnormal responses secondary to the child's extreme abnormal behaviour which is very difficult to manage without support.

Differential diagnosis

There are five syndromes which are to some extent similar to autism, but there are subtle or some differences between these conditions and autism. They are as follows:

1. *Autistic like syndrome with severe mental retardation* (MR)

About half of children with MR show autistic-type symptoms. However, autism needs to be differentiated from mental retardation, since in MR, there is poor development of speech and to some extent social behaviour. Repetitive behaviour is not uncommon in MR, and may be mistaken for obsessive compulsive phenomena of the autistic disorder. However, most behaviour of mentally retarded children accords with their mental age but it is not the case in autism.

2. *Disintegrative psychosis*

This autistic-like syndrome occurs in children with normal intelligence. It is also called Heller's syndrome or dementia infantalis and has been classified as a pervasive developmental disorder not otherwise specified in DSM–III–R, but ICD-10 separates it from autism. It is really a collection of disorders which develop rarely in children after a period of normal development, at the age of three to four years. The condition usually follows some minor physical disease such as a common cold or psychological stress (for example, separation from parent, or fear of an animal). In this disorder, the prodromal symptoms are irritability, anxiety, overactivity and restiveness. Then, acutely or gradually they lose all of their mental abilities, even all of their speech, show severe intellectual deterioration, loss of social skills, loss of general interest in objects, and develop mannerisms and stereotypes. They may urinate or defaecate on the floor, and they show most of the psychiatric features of autism. Often, after several months of affliction, there is a plateau followed by a limited improvement. In some cases, the condition is persistently progressive and is later associated with gross motor abnormality and epilepsy. These are usually due to known neurological diseases, such as lipoidoses or leucodystrophies (see chapter 32).

In girls, Rett's syndrome may be the cause of this disorder. This condition is associated with progressive dementia, loss of facial expression and social communication, loss of purposeful hand use, chronic hand washing movements, ataxia, stereotyped movements, and severe growth problem.

In some cases, the cause is unknown, without evidence of brain damage, especially if it has an early onset at about 2½ to 3 years.

3. *Later onset autistic-like syndrome*

These disorders include both Asperger's syndrome and schizoid disorder. In Asperger's syndrome, there is a lack of empathy, a disturbance in communication, and often morbid attachments to unusual objects and restricted intellectual interests such as a bus or train time table, astronomy, calendar, etc. However, it is not associated with language deficits. Some authors include Asperger's syndrome in schizoid disorder.

4. *Schizophrenia-like syndromes in childhood*

These disorders develop in early or middle childhood; most are schizophrenia. They develop after six years of age and accompanied by psychotic symptoms similar to adult schizophrenia (see chapters 32, 33).

5. *Very severe specific developmental receptive language disorder*

In this disorder, language, cognition and behaviour are different from autism. However, there is a small group of children with mixed features. Some of them show severe social and behavioural abnormalities when they get older. Some studies of these children show that many of them exhibit autistic symptoms. However, there are differences. In receptive language disorder, there is no proponderance of boys and girls, the prognosis is better, the cognitive disability and socioemotional and behavioural abnormalities are less severe than autism. In particular, they do not show the severe disturbances in their relations to others which are found in autistic children.

Other disorders

Hearing impairment may simulate autism in infancy due to lack of auditory response and lack of speech, which is also a common finding in autism. However, in hearing defects, there are no other symptoms of autism. Although deaf children lack speech, they try to communicate by vocalisation, gestures, postures and other means of communications.

Very anxious or very shy children may avoid visual contact but, they have no other major psychiatric symptoms that could be similar to autism.

Occasionally blind children, particularly with Leber's congenital amaurosis, may also suffer from autism (associated with optic atrophy, disseminated sclerosis, spasticity of muscles, disorder of gait, spinocerebellar disorder, occasionally mental retardation and epilepsy). On rare occasions other illnesses are associated with autistic symptomatology.

Investigations

Complete physical, neurological and laboratory investigations need to be done to find any treatable causes of autistic disorder.

Laboratory studies for amino acids may show phenylketonuria (PKU) which is a treatable condition if it is discovered during the first six weeks of life. Even after the age of six weeks treatment diminishes the severe behaviour disorder which is associated with PKU. Other tests, for example, leucocyte, enzymes, will show rare diseases. Computerised tomography (CT) scan of the head may show calcification in the brain in 'tuberous sclerosis'.

An electroencephalogram (EEG) may show abnormality particularly if the child is suffering from epilepsy. In infantile spasm, EEG shows a specific abnormality—'hypsarrhythmia'. Some children with infantile spasm recover with medications such as corticosteroid, or adrenocorticotrophin hormone (ACTH).

Chromosomal studies are also indicated to rule out fragile X syndrome, which is one of the associated factors in autism.

Other investigations such as positron emission tomography (PET) and magnetic resonance imaging (MRI) of the brain may be done as complementary to other investigations. MRI may show underdevelopment of the cerebellum in non-retarded autistic children. An electroretinogram may show decreased function of the rods (light sensitive structures) in the retina of the eyes.

Treatment

Although medication is not the first line of management in autism it may be used for severe behaviour disorder or any associated psychiatric disorder. Usually psychotropic drugs help these aspects of their disorder to some extent. Phenothiazines (for example, chorpromazine, thioridazine; and fluphenazine) reduce general behaviour disorders. Haloperidol is helpful for self-injurious behaviour disorders. Lithium Carbonate can decrease dramatically self-injurious behaviour (for example, self-biting, head banging) and aggressive behaviour (see chapters 56, 57).

A problem with medication for these children is that many of them show idiosyncratic reactions shortly after the use of medication. Thus, they may become extremely restless and distressed, with crying and screaming which is really unbearable for their parents.

Despite some workers' claim about the efficacy of some drugs, such as megavitamin therapy (many times higher than usual dosage) in treatment, particularly, vitamin B6 and fenfluramine, the efficacy of these drugs have not been confirmed by rigorous research. There are rare cases where improvement has been reported by megavitamin therapy and in some cases with fenfluramine.

The best available management for autism is *education* by expert people. It has been shown that education and behaviour therapy based on operant conditioning can help to a great extent in all aspects of disabilities such as language, speech, social behaviour and obsessive compulsive phenomena.

Abnormal behaviour should be abandoned, otherwise this interferes with learning. Any positive learning should be rewarded. Individual teaching is necessary in the beginning. A special school is very helpful for autistic children to attend during the daytime, but some children need to stay in a residential unit. Parental cooperation, motivation and their participation are necessary in education. Since autistic children can not easily generalise their learning experiences from one situation to another situation, parents should continue teaching them at home. For this purpose, the educator should gradually teach parents the principles of learning when he tries to educate the autistic child. This is the best method of educating for any person with a learning disorder.

Education is used for the following purposes:
1. Reduction of useless behaviour such as headbanging, whirling, hands flapping, etc.
2. Establishment of useful behaviour such as communication with others, self-care, etc.
3. Improvement of speech and cognition.
4. Strengthening of sensory abilities and perception.
5. Improvement of coordination.
6. Teaching of lessons in the classroom.

For education, the following points must be considered:
1. Establishment of a good relationship with the child, if possible.
2. Existence of a very well organised and highly structured program.
3. Development of a specific and individualised program for each child.
4. Reduction of inappropriate external stimuli in order to increase attention.
5. Participation in group activities.
6. Normal progression of development in *all aspects* to be encouraged.

7. Cooperation of all concerned professional people and parents and siblings.

Parents and siblings need professional help, since they suffer a great deal of distress. In many developed countries, parents have established an Autistic Association with the help of professional experts and this provides assessment, treatment and support services for children with autism and their families.

Course and prognosis

In untreated cases, the course of autistic disorder does not fluctuate very much. However, autistic children may lose some of their symptoms as they grow older, usually in adolescence. They may improve to some extent with appropriate treatment. Nearly all autistic children will need life long support, but about one in three are able to live in the community as adults with minimal supervision. Some find useful and enjoyable occupations. Others will require varying degrees of social support throughout their lives. However, the general long term picture for autistic children is much more hopeful now due to the better management of autism over the past two decades. Good prognosis depends on reasonable intellectual skills and the presence of speech before the age of five or six years.

Further Reading

Rutter M, 'Infantile Autism and Other Pervasive Developmental Disorders', in *Child and Adolescent Psychiatry: Modern Approaches*, 2nd edn (ed Rutter M and Hersov L), Blackwell Scientific Publication, Oxford, 1985, pp 545–66.

Rutter M and Schopler E, 'Autism and Pervasive Developmental Disorders: Concept and Diagnostic Issues', *Journal of Autism and Developmental Disorders*, Vol 17, No 2, 1987, pp 159–86.

Chapter 11

Learning disabilities

H Salimi Eshkevari

Specific learning disorders are persistent and life long disorders, except for those which are due to a maturational delay. Although they are not classified as mental disorders, they are strongly associated with psychiatric illnesses. Specific reading retardation was found in 4 per cent of ten year olds in a survey of children in the Isle of Wight (United Kingdom) and was found to be twice as common in inner London. In the United States of America during 1985 to 1986 learning disability was found in 4.73 per cent of all students surveyed; and academic under-achievement was found among 20 per cent. The reasons for underachievement include mental retardation, emotional disorders and specific learning disabilities.

Definition

Specific learning disabilities are disorders in one or more of the basic psychological processes which are involved in understanding or in using written or spoken language. They may manifest themselves in deficits in thinking, listening, speaking, writing, spelling or arithmetic. Deficits due to visual, auditory, or motor handicaps and emotional, neurological or environmental factors are excluded. In DSM-III-R, specific learning disabilities are included under the term 'Specific Developmental Disorders'. A diagnosis of specific learning disorder should be based on the results of standardised, individually administered psychological tests that measure both intellectual skills and impairments.

Classification

Specific learning disabilities are classified as the following:
1. *Academic (learning) skills disorders*
(a) reading disorder
(b) writing disorder
(c) arithmetic disorder
(d) language and speech disorders
2. *Motor skill disorders* (see chapter 65).

Specific reading retardation

In this condition, reading achievement is substantially below the level that could ordinarily be expected for the child's level of schooling and intelligence. On psychological tests for IQ, such as the Welchsler Intelligence Scale for Children (WISC), specific reading retarded children produce a lower verbal IQ than performance IQ. Language and speech disorders are strongly associated with reading retardation. Poor motor control often exists in these children. Social environment is also important in the attainment of reading. Parents who place a high value on education and provide a stimulating intellectual environment for their children by talking to them and reading books with them help to develop their childrens' reading skills. However, specific reading retardation occurs in many social environments.

Factors associated with reading retardation

One third of speech retarded children are also impaired in reading and spelling; and reading retardation occurs in some children with speech delay and with articulation defects.

Defects in visual–spatial motor coordination are not significant causes of reading retardation in school aged children, although they may be of significance for the very young child beginning to read letters. For this reason visual–motor training is not helpful for the improvement of reading.

Brain impairment is often associated with reading difficulty. High rates of reading difficulty are found among children with cerebral palsy, independent of otherwise normal intellectual functions. Many children with epilepsy also show reading retardation. Localised head injury, especially if it involves the left cerebral hemisphere, is likely to cause reading difficulties.

It is claimed that smoking during pregnancy can cause low birth weight, which in turn, is associated with reading difficulty when measured at the age of seven years, however, this association is weak. Low level lead poisoning may affect intellectual functioning in children and consequently, reading. However, it is not entirely clear whether lead poisoning or the lower social class, from which many lead affected children come, affects reading in lead poisoned children. The role of genetic factors in reading retardation is also not clear. However, the familial pattern of most severe cases of reading disability is compatible with a recessive mode of genetic inheritance. Lag in the maturation of left cerebral hemisphere is another possible cause of reading disability, that is, the left cerebral hemisphere develops slower than the right hemisphere in poor readers. It has also been suggested that isolated reading disorders may result from biologic variation of brain development during the prenatal period.

Overall, it can be said that the biological basis of reading disabilities is that there is:
1. a preponderance of males (3.5 to 1 ratio);
2. frequent speech and language delays or anomalous speech production such as stuttering and/or disorder of articulation;
3. a higher proportion of specific reading retardation in near relatives;
4. slight increase in the number of affected children who are left handed.

These factors suggest a biological basis in cerebral lateralisation. However, the presence of biological factors does not rule out the importance of the environmental elements, since biological impaired children may be more vulnerable to environmental adversities.

An electroencephalogram of poor readers differs from that of good readers, but there are no specific features, rather an immature pattern. Positron emission tomography (PET) shows decreased activity in the left hemisphere of people with specific reading retardation, but increased activity, bilaterally, in the mid temporal cortex.

Specific spelling retardation

In spelling retardation, written language skills are normally below the level that could be expected for the child's level of schooling and intelligence. Although reading and spelling are related, there are marked differences in the two skills. The essence of writing is the representation of speech sounds into corresponding letters. There are two stages in spelling:
1. From the sound of a word, one or more graphic representations are generated (such as 'sea' and 'see', etc).
2. The correct graphic representation is chosen according to information about the sequence of letters in the word (for example, 'sea' has a similar sound to 'see', but their meanings are different).

However, this correspondence is not the only factor in the English language. There are also some additional rules and word specific information necessary for the acquisition of spelling for example, many different words may represent the same meaning for example, nice, good, etc.

Mathematical difficulties

For mathematical skills, children need to be able to classify or group objects, for example, all cars together or all round objects together, then they must develop an understanding of numbers.

Mathematical difficulties have not been studied very much up to now. It has been estimated that this affects about 6 per cent of school children. Low general intelligence, poor teaching and excessive anxiety may affect learning maths. Spatial deficits are associated with poor maths ability and in these cases neurophyschological tests suggest these may be linked with deficits in the right hemisphere parietal lobe.

Some of the problems of children with maths disorders or difficulties are associated with deficits in their perception of spatial relationships, namely, up–down, top–bottom and near–far. Such children are also unable to work adequately with puzzles or to count objects in a series and cannot easily perceive objects in groups. There may also be related language problems such as an inability to understand the meaning of 'plus', 'minus' or 'take away'. Memory is also disturbed in children with mathematical disability and often they cannot remember computation facts (time tables) easily.

Neurological examinations may show slight nervous reflex and coordination asymmetries and difficulties in right and left orientation. Unlike specific reading disorders, in mathematical retardation the male to female ratio is equal.

Assessment of reading difficulty

Reading ability is tested by many standardised reading tests. This is dealt with in chapter 61. However, we should note here that there are different opinions on calculating reading and spelling abilities. Some authors believe that reading should be assessed according to chronological age (CA) or grade level. A difference between CA and reading age (RA) or a ratio between RA/CA represents the index of reading difficulty or retardation. However, these are arbitrary limits for reading retardation. Most workers agree that a half a year behind in first grade, a year behind in second grade and so forth, should indicate reading retardation. Other investigators believe that it is better to take into account the ratio of attainment age to expectancy, that is, $\frac{MA + CA + Grade\ Age}{3}$. Others use the difference between IQ and a standardised reading score.

However, most workers believe that IQ and reading do not run in parallel and it is therefore necessary to determine individual reading achievements on the basis of observed scores between the average educational attainments in the general population of the same aged children of average intelligence. Achievement in reading more than two standards below the average is considered a very considerable disability. Since reading disability is often associated with spelling disorder, the latter should always be tested for too.

Differential diagnosis

Specific reading disorder should be differentiated from general backwardness in reading. This is associated with general backwardness in most learning areas. It occurs in both girls and boys nearly equally. In specific reading disability, the number of boys to girls is 3–4:1 and it is not usually associated with any particular type of brain disorder, but is associated only with language and speech disorders.

Psychiatric disorders and reading difficulties

There is a strong association between severe specific reading disability and psychiatric disorder, especially conduct disorders. A quarter of the children with specific reading retardation show anti-social behaviour. Conversely, a third of children with conduct disorder have reading retardation (compared with 4 per cent in the general population). However, this association does not apply for conduct disorders which develop in adolescence.

The association of reading disorders and childhood conduct disorders appears to rest on the failure of reading retarded children to achieve at school, with consequent frustration. They develop low self-esteem, antagonism to school, and emotional problems. Improvement in schooling usually reduces the behavioural problems. In some cases, conduct disorder precedes reading retardation and there is a possibility that both conduct disorder and reading retardation have a common aetiology in terms of social, familial or temperamental factors. Impulsive children who have poor learning strategies show reading retardation.

There are many other symptoms which may develop due to educational failure. These include avoidant reactions, anxiety and phobic responses, somatic complaints, sensitivity and suspiciousness; and depression with irritability and aggression. Clowning may serve as a way of controlling feelings of inadequacy, lack of worth and disruption in the classroom. Difficulties in social relationships include a lack of friends and loneliness, with an inability to achieve friends, or poor communication with peers.

Family problems may also occur as a result of the child's learning disabilities. It can be very stressful for parents to have a child handicapped in this way. Parents may deny their child's educational problems and become angry with the school authorities or the child, or they may themselves feel guilty. Denial of problems may cause negative feelings in the child, who senses that his parents cannot accept him and his difficulties. Siblings may show low self-esteem, especially if they go to the same school. They may get angry because of the extra attention needed by the learning disabled child.

Mathematical difficulty and psychiatric disorders

Children with mathematical disorders have intact oral vocabulary but they generally use it rigidly, ineffectively, socially inappropriately and/or nonprosodicly. They cannot appreciate humour and have difficulty in inferential thinking. These children have deficits in measuring social distance, or in 'reading' people, especially at an emotional level, and their interpretation of other people's facial expressions and gestures is impaired. Such children consequently are perceived as eccentric and may evoke negative social responses in others.

Intervention and remedial education

Educational help is necessary for learning disabled children. Treatment of any psychiatric features is a prerequisite. Family counselling should include full information about the child's educational and psychosocial problems. Results of the evaluation of the child must be shared with him and the family. Parents should be aware of the child's abilities as well as his disabilities. Parents should be discouraged from doing tasks for their children. It is better that parents assist their children in organising their work. Teaching should be based on metacognition, that is, teaching learning disabled children how to learn.

The teaching environment must not be discriminating. Learning disabled children should share their education with other children in a normal classroom. In the regular classroom, a special education teacher, who relates to the learning disabled child may serve as a consultant and provide materials for the child. A resource room may be available for such children, receiving special teaching there, for a portion of the day. In these rooms, only a small number of children attend (around 4–6 at a time). More individual programs and one to one education are useful for severely reading disordered children, who need intensive individualised programs for many years.

Many education procedures such as repetition, allotting longer time for the completion of work, providing more examples and reviews, introducing the work more slowly, and expanding the background information with more work on vocabulary are useful for the education of learning disabled children. Multisensory methods utilising sound, vision, speech and tracing, are effective for improvement of reading. Decoding skills, learning synthetic phonics and developing recognition of the whole words are also useful. Sequencing skills can be improved by training.

Reading retarded children can benefit from exercises that emphasise the concept of phonemes by listening and speaking, but 'look and say' methods do not seem to be very useful. The child's cognitive skills or thinking processes should be used for learning. Children can be helped to ask themselves questions and answer them by organising their thoughts and using their past experiences. For the improvement of spelling, the child should pay attention to letter by letter, and then words.

Medication

Medication does not affect reading directly; however, one of the psychostimulant drugs (Methylphenidate) may enhance educational performance by improving attention.

Prognosis

In most cases, without help, reading and spelling disabilities (except in maturational delay) persist throughout life. Reading retardation may show some spontaneous improvement, but spelling difficulties usually remain unchanged. Also, associated psychiatric disorders are unlikely to improve, and they interfere with social and personal development. Consequently, these children can face frustrating unemployment, or unsatisfying occupations. Maths difficulty seems to affect childrens' futures less than reading difficulty.

Conclusion

Reading disability is strongly associated with psychiatric disorders. Educational help is effective to some extent. Psychiatric intervention in the form of individual therapy as well as family counselling and/or family therapy is often indicated since the child's learning disability has complex personal and family ramifications.

Further Reading

Baker L and Cantwell D P, 'Developmental Arithmetic Disorder', in *Comprehensive Textbook of Psychiatry*, 4th edn (ed Kaplan H I and Sadock B J), Williams and Wilkins, Baltimore, 1985.

Duane D D, 'Neurobiological Correlates of Learning Disorders', *Journal of the American Academy of Child and Adolescent Psychiatry*, Vol 28 No 3, 1989, pp 314-18.

Frith U, 'Reading and Spelling Skills', in *Scientific Foundation of Development Psychiatry* (ed Rutter M), 1980, Heinman Educational, London, pp 220-9.

Lerner J W, 'Educational Intervention in Learning Disabilities', *Journal of the American Academy of Child and Adolescent Psychiatry'*, Vol 28 No 3, 1989, pp 326-31.

Rutter M and Yule W, 'Reading and Other Learning Difficulties', in *Child and Adolescent Psychiatry*, 2nd edn (ed Rutter M and Hersov L), Blackwell Scientific Publication, Oxford, 1985, pp 444-64.

Silver L B, 'Learning Disabilities: Introduction', *Journal of the American Academy of Child and Adolescent Psychiatry*, Vol 28 No 3, 1989, pp 309-13.

Silver L B, 'Psychological and Family Problems Associated With Learning Disabilities: Assessment and Intervention', *Journal of the American Academy of Child and Adolescent Psychiatry*, Vol 28 No 3, 1989, pp 319-25.

Chapter 12

Encopresis

R Kosky

Encopresis, or faecal soiling, is a symptom which many people find objectionable, and can result in the sufferer being ostracised and victimised. Faeces are passed into the clothes rather than the toilet. This can happen during the day or at night. It is a specific developmental disorder.

Most children achieve continence of faeces by four years of age and should have bowel control in time to attend school. Encopresis, thus, usually has onset after the age of five to six years. Should soiling occur after this time, mental retardation, autism, other developmental disorders or physical causes such as anal fissure (which causes pain on defaecation), Hirschsprung's disease, (a rare condition where the normal neuro-muscular ability to contract the colon is lost), spinal cord damage, brain damage, severe infection, toxaemia, and acute or chronic sexual abuse should be considered. Soiling can also occur as an adjustment reaction to stress, in which case it is usually temporary.

About 2 per cent of boys and less than 1 per cent of girls in the general population soil at least once a week at seven years of age. These figures fall slightly with increasing age. Soiling is a persistent problem in most untreated cases.

Clinical picture

There are basically four types of soiling.

1. Training

Some soilers are *poorly trained* or are trained to inappropriate standards. In these cases the fault lies with the parents who do not teach their children how to use the toilet. However, it should be noted that in some remote rural communities, toilets may not be readily available and toileting may not be considered a high priority.

2. Retention

Other soilers, have good bowel control but *retain faeces.* These children may go for weeks without defaecating. As the faecal mass builds up in the bowel it becomes distended, often visibly distending the abdomen. Faecal fluid and faecal material dribbles around the mass and out of the anus, soiling clothing.

These children are often found to be stubborn, inflexible and rather obsessional. They are usually in conflict with their parents, and resist their desires for appropriate toileting. The parents themselves are often inflexible and obsessional and may place undue emphasis on early and rigid toilet training. Basically, the situation is a battle of wills. The parents cajole, plead, bribe, and punish in their attempts to persuade the child to give in. This is extremely exasperating for them and worrying. The more emotional the parents become, the more rewarded the child gets for his stubborn retention, as the greater his power over them seems. However, the situation is also anxiety provoking for the child as he realises that he has no control over these essentially destructive feelings and also sees his parents losing control.

In these cases the clinical picture is always of a chronic situation beginning early in life. The underclothes are regularly soiled and many means—diet, laxatives, buying potties, fitting toilets, games on the toilet, rewards and punishments—have usually been tried to induce the child into regular defaecation, but without any lasting success. While laxatives can have temporary success, the retention and accumulation of faeces usually begins straight away. In some cases, surgical removal of the faecal mass has been undertaken because of the fear that the bowel would become impacted.

These children may appear to be ashamed of their soiling and hide their soiled clothes, although this just succeeds in creating dirty areas around the house and infuriating and frustrating the parents further.

They are often intelligent children with good academic records. However, their symptoms keep them apart from other children who understandably, cannot tolerate the smell. As a result, children with chronic retentive soiling fail to learn adequate social skills and often seem immature.

3. Aggressive soiling

In these cases, soiling is associated with anger. These children, unlike the retentive soilers, usually come from chaotic family and social backgrounds. Inconsistency and disorganisation are characteristic of their families and their lives. Often they are subject to inconsistent, occasionally violent punishment. The soiling can be seen as an expression of aggression and retaliation. It is often associated with faecal smearing and sometimes, in older children, this occurs in public places. These children are also likely to be aggressive in other ways. They do poorly at school and mix poorly with their peers. They may bully younger children.

4. Regressive soiling

The clinical picture in these cases is of many features of inappropriate 'infantile' behaviour including baby talk, clinging to parents, infantile demands for feeding (even breast feeding), refusal to sleep alone, immature play and, sometimes, requests for nappies.

This type of soiling usually follows a severe stress but it is not uncommon in young children who have just encountered a baby sibling. The loss of the mother's attention, which is now focused on feeding and caring

for the new baby, may produce attention-seeking behaviour in the older sibling with imitation of the baby's behaviour.

Investigation and treatment

It is important to eliminate the possibility that the soiling may be due to a physical cause. This will require a thorough physical examination. Abdominal and rectal examination may be necessary. The possibility of sexually-transmitted diseases should be kept in mind. X-rays of the abdomen may establish the size of faecal masses.

Physical treatments such as exercise, a good high fibre diet, appropriate fluids, plus the long term administration of laxatives (such as Senokot) may be sufficient. Suppositories and enemas are not usually recommended. If the above regime does not work, hospitalisation is appropriate.

In hospital, it is important to establish a toileting routine. The child should go to the toilet about 20 minutes after each meal and remain there until he passes faeces or a reasonable time has elapsed. Nursing staff must not be tempted into getting emotionally involved as, if they do, they are likely to repeat the 'battle of wills' with which the child engaged his parents. They should not become punitive or hostile.

Most children who soil become clean within a few weeks in a hospital situation. The staff must, of course, work with the parents so that a more facilitating and maturing relationship between the child and the parents can be developed. Some attention usually needs to be given to the child's social skills and this can occur in hospital or on a day hospital or outpatient basis.

The same regime or retoileting is also appropriate for aggressive soilers. However, the problem here is usually their behaviour. Firm and consistent limit setting is essential. It is not until the child has internalised some control over his impulses and behaviour, that the soiling also will come under control. Attempts to change the family are often unrewarding and substitute care may be necessary.

Regressive soiling must be considered a rather severe instance of regressive behaviour in the face of stress. It is essential to identify the source of stress and to modify it. Individual psychotherapy with the child and/or family therapy may be appropriate to help re-establish appropriate developmental levels.

Outcome

The response to treatment is good and up to 75 per cent of chronic soilers are able to develop adequate toileting patterns. Untreated cases have a poor prognosis and although the soiling may cease in adolescence, many of these young people go on to express their aggression by other antisocial ways. The retentive soiler may develop life-long preoccupation with bowels and diets, and may develop eccentric habits.

Further Reading

Bellman M, 'Studies on Encopresis', *Acta Paediatrica Scandinavia*, Suppl 170, 1966.

Berg I, Forsythe F, Holt P and Matts J, 'A Controlled Trial of Senokot in Faecal Soiling Treated by Behavioural Methods, *Journal of Child Psychology and Psychiatry*, Vol 23, 1983, pp 543–9.

Hersov L, 'Faecal Soiling', *Child and Adolescent Psychiatry: Modern Approaches*, (eds Rutter M, Hersov L) 2nd ed, Blackwell Scientific Publications, Oxford, 1985.

Parks A, 'Anorectal Incontinence', *Proceedings of The Royal Society of Medicine*, Vol 68, 1975, pp 21–30.

Vaughan V C, McKay R J and Nelson W E, *Textbook of Paediatrics*, 10th edn, W B Saunders, Philadephia, 1975.

Chapter 13

Nocturnal Enuresis

J Bollard

Definition

Functional nocturnal enuresis is defined as involuntary passing of urine during sleep, beyond the age of about four years, and in the absence of physical cause. A more common term for this condition is 'bedwetting'.

Clinical features

Two types of bedwetting are often distinguished; a *primary* form in which the child has never achieved complete night-time bladder control; and a *secondary* or acquired type which is characterised by a previous period of control (usually a period of more than 12 months) followed by a return to regular night-time wetting. It is often assumed that these two forms have different causes, with secondary enuresis more likely to be accompanied by evidence of psychological stress. This distinction appears to matter little in respect of prognosis, since most cases of enuresis categorised as primary or secondary appear to respond to treatment in essentially the same way.

Patterns of bedwetting vary from children who wet the bed several times each night, to others who wet only occasionally, and still others who wet heavily, but in sporadic bursts. There is no strong consensus with regard to the minimum frequency of bedwetting before a child should be regarded as enuretic.

Bedwetting runs in families. Studies have found between 70 to 80 per cent of children to be enuretic when both parents had a past history of enuresis. Concordance for enuresis between identical twins has been found to be double that for fraternal twins.

Prevalence

Prevalence figures indicate that bedwetting is common. Ten to fifteen per cent of five year olds wet the bed regularly, 5 to 6 per cent of ten year olds, and 2 per cent of teenagers. Thereafter, about 1 per cent of cases continue into adulthood. Bedwetting is somewhat more common in boys than girls up until the age of 11 years, the ratio being approximately 3:2.

Aetiology

It is unlikely that there is a single cause for bedwetting, since in any large group of enuretic children, one finds considerable variability in terms of bedwetting frequency, functional bladder capacity, the presence of diurnal incontinence, ease of arousability from sleep, motivation to become dry, and so on.

Physical factors

Bedwetting caused by organic disease is rare, probably constituting no more than 5 per cent of the total enuretic population. Bedwetting may occur in association with an infection of the urinary tract. It may be secondary to the excessive production of urine caused by diabetes mellitus, or certain kidney diseases. The likelihood of an association between night-time bedwetting and organic disease is increased if daytime enuresis is also present. Incontinence may also be associated with conditions such as spina bifida, nocturnal epilepsy, and physiological abnormalities of the bladder. These conditions, although uncommon, highlight the need for an adequate medial examination of the child who wets the bed.

Parents often report these children to be unusually heavy sleepers, and view this as the cause of the child's problem. In spite of such strong anectdotal evidence however, clinical observations and empirical studies have produced conflicting results about the relationship between depth of sleep and bedwetting. Bedwetting is associated with a particular stage of deep sleep (as measured by electroencephalography (EEG) recordings), but it is better regarded as a failure to arouse from sleep in time to control the bladder. This explanation fits with effective forms of treatment for the majority of bedwetters (that is, the bed-pad and alarm device) which derive some part of their success from their capacity to improve the arousability of the child.

Functional bladder capacity is a term used to refer to the volume of urine retained in the bladder before voiding, rather than the actual size of the bladder. There is now a considerable body of evidence to show that on average, enuretic children have smaller functional bladder capacities than non-enuretic children of the same age, thus supporting the notion that bedwetting is the result of under-developed functional bladder capacity. However, the nature of this relationship is not clear. Low functional bladder capacity, as measured by frequency of urination during the day, is not a reliable index of a child's night-time capacity to exercise control over the bladder. Many children can display frequent urination during the day, but can be nevertheless dry at night. Furthermore, training procedures designed to distend the bladder, thereby increasing functional bladder capacity, by what is known as 'retention control training' have only been partially successful in eradicating bedwetting.

Emotional factors

Some mental health professionals regard bedwetting as merely a surface indicator of some underlying state of emotional disturbance. Psychoanalytical theorists have offered a number of explanations for bedwetting such as a substitution for repressed sexual drive. However, general population surveys have indicated that while there is an association between enuresis and some psychological disorders, particularly the common neurotic and conduct disorders, the majority of enuretic children are well-adjusted. Even when an enuretic child displays signs of emotional disturbance, these are not necessarily proof of a psychogenic origin, since the disturbance may be secondary to the enuresis itself. It is not difficult to imagine how persistent bedwetting could result in lowered self-esteem, restricted social interaction and consequences that could upset the child. In other words, psychological disturbance may be caused by the enuresis, rather than the other way round.

As urine is collected in the bladder, the muscle tone in the bladder is repeatedly adjusted to allow larger volumes of urine to be stored. When the volume of urine exceeds about 200 mls in a normal adult, nervous impulses arise from the bladder wall triggering reflex urination. This action involves strong rhythmical contractions of the bladder followed by relaxation of the sphincters at the opening of the bladder, and ultimately, the passing of urine.

Bladder control is established in the following sequence. Between one and two years, most infants will gradually achieve an awareness during the day of increasing bladder tension as the bladder fills. By about three years of age, most children have learned to tense the muscles in the crutch, thereby being able to hold on to a full bladder for some time before voiding. By about four years of age, most children can start and stop the urinary stream at will, when pressure inside the bladder is high, and by six years of age, the same ability is present in response to almost any degree of bladder filling.

For the achievement of nocturnal bladder control, the child learns to transfer control over urination to the sleeping state. In other words, the child learns to perceive the stimuli arising from a filling bladder during sleep and responds by either contracting the sphincter at the bladder outlet, thereby holding on throughout the night, or if the pressure within the bladder becomes too great, waking and going to the toilet. Failure to learn the above process results in bedwetting.

The means by which one learns the association between a full bladder and sphincter contractions is not clearly understood. Some authors have argued that the practice of 'lifting' during the night for toileting teaches the appropriate response, but clearly many, if not most children, seem to acquire nocturnal bladder control spontaneously.

Initial investigations

Before embarking on any form of therapy, it is necessary to perform a number of medical and psychological investigations.

Medical screening

As noted above, while it is actually quite rare for bedwetting to be caused by organic disease, it is nonetheless essential that every bedwetter identified as needing treatment must first be examined by a medical practitioner. Initial medical assessment should include a detailed history and physical examination, and the child's growth velocities as the latter would be markers for possible renal failure. Analysis of urine is regarded as mandatory. Additional radiologic or other investigations generally would not be required unless a physical abnormality is apparent from the initial checks, or the child failed to respond to treatment.

Psychological investigation

A psychological assessment usually involves interviewing the child and at least one parent. Areas of interest include the child's history and pattern of bedwetting, the presence of any personal, social or environmental circumstances which might have resulted in stress, whether other problems with bladder or bowel control are present, such as excessive urgency and/or frequency of urination or daytime enuresis and encopresis, and any family history of enuresis. In addition, specific fears that may be related to bedwetting, such as fear of the dark or toilet phobia, should be identified. The child's own reaction to the bedwetting and the impact of this reaction on self-esteem, confidence and motivation to become dry, should be explored. If any of the

above problems are uncovered, then, they may need therapeutic intervention, in addition to the direct treatment of the bedwetting.

Treatment

Modern day treatment approaches can be reduced to three categories: simple behavioural measures, medical intervention and conditioning treatment involving the bedpad and buzzer. It should be noted that in some cases simple reassurance that the child will outgrow the problem may be all that the child and parents need.

Simple behavioural measures

Most parents of bedwetters at some stage, prior to seeking treatment, will have utilised the practice of waking or lifting the enuretic child during the night, for toileting. This method can result in a reduction in bedwetting frequency while it is practised, but it involves little 'training' and when the procedure is ceased, most children revert back to their pre-existing bedwetting frequency. Restriction of fluid intake (for example, no drinks after the evening meal) is another common practice. Star charts and other reward systems are often recommended as helpful, especially for younger children. These strategies have been shown to reduce bedwetting frequency, but their effectiveness tends to wear off. There is also a risk that reward systems can elevate anxiety or sense of failure when they do not work, though this problem can be overcome by sensible reassurance. Punishment techniques especially those involving physical punishment, have rarely been demonstrated to be an effective cure of bedwetting, and may in fact exacerbate the problem.

Overall, some of these simple behavioural measures are worthwhile 'first-up' strategies since they are relatively easy to implement and may result in a reduction of bedwetting frequency, however, their success rate in terms of complete cessation of bedwetting symptoms is not high.

Medical treatments

Of the wide range of medications used to treat bedwetting, only the tricyclic anti-depressants have been consistently found to be better than placebo, the most commonly used and extensively studied medication being Imipramine. This is not to suggest that enuretic children are depressed, nor that the therapeutic effects of the drug for enuresis are related to its anti-depressant properties. Such drugs possibly work by increasing arousability from sleep, and their anti-cholinergic properties may also act at the level of the bladder and sphincter. However, scientific evidence relevant to these explanations is inconclusive.

Imipramine and similar tricyclic anti-depressants usually reduce bedwetting frequency, with improvement typically being found during the first weeks of treatment. However, not infrequently, further improvements are not made, with bedwetting incidents levelling out at perhaps two or three nights per week. Complete initial remission is usually obtained for less than 50 per cent of those cases treated with Imipramine, and relapse tends to occur immediately following withdrawal of medication. Further shortcomings of such medication include the possibility of Imipramine side effects such as reduced concentration, restlessness, increased irritability and more serious toxic effects (see chapters 56 and 57).

Conditioning treatment

Conditioning treatment is based on the belief that the problem is due to a failure to learn the response of sphincter inhibition during sleep. This 'habit deficiency' is considered to be the consequence of inadequate environmental conditions for bladder training and/or other factors that would impair learning, such as abnormalities within the central nervous system, particular sleep characteristics, lower intelligence, and in some cases, high anxiety or nervous tension. Treatment is derived from the theory that achieving continence requires the initial learning (in the case of primary bedwetting) and re-learning (in the case of secondary bedwetting) of the disciminative cues that permit the inhibition of urination until appropriate toileting is possible (see chapter 61).

The 'standard' conditioning treatment involves having the enuretic child sleep on a urine-sensitive pad which is connected to a loud bell or buzzer. When a bedwetting occurs, the loud alarm is triggered, thereby causing the child to awaken and urination to cease. The child is then required to complete the act of micturition in the toilet before drying the detector pad, re-setting the alarm and retiring to bed again. As this procedure is repeated, the child eventually learns to contract the bladder sphincter before urination begins, thereby maintaining a dry bed. The modern bed-pad and buzzer device is operated by a low voltage battery and is completely safe. Bed-pad and buzzer devices are very effective in arresting bedwetting. On average, bedwetting ceases in about 80 to 90 per cent of cases treated by standard conditioning, with the duration of treatment ranging from five to 12 weeks. This method has been shown to be more effective in arresting bedwetting than drug therapies, various forms of counselling or psychotherapy, encouragement and exercises aimed at increasing functional bladder capacity.

The biggest shortcoming of the standard conditioning procedure is the substantial number of children who resume wetting the bed after achieving an initial period of dryness. Relapse rates of approximately 40 per cent can be expected following standard conditioning. Countermeasures to relapse have generally followed two strategies: an intermittent schedule of alarm presentations (for example, alarm following 50 per cent or 70 per cent of bedwetting events) and over learning (that is, increasing the child's fluid intake towards the end of treatment). Both strategies have been shown to reduce relapse rates somewhat following conditioning treatment. However, this reduction appears to be at the expense of increasing the duration of treatment time to achieve initial dryness. Fortunately, children who do relapse following standard conditioning treatment respond well to a second treatment and the probability of further relapse is low.

Conclusion

Nocturnal enuresis, or bedwetting, is one of the most common of all childhood disorders.

Various explanations and associated treatments for bedwetting have been advanced. The approach emphasised here is based on the theory that for most children who wet the bed, this is simply a consequence of a failure to learn appropriate control of the bladder during sleep. The treatment of choice is the bed-pad and alarm procedure. Treated by this method, with appropriate equipment and close therapist supervision, the complete arrest of symptoms can be expected in 80 to 90 per cent of enuretic children. Of these children who achieve initial arrest of bedwetting, approximately 40 per cent will relapse within a two year follow-up period. However, for relapsers, a second treatment with the bed-pad and buzzer procedure is usually sufficient to resolve the problem completely.

Further Reading

Bennett-Johnson S, 'Enuresis', in *Clinical Behaviour Therapy and Behaviour Modification*, (ed Daitzman R J), Garland STPM Press, New York, Vol 1, pp 81–142.

Bollard J and Nettelbeck T, *Bedwetting: A Treatment Manual for Professional Staff*, Chapman and Hall, London, 1989.

Kolvin I, MacKeith R C and Meadow S R, *Bladder Control and Enuresis*, Lippincott, Philadelphia, 1973.

Lovibard S H and Coote M A, 'Enuresis', in *Symptoms of Psychopathology* (ed Costello C G) Wiley, New York, 1970, pp 373–96.

Smith P S and Smith L J, *Continence and Incontinence*, Croom Helm, London, 1987, pp 123–73.

Chapter 14

Personality Disorders

J Grigor

The concept of personality disorders is one which has proved intellectually vague and it has been difficult to achieve any consensus among authorities in mental health, welfare or the law about what exactly the term means. Cameron has written that: 'Under this general heading the official classification has made an heroic attempt to gather together under one large tent a number of miscellaneous disturbances. Most of them are highly important in behaviour pathology. Unfortunately the result has been rather to confuse than to clarify.'

It was generally agreed that what distinguished personality disorders from emotional disorders (or neuroses) was that, in the former case, patients experienced only minimal feelings of anxiety or depression. However, more recent work has suggested that many persons who have 'personality disorders' do feel uncomfortable, even distressed, by the many personal inhibitions and restrictions which result from the particularly one sided pattern of behaviour which dominates their personality structure.

In essence, in personality disorders some distortion of the personality develops early in life and persists as the characteristic features of that person and the way in which he copes with the environment. In chapters 2 and 3 the early developmental influences on personality are discussed in detail. All individuals are born different because of their *genetic* component and the experiences of their *intrauterine* life. The *parents' expectations* and attitudes towards their baby and their knowledge and *skills* concerning parenthood will influence how they respond to the baby whose *temperament* in turn may shape those

responses. During early life the *family influences* are paramount. Impairment of attachments to parents can lead to lasting problems in personality. Over-anxious attachments may lead to an over-anxious child. Failure of attachments may lead to an affectionless young person. Disruption of attachment due to separations and losses can lead to a chronically angry or a persistently depressed young person. Parents who carp and criticise and demand conformity may lead to a child developing a reciprocal acceptance and becoming overconforming and seemingly accepting of, even inviting, criticism. Parents may keep a child in a state of infantile dependency which can persist as a lifelong pattern, so that the person always seeks out situations of dependency on others.

Later in childhood, *school* and *peers* can have significant influences on development. These influences may counteract adverse family influences. For instance, a child of loveless parents may meet someone who takes an interest in him and encourages him in a positive way. School and organisations such as Guides and Scouts offer the child wider social experiences than had hitherto been available in the family. These *sociocultural* influences probably become paramount during adolescence when the young person may begin to break away from the values and attitudes of parents. Psychoanalytic concepts of personality development are discussed in chapters 2 and 58.

There are, of course, 'many rooms in God's house' and there is a place in our society for many varieties of people. Moreover, as Cameron points out, unquestioning conformity, self-effacement, suffering and dependence are often acceptable and, sometimes, highly valued by society. Many people with personality traits of this type are admired because they are able to do good things for society. People who are eccentric and dramatic may also be creative. Obsessiveness may be an attribute in certain occupations which involve danger and safety. There are many other examples. It is only when the personality needs are carried to extremes and the qualities turn into demands on others who do not want them and who do not 'gain in warmth and understanding from them' that we would see them as disorders rather than virtues.

The current systems of classification of personality disorders in DSM-III and ICD-9 reflect long standing clinical experience rather than any scientific–rational basis. The ICD-9 classification refers to personality disorders as 'deeply ingrained maladaptive patterns of behaviour'. These are usually evident by adolescence. The DSM-III classification refers to 'inflexible and maladaptive' personality traits which are 'enduring patterns of perceiving, relating to, and thinking about the environment and oneself'. There are eight main types of personality disorders listed in ICD-9: paranoid, affective, schizoid, explosive, anancastic, hysterical, asthenic and antisocial. In DSM-III, there are 11 main types. For simplicity the DSM-III types will be discussed in this chapter. It should be noted, however, that disturbances of mood, frequently involving anxiety or depression, are common and may even be the individual's chief complaint.

The frequent overlap in symptoms found in clinical and research studies of personality disorders has led to a tentative grouping into three main clusters which share common traits. *Cluster A* includes personalities which are odd and eccentric. *Cluster B* includes dramatic, emotional and erratic personalities and *Cluster C*, anxious and fearful personalities.

Cluster A disorders

This includes paranoid, schizoid and schizotypal personality disorders which are characterised by mistrustful, suspicious and sensitive interpersonal relationships.

The *paranoid personality disorder* is characterised by a pervasive and unwarranted suspiciousness, mistrust of people, and hypersensitivity. Such people frequently will not accept the decisions of the law, leading to persistent, unnecessary or inappropriate litigation. People with paranoid personality disorder may come into conflict with the law by committing acts of violence, including murder, usually in a temper or associated with alcohol. Morbid jealousy (the 'Othello Syndrome') may be an extension of the paranoid personality, but is also found among alcoholics, in drug psychoses and in paranoid schizophrenia.

People with paranoid personality disorders appear cold to others, lack humour, are easily slighted and avoid intimacy. They may decompensate into a depressed state under stress and to avoid this, they may keep to themselves or focus on mechanical pursuits and interests.

People with *schizoid personality disorder* have similar defects in their capacity to form social relationships. They lack warm feelings for others and are seemingly indifferent to praise or criticism. They may be distinguished from people with avoidant personality disorder, who do have a genuine desire for social relationships, but are inhibited by their hypersensitivity to rejection by others. At times, the distinction between schizoid personality disorder and avoidant personality disorder may be difficult and perhaps, in future classifications, one category might be deleted. Schizoid personality disorder is, however, not related clearly to schizophrenia. People with this personality disorder live alone with few material possessions, avoid social contact and lead generally quiet and inoffensive lives although some may end up on skid-row. Schizoid persons may present with minor offences related to their low socio-economic status, but they are seldom referred for psychiatric assessment.

Drug therapy is not usually indicated. Traditionally, such patients have been treated with long term psychotherapy and recently, with social rehabilitation.

People with *schizotypal personality disorder*, in contrast, have peculiar ideas and odd behaviours as well as problems with inter-personal relationships. The differential diagnosis from alcohol and drug psychoses, borderline personality disorder and schizophrenia may be difficult. Such people commonly feel that others talk negatively about them and are anxious in social situations. Their speech is commonly disjointed, idiosyncratic or vague. They may become preoccupied with magic, extra sensory perception or clairvoyance and their affect is restricted and sometimes inappropriate. The condition is not uncommonly found among the first degree relatives of people with schizophrenia.

Cluster B disorders

These include antisocial, histrionic, borderline and narcissistic personality disorders and are characterised by unpredictable and 'dramatic' behaviour patterns.

The essential feature of the *antisocial personality disorder* is a long history of behaviour which shows a disregard for social obligations, a lack of feeling for others, and is sometimes violent and frequently unlawful. It is often evident in childhood and persists into adult life. The behaviour is not due to mental retardation or other psychiatric illness. In childhood, lying, stealing, fighting, cruelty, truancy and resisting authority are typically present. Characteristically, people with antisocial personality disorders project blame on to others for their actions. However, there is often subjective personal distress, with evidence of anxiety and depression.

In adolescence, aggressive sexual behaviour and substance abuse are frequently found. In adulthood there is difficulty in maintaining employment, in functioning responsibly as a parent or in accepting social rules. The behaviour is not readily modified by experience, including punishment but the more flagrant aspects tend to diminish after middle age.

Substance abuse is a frequent complication. Attention deficit disorders in childhood often predate the antisocial behaviour. However, modelling on antisocial parents or the experience of harsh rejecting, punitive parental attitudes are significant contributing factors.

Other factors include the experience of separation from, and losses of, parents. The disorder is more common in males than in females and occurs in about 3 per cent of men and nearly 1 per cent of women in the general population.

A central feature of antisocial personality disorder is a failure in the capacities for guilt, loyalty and empathy. This feature is excluded from DSM-III, not because of its lack of validity, but because it requires a judgment which may vary from clinician to clinician. Schneider described people with this disorder as 'affectionless' or 'feelingless', that is, people who are indifferent to the needs and sensibilities of others. Different authorities have noted the superficial charm of some antisocial people. Some have noted features of unreliability, untruthfulness and the poorly integrated nature of their sexual lives. They may come to the attention of the law because of stealing and driving offences, social security fraud and shoplifting. Their crimes are often characterised by a disregard for consequences and a callousness about the victims.

Treatment for antisocial people is commonly unsuccessful. It is frequently dependent on social, institutional, financial and sometimes, legal constraints and by the availability of resources. It is also dependent on patient's motivation. Antisocial people rarely volunteer for treatment. The disorder is not responsive, in the long term, to medication. Long term intensive psychotherapy is sometimes advocated as a primary treatment, although supportive psychotherapy is more appropriate and can be useful for symptom relief and the prevention of breakdown under stress. Hospitalisation is inappropriate unless a special multi-disciplinary and comprehensive program, preferably court enforced, is available. Such programs are not routinely found in Australia. They are expensive, time consuming, require great consistency, firm limit setting, experienced staff and predictable responses to infractions of rules. It is sometimes possible to introduce such programs within prisons, but the long term benefit is unclear.

Antisocial behaviour secondary to other psychiatric disorders will respond to the treatments indicated for the primary diagnosis. Carbamazepine may be useful for certain forms of recurrent, possibly seizure-related assaultiveness. Hormone treatment can decrease sexual aggression in appropriately informed and motivated patients who have unacceptable sexual behaviour. Lithium carbonate may reduce the tendency for some people to fight while in a prison setting.

The person with a *histrionic personality disorder* has overly dramatic and intensely expressed behaviours in the context of shallow, demanding interpersonal relationships. Such people are quick to form relationships, but they are egocentric, inconsiderate and insensitive. They seek constant personal reassurance because of chronic feelings of insecurity and can make suicidal threats to attract attention and meet their needs for dependency. Typically, they are interesting, even alluring people who often exhibit a range of sexually enticing behaviours, are prone to mood disturbances and complain of poor health. The disorder is probably more frequent in females than males and shows a familial pattern. It may overlap with borderline personality disorder, antisocial personality disorder and somatisation disorder.

People with histrionic personalities may come to the attention of the law through some aspect of attention seeking behaviour, such as shoplifting. They may periodically use drugs and alcohol and become dependent on these substances. They may respond to short or long term psychotherapy. Depressive symptoms may occur from time to time, and require tricyclic antidepressant medication.

The central feature of the *borderline personality disorder* is significant instability in a number of areas of personality function including interpersonal behaviour, perception and mood. It is often associated with impulsive and unpredictable behaviour, which is potentially self damaging. Originally, conceived as lying on the borderline between neurotic and psychotic disorders, the concept of the borderline personality later was expanded to include various forms of personality disorder thought to be related to schizophrenia. However, people with borderline personality disorders rarely go on to develop schizophrenia. Transient depressions, intense angers, loss of temper, impulsiveness and unpredictability are common. There may be an excessive interest in gambling, promiscuity or shoplifting. There may be crises of sexual identity, episodic drug and alcohol abuse and drug overdose or self mutilation. There is usually an extensive psychiatric history, a variety of diagnoses and little evidence of therapeutic success. On the positive side, there may be lengthy periods of responsible behaviour between episodes.

There may be a genetic relationship between borderline personality disorders and affective disorders. Treatment response to monoamine oxidase inhibitor drugs also suggests a common biologic factor.

Supportive psychotherapy, coupled with firm setting of limits on behaviour, is an effective treatment. Others advocate a more intensive, explorative psychotherapeutic approach, confronting and clarifying pathological defences, perhaps in an in-patient setting geared for longer term care. Group therapy may be a useful adjunct.

The final disorder in the Cluster B 'dramatic' group is the *narcissistic personality disorder*. Such people have a sense of self importance, need admiration and constant attention and are exhibitionistic. The meaning of the term 'narcissism' remains controversial. The category is not based on any empirical work and the validity of the criteria remains unknown. For the present, the diagnostic criteria include strong reactions to criticism, exploitation of others to achieve their own needs, a belief that their problems are unique, a sense of entitlement and a lack of empathy for others. However, they are frequently depressed, their self-esteem is fragile and relationships with others are impaired.

Cluster C personality disorders

This cluster includes the avoidant, dependent, obsessive compulsive and passive agressive personality disorders which are characterised by anxious or fearful relations with others.

The person with an *avoidant personality disorder* is timid and shy, easily hurt by criticism, lacks friends, is reticent in social situations, and is easily embarrassed or anxious in front of others.

As a consequence, they are frequently

depressed, develop social phobias, exaggerate the risks or dangers of commonplace social events and are distressed by their lack of ability to relate comfortably with others.

The person with a *dependent personality disorder* is submissive, has difficulty in making simple decisions, is easily hurt, relies over-much on others and lacks self confidence. These features interfere with social and occupational functioning. Depression is again a common complication.

Those with a *compulsive personality disorder* have a restricted ability to express warm and tender emotions. Perfectionism interferes with their ability to complete tasks and they are preoccupied with details, rules, schedules and lists, and excessively devoted to work to the detriment of personal pleasure. At the same time, they remain indecisive and avoid or prolong decision making, yet insist that others submit to their way of doing things.

The disorder is relatively common and more frequently seen in males. It has a tendency to run in families. In ICD-9, the disorder is called anancastic personality disorder and excessive conscientiousness, perfectionism and a need for repeated rechecking are features which are emphasised in this category.

The person with a compulsive personality seldom seeks treatment. Occasionally, episodes of acting out behaviour may be associated with criminal behaviour. More frequently, such people are seen in divorce courts because of the effects of their rigidity and intolerance on their partners. Medication is not indicated but psychotherapy, where accepted, is often useful.

The person with a *passive aggressive personality disorder* indirectly and passively resists social and occupational demands by procrastinating or becoming sulky, irritable or disruptive if asked to do something, by working deliberately slowly or poorly on a task, by apparently 'forgetting' obligations or obstructing and criticising in other ways. They lack self confidence, are basically dependent and frequently become depressed or substance abusers.

Explosive personality disorder remains in the ICD-9 classification but is categorised in DSM-III-R under disorders of impulse control. Such people are characterised by sudden, unexpected, violent outbursts under minimal provocation.

Two further categories or personality disorder have been recently proposed, to facilitate further systematic clinical study and research. These have tentatively been named sadistic personality disorder and self-defeating personality disorder.

The central characteristic of the *sadistic personality disorder* is a pervasive pattern of cruel and aggressive behaviour, beginning by early adulthood and directed at more than one person. Such people are physically cruel, humiliate and demean people publicly, inflict harsh discipline or take pleasure from the suffering of others and are fascinated with violence, weapons, injury and torture.

Although not to be confused with sexual sadism, the characteristics of this disorder are recognisable in many people in prisons or before the court, including family courts. Currently, many such persons also fulfil the requirements for antisocial personality disorder. Treatment efforts have so far provided disappointing.

The *self-defeating personality disorder* embraces the concept of the masochism. The concept relates to a pervasive pattern of self-defeating behaviour beginning in early adulthood and not restricted to periods of depression or as a response to physical, sexual or psychological abuse. The diagnosis requires the repeated occurrence in a variety of social contexts of a number of the following: a deliberate choice of persons, or situations, that leads to disappointment when better options are clearly available; behaviour deliberately leading to criticism by others; refusal to take advantage of opportunities for pleasure or to respond to people who care; failure to complete tasks within abilities, excessive unsolicited self sacrifice or rejection of attempts to be helped by others.

Such patients often arouse anger in those who try to help them. They fail to keep appointments, do not seek legal assistance and seemingly welcome punishment, which generally only reinforces their feelings of worthlessness.

Exclusion of depressive illness and abuse by others is important and a careful history may throw some light on the genesis of such behaviour. Psychotherapy is the treatment of choice, recognising that the patient will be adept at refusing or negating help.

Treatment issues

There is frequently a distinction made between personality disorders that can be treated and those that cannot. Poorly motivated, often hostile individuals who frequently have difficulty recognising that their personality is contributing to their social adaptation, do not attract enthusiasm from clinicians. Where their treatments are also of apparently low benefit and are seldom specific, then such pessimistic therapeutic views may be reinforced. It is all too easy for such people to be relegated to categories outside the province of treatment.

Nevertheless, considerable time is spent by clinicians endeavouring to treat people with personality disorders. Moreover, the treatment favoured by psychiatrists is insight oriented psychotherapy and this requires a substantial number of treatment hours. It is easy to criticise psychiatrists for their seemingly futile work in this area. However, clinical practice suggests that psychotherapeutic treatment approaches frequently provide positive support for many individuals and enables them to maintain stability and meet work and family commitments and frequent crises and breakdowns. These benefits are not readily quantifiable in research analyses.

As indicated previously, various modalities of treatment have been suggested for a number of personality disorders. The existing categories of disorders are still tentative and evolving, and several cannot be said to be well established. Treatment must also reflect the clinical heterogeneity of the disorders and the breadth of the range of the clinical problems that are presented in individual cases.

Overall, the principal general treatment modalities include insight psychotherapies, supportive psychotherapies, behavioural therapies, family and couple therapies, group therapies, somatic therapies and residential treatments.

Several major developments in the last 20 years have created a new interest in treatment. The first has been the enthusiasm for psychosical initiatives, such as residential placements in therapeutic communities for adolescents with poor impulse control or with antisocial personality disorders. Secondly, there has been a fresh focus on long term explorative psychotherapy, both at outpatient and inpatient level, for these young people.

Impetus for treatment has also come from biological studies, leading to a revival of interest in biological treatments. Pharmacotherapies are now being explored more systematically in order to alleviate specific symptoms or to reduce general arousal.

A major development has been in the classification system of DSM-III in 1980 and DSM-III-R in 1987. Despite the continuing overlaps and the arbitrariness of such classification, it has enabled more controlled, systematic and standardised research which can be focused on therapeutic issues.

Conclusion

It will be clear from the descriptions above that many people with personality disorders, whatever mask they show to the world, can suffer considerably. Moreover, their interpersonal and social difficulties affect the health and well-being of others. They usually fail to achieve expected employment goals and have defective interpersonal relationships. They are over represented in the criminal justice system, frequently become depressed and sometimes exhibit transient psychotic behaviours.

They are also under-diagnosed and under-treated. Studies in the United Kingdom show that general medical practitioners and psychiatrists underestimate the prevalence of people with personality disorders in their practices.

This chapter indicates that there is a renewed clinical and research interest in these disorders and that there are broad treatment strategies under evaluation. The health professionals should be able to apply balanced management approaches and become less frustrated and angry with people who frequently behave in self destructive and negative ways. The possibility of accompanying depression is always worth considering. Evaluation of possible brain damage may assist in focusing treatment. Supportive psychotherapy is usually helpful and referral to a psychiatrist may help clarify diagnostic issues and focus on treatment plans.

Further Reading

Andrews G and Hadzi-Pavlovic D, 'The Work of Australian Psychiatrists', *Australian & New Zealand Journal of Psychiatry*, Vol 22, 1988, pp 153–65.

Cameron N, *Personality Development and Psychopathology*, Houghton Miffin and Co, Boston, 1963.

Casey P R and Tyrer P, 'Personality Disorder and Psychiatric Illness in General Practice', *British Journal of Psychiatry*, Vol 156, 1990, pp 261–5.

Chodoff P and Lyons H, 'Hysteria, the Hysterical Personality and Hysterical Conversion', *American Journal of Psychiatry*, Vol 114, 1958, pp 737–60.

Drake R E and Vaillent G E, 'A Validity Study of Axis II of DSM-III', *American Journal of Psychiatry*, Vol 142, May 1985, p 5.

Frosch J, *Current Perspectives on Personality Disorders*, American Psychiatric Press Inc, Washington DC, 1983.

Gayford J J and Jungawalla H N K, 'Personality Disorder According to the ICD-9 and DSM-III and Their Value in Court Reporting', *Medical Science Law*, Vol 26, 1986, p 2.

Klein D F, 'Psychopharmacological Treatment and Delineation of Borderline Disorders' in *Borderline Personality Disorders: The Concept, The Syndrome, The Patient*, (ed Hartocollis), International Universities Press, 1977.

Lilienfield S O, et al, 'The Relationship of Histrionic Personality Disorder to Antisocial Personality and Somatisation Disorders', *American Journal of Psychiatry*, Vol 143, June 1985, p 6.

Russell D D, 'How Useful a Diagnosis is Borderline Personality Disorder', *British Medical Journal*, Vol 294, 1987, pp 265–6.

Schneider K, *Psychopathic Personalities*, 9th edn, Vienna, 1950, translated by M W Hamilton Cassell, London, 1958.

Widiger T A and France A, 'Axis II Personality Disorders: Diagnostic and Treatment Issues', *Hospital and Community Psychiatry*, Vol 36, June 1985, p 6.

Part 4

Assessment and Classification

Chapter 15

Interviewing 1: Children

G L Carter

The psychiatric interview with a child has some similarities to and some differences from the psychiatric interview with an adult patient.

As with adults, the interviewer needs to elicit and record pertinent data which will allow a diagnostic formulation and management strategies to be developed, and to understand the child in a developmental, family, educational and social context. The patient and family need to have the opportunity to explain the nature of the problem and its origins in their own terms, and to indicate the type of assistance they may require or expect. The initial psychiatric interview, or series of interviews, has to resolve an important initial conflict. This is the need for information (for the clinician) versus the need to allow the child (and the family) to convey their sense of meaning about the problem and its possible solutions. This conflict is common to most initial psychiatric interviews and perhaps the most obvious aspect of its resolution is in the developing therapeutic alliance between the clinician and the child.

The main difference between interviewing adults and interviewing children concerns the referral process itself. Children only rarely request treatment for themselves. They are usually referred either by one or both of their parents, or at the suggestion of their teacher or a doctor. Secondly, the child is developing at a rapid rate, in the context of a family environment. This is again different to the usual adult patient where development is occurring much more slowly and in a number of different contexts, of which the family of origin may not be the one most immediately

relevant. This difference has implications for the interviewer in regard to the relevance of the information required, as well as the process by which it might best be obtained.

One of the most important features is the rapid rate of development of the child and the considerable variations in cognitive, social and emotional levels which are encountered in the normal child. In the cognitive area, this is most easily seen in the level of verbal communication. Simply put, the younger the child, the less he is capable of using language effectively. However, a child's understanding of the important aspects of his environment may be expressed more in non-verbal ways than that of the adult patient. The child's ability in conceptual and abstract thinking develops and this increasing complexity with age needs to be taken into account in the interview process. The most obvious practical implications for this is that children often communicate their thoughts and feelings in a symbolic, non-verbal way in behaviour and play. Likewise, children differ greatly in their levels of socialisation. Children under five years of age will rarely stay in a room with an interviewer who is a stranger unless a parent is present with them.

Background information

The process of the psychiatric interview with the child commences with the initial contact by the referral agent, and concludes with the report of the interviewer's findings.

It is necessary to obtain information from the referring agent about the nature of the problem, its duration, and the circumstances or context in which it had its onset or most frequently occurs. It should also be established if there are any associated features. Relevant background information about the child's family structure and changes in the family are also essential. Information about obvious precipitants of the current problems, particularly where it is an acute one, should also be sought. It is also important to obtain some information about the level of the child's academic function, behaviour at school and home, and peer relationships. A report from the teacher is often extremely useful, and parents should be asked to bring report cards to the interview.

An understanding also needs to be sought as to why the referral is being made at this particular time (particularly where the problem is a more longstanding one), as well as the expectation by the referring agent of the form of assistance they may be seeking or would be prepared to accept. Most simply put, this should include whether an opinion alone is required, or whether the opinion is sought in conjunction with recommendations about management.

It is also useful to determine the urgency of the assessment. Very urgent cases include those where there is a risk of self harm, harm to others, or a need to protect the child from others.

The interview

The child can be seen individually or in the presence of family members. It is not uncommon for an initial assessment to consist of a number of interviews with child and parents. In general, it is better to see the child first, as this provides the opportunity to obtain the child's story and allows him to speak about his distress. Obviously, young children will need to have a parent with them. Adolescents usually resent not being seen first.

Flexibility needs to be maintained in the assessment process. For example, the child may experience intense anxiety in inter-personal relationships, particularly with adults, and it may be necessary to shorten the sessions with the child accordingly. Families may have to travel long distances to attend appointments, or may have to make complicated arrangements with their employers in order to obtain time off. In such circumstances, it may be important to extend the duration of the initial family interviews.

When there are immediate concerns about the child's safety or the safety of others, it will be essential to establish the nature of the risk at the first interview, as well as to arrange appropriate management strategies designed to secure the safety of the individual(s) involved.

If there is no immediate urgency, it is possible to have several days or a week between each of the initial appointments. This may allow time for the interviewer, the child, and family to reflect on the material of the first interview, and to begin to assimilate and integrate the information. This also enhances the belief that the problems experienced by the child and family are important and need to be considered in depth before making decisions about intervention.

A number of different physical settings are possible for the psychiatric interview of a child. Purpose-built interview rooms for children are often playrooms. The playroom setting is usually equipped with children's needs in mind. These include the physical dimensions of the room, height of door handles, tables and chairs appropriately sized, and so on. An ordinary office may be adapted by adding toys and other items of equipment. A hospital bed or wardroom may also be used as a setting for interviewing children. Ensuring privacy under these conditions is difficult, but efforts should be made to do so within the physical limitations of the setting. In all cases, the general considerations of privacy, space, and reasonable protection from interruptions are crucial. Play materials may be employed as adjuncts to interviewing children. Careful consideration should be given to the provision of these, as well as appropriate furniture for children. This is an important acknowledge-ment to the child that the interviewer is prepared to understand the child's perspective and to communicate at a non-verbal level. In the family setting, it also helps to offer an important model of behaviour for adults in communicating with children and in understanding a child's point of view.

Toys which have clearly set rules of their

own (for example, board games), or sophisticated toys with 'a life of their own' (computer and video games) are not usually suitable for these occasions. Cheap, simple play materials, such as plain drawing paper, crayons, coloured pencils or felt pens, a doll family and doll house, modelling clay, scissors and glue are better. Small human doll figures are essential.

Interviewing the child

It is rarely useful or appropriate to interview children of five years or younger individually. Children aged six to eleven years may benefit from an individual assessment and may be able to utilise this contact quite effectively. The decision regarding an individual assessment for children in this age group may be determined by several factors. These include the child's ability to separate from parents and meet with a relatively unknown adult, and the ability of the child to communicate their thoughts and feelings.

Techniques utilising a verbal, as well as non-verbal, approach may be required. Generally, an adolescent can participate in an entirely verbal interview process, whereas younger children may well be more comfortable with drawing and play tasks where the bulk of the verbal interaction is carried on by the interviewer.

Some indications should be given to the child about the level of confidentiality that might reasonably be expected. The issue of confidentiality is often a complex one in regard to the child. It is rarely the case that the absolute rules of confidentiality applied to adult patients will be exercised with the child patient. It may be useful to explain to the child that although it will be important for his parents to understand some of the main themes and ideas arising from the individual assessment, the detail of what he says will be kept confidential. The interview can then proceed to more direct questions concerning the presenting problems of the child.

For the child who finds this process quite difficult or anxiety provoking, it may be useful to explain that he is not being punished, nor is the child in trouble in any way with the interviewer. Children suffering from emotional or behaviour disorders often feel that authority figures only see them because they are 'in trouble' and in imminent danger of being punished. It may also be useful to explain that many children have worries or thoughts that they may find difficult to express to other people. The interviewer should attempt to communicate that this experience for children is not unusual, and also convey the impression that such difficulties can be overcome. Sometimes it is helpful to communicate by speculating in an empathic way about the current feeling state of the child. For example: 'I guess you may be feeling rather angry or upset today and that may make it hard for you to think of something to say'.

For younger children, where verbal interaction is less meaningful, it may be useful to allow free play with the toys or materials previously described.

Spontaneous play with the younger child may be encouraged at some point in the individual interview. Family figures, farm animals, toy soldiers, and other simple play materials may be used to elicit children's anxieties, fears, and fantasies. The use of spontaneous play and simple play materials may also be quite effective with the older child who still finds the experience of verbal interaction with a strange adult too difficult.

Interviewing the family

Interviewing the family is usual in many branches of medicine and psychiatry. There are a variety of different approaches to this, but some of the common features of each are as follows.

An introduction of family members to the interviewer is an obvious first step. This should allow direct enquiry by the interviewer of the names, ages, and occupational or school placement of each of the family members. Interviewers should also take the opportunity to introduce themselves by name. The family should then be invited to explain their view of the problem and to express the expectations they may have for assessment and treatment. The family's need to describe the problem and its context in their own terms needs to be balanced against the interviewer's need for specific information. During the first interview, the initial part of the session should be used by the family to tell their story. The later part of the interview may be more usefully spent pursuing the specific informational needs of the interviewer which have not been satisfied. There is usually a considerable degree of overlap between these two processes. The interviewer's task during this initial interview is to begin to lay down the basis for a therapeutic alliance with the whole family, and to avoid forming an exclusive alliance with any individual or subgroup of the family (for example, parents, siblings, or parent–child alliances that exclude other family members).

It is important for the interviewers to allow and, at times, draw attention to children's communication of their perspective on the family or the presenting problem, as well as spending time listening to the adults.

While attending to the content of the interview, the interviewer also needs to assess the nature of the relationships between family members and particularly how the child reacts to his parents, whether, for instance, their interactions are anxious, fearful or warm and attentive.

The interviewer may also attempt to establish whether there are concerns about other members of the family besides those of the referred child. These may be raised spontaneously by the family or may occur as the result of the interviewer's direct enquiry.

The interviewer must obtain certain basic information from parents, including the nature of the problem, its duration, and the setting or context in which it occurs. The presence of other problems or associated features should also be sought. The family's views on the 'causes' of these problems should be explored.

Such apparently causal factors may be more correctly regarded as precipitating factors which 'trigger' the problem, or perpetuating factors which tend to maintain it but do not necessarily initiate it. Other seemingly casual factors may have merely a predisposing influence. That is, they may simply act to make the child or family more vulnerable to the emergence of the problem they are describing.

Where the interviewer forms hypotheses about any of these three types of casual factors, they may be tested by stating them to the family at an appropriate moment.

Information about the child's past medical and psychiatric health, and the family's history of psychiatric and medical health should also be obtained. The use of medications, alcohol, and other substances by family members should be determined. The child's developmental history including circumstances of the pregnancy, delivery, neonatal period, and developmental milestones, especially for walking, language, play, toileting skills, and school achievement, should also be obtained.

Enquiries need to be made about the child's current level of function at school, at home, and with friends.

The parents' developmental histories should be obtained. A history of the development of the marital relationship can be usefully included in this developmental history of each parent.

It is also important to obtain some information which allows the interviewer to form some assessment of the child's personality strengths and successes. This information is often more easily obtained once the family feels it has had an opportunity to describe the distress or the disabilities of individual members. On the other hand, some families may prefer to detail strengths and successes initially, before they are able to present details they feel have negative connotations.

Information should be sought about what other treatment agencies and interventions have been employed in the past, as well as those which might be currently used.

It is essential for the interviewer to perform a mental state examination. The information necessary to complete such an examination is usually obtained during the process of the interview itself. At times, it may be necessary to test particular skills in a more precise manner and, where this is the case, it might best be left until near the end of the individual session.

The mental state examination should be recorded using the following headings:

Appearance. This may include reference to clothing, grooming, gender attributes, and facial expression. Abnormalities of appearance should also be noted.

Behaviour. This may include the general level of activity, the goal directedness and persistence of behaviour, as well as detailing the content of the behaviour in terms of the materials used and the manner in which these materials were used. Description of the pattern of play and its appropriateness to the child's age is useful. The child's participation in particular activities, hobbies or sports should be noted. Similarly, any activities which are disliked, avoided or which present challenges which cannot be mastered by the child are important. Abnormalities of behaviour, such as rituals or stereotyped actions, should be recorded.

Mood and affect. Specific enquiry as to the current mood state of the child should be made. Some attempt should also be made to elicit changes in mood over time that the child can describe. The interviewer should also attempt to observe and record the child's current mood, its range and appropriateness.

Motor function. The gait, posture, level of muscular tension, and the presence of any tics, mannerisms or abnormal involuntary movements should be noted. Clumsiness and uncoordination should be specifically sought and recorded if present. Some objective assessment of gross motor and fine motors skills should also be made and recorded.

Sensorium. The level of concentration and alertness should be noted, including any fluctuation in these functions. Some attempt should be made to quantify the length of time a child can concentrate on any given task. In order to maximise the child's performance in this area it may be necessary to select a task that the child is particularly interested in, as well as to provide considerable encouragement within the interview relationship. The child's sleep pattern should be noted. Any abnormalities of sleep, including insomnia, nightmares, night terrors, and/or somnambulism (sleep-walking) should be noted (see chapter 2).

Cognitive function. The ability to understand simple auditory or visual instructions or commands is an important component of the examination. The ability to recognise and reproduce simple shapes, numbers and letters may also be assessed. Any abnormalities of perception (for example, illusions, hallucinations, depersonalisation, hyper-vigilance) should be noted.

This should also include an assessment of the child's level of general knowledge and, where possible, specific cognitive skills (for example, mathematics, reading, and writing). Conceptual capacities, including notions of causality, morality, and the passage of time may be usefully tested and recorded. Memory functions for names, places, times and dates in both the short and long-term should also be established.

Language. The child's ability to comprehend verbally presented material and to express his own thoughts and feelings verbally must be recorded. Non-verbal communication skills, including eye contact, facial cues, head nodding, head shaking, pointing, and the like, should be assessed. Abnormalities of the motor aspects of speech and, where they occur, any specific disorders of language or thoughts should be recorded.

Thoughts. The form of the child's thinking should be recorded, as well as the content of his thoughts. Any specific abnormalities of the form of thought (for example, thought blocking, circumstantiality, flight of ideas), and specific disorders of content (for example, delusions, confabulations, obsessions) should also be noted.

Self concept. This should include the ability of the child to view himself as separate from others. It may be expressed in terms of the child's relationships with others, his hopes or aspirations for the future, and the capacity to view situations from the viewpoint of other people.

Insight and judgment. To what extent does the child recognise some problems? Does the child ask for help, or comply with the adults' requests for help? Is the child able to identify his own feelings and thoughts? Can the child relate these internal experiences to his subsequent behaviour? Is the child able to identify the internal experiences of other people?

Relationship with the interviewer. The nature of the developing relationship with the interviewer should be recorded. For example, does the child ignore the presence of the interviewer altogether whilst engrossed in play activity? Alternatively, does the child attempt to gain the interviewer's ideas for activity so that he can comply with the interviewer's perceived needs?

Physical examination

Wherever physical symptoms exist or disturbance of psychological function is suggestive of physical disease, a physical examination is mandatory. For children with complaints that are seemingly non-physical in nature, a simple neurological examination, including morphological features, facial movements or asymmetries, eye movement, coordination tasks, grip strength, fine motor control, gait, posture, balance, and hearing tests should be done.

Where conditions of time, space, equipment, or privacy are not appropriate to complete a full physical examination, this should be arranged for a future time where these facilities are available.

Conclusion

Interviewing children involves skills and techniques which differ in some ways from those commonly used with adults. A clinician involved with children should be able to use non-verbal communication skills, recognise the complexities of emotional, cognitive and social development, form a therapeutic relationship with a child who does not directly request assistance, and acknowledge the complexities of confidentiality in such a setting. Assessment of children also offers the clinician an opportunity to develop his existing interview skills in the individual and family settings, where understanding the developmental and intrapsychic aspect of each individual and the interpersonal relationships between family members is central to the understanding of a 'presenting problem' in any individual member. Traditional skills of history taking, observation of phenomena, diagnostic reasoning and management planning are also relevant for children, and so the opportunity exists for these skills to be enhanced by the clinician when interviewing children and their families.

Further Reading

Axline V M, *Play Therapy*, 3rd ed, Ballantine Books, New York, 1969.

Barker P, 'Addessing Children and Their Families', in *Basic Child Psychiatry*, 5th ed, Blackwell Scientific Publications, Melbourne, 1988.

Chess S and Hassibi M, 'Assessment', in *Principles and Practice of Child Psychiatry*, 2nd ed, Plenum Press, New York, 1986.

Simmons J E, *Psychiatric Examination of Children*, 4th ed, Lea & Febiger, Philadelphia, 1987.

Chapter 16

Interviewing 2: Adults

R D Goldney

At any one time no less than ten per cent of the general population have sufficient symptoms to warrant a psychiatric diagnosis. This does not necessarily mean that all such persons require treatment, but it does indicate that all health care professionals should be aware of the prevalence of psychiatric illness in the community and possess sufficient skills to establish whether or not patients have psychological problems.

Formal psychiatric interviewing is both time consuming and personally demanding, and no clinician should feel obliged to pursue in depth psychiatric assessment if he does not have the time, temperament or training to commit to this task. However, all should be aware of a number of broad principles which apply for interviewing, no matter what the depth of enquiry individual clinicians will embark upon. The most important of these is that psychiatric interviewing is not simply a matter of uncritically listening to what patients say. Rather, it involves continuing appraisal and modifications of the patient–clinician interaction, right from the moment that the initial assessment has been scheduled.

Clinicians should approach the initial interview with a view to fulfilling the following two tasks. The first is to establish whether or not a patient has sufficient signs and symptoms of psychological illness to formulate a diagnosis. The second is to ensure that the interview itself is therapeutic and that the patient is left with a clear understanding of whether or not further assessment and/or therapy is necessary and what this may entail.

Before noting the structure of the psychi-

atric interview, it is pertinent to examine some of the issues which can influence both patient and clinician as well as pointing out a number of different techniques which can be employed.

General considerations

Although psychiatrists would like to think that there is now little stigma associated with psychiatric consultations, the reality is that many patients are still quite apprehensive when speaking about their emotional problems with any professionals, let alone a psychiatrist. Furthermore, patients have expectations and fantasies about therapists, and factors such as the age, sex and nationality of the clinician can be influential in either promoting or inhibiting rapport.

The physical setting of the interview is important. In hospitals one may have little choice but to conduct an interview either at the bedside or in a rather sparse office situation. However, at the very least it is important to have as little as possible in the way of furniture between oneself and the patient. Thus, a broad desk between patient and clinician is hardly conducive to a free expression of feelings. It is also pertinent to note that in the private practice setting ostentatious opulence in furnishings will be perceived as unduly provocative by some patients. It is probably most therapeutic to have relatively neutral furniture, the neutrality being important in the sense that it does not intrude into the therapeutic relationships. Thus, an overly spartan or opulent consulting room can provoke comment and feelings in patients, taking up valuable contact time in essentially non-productive issues.

The clinician's dress can also become an issue if it is too casual or too flamboyant and the optimum mode of dress, in common with furnishings, is that which is essentially neutral and does not intrude into the therapeutic situation.

The introduction to patients is sometimes effected by a receptionist ushering a patient into one's consulting room, but a more acceptable method of introduction is for the clinician to introduce himself in the waiting room. This implies an approachability and openness which can help break down barriers and facilitate the disclosure of emotionally laden material. A handshake can also yield valuable information, as it not only is a method of encouraging confidence, but it also can reveal the clammy palms or bitten nails of the anxious patient.

The mode of address from clinician to patient is also important. For adults the formal Mr, Mrs, or Ms is preferable to using first names, as the latter can promote infantilism and dependence and suggest inappropriate intimacy. Furthermore, it is not usual for patients to use the clinician's first name and by retaining a formality, a sense of professionalism and neutrality is preserved and the focus of attention remains on the problem which the patient is about to present.

The use of notes is often queried, as some would argue that it may impair the flow of information from patients. Whilst this is possible, a lack of notes may imply to some patients that what they are saying is not of importance. Patients accept the fact that professional persons cannot remember everything that is said unless it is written down, and a balance between writing notes and listening intently with full eye contact must be struck. It is fair to ask patients if they mind if notes are taken, and having gained their permission then one must ensure that this does not intrude into the ready flow of information being given. It should be noted that if permission is denied, it is a valuable piece of information, suggesting a particularly sensitive, possibly even paranoid, patient.

There are a number of techniques which facilitate the flow of information from patients. The use of silence indicates a willingness to listen, and simply nodding one's head or making comments such as 'Mmm' and 'I see' can also encourage disclosure of emotionally charged information. If these simple techniques are not effective, the reiteration of several words which patients have used can stimulate a flow of conversation. The clinician should always be willing to seek clarification by acknowledging that he may not understand exactly what has been said and that it is important to do so. In a sense the clinician throws himself at the mercy of the patient to clarify events in order that both clinician and patient can seek understanding.

The psychiatric interview is not a simple, passive receipt of information but a two-way process whereby the clinician subtly influences the flow of information. One may have to intrude directly into a patient's flow of conversation at times, and this can be done by making comments such as 'I know what you are saying is important, and we can come back to that, but I would like to change the subject if I may to that of your family/work, etc'. Very few patients resent such interventions and, just as was noted in relation to patients who reject the use of notes, those who object to such structuring are giving the therapist important insights about their mental state.

The acceptance of patients' expression of emotion is also a powerful tool in facilitating further catharsis. Patients may be embarrassed when shedding tears, and the inexperienced clinician may also be embarrassed, hastening to reassure the patient they should not be upset. Rather than that, an empathic statement such as 'Talking about that seems to upset you', with the proffering of tissues, is likely to be interpreted as encouraging and accepting of the emotion, with further catharsis likely to ensue.

In recording the history it is useful to insist on patients specifying dates for certain events, as by providing anchor points to their life one can check on whether or not school, work and marital history has been given forthrightly or perhaps glossed over. It is by seeking precision in dates that the clinician can seek out events in a history which might otherwise not have emerged. Thus occasionally patients may have had a brief but disastrous initial marriage or there may have been an absence from the work place because of previous illness, prolonged unemployment, or even imprisonment. It is only by careful attention to dates that such psychologically important events can sometimes be elicited.

Structure of the interview

In order that enquiry is made about all areas of a patient's functioning it is important that the clinician is able to complete a relatively structured interview. With some disturbed patients this may be difficult, if not impossible, but the very act of attempting to exert structure and failing is in itself of significance in the formulation of a patient's condition.

The presenting problem

At the beginning of the interview it is courteous to ask if the patient is comfortable and to ensure that factors such as direct sun glare or the presence of a draught do not distract the patient. It is useful to explain what you know about the referral and indicate that it is important to hear from the patient himself. If a patient has attended only to please someone else, it can be stated that they have fulfilled their commitment—to attend—and that it is up to them if they wish to take the opportunity of talking further. This indicates that the clinician is interested in what that individual has to say, not what others may have said, and few patients opt out with this approach.

After having established the patient's initial comfort it is important to ask open-ended questions such as 'How can I help you?' or 'What led up to your seeking help?' If the patient has indicated that he did not wish to attend, a question such as, 'I wonder why your wife/husband suggested you should come and seek help' usually elicits a response. The majority of patients respond to such open-ended questions, and then when general reasons for presentation have been established, more specific closed questions can be used to delineate specific symptoms of certain psychiatric disorders.

Some patients find it difficult to describe the onset of problems, and a useful technique is to ask when they last felt 100 per cent well. It is important to elicit the precise details of the onset of symptoms, and this may require a minute by minute recall of the chronological sequence of significant events leading up to the present.

When patients speak of other people it is important to be sure exactly what the relationship of the patient to that other person is or has been. Seeking clarification of such relationships will not be considered intrusive by patients. Rather, it will be an indication that the clinician wishes to obtain as clear a picture of the circumstances of their life as possible. If patients are reluctant to acknowledge symptoms and behaviour themselves, it can be useful to ask them what other people may have said about them.

Having established the reasons for referral and the history of the current problem, it is imperative that specific questions be asked about symptoms of the major psychiatric illnesses. Thus questions related to mood disturbance, sleep pattern, gastrointestinal functioning, sexual feelings, concentration and thought processes must be asked.

Family and personal history

The establishment of a family and personal history should then be undertaken. Demographic details and the patient's perception of their parents' and siblings' personality and health can give an indication of the presence of psychiatric illness within the family. Furthermore, the position of the patient within the family may be of significance, particularly for the first or last born, or those born after miscarriages, stillbirths or the deaths of siblings, when, for example, they may have been either neglected because of parental depression or, conversely, overprotected because of parental fear of further losses. Marital and work histories of parents and siblings can give an indication of the family's work ethic and ability to form interpersonal relations.

In gaining a personal history it is wise to start pre-natally and enquire whether or not conception was planned. Specific details associated with the perinatal period can give an indication of whether or not effective bonding may have occurred at that critical period of time. Enquiry about their mother's health immediately post-partum is also useful in that if there has been a puerperal illness this can indicate both that there may be an hereditary component to their illness and that their early parenting experience may have been less than optimal. Early separations through parental illness or divorce can also be associated with psychological illness in adult life and should be sought.

Academic achievement and work record should be recorded in some detail, as that gives a clear indication of not only the patient's intellect, but also their ability to form interpersonal relations with authority figures and their peers.

Details about a patient's psychosexual development can be approached in a neutral manner by asking the age of onset of puberty, and then how their sexual information was gained. Subsequent questions such as 'tell me about your special friends' then allow patients to speak of both homosexual and heterosexual relationships.

Information about a patient's marriage, including the presence of children, should be carefully noted. It is particularly useful to ask whether or not there have been other pregnancies which may have resulted in termination of pregnancy or miscarriage. Furthermore, early infant deaths are sometimes glossed over by patients and it is only by specific questioning that details of such deaths may sometimes emerge.

In the older patient it is important to determine whether or not their children have reawakened fears and fantasies that the patient may have had in their own early years. The attitudes of patients, particularly women, to the adult children leaving home should also be established. In later years retirement may be a potent cause of depression as many men and women find it difficult to give up their careers without any substitute activities.

Past medical and psychiatric history

At some stage in the interview it is necessary to ask about past medical and psychiatric history. Some illnesses are particularly feared, such as cancer and epilepsy, as well as some psychiatric conditions. The use of medication should also be elicited as there are a number of drugs which may contribute to psychiatric syndromes. Furthermore, the use of alcohol and other drugs of dependence may also be of importance in the genesis of some conditions.

Mental status examination

Mental state assessment is of crucial importance in the psychiatric interview, being analogous to the physical examination in general medicine. Whilst the experienced clinician will have already formulated a number of different components to the mental status assessment in the course of obtaining clinical and demographic data, it is useful to have a schema of assessment. The following is one such format.

Appearance. The appearance of the patient should be recorded. Apart from such details as height, weight and complexion, information about hairstyle and dress as well as distinguishing features such as the presence of spectacles, tattoos and jewellery should be noted. Flamboyant, inappropriate dress may be indicative of a personality disorder or psychotic illness, whereas an unkempt appearance could suggest a disorganised psychosis or a dementing illness. The fastidiously dressed person usually has obsessional personality traits.

Behaviour. The patient's behaviour may indicate psychiatric illness. Thus, the agitation of severe anxiety or depression may be marked and the inappropriate behaviour of moving intrusively around the room, perhaps interfering with items on one's desk, can indicate a degree of disinhibition consistent with either a brain disorder or a psychotic illness. Some patients may appear to respond to auditory hallucinations appearing from various parts of the room, and such reactions should evoke careful questioning. Facial grimacing or tics are also indicative of certain psychiatric conditions or drug reactions.

Conversation. Assessment of the patient's conversation is imperative, as if there is a disorder of the form or content of speech, this indicates thought disorder which may be of great significance in diagnosis. A normal thought form allows for a logical and sequential presentation of history. A retardation in the flow of thoughts and conversation indicates depression, and this is in contrast to the overactivity of thoughts, referred to as flight of ideas, seen in hypomania. A markedly circumstantial presentation, with frequent elaborations of detail and delay in reaching the point is suggestive of an obsessional personality. Loosening of associations of ideas, where thoughts flow from one idea to another with no logical connection is typical of schizophrenia, and the terms 'knight's move' or 'tangential thinking' are sometimes used to describe this. This can become more marked with clang associations, where words with similar sounds but unrelated meaning are juxtaposed, and thought blocking, where there is an abrupt cessation in the train of thought. In extreme cases this can lead to incoherence, verbigeration or word salad, where thought and speech is so disordered that ideas run into each other in a totally disorganised manner. This is occasionally seen in severe schizophrenia or mania, and it may be difficult to distinguish these conditions.

Disorders of thought content can vary between simple preoccupations to severe delusions. It is normal to be preoccupied with one's thoughts occasionally, but if these become pressing such thoughts are termed over valued ideas. When thoughts intrude repeatedly into consciousness, and can not be dispelled, they are termed obsessional ruminations, and these are typical of obsessive-compulsive disorders and depression. The content of depressive obsessional ruminations is frequently that of guilt about real or imagined misdemeanours in the past. Phobias are unfounded fears of specific objects or situations, and such fears persistently intrude into the patients' consciousness in a manner similar to obsessional ruminations.

Delusions are a specific disorder of thought content and are false beliefs held in the face of logical argument to the contrary and foreign to that patient's socio-cultural background. Delusions may be encapsulated to a small area of a patient's functioning, such as

in delusions of parasites or germs, or they may be quite systematised to explain all aspects of life. Sometimes a patient may suddenly feel as if everything is understandable and explained by certain events in his life, and this is referred to as the crystallisation of the paranoid pseudocommunity. There may be delusions of persecution, typical of schizophrenia; delusions of grandeur, suggestive of mania; and delusions of guilt, nihilism and poverty, often observed in severe depression. Ideas of reference are those in which patients believe that remarks or actions of others in their lives, or of radio or television personalities, have specific meaning for them.

Affect or mood. Observation of the patient's affect or mood can give an indication of the elation associated with hypomania, the depression of affective disorders, and the serene lack of concern (sometimes referred to as la belle indifference) of a conversion reaction. Other disorders include the inappropriate affect indicative of schizophrenia, where a patient's mood is not congruent with the topic of conversation, and the rapid fluctuation or lability of mood of organic brain disorders.

Perception. Hallucinations are sensory experiences made in the absence of external stimuli. When these occur in a clear consciousness with no memory disturbance they are very suggestive of psychotic illnesses, particularly schizophrenia. Auditory hallucinations, with voices arguing or commenting on one's actions are the most common, but hallucinations may occur in any of the senses, including vision, hearing, taste, smell and touch.

The term pseudohallucination is used when the patient retains insight into the unreality of the perception, and these are sometimes experienced in bereavement, with the transient belief that the dead person is still present, or in patients with markedly histrionic personalities who describe events in a particularly vivid manner.

Illusions are errors of perception, such as the misinterpretation of shadows as threatening figures, or of simple spots on walls as insects. Illusions are common in brain syndromes such as *delirium tremens.*

Cognitive function. The assessment of cognitive functioning is crucial, particularly in the establishment of a brain syndrome. Each clinician should have a formal procedure whereby memory is tested and it is wise to use parts of a standard instrument such as the Mini Mental State examination (Folstein et al, 1975). It is only by using methods of assessment which are generally utilised by one's colleagues that useful sharing of information can be achieved. At the very least, questions related to memory and orientation should be recorded, as well as the ability to attend to a simple arithematical task such as the serial subtraction of 3 from 20. Indeed, the latter task can be used not only as a test of attention, but also as a test of motivation and cooperation, as unless the patient has clouding of consciousness, it should be within the capability of most subjects.

Intelligence and insight. Finally, it is pertinent to make comment on the general level of intelligence of the patient and also on the degree of insight exhibited in relation to their condition. Insight can be considered in two ways. First, whether or not the patient acknowledges that he has an illness; and second, whether or not the patient has awareness of their problems and as to why their symptoms may have occurred at this point in time.

It cannot be emphasised enough that it is important to record mental state observations carefully. The presence, albeit transient, of definite examples of thought disorder or hallucinations are as significant in psychiatry as are, for example, the recording of heart murmurs in cardiology or abnormal tendon reflexes in neurology.

Additional information

It is often valuable to have corroborative information from significant other persons in the patient's life. Furthermore, information from other clinicians who have treated the patient in the past should be sought. The patient's permission must be given in order to seek such information, and in speaking with these other people it is wisest to have the patient present at the time.

Concluding the interview

Concluding the interview is not always easy. Even though the interview will generally last 45 to 50 minutes, important information may still not have emerged. Indeed, some patients find it difficult to reveal significant information until near the end of interviews, and in a sense this slow release of information can be used to control the interview. One may have to indicate that such information is important and warrants further interviews, rather than prolonging the initial assessment.

It is fair to note that prolonged interviews have little to recommend them. The clinician's attention span is finite, and it is better to schedule a second session than to be frustrated by imposing on one's subsequent time commitments. Indeed, whilst a prolonged interview can result from the degree of the issues involved, more often than not it is an indication of poor control by the clinician, albeit because of a particularly discursive historian. However, this in itself is another positive feature in diagnosis, with over-inclusive circumstantial presentation indicating an obsessional personality; voluble rapid wide ranging speech suggesting hypomania; and disjointed thought disordered discourse indicative of schizophrenia.

At the conclusion of the initial interview the clinician should have a reasonable understanding of the patient's condition and what should be done in order to pursue further assessment and/or therapy. This understanding should be conveyed to the patient both by being generally reassuring and by giving a brief conceptualisation of the main issues involved in leading to the patient's condition. This almost invariably provides a considerable sense of relief.

If further assessment or therapy is indicated, the procedures for this should be carefully explained, and the ordering of investigations requires a clear commitment to provide results. Details of treatment such as the frequency of contact, the nature of that contact and a description of the therapeutic course and side effects of medication must also be given.

Many patients are reluctant to commit themselves to treament, be it psychotherapy or medication, after the initial interview. This is not unexpected in view of the wide ranging nature of the initial psychiatric interview, and many experienced clinicians schedule a second session in order to clarify significant factors in relation to the patient's condition and its treatment in order that both they and the patient fully understand where treatment may be progressing. This is certainly better than effecting premature closure on issues which may well become more complicated than was immediately apparent.

Presentation of data

Although the prime purpose of the initial psychiatric interview is to establish a relationship with the patient in order to determine whether or not a psychiatric diagnosis is warranted, and, if so, what treatment may be offered, it is important that the information obtained can be presented to one's colleagues. The sharing of information is the essence of good clinical practice, and just as other clinical skills require practice, so does the presentation of a concise, logical psychiatric history and formulation.

In presenting data it is important to have a succinct presentation of the basic reasons for referral, the issues involved and the symptoms which have emerged. A diagnosis is then made and a formulation, which examines the patient's illness in the context of his family and personal history is then provided.

Diagnosis

The diagnosis is essentially a symptom pattern recognition exercise and has a number of components. The usual manner of presentation of diagnosis is that which has been employed by DSM–III–R.

In addition to arriving at a diagnosis, more often than not differential diagnoses or alternative hypotheses will be considered, even if only to exclude them later as a result of either physical investigations or further information gained in psychotherapy.

Formulation

The formulation summarises the different areas of the patient's life which can be

hypothesised to have contributed to the current illness. It is presented by commencing with perinatal issues and whether or not familial factors could be involved, and then childhood experiences with siblings and with others at school and later in the workplace can be referred to, as can the achievement of sexual development. Then important persons in adult life can be introduced, with an indication given of how the patient's interpersonal relationships have resulted in or interacted with their condition.

The following hypothetical example is provided in order to illustrate the presentation of the main reasons for referral, the diagnoses and the formulation in conceptualising the overall problem of a patient.

Mr A is a 35 year old man who separated from his wife three months ago and who presented with a a six week history of depressed mood and excess alcohol use. There were not other significant symptoms of depression and his mood disturbance and alcohol abuse appeared to be related to his difficulty coming to terms with his separation and his inablity to relate to others.

Mr A's Axis I diagnosis is that of an adjustment disorder with depressed mood as well as substance abuse disorder (alcohol). The Axis II diagnosis is that he demonstrated dependent and schizoid personality traits. The Axis III or organic diagnosis is that of cirrhosis of the liver. The Axis IV diagnosis is that the psychosocial stressors appeared to be severe with him having recently separated from his wife and the Axis V, level of adaptive functioning, is poor in that he is unemployed and living in social isolation in relatively impoverished circumstances.

The formulation of Mr A's problems is as follows:

Mr A was an unwanted child, conceived before marriage by a mother who was alcohol dependent. His mother was depressed following his birth, and this could have made early bonding more difficult. Furthermore, his mother had three other children in the next five years and one could postulate that he may not have received adequate parenting, as not only did his mother have four children aged five years or under, but his father was a seaman and absent for long periods of time. There were no other parent surrogates.

Mr A's school record was poor, as was his work record, with difficulties relating to authority figures. At the age of 18 he married a woman aged 28 who had three children, and he perceived her more as a mother figure than a wife. There were not further children by that marriage and he thought he may have been sterile. However, he did not seek medical advice. His sexual relations with his wife were marked by frequent impotence, although he was able to engage in extra-marital affairs.

Relations with his wife deteriorated, he said due to his heavy drinking, and he separated from her three months ago. Since then Mr A has lived in a city boarding house, although he had a brief hospital admission for haematemesis. The loss of his wife and the loss of his physical health, which is probably related to alcohol abuse, appear to have precipitated an adjustment disorder with depressed mood and underlying this is his substance abuse disorder, that of alcohol.

The above formulation not only provides the diagnoses, but also some understanding as to why Mr A has developed his psychological condition at this point in time. By providing such a formulation, data is not only conveniently conveyed to one's colleagues, but also a framework of the areas of emotional importance in the patient's life is established and the issues delineated can be pursued in psychotherapy.

Conclusion

Far from merely listening to patients, psychiatric interviewing demands close attention to many different facets of the patient/clinician interaction. It is time consuming, requires a critical use of one's own faculties, and should not be pursued by those who lack interest in this task.

The well controlled psychiatric interview allows the clinician to create order and understanding out of the patient's presenting problems. This can be conveyed to both colleagues and patient, and provides the basis for continuing therapy.

Further Reading

American Psychiatric Association, *Diagnostic and Statistical Manual of Mental Disorders* (third ed, revised), American Psychiatric Association, Washington, DC, 1987.

Folstein M F, Folstein S E and McHugh P R, ' 'Mini-Mental State': A Practical Method for Grading the Cognitive State of Patients for the Clinician', *Journal of Psychiatric Research*, Vol 12, 1975, pp 189–98.

Goldney R D and McFarlane A C, 'Assessment in Undergraduate Psychiatric Education', *Medical Education*, Vol 20, 1986, pp 117–22.

Leff J P and Isaacs A D, *Psychiatric Examination in Clinical Practice*, Blackwell Scientific Publications, Oxford, 1981.

Nurcombe B, *The Clinical Process in Psychiatry*, Cambridge University Press, Cambridge, 1986.

Chapter 17

Classification: General

G Mellsop

All species who can make decisions, classify. Almost every noun in the English language embodies the recognition of a class of objects. Psychiatric classification involves the identification of features that are common to some patients but not to all, and grouping these features into categories. In each case, with the primary diagnosis we seek to classify the disorders, not the patients.

There are several particular difficulties in the classification of psychiatric disorders. The first is that in our efforts to interpret and understand we are using that very function, the mind, which is itself being observed. Secondly, we are dealing with dysfunctions of a particular organ, the brain, the evolution of which most distinguishes man from all other species. As a result there are unlikely to be helpful animal models. In other words, we are attempting to categorise disorders of those functions which make homo sapiens sapient. Thirdly, we need to accommodate quite diverse concepts. Some people present with disorders attributed to obvious brain pathology, others with developmental delay, others with temporary dysfunctions which clearly have an obvious onset (involving a decline from a previous level of normal functioning) and still others with dysfunctions which have been an integral part of the person, most of their life. The fourth major problem is that psychiatry is a very young science and, as yet, much is unknown.

At present, the classificatory systems for mental illness and disorders most widely used utilise a strategy known as numerical taxonomy. Here, the classificatory process is on the basis of the sharing of characteristics by people who are grouped together. These characteristics can be quite culture dependent, rather than 'natural' like the classification system developed by Linnanaeus for plants.

Why classify

There are very good reasons to attempt a classification in clinical situations where people present with significant behavioural or psychological distress. People come to health professionals because they want some relief, help or change. While each person is unique, the assumption underlying a classification is that there will be some features shared in common with others. Classification enables an efficient allocation of treatment, and allows a prognosis to be given. Classifying illnesses helps clinicians to communicate with each other, with students, and with other interested persons. Furthermore, the search for rational treatments depends on classifying symptoms in order to establish common causes and predictable natural histories.

How to classify and diagnose

The uniqueness of each individual can be assessed in a number of ways. Biologically, it can be done by the process of deoxyribonucleic acid (DNA) analysis. Within the field of psychiatry it can be attempted by seeking to understand the person. The process of understanding is a very important part of the assessment procedure in psychiatric practice and is most clearly demonstrated in psychiatric formulation of a person's problems. This is based on data from their culture, family, development and life circumstances (see chapter 16). In contrast, the process of classifying disorders is based on the symptoms complained of by the person, the signs they exhibit, the time course of these symptoms and signs, the results of a physical examination and laboratory investigations and the response to treatment. Unfortunately, it has not yet proven possible to develop a reliable classification system based on known causes of mental illness.

The reliability of any classification of disorders will be influenced by variations in the criteria used and in the information available. Information depends upon what the person allows the clinician to know. Variance will depend on how clinicians use that information. The development of the present psychiatric classificatory systems has placed much emphasis on achieving reliability between clinicians and 'across time' in test-re-test situations.

Classification in practice

The World Health Organisation has considered as one of its responsibilities the provision of a comprehensive classificatory system for all diseases for all the countries of the World. These are the International Classifications of Diseases (ICD). Psychiatric illnesses have only been represented with useful glossaries in recent years. The clinical modification of the ninth edition (ICD-9) provides the basis for the official recording of psychiatric illnesses in Australia and New Zealand. It will be replaced by ICD-10 in the early 1990s.

Although the ICDs provide the basis for the official statistics in most countries, many clinicians have found recent versions of the Diagnostic and Statistical Manuals of mental disorders (DSMs) developed by the American Psychiatric Association to be more useful. In 1980 the third version of the DSM-III was published. It represented a major advance in concepts and practice, seeking greater reliability and utility. This system has undergone one further published modification, DSM-III-R (1987).

Both ICD and DSM systems operate on similar principles. They are multiaxial classifications and the idea of this is to convey a lot more useful information about a person and to ensure a more comprehensive, formal assessment. This allows more precise matching of treatments and progress with signs and symptoms.

The five axes used in DSM-III-R are as follows:

1. Axis I, the clinical syndromes. This classification of the primary illness corresponds to what doctors usually think of as the diagnosis. For example, diagnostic labels which might appear here include schizophrenia, major depression or obsessive compulsive neurosis.

2. Axis II, which includes developmental disorders and personality disorders. These generally have their onset in childhood or adolescence and persist in adulthood. Personality disorders are most clearly seen in the context of interpersonal relationships and are regarded as lifelong, maladaptive patterns of behaviour. In some cases they may represent the only applicable diagnosis, or they may provide a complementary assessment to the Axis I label. No matter what primary illness diagnosis a person has on Axis I, they may well have the personality difficulties which are described by Axis II which are relevant to their presentation and to their management. The type of personality can exert a considerable influence on a person's commitment to, or participation in, their management.

3. Axis III which deals with any concomitant physical illnesses which may be relevant to the person's presentation or management. A person with cancer and depression has a different problem from the person whose body is healthy and yet who is depressed.

4. Axis IV deals with stressors in a person's life. This axis arose out of the many years of psychiatric research into the relationship between life events and the development of psychiatric difficulties.

5. Axis V is to do with a person's social and functional adjustment to life. This axis draws attention particularly to the person's normal psychological assets and to their best level of functioning. The implication here is that a person's management may well benefit

enormously from taking into account aspects of their mental functioning rather than just concentrating on the morbid features. In addition, if a person is suffering from an illness, it is unlikely that treatment will return them to a functional level greater than their previous best.

The second major advance with DSM-III-R was the development of specific operational criteria for the diagnostic categories. These are described more fully in chapters of the DSM-III-R. In essence, the idea was to make it quite clear that specific criteria were required before diagnosing a particular illness. The aim was to reduce clinician's variance as a contributor to diagnostic unreliability. The criteria vary from the objective (for example, age) to those requiring clinical judgement (for example, restricted expression of affect).

For a particular illness, for example, criteria A, B, C, D and E may have to be met. In A, a person might have to have a described phenomenon (for example, to feel persistent anxiety for at least six months). Within B they might have to have any three of five described symptoms, without a 'sine qua non'. C and D might be temporal or demographic criteria (for example, they must be under the age of 65 and female), and E might be an exclusion criterion (for example, not suffer dementia).

The remaining two principles which affect the structure of DSM-III-R are that it is claimed to be relatively free of theoretical bias. Assignment to the diagnostic classes does not necessarily imply aetiology but means that the person simply exhibits the characteristics which allow one to apply the label to their disorder. To some extent the system remains hierarchical, in that, where severe illness (for example, dementia) is diagnosed, it is usually assumed to explain the symptoms which might otherwise meet the criteria for a more minor illness (for example, dysthymia).

While the DSMs have proven a very useful development and a boost to the cause of reliable diagnosis, they should be seen as only one step on the way to the most optimal classification system. The categories used closely parallel those in the ICD-9-CM. The diagnoses are not to be regarded as natural entities, but rather the most reliable diagnostic statements for the purposes of communication and planning treatment that we can currently conceptualise.

Summary

Human thinking relies heavily on the process of classification. In clinical psychiatry a reliable and valid classification of disorders is essential for rational decision making. The International Classifications of Disease (ICD) acknowledged the central position of the diagnostic process but the advent of DSM has provided a more comprehensive and reliable classification of patients' problems due to its multiaxial approach, and its specific operational criteria. Future developments are likely to focus on defining groups more in terms of aetiology and treatment response, and so enhance classification validity.

Further Reading

Ellis P M, Welch G, Purdie G L and Mellsopp G W, 'Australasian Field Trials of the Draft ICD-10, *Australian & New Zealand Journal of Psychiatry*, Vol 24, No 3, 1990, pp 313-22.

Fernando T L U, Mellsop G W, Nelson K, Peach K and Wilson J, 'The Reliability of Axis V of DSM-III', *American Journal of Psychiatry*, Vol 143, 1986, pp 752-5.

Jablenskey A, 'Methodological Issues in Psychiatric Classification', in *Psychiatric Classification in an International Perspective*, (ed Sartorius N, Jablenskey A, Cooper J E and Burke J D), *British Journal of Psychiatry*, Vol 152, 1988, Suppl 1, pp 15-20.

Mellsop G W, 'Developments in Diagnosis in Psychiatry', *New Zealand Medical Journal*, Vol 96, 1983, pp 1010-13.

Mellsop G W, Varghese F T, Joshua S and Hicks A, 'The Reliability of Axis II of DSM-III', *American Journal of Psychiatry*, Vol 139, 1982, pp 1360-1.

Sartorius N, 'International Perspectives of Psychiatric Classification', in *Psychiatric Classification in an International Perspective*, (ed Sartorius N, Jablenskey A, Cooper J E and Burke J D), *British Journal of Psychiatry*, Vol 152, 1988, Suppl 1, pp 15-20.

Chapter 18

Classification: Childhood and Adolescence

J M Rey

While DSM-III-R and ICD-9 conceptualise mental disorder as a behavioural or psychological syndrome, the boundaries between what is considered normal and abnormal are not sharp. These boundaries are more blurred in childhood and adolescent disorders because abnormalities in this age group need to be considered against the background of ongoing development. Many behaviours that are deviant at one stage of development are normal at other stages. Moreover, abnormalities are usually responsible for a failure to achieve appropriate developmental goals rather than producing intrinsically pathological phenomena such as hallucinations or delusions. As a consequence, the differences between what is normal and abnormal are more vague than is usually the case with adult psychiatric disorders.

Take, for example, this case: When *Judy* began attending school at the age of five years it meant a quite dramatic change for her family, particularly for her mother who relied on Judy a good deal for companionship—she was the youngest child and the only one remaining at home. The parents expected some difficulties because Judy did not usually react well to separation from her mother and was a shy and wilful girl who threw tantrums when she could not have her way. Reality, however, surpassed their worst fears. Apart from reluctance to go to school and a good deal of crying *Judy* refused to speak. Initially parents and teachers dismissed this behaviour as a 'reaction' to her beginning school. However, concerns mounted when after a few

weeks *Judy* still remained silent at school.

Does *Judy* have a psychiatric disorder or can her problems be considered a normal (but extreme) reaction to her beginning school? Does she have a language or intelligence problem? Is she emotionally disturbed or autistic? Does she lack social skills? Is she abused or deprived? What can be done to help her? What is her prognosis? These are some of the questions that may be asked when such a problem arises. Experience of similar cases may help to explain whether *Judy*'s reaction is normal, what type of interventions may help, and what is likely to be the prognosis.

Some developmental clinicians find it difficult to use traditional classifications because their focus is on the child as a carrier of family pathology and because they see classifications as not capturing the complex interactions usually observed in child psychiatry. There is little doubt that the multiple aspects of a child's behaviour require a variety of assessment procedures (psychometric, educational, family functioning etc) which need not converge on a single categorical construct for each child. In this context a multiaxial model of classification is likely to be the most useful.

Categorical and dimensional classifications

Some classification systems are categorical, that is, they conceptualise psychiatric disorders as distinct clinical entities, discontinuous from normal, and characterised by a series of symptoms that tend to occur together, having a known course, outcome and response to treatment. Here, there is a qualitative distinction between having and not having a disorder.

Dimensional systems, on the other hand, conceptualise disorder as the extreme of a trait or of a dimension of behaviour, and the difference between normality and abnormality is seen as quantitative, a matter of degree. For example, body weight is a continuous dimension. The extremes, the very overweight and the very thin may be pathological, but their differences from normality are only a matter of degree.

In practice, both categorical and dimensional models have advantages and shortcomings and most recent classifications, such as DSM–III–R and ICD–9, tend to make use of both.

Multivariate classifications

The main approach to classification in child psychiatry has been dimensional. The system used is called multivariate analysis. This is done by collecting (often using questionnaires) a series of symptoms or behaviours that are rated as present for a given child. Data from many children are then analysed using complex statistical techniques to ascertain groups of symptoms that tend to occur together or are linked.

Despite substantial methodological differences, most of these studies have shown the existence of two groups of symptoms. The first, called internalising or overcontrolled, is characterised by symptoms such as fearfulness, sadness, worry and physical complaints. This group comprises children with various emotional disorders. The other group, called externalising or undercontrolled, is characterised by behaviours such as aggression, overactivity, disruptiveness, defiance and untruthfulness, reflecting a conduct disturbance dimension.

These studies, however, have shortcomings, the main one being that they are completely dependent on the quality of the measures used and the populations studied. Another difficulty is that there are no clear rules on how to combine information from different sources

(parent, child, teacher) which often disagree.

An example of this approach to knowledge about childhood disorders is the Child Behaviour Checklist designed by Achenbach and Edelbrock. This questionnaire has two parts, the first one dealing with the child's participation in activities and school performance and yields ratings on three scales of social competence. The second part has 113 items (for example, 'argues a lot', 'fears going to school') which are rated as O ('not true'), 1 ('somewhat true') or 2 ('very true'). These yield ratings on a series of scales of specific behavioural dimensions. When scores in each scale are above a cut-off point, they are considered indicative of disorder. The result is a profile which shows the dimensions in which the child's behaviour is abnormal, when compared to large numbers of other children (see chapter 71).

The DSM–III–R classification of childhood and adolescent disorders

This is primarily a categorical classification. DSM–III–R includes disorders that usually appear and are first evident during infancy, childhood, or adolescence. However, it cannot be forgotten that there are other disorders which may occur during this age period such as depression, schizophrenia, adjustment disorders, sexual disorders etc which are found in the adult section of this classification.

The multiaxial classification has already been presented in the previous chapter. However, the application of DSM–III–R Axis I and II in child psychiatry is illustrated below.

Axis I disorders

Disruptive behaviour disorders are characterised by behaviour that is socially disruptive and often more distressing to other people than to the individuals themselves. This class corresponds to the externalising or undercontrolled syndromes of the multivariate classifications.

The *anxiety* disorders of childhood and adolescence have the main clinical feature of anxiety in adults and the most typical is separation anxiety. Some children, however, may suffer from obsessive compulsive or phobic disorders which are described in the adult section.

Disturbances in eating behaviour are included under the section of eating disorders. *Anorexia* and *bulimia nervosa* are the most common. *Pica* refers to a pattern of eating non-nutritive substances such as plaster, hair or cloth. *Rumination* is characterised by repeated regurgitation of food.

Disorders in which there is an incongruence between the assigned sex and the individual's perception of his or her own gender identity are classified as *gender identity* disorders. These disorders are characterised by intense distress about the assigned sex and desire to be of the other sex. By contrast, the essential feature of *identity* disorder is distress about aspects of the individual's identity such as long term goals, sexual orientation and behaviour, moral values, career choice etc.

Tic disorders are characterised by the presence of involuntary movements of the body when there is no physical cause for these. Tics can be defined as abnormal, rapid, repetitive and involuntary movements or verbalisations that are experienced as irresistible but can be suppressed to some extent and for varying lengths of time. The most typical of these is *Tourette*'s disorder which is characterised by multiple motor (eye blinking, grimacing) and one or more vocal tics (grunts, coughs, sniffs). On occasions these individuals also show coprolalia, the irresistible urge to utter obscenities. The onset of this disorder is usually before the age of 14 years and can be quite incapacitating (see chapter 67).

The elimination disorders are characterised by the voiding of urine (*enuresis*) or the passage of faeces (*encopresis*) in inappropriate situations after an age at which toilet training is expected (at least four years). *Cluttering* and *stuttering* are disorders of speech. Cluttering is characterised by pauses and bursts of speech that make speech difficult to understand; when there are frequent repetitions or prolongations of sounds and syllables it is called stuttering. *Elective mutism* is characterised by persistent refusal to talk in one or more major social situations, such as the case of *Judy* described above.

Reactive attachment disorders are charac-

terised by markedly disturbed social responses that begin before the age of five years. This takes the form of excessive familiarity with strangers or failure to respond appropriately to social situations. In some severe cases there is lack of weight gain (failure to thrive).

Axis II disorders

This axis includes disorders that persist in a relatively stable form from childhood into adult life without remissions or exacerbations. In adults, Axis II contains mainly personality disorders. In childhood and adolescence, however, the disorders that entail disturbances in the acquisition of cognitive, language, motor or social skills are classified in this axis. The main examples of those are mental retardation, pervasive developmental disorders and specific developmental disorders.

In the *pervasive developmental* disorders there is a qualitative impairment in the development of social interaction and of verbal and non-verbal communication skills. The most typical example of these disorders is *autism* (see chapter 10).

Specific developmental disorders, on the other hand, are characterised by inadequate development of specific academic, language, speech and motor skills. Some examples of these are *developmental articulation disorder* (failure to make correct articulation of speech sounds at the developmentally appropriate age), *developmental reading disorder* (see chapter 11), also called 'dyslexia', and *developmental coordination disorder* (clumsiness).

Conclusion

Classification systems in child psychiatry are still not well developed. Clinicians need to be acutely aware of the close relationships between the child and the environment, particularly the family, and the effects that family, school etc have on the child's behaviour. Furthermore, symptoms need to be seen in a developmental framework. For classification to be helpful, diagnosis should be made only after careful assessment of all these factors.

Further Reading

Achenbach T M, *Assessment and Taxonomy of Child and Adolescent Psychopathology*, Beverley Hills, CA, Sage, 1985.

Achenbach T M and Edelbrock C, *Manual for the Child Behaviour Checklist*, Burlington, VT, University of Vermont, Department of Psychiatry, 1983.

American Psychiatric Association, *Diagnostic and Statistical Manual of Mental Disorders*, 3rd ed, rev, Washington, DC, American Psychiatric Association, 1987.

Rey J M, 'DSM–III–R; Too Much Too Soon?' *Australian and New Zealand Journal of Psychiatry*, Vol 22, 1988, pp 173–82.

Chapter 19

Biological Investigations

J Kulkarni, D Copolov and N Keks

Laboratory investigations are standardised, technical procedures used to quantify or identify variables. They usually indicate or mark the presence of underlying pathophysiological processes. In this way the term laboratory 'marker' is often synonymous with laboratory 'test'.

Recent developments in medical technology coupled with the acceptance of operational criteria for classification of psychiatric diagnoses (such as DSM–III) have led to a 're-medicalisation' of psychiatry. As a result, laboratory investigations are able to assist with the confirmation of clinical impressions and ongoing management of mental illness.

History

Early attempts to link psychopathology with biological markers can be found in the writings of Plato and Hippocrates. Plato equated mind with soul and while searching for its location, recognised the need to view disease as an holistic entity with interplay between the psyche and soma. The following quote demonstrates this view: 'As it is not proper to cure the eye without the head, nor the body without the soul, neither is it proper to soothe the soul without the body.' (Plato 312 BC, quoting Socrates). Hippocrates in the fourth century BC equated brain dysfunction with mental illness and subsequent centuries saw increasing attempts to localise mental dysfunctions in the brain. By the 1800s attempts at developing quantifiable 'laboratory data' as an aid to treating the mentally

ill can be found in Gall's system of phrenology.

The discovery of serological tests for central nervous system syphilis in the early twentieth century made a great impact on the diagnosis of mental illness. During the 1940s and 1950s psychiatrists adapted procedures used by their neurological colleagues such as lumbar puncture with cerebrospinal fluid chemistry, electroencephalography and pneumoencephalography to assist in the diagnosis of mental illness. Other important tests used in psychiatry in the late 1950s–1960s include the measurement of copper and ceruloplasmin levels to detect Wilson's disease, porphyrins for porphyria, serum metal levels for heavy metal poisoning and thyroid function tests.

In recent times, the 'explosion' in technology has provided new brain-imaging tools such as positron emission tomography scans, nuclear magnetic resonance imaging and electro-encephalographic spectral topography. Advances in, for example, radioimmunoassay techniques currently allow measurement of very small hormonal and neuropeptide concentrations, thus permitting indirect examination of an important component of central brain function.

Uses for laboratory tests in psychiatry

A thorough history and detailed physical and mental state examination must precede laboratory investigations and provide valuable direction for the use of testing procedures.

The most obvious use for laboratory tests

in psychiatry is in making or confirming a diagnosis (see Table 1). Investigations can assist the clinician in determining whether psychiatric symptoms arise from primary or secondary psychiatric disorders. The latter term is used to describe physical illnesses that produce psychiatric symptoms and thus mimic primary psychiatric disorder. For example a patient suffering from what appears to be a major depressive illness may in fact have hypothyroidism causing the symptoms of depression. Also, a large number of patients with psychiatric disorders have co-existing physical diseases that need investigation and treatment.

Another important area for the use of laboratory tests is with ongoing management of the psychiatric illness. Careful monitoring to prevent the development of physical complications of the treatment of the psychiatric disorder may be assisted by laboratory tests. For example, patients receiving lithium treatment for affective disorders need ongoing monitoring of the potential complications of the drug as well as its therapeutic efficiency, which is dependent on blood levels. Patients with psychiatric disorders leading to altered food or water intake (for example, anorexia nervosa and schizophrenia) may need careful metabolic monitoring.

Table 1. Summary of the uses of laboratory tests in psychiatry

Diagnostic aids to determine:

Causal physical disease (eg patient presents with hallucinations and delusions due to neurosyphilis)

Concomitant physical disease (eg patient presents with personality disorder and also needs management of hypertension)

Contributing physical disease (eg patient presents with depression as a reaction to recent myocardial infarction)

Consecutive physical disease (eg patient presents with problems of malnutrition as a result of having anorexia nervosa)

Management aids to assist with:
- Determination of **severity** of illness
- Prediction of **outcome**
- Choice of **treatment**
- **Monitor** ongoing treatment

Types of laboratory tests in psychiatry

In general, laboratory investigations used in psychiatry can be divided into the following groups.

1. Brain imaging tests, for example: computerised tomography positron emission tomography (see chapters 20 and 21).

2. Biochemical tests, for example: enzyme assays, platelet chemistry, drug level estimations.

3. Psychophysiological tests, for example: eye-movement studies, electro-encephalography, speech sound analysis (spectography).

4. Neuroendocrine tests, for example: basal assays of hormones such as cortisol, growth hormone, prolactin, challenge tests such as the dexamethasone suppression test.

5. Genetic tests, for example: chromosomal studies, linkage studies.

6. Pharmacological challenges, for example: amytal interview, lactate infusions.

7. Microbiological tests, for example: cultures of urine, sputum, blood to identify bacterial infections, human immunodeficiency virus (HIV) testing for AIDS.

8. Haematology, cytology and anatomical pathology tests, for example: blood films, haemoglobin testing for nutritional status, histopathological examination of tumours for malignancy.

9. General radiological services, for example: plain chest x-rays for infections, neoplasms.

10. Cardiology investigations, for example: electrocardiograms to monitor heart function.

11. Other investigations, for example: gastroscopy to detect peptic ulcers.

The tests grouped under headings numbered 2 to 6 inclusive are representative of laboratory tests for psychiatric disorders that are almost exclusively research-orientated. The remainder are important tests in screening for physical disease in psychiatric patients.

Neuroendocrine tests in psychiatry

Neuroendocrine tests in psychiatry involve measurement of hormones released and regulated by the hypothalamic-pituitary-adrenal axis. The rationale underlying the neuroendocrine strategy is that limbic regions of the brain such as the amygdala, septum, hypothalamus and hippocampus are involved in controlling appetite, sleep, psychomotor activity, reward and reinforcement, memory, anger, pleasure and autonomic activity. Many psychiatric disorders are characterised by disturbance of these functions and since the limbic system regulates the neuroendocrine system, it is logical to measure changes in hormonal output during periods of psychiatric illness. This strategy thus provides an indirect view of limbic activity, and has been referred to as 'a window to the brain'.

Perhaps one of the best known neuroendocrine tests in psychiatry is the dexamethasone suppression test (DST), which was developed as a potential laboratory marker for depression. This test involves the measurement of blood cortisol levels. Cortisol is a steroid hormone secreted by the adrenal gland in response to adrenocorticotrophic hormone (ACTH) which is secreted by the anterior pituitary gland. ACTH secretion is in turn controlled by corticotrophin releasing factor (CRF) which is secreted by the hypothalamus. Feedback loops exist whereby cortisol interacts at both the pituitary and hypothalamic levels to inhibit release of ACTH and CRF. Several researchers noted increased cortisol production in patients with depressive disorders, and a proposed connection between limbic system (the hypothalamus in this case) dysfunction and depressive illness was made. Using this basis, a challenge test already used in endocrinology, the dexamethasone suppression test, was modified to test for the presence of distribution of cortisol production which was taken as a marker of severe depression. Dexamethasone is a synthetic glucocorticoid which in normal individuals exerts negative feedback at the level of the pituitary. By mimicking the effect of cortisol it suppresses the production and release of cortisol from the adrenal gland. In a study of depressed patients, 50 per cent had high blood cortisol levels after dexamethasone administration which meant that dexamethasone had failed to suppress cortisol production in these patients. This is called a 'positive DST' and implies overactivity of the hypothalamic-pituitary-adrenal axis. It was, in fact claimed that the DST was a highly specific marker of melancholia or severe drepression, however other studies of the DST in severe depression have found great variability in the results of this test.

Other neuroendocrine tests in psychiatry

In recent times many neuroendocrine tests have been described in attempts to identify markers of affective disorders and schizophrenia. Basal levels of growth hormone, prolactin, gonadotrophins, thyroid hormones and various peptides have been widely assayed. Challenge tests have also been widely used when slight or no differences are detected between normal and patient populations. In this technique, a small amount of a chemical is used to 'challenge' secretion of the hormone which is then measured over a period of time. For example, growth hormone secretion from the pituitary gland has been measured after using drugs such as amphetamines or clonidine as challenges. Although a large number of tests measuring aspects of the hypothalamic-pituitary-adrenal axis as well as thyroid and gonad function can be listed, none have current clinical applicability and are in relatively early stages of research. However, it is important to be aware of these tests as they may become valuable clinical tools in the future.

Investigation of the psychotic patient

A psychotic state is not specific to any particular diagnosis and can be associated with an underlying medical disease as well as a variety of psychiatric disorders. In order to make a diagnosis in the case of psychotic conditions such as schizophrenia, the clinician must exclude the possibility that physical factors may be causing the hallucinations or delusions by performing appropriate examinations and laboratory investigations where necessary. As with other psychiatric disorders, there are a large number of physical agents and diseases that can produce psychotic states. Some of these conditions are listed in Table 2.

Table 2. Medical disorders associated with psychosis

Toxins—Exogenous
Amphetamines
Cocaine
Hallucinogenic substances (LSD, PCP (Phencyclidine), Mescaline), Cannabis
Alcohol (halluciosis, withdrawal states including delirium tremens)
Barbiturates (intoxication, withdrawal)
Steroids
Anticholinergic drugs
Heavy metals (lead, manganese, mercury, thallium)

Infections
Viral encephalitis (Herpes, HIV)
Meningitis: viral or bacterial
Syphilis
Subacute bacterial endocarditis
Slow virus disorders (Creutzfeldt—Jakob disease)

Metabolic—Endocrine
Thyroid disorders (Hypo/hyperthyroidism)
Adrenal disease (Addison's/Cushing's disease)
Porphyria
Electrolyte imbalances/diabetic ketosis
Parathyroid disorder
Post-partum psychosis

Space-occupying lesions
Subdural haematoma
Brain abscesses

Nutritional deficiencies
Niacin: Pellagra
Thiamine: Wernicke-Korsakoff's syndrome

Vascular abnormalities
Collagen disorders
Aneurysm
Intracranial haemorrhage

Cerebral hypoxia
Secondary to decreased cardiac/respiratory output or blood loss

Miscellaneous
Seizures
Wilson's disease
Huntington's disease
Normal pressure hydrocephalus
Multiple sclerosis

Source: Adapted from Sederer L I, *Inpatient Diagnosis and Treatment of Schizophrenic Disorders*, Williams and Wilkins, Baltimore, p 45.

Case example

A 20 year old single university student was admitted as an involuntary patient to a psychiatric hospital. She was recommended for admission by her local doctor who made a provisional diagnosis of schizophrenia. The patient had a four week history of believing that a member of a rock band was in love with her and communicating with her via television programs. She also heard the musician's voice at times stating his love for her. The patient had attended university classes up to six weeks prior to hospitalisation and had a good academic record as well as a background of stable social relationships.

On admission to hospital, she was noted to have great difficulty finding her way about the ward even after repeatedly being shown around by the nursing staff. She was preoccupied by her thoughts and often smiled or laughed inappropriately to herself. She required constant attention from the nursing staff and had a tendency to wander off the ward.

There was no abnormality on physical examination or routine laboratory tests but an EEG was abnormal. Subsequent neurological investigations revealed that the patient was suffering from encephalitis caused by the Herpes Simplex virus. Following treatment with anti-viral agents she made a good recovery over the following three weeks and returned to University where she completed the semester.

Table 3 lists some of the laboratory tests which may be used in the investigation of psychiatric disorders in which causal physical factors are suspected.

Investigation of the patient with affective symptoms

As with the psychoses, depression and mania may be caused by physical factors (see Table 4) as well as being manifestations of primary disorders of mood (see chapter 28).

Case example

A 48 year old married librarian presented with a 12 month history of worsening depression.

She detailed symptoms of depression, lack of energy, loss of interest, tearfulness and insomnia. She had no taste for food and was eating less than usual, but had gained weight. She had been treated with antidepressants over the past few months by her local doctor. Her local doctor became concerned about suicidal ideas she expressed and referred her to the clinic.

On physical examination, she was noted to have a very slow pulse, slow ankle and knee reflexes and a rather deep, husky voice. As part of the laboratory investigations performed, thyroid function tests were done.

Table 3. Laboratory tests for investigating psychosis

Biochemistry
Electrolytes (sodium, potassium, chloride, calcium, magnesium) serum urea and creatinine (to detect renal dysfunction)
Liver function tests
Thyroid function tests
Blood glucose
Urine and blood drug screen
Urine analysis (microscopy and culture)

Haematological
Full blood examination (including erythrocyte, sedimentation rate and white cell count)
Iron studies/serum vitamin B_{12} and folate levels

Infectious diseases screen
Syphilis testing
HIV (AIDS) testing
Hepatitis screening
Paul Bunnell test (for glandular fever)

Radiological studies
Chest X-ray
Brain CT scan

Electrocardiogram

Electroencephalogram

Lumbar puncture with microscopy, culture and immunological studies of the cerebrospinal fluid

Serum copper/ceruloplasmin levels (to detect Wilson's disease)

Serum zinc, lead, mercury (if heavy metal poisoning suspected)

Brain imaging with MRI/cerebral angiography

Respiratory function tests

Results of these revealed that the patient had an underactive thyroid gland. She was treated with replacement thyroid hormone and the depressive symptoms as well as the physical signs of thyroid disease disappeared.

Table 4. Physical causes of affective symptoms

Endocrine disorders
Hypothyroidism
Hyperthyroidism
Hyperparathyroidism
Cushing's syndrome
Addison's disease

Anaemias
Iron deficiency
Vitamin B_{12}/folate deficiency

Infective
Post-influenza
AIDS
Infectious mononucleosis
Brucellosis

Neurological (see chapters 20 and 21)
Multiple sclerosis
Parkinson's disease
Intracranial tumours
Cerebral systemic lupus erythematosus
Syphilis
Epilepsy

Drugs
Antihypertensives
Steroids
Barbiturates
Prolonged use of amphetamines
Opiates
Cocaine (may induce manic states)

In making a diagnosis of affective disorder, it is important to determine whether the disorder is primary or secondary to underlying physical factors.

As well as performing tests to exclude physical causes of affective disorder, it is very important to perform laboratory tests to monitor potential side-effects of treatment. Lithium therapy is a particularly important example. It must be monitored very carefully with serial estimations of serum lithium levels because abnormally high levels can adversely affect the central nervous system, thyroid, heart, bone-marrow and kidneys. Before commencing lithium treatment a thorough physical examination followed by the laboratory investigations listed should be undertaken:

1. *renal function tests*
   serum electrolytes, urea, creatinine and urine osmolarity
2. *haematological*
   full blood count
3. *thyroid function tests*
4. *electrocardiogram.*

After stabilisation of the lithium dose, regular monitoring of serum lithium, as well as thyroid and renal function is vital.

Investigation of the patient with anxiety disorders

The symptoms of anxiety can be relatively non-specific and are commonly found as part of other disorders such as depression, or secondary to physical diseases. As with other psychiatric disorders there are a number of physical conditions that can mimic the symptoms of anxiety states (see chapter 27).

Case example

A 28 year old single secondary school teacher presented to a casualty department of a general hospital after experiencing episodes of palpitations, chest pain, choking, trembling and sharpness of breath associated with intense anxiety. He had three attacks of these symptoms over two weeks, and the attacks each lasted for approximately thirty minutes. These symptoms were thought to be due to heart disease but no physical cause was found. When the history of his condition was reviewed, it was clear that a significant precipitating factor was the death of his grandmother three weeks before. The patient had been raised by his grandmother after being abandoned by his own mother at an early age. He never knew his father. A diagnosis of panic disorder was made and the patient was treated successfully with a combination of medication and psychotherapy aimed at helping him resolve his grief.

This patient's case illustrates the importance of balancing careful history taking with thorough physical examination and investigations, when evaluating patients presenting with psychiatric symptoms (see Table 5).

Table 5. Possible differential diagnoses for anxiety disorders

Endocrine disorders
Hyperthyroidism
Phaeochromocytoma
Insulinoma
Pituitary/hypothalamic tumours
Carcinoid syndrome

Neurological disorders
Temporal lobe epilepsy
Meniere's disease
Transient ischaemic attacks
Brain tumours

Respiratory disorders
Acute asthma
Respiratory infections
Chronic airways disease
Respiratory tumours

Cardiovascular disorders
Myocardial infarction/ischaemia
Arrhythmias
Valvular disease

Drug abuse (withdrawal or intoxication)
Alcohol and benzodiazepine withdrawal
Opiate withdrawal
Hallucinogens (eg LSD cocaine, amphetamines and cannabis)

Gastroenterological disorders
Crohn's disease
Ulcerative colitis
Infective disorders
Tumours of gastro-intestinal tract
Irritable bowel syndrome

Laboratory tests for the investigation of drug abuse

Many psychiatric illnesses can be mimicked by various drugs, as well as precipitated by drug abuse (see chapter 43). Therefore, the investigation of most psychiatric disorders must include comprehensive drug screening.

Problems with using drug screens

The choice of body fluid and estimated time after use are often key factors in determining the success of drug detection. To maximise success, we must carefully consider, how long the drug stays in the body, whether it is broken down quickly into metabolites, and whether to examine saliva, spinal fluid (CSF), serum, urine or whole blood.

Tests in current use for the detection of drugs involve techniques such as chromatography, enzyme immunoassay, radioimmunoassay and mass spectometry. Combinations of these techniques are used to detect drugs in specifically chosen body fluids. For example, opioids (heroin, morphine) are best detected by examining blood or urine during an acute intoxication phase, but urine tests yield better results in suspected opiate withdrawal states. In the latter case, opiates may be detected in urine up to 72 hours after the last dose. Other drugs such as phencyclidine, amphetamines and cocaine can also be detected by examining blood or urine during the intoxication phase. It is currently difficult to accurately detect the presence of hallucinogens (such as LSD), although some laboratories are able to assay hallucinogen levels in blood and urine.

Conclusion

The importance of performing laboratory tests to assist in the diagnosis and ongoing management of psychiatric disorders cannot be over-emphasised. However, with escalating costs of medical care, laboratory tests should be carefully considered in the context of a thorough history and physical examination, thereby preventing the ordering of unnecessary 'routine' screens.

While it is clear that laboratory tests will play a greater role in the future practice of psychiatry, it is important to recognise the potential adverse effects of such progress. Experience in other medical specialties is that the extensive use of laboratory tests may lead to a loss of clinical skills. Thus, psychiatrists are provided with a greater opportunity to learn from the experience in other medical disciplines by ensuring that advancing technology is put to good use by carefully balancing the use of laboratory tests with clinical skills. Such a well integrated and complementary approach would provide the patient with optimal care.

Further Reading

Caroll B J, Feinberg M and Greden J F, 'A Specific Laboratory for the Diagnosis of Melancholia, Standardisation, Validation and Clinical Utility' *Archives of General Psychiatry*, Vol 38, 1981, pp 15-22.

Greden J G, 'Laboratory Tests in Psychiatry' in *Comprehensive Textbook of Psychiatry*, Vol 2, 4th edn, (ed Kaplan H I and Sadock B), Williams and Wilkins, Baltimore/London, 1985.

Korany E K, 'Morbidity and Rate of Undiagnosed Physical Illness in a Psychiatric Clinic Population', *Archives of General Psychiatry*, Vol 35, 1979, pp 414-19.

Sederer L I, *Inpatient Diagnosis and Treatment of Schizophrenic Disorders*, Williams and Wilkins, Baltimore, 1983, pp 42-63.

Verebey K, Martin D and Gold M S, 'Drug Abuse: Interpretation of Laboratory Tests', in *Diagnostic & Laboratory Testing in Psychiatry*, (ed Gold M S, Pottash A L C), New York, Plenum Press, 1985.

Chapter 20

Neurological Investigations

R Burns

The extent of any neurological investigations in patients with psychiatric symptoms depends on the degree of clinical suspicion that an organic disease might be present. Neurological investigations in psychiatric patients should not be necessary unless there are coincidental neurologic symptoms and signs. In practice, of course, it is sometimes difficult to distinguish psychiatric from neurological disease; sometimes they co-exist. Evidence for organic neurological disease is largely determined by the history and, to a lesser extent, the examination. If there are signs of a neurologic deficit, this usually reinforces the need to look further. Hence, before any investigations are requested, it is mandatory that a full medical history is obtained and that a complete physical examination is made. For a full neurological history and examination, it is essential to obtain the opinion of a neurologist.

The purpose of any investigation should be to test an hypothesis which enables a correct diagnosis to be made. This, in turn, will lead to appropriate treatment, and both patient and family can be given a more accurate prognosis.

While this chapter will deal essentially with neurological investigations, it must always be borne in mind that virtually any medical disease can masquerade as a psychiatric illness or have associated psychiatric symptoms, and hence any medical investigation might be necessary depending on the level of clinical suspicion. If the patient is confused or drowsy, or if there is no adequate explanation of the psychiatric symptoms on the basis of the psychiatric history or if the evolution and nature of the symptoms suggest there might be some organic disease present, the following tests might need to be considered:

1. A complete blood picture, for example, looking for anaemia or polycythaemia.
2. Serum electrolytes, for example, looking for hyponatraemia, hyper or hypocalcaemia, uraemia and hypoglycaemia.
3. Blood gases, for example, looking for hypoxaemia or hypercapnia.
4. Serum drug levels, for example, anticonvulsants, digoxin, theophylline.
5. Serological tests for syphilis and HIV infection.
6. Serum B–12 and folate levels.
7. Thyroid function tests.
8. Chest radiographs, for example, looking for a primary lung cancer.
9. An echocardiogram, for example, looking for evidence of an atrial thrombus or atrial myxoma.

Even this list is not exhaustive and for example, in some instances, it might be necessary to perform specific immunological tests on the serum to look for lupus erythematosis which can present with psychiatric symptoms or it might be necessary to attempt to measure certain heavy metals in blood, urine or tissue, particularly if there is an appropriate occupational history (see also chapter 19).

Specific neurological investigations

Lumbar puncture and examination of the cerebrospinal fluid (CSF)

This test is now basically used to look for evidence of central nervous system (CNS) infection or subarachnoid bleeding. It rarely provides diagnostic information in the chronic psychiatric patient. But in the setting of an acute psychiatric illness, especially when there is a history of headache, vomiting and neck stiffness which might raise the possibility of bacterial meningitis, herpes simplex or some other form of encephalitis or subarachnoid bleeding, diagnostic information may be found.

Electro-encephalography (EEG)

A resting scalp EEG getting the patient to hyperventilate and with photic stimulation, is a simple and safe test. But it provides only limited information which is rarely diagnostic. Its main use is in the differentiation and categorisation of the various epileptic disorders. It may show some moderately specific changes in some of the rarer forms of dementia (sub-acute sclerosing pan-encephalitis (SSPE) in childhood, and Creutzfeldt-Jacob disease in adult life). The EEG may show diffuse generalised abnormalities in the metabolic encepha-lopathies. It is not regarded as a reliable tool to establish focal disease of the brain. Sphenoidal EEG recordings are not used as a routine in psychiatry but they may help to establish a more precise focus when investigating the suitability of a patient with complex partial seizures for neurosurgical treatment. Video EEG monitoring is becoming increasingly used in neurology clinics. Its particular use in psychiatry is to help differentiate pseudo-seizures from true seizures.

Computerised tomographic scanning of the brain (CT scan)

This test is becoming so widely available now that in some centres it is regarded as a 'routine' investigation (see chapter 21). But most would agree that the yield is low if the test is performed in this way and the principle of ordering the test to confirm an hypothesis should apply equally for a CT head scan. It will reveal structural diseases of the brain, especially supratentorial lesions and therefore conditions which might present psychi-atrically. This includes primary and secondary brain tumours, hydrocephalus, cerebral

abscess, herpes simplex encephalitis, cerebral infarcts, haematomas, both intracerebral and subdural, and cystic lesions of the brain. A CT head scan will reveal cerebral ventricular dislocation and cortical sulcal widening—findings consistent with many atrophic processes such as Alzheimer's disease—but correlation with the clinical state is often poor. The scan can be normal in patients with Alzheimer's disease and Huntington's disease. Features consistent with 'atrophy' may in fact be a normal variant, especially in the elderly.

Magnetic resonance imaging (MRI)

The MRI scan is especially helpful in detecting diseases of white matter, namely multiple sclerosis (see chapter 21). It will show small lesions within the temporal lobes and posterior fossa such as brain stem gliomas. Very occasionally primary brain tumours will be revealed by an MRI scan which have not shown on routine CT scanning. Like many investigations, interpretation of MRI abnormalities deserves caution, as white matter lesions can be seen in the elderly which have no clinical significance. In addition, the MRI scan may reveal unsuspected asymptomatic lesions such as vascular malformations.

Other investigations

Plain radiographs of the skull are rarely necessary now, particularly when a CT scan is available.

Cerebral angiography is mainly used now to detect extracranial vascular disease and intracranial aneurysms and therefore is not likely to be required in the routine psychiatric setting.

Radioactive isotope studies are not used as a routine diagnostic interpretation now for neurologic diseases.

Positron emission tomographic (PET) scanning is used in a few specialised centres as a research tool and in the assessment of patients with epilepsy who might be suitable for surgical intervention, but not as a routine investigation (see chapter 21).

Electromyography (EMG) is helpful in the assessment of weakness and will usually enable one to differentiate between primary muscle disease and denervation atrophy. It may be helpful in excluding these diseases in patients who have weakness of psychological origin. Single fibre EMG and repetitive nerve stimulation studies will aid in the diagnosis of those patients with fatigable weakness such as myasthenia gravis and the myasthenic syndrome which can masquerade as a psychiatric disorder.

Nerve conduction studies can be of assistance in the diagnosis of localised and generalised diseases of peripheral nerves.

Evoked potentials, namely the stimulation of peripheral nerves, the visual pathways or the auditory pathways and recording their central potentials, are commonly used now. These include the visual evoked responses, the brain auditory evoked responses and somatosensory evoked responses. Delay in signal and abnormal wave forms indicate the presence of disease, particularly that of white matter, although these tests do not provide diagnostic information as such.

Further Reading

Adams R D and Victor M, *Principles of Neurology*, 4th ed, McGraw Hill Book Co, New York, 1989.

Chapter 21

Brain Imaging in Psychiatry

E Gordon and D Copolov

A number of technologies have emerged since the early 1970s that examine different aspects of the structure of function of the human brain. These technologies have two elements in common. Firstly, utilisation of the processing speed of computers to acquire the information and secondly, the synthesis of these measures into a pictorial representation or image of the brain.

To obtain an image of the brain, data is recorded simultaneously from many sites over the brain. This information is converted by computer into a synthesised image. The specific measurements which are recorded are converted into an array of numbers in a two dimensional grid (for example, of 64 [x axis] by 64 [y axis] pixels (the degree or extent of clarity of coloured image) on a computer monitor). For any of the 4096 pixels that do not correspond with an actual measurement of brain function, a value based on the surrounding numbers is mathematically determined. Each number in the array is then assigned a corresponding shade or colour— the highest measurement will be accorded the brightest colour in the scale, thereby generating a colour image of the entire brain.

Brain imaging is increasingly applied in psychiatry for both clinical evaluation and research of the underlying neural mechanisms of mental illness. The findings obtained from the potentially powerful techniques of brain exploration are still very preliminary.

Computed tomography (CT) and magnetic resonance imaging (MRI) provide detailed scans of brain *structure* that are relatively unambiguous to interpret. These scans, however, provide little information about changes in neuronal metabolism, information processing, brain chemistry or drug activity. Such phenomena can only be assessed by the examination of brain *function*.

The aim of this chapter is to explore the most contemporary and relevant developments in brain imaging. Two themes will be addressed. Firstly, we describe how these technologies work and provide a summary of the findings in psychiatric disorders thus far. Secondly, we address the limitations in the use of these technologies and look to the future directions in the exploration of brain dysfunction in psychiatry.

The modern technologies of brain imaging

In describing the technologies and findings obtained with their use, the methods are divided into those which image brain structure and those which image brain function. These various techniques are listed in Table 1.

1. Structural brain imaging

(a) *Computed tomography (CT)*

The era of brain imaging began in 1973 when Hounsfield introduced the first structural imaging technique, that of computed tomography. In this technique X-rays are passed through the brain on to an arc of detectors that swing around the head. Hundreds of thousands of X-ray measurements are registered by the detectors, from which a reconstruction of a two dimensional image of the brain's structure is undertaken. CT scanning allows the

Table 1. The spectrum of brain imaging systems employed in psychiatry

STRUCTURAL BRAIN IMAGING

Computed tomography (CT)
• Provides images of tissue density in slices of the brain

Magnetic resonance imaging (MRI)
• Reflects the distribution of naturally occurring elements in the brain

FUNCTIONAL BRAIN IMAGING

Electroencephalography (EEG)
• Recording discs on the scalp allow the measurement of the brains ongoing electrical activity

Event related potentials (ERPs) [1]
• Reflects the brains electrical processing of specific stimuli (eg a sound or word)

Magnetoencephalography (MEG)
• Reflects the magnetic fields which surround electrical signals in the brain, and accurately locates the sources of these electrical signals

Radioisotope methods

Regional cerebral blood flow (RCBF)
• The washout from the brain of a radioisotope (usually Xenon-133) reflects the cerebral perfusion (and hence gross metabolic activity) over a number of minutes
Primarily cortical activity of brain function is obtained

Single photon emission computed tomography (SPECT)
• Single photon nuclides, which are not normally metabolised in the brain are measured
A rotating gamma camera allows cortical as well as sub-cortical information of the brain function to be visualised

Positron emission tomography (PET)
• Positron emitting nuclides are used to reflect the metabolic rate of substances (such as oxygen and glucose) that are normally metabolised in the brain. Precise images of biochemical as well as drug activity, are obtained in cortical and subcortical areas of the brain

identification of the cerebral ventricles and some anatomically distinct bodies such as the basal ganglia. It can, to a certain extent, differentiate grey from white matter.

CT application is in the diagnosis of specific, gross brain pathology such as tumours and haemorrhages. Studies suggest that between 5–25 per cent of all psychiatric in-patients referred for CT scans have definite abnormalities. Focal CT abnormalities may occur as frequently as 1 in every 200 unselected psychiatric in-patients and over ten

per cent of psychiatric patients' management is influenced by CT scan findings. The most cost-effective indications for ordering a CT scan in psychiatry include cases of delirium, dementia, psychosis of unknown cause, a movement disorder of unknown aetiology and the first episode of major depression or personality change over the age of 50 years.

A number of studies have demonstrated that a sub-group (approximately 10–20 per cent) of schizophrenic patients have larger cerebral ventricles and cortical sulci than normal subjects of the same age. It is hypothesised that these ventricles and sulci enlarge to take up that space occupied by brain tissue which in schizophrenia has atrophied. Some studies report that when atrophy exists, it is especially evident in the frontal part of the cerebral hemispheres.

Similar brain abnormalities are not only found in schizophrenia but also they have been found to occur in normal ageing, in many dementias and in some patients with affective disorders. In this last group, patients with atrophy have been shown at follow-up to have an increased rate of mortality compared with patients who have no atrophy. That severe atrophy is associated with poor prognosis is actually one of the consistent CT scan findings.

(b) *Magnetic resonance imaging (MRI)*

In 1977, four years after the introduction of CT scanning, the first magnetic resonance images of the human body were reported. MRI provides a superior resolution of grey:white matter in the brain than a CT scan. MRI does not use ionising radiation. It involves aligning the brain's hydrogen nuclei in a high strength magnetic field, then deflecting the nuclear alignment with a rapidly alternating radiofrequency pulse which is applied at right angles to the magnetic field. When the radiofrequency pulse is switched off, the nuclei emit energy as they return to their previous alignment. This energy is registered by radiofrequency coils and can be used to create an image in any plane.

MRI is preferable to CT for patients in whom abnormalities in certain anatomical regions are suspected. The search for focal lesions giving rise to seizures, for

[1] See Figure 1 following p 148.

demyelination as in multiple sclerosis, or for abnormalities in the temporal lobe or posterior fossa region are best conducted with the aid of MRI.

2. Functional brain imaging

It is helpful to consider these in two main groups. The first group consists of those methods which detect inherent brain function and are able to do so in time envelopes as brief as milliseconds (thousandths of a second). Included in this category are the computerised mapping of quantative EEG, event related potentials, and magneto-encephalography.

The second group of functional imaging techniques involve the use of radioisotopes, which are inhaled or injected intravenously. In the brain the radioisotopes emit gamma rays which are detected by the surrounding gamma ray detectors—the higher the gamma ray count, the more active is the function in that region of the brain. Using radioisotope technologies brain function cannot be measured in time envelopes shorter than a few minutes. The radioisotope dependent technologies include regional cerebral blood flow, single photon emission computed tomography and positron emission tomography.

(a) The electro-encephalogram (EEG)

The EEG is a non-invasive measure of the brain's electrical activity. It is recorded using electrodes on the scalp and is a process which therefore involves little inconvenience for the patient.

The most common clinical application of the EEG in psychiatry is to determine the presence of epilepsy. Temporal lobe seizures, for example, may give rise to a variety of transient psychiatric symptoms such as hallucinations, obsessional thinking and alterations of mood. The diagnostic distinction between epilepsy and schizophrenia is of course vital for appropriate management.

In schizophrenia, the more common reported EEG brain abnormalities include more slow wave activity in the frontal parts of the brain and more faster rhythms posteriorly. The hypothesis that a specific sub-group of schizophrenia is associated with dysfunction of the left hemisphere has also found some support in EEG studies.

In depression, sleep abnormalities are considered to reflect a larger disturbance in biological rhythms. The most consistent sleep EEG finding in depression is of short rapid eye movement (REM) or dream sleep latency (the time from the onset of sleep to the onset of REM) in cases of severe major depression. A number of studies have also investigated the effect of medication on EEG sleep patterns. These studies have been undertaken in an attempt to obtain objective neuro-physiological evidence of changes in brain function due to antidepressant and lithium therapy. Such therapies result in changes in the EEG towards normality.

(b) Event related potentials (ERPs)

Unlike EEGs which reflect the electrical activity that goes on continuously in the brain, an ERP reflects the brain's transient electrical response (in milliseconds) to a discrete stimulus. However these electrical responses are small in comparison to the EEG and so the stimulus needs to be presented a number of times and the responses are averaged. Averaging the random EEG flattens it out to an approximately straight line whereas the ERP stands out in summation. The ERP is seen as a sequence of negative (N) and positive (P) voltage peaks and troughs.

The early components (less than 50 milliseconds) of ERPs are studied to evaluate the integrity of the sensory pathways (for example, the visual system). The later components of the ERP reflect stages of information processing, processes of attention and aspects of decision making, such as distinguishing novel from commonly occurring stimuli.

No consistent results from the ERP findings have illuminated the underlying dysfunction in schizophrenia. Theories of schizophrenia include disturbances in attention and abnormalities of information processing. Both may be reflected in the components of ERPs in people with schizophrenia.

ERP components at almost all stages of information processing suggest dysfunctional processing in schizophrenia. There is also some evidence that in children with a high

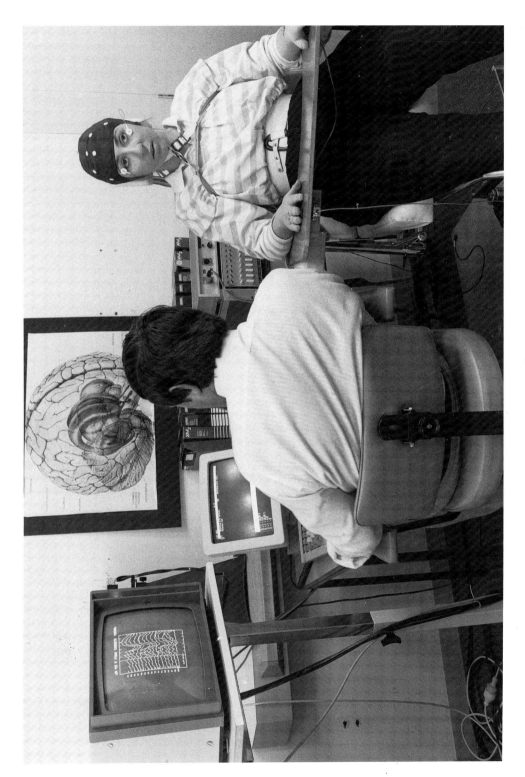

Figure 1. *ERP laboratory in the Cognitive Neuroscience Unit, Westmead Hospital.*

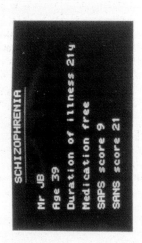

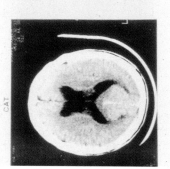

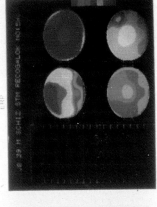

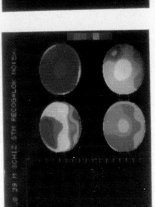

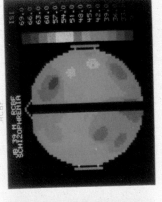

Figure 2. *Different and complementary measures from the brain are undertaken on the same subject shown in Fig 1 in order to obtain a more comprehensive assessment of the overall status of brain function than that provided by a single measure in isolation. From left to right above— CT, eye tracking, ERP (electrical brain function in thousandths of a second), RCBF (blood flow over a number of minutes) in the same schizophrenic subject, showing both central atrophy and diminished RCBF.*

genetic risk of developing schizophrenia, similar findings occur.

ERPs also have a role in the exploration of brain function in depression. A number of theories suggest that depression may be caused or maintained by specific cognitive defects. These have not been tested using biological measures. ERPs may provide a neurophysiological means to test these theories of specific cognitive dysfunction. Preliminary approaches in this regard have not found consistent ERP changes specific to depression.

(c) Magnetoencephalography (MEG)

Magnetoencephalography makes use of the principle that a magnetic field surrounds every electrical current. Magnetic fields are not distorted by biological tissues such as the scalp and are not volume conducted as are electrical signals. The magnetic fields which surround electrical currents in the brain thus emerge from the brain close to their source of origin and relatively undistorted.

The pattern of magnetic fields may be measured by a superconducting quantum interference device (SQUID) which is linked to magnetic sensor coils that are placed just above the scalp. The distribution of the magnetic fields measured outside the head is converted by computer into an image which indicates the location of their sources within the brain.

Full head (100 channels or more) systems that measure the distribution of magnetic fields emerging from the brain are likely to be available by 1992. Magnetoencephalography seems likely to provide us with the means to locate with a high degree of accuracy the generators of ERP components and EEG rhythms and may help us determine the neuronal networks within the brain of those electrophysiological abnormalities which have been found in psychiatric disorders.

(d) Regional cerebral blood flow (RCBF)

In the oldest method RCBF is indirectly measured using inert gamma emitting substances such as Xe 133. Following inhalation or intravenous injection, the gas saturates the brain and over the ensuing minutes is washed out from the various brain regions at a rate proportional to the blood flow to those regions. The disappearance of the isotope is measured by stationary gamma ray detectors and information about cortical blood flow is provided.

In schizophrenia most studies have used RCBF in chronic patients and have shown normal global flows, but a relative reduction in blood flow to the frontal regions of the brain at rest, particularly on the left, has been noted. One controlled activation study employed a task (the Wisconsin card sorting test) that provided evidence of a specific failure to activate the dorsolateral prefrontal cortex in patients with schizophrenia. Other studies have found a paradoxical increased activation of the left hemisphere compared to normals, during a spatial right hemisphere task. These studies provide tentative evidence of dysfunctional activation profiles of the frontal lobe and left hemisphere in schizophrenia. It has not yet been determined whether specific dysfunctions are associated with different sub-groups of schizophrenia.

A number of studies have assessed blood flow at rest in patients with depression. A small number of these studies show a generalised low metabolic rate in the brain in this disorder with reduced activation of the right hemisphere in some depressives compared to normals. Case studies of patients have shown elevated RCBF in the right hemisphere during the manic phase of manic-depressive disorder, with subnormal symmetrical flows after recovery.

(e) Single photon emission computed tomography (SPECT)

Single photon emission tomography provides information about both cortical and subcortical perfusion. SPECT utilises a gamma counter which rotates around the head, thereby allowing a tomographic reconstruction to take place according to principles similar to those previously discussed for CT scanning. Whereas Xe 133 used in RCBF studies has a fast washout, the isotopes used in SPECT are labelled to substances that are not normally metabolised in the brain (for example Iodine 123 labelled amphetamine). These substances are trapped in the brain in concentrations proportional to regional cerebral perfusion. This trapping of the isotopes allows the rotating gamma counter to obtain a 'freeze-frame' picture of the blood flow distribution of the brain.

SPECT studies have shown a bilateral hemisphere dysfunction in schizophrenia and hypometabolism (greater in the right than the left hemisphere) in depression.

SPECT systems will be more accessible than PET systems for the foreseeable future and much hope in psychiatry research and clinical practice is vested in the possibility that this technique may ultimately provide information regarding neurochemical abnormalities and the distribution of drug activity in psychiatric disorders.

(f) Positron emission tomography (PET)

Positron emission tomography is the most powerful of the radio-isotope functional neuroimaging systems. When emitted from their parent atoms positrons collide with electrons leading to the creation of a pair of gamma rays which are given off in opposite directions. The points of coincidental emission, detected by rings of gamma detectors, are used to construct images reflecting the distribution of the brains' activity much more accurately than SPECT.

Not only can PET measure cerebral blood flow but, unlike SPECT, it can also assess cerebral metabolism measurement via the measurement, for example, of oxygen and glucose consumption. It does so by tagging positron emitting isotopes to compounds (such as 2-deoxyglucose) which are metabolised in the brain. Additionally, PET allows the measurement of protein synthesis and can also facilitate imaging of drug binding sites in the brain.

The PET measures of brain metabolism (primarily deoxyglucose) in schizophrenia have tended to show a diminished frontal distribution of glucose metabolism in a sub-group of chronic patients. However, contradictory findings are evident particularly in acute schizophrenic patients who tend to show hypermetabolic states. An example of the manner in which PET may improve our understanding of the interrelationship between symptom relief and medication is a study that has shown that 80 per cent of dopamine receptors in the corpus striatum needed to be occupied by an antipsychotic drug before symptom relief was evident.

PET studies of glucose metabolic rate in patients with depression show diminished cortical activity in unipolar and increased activity in bipolar depressives compared to normal controls. A sub-group of patients with unipolar depression showed a lower glucose metabolism in the right compared to the left hemisphere. However, methodological limitations, unstandardised implementation of these studies and contradictory results render these findings preliminary and tentative.

With the commonly used positrons namely carbon, nitrogen, hydrogen, fluorine and oxygen, almost any biomolecule (or drug) can be labelled and information concerning their specific sites of activity in the brain may be obtained. However, PET is a very expensive technology that requires a cyclotorn (a particle accelerator) close to the laboratory since positrons have short half-lives of, at most, a few hours. These limitations restrict the use of PET to specialised centres.

Problems and future directions

Most of the effects using the brain imaging technologies we have discussed above have been to examine the correlation between measures of brain function and specific psychiatric disorders, in an attempt to uncover biological markers that might aid in diagnosis. A more challenging approach concerns the attempt to use these technologies to determine the specific mechanisms underlying brain functioning and its dysfunction in psychiatric illnesses.

Despite the encouraging preliminary findings, the assessment of higher order brain processing in psychiatric disorders is still embryonic and it is not surprising that this endeavour has failed to yield any reproducible patterns of dysfunction thus far. This could be due to at least three reasons. Firstly, specific hypotheses may be insufficiently clear in the application of imaging technologies. Secondly, methodological limitations are evident in the majority of studies. Thirdly, simplistic approaches tend to be employed in the analysis of brain function.

These limitations are currently being addressed by most neuropsychiatry units. Many studies are now incorporating more standardised diagnostic workups with consideration given to determining diagnostic sub-groups, assessing symptom profile in addition to the patients' diagnosis and controlling for the effects of medication. The diagnostic sensitivity and specificity of brain imaging technologies has not yet been systematically determined. Furthermore, in an illness such as schizophrenia, there is no reason to believe that any currently used diagnostic categorisation of a particular group of symptoms and illness course, such as DSM–III–R schizophrenia, represents a homogenous neurobiological entity which can be confirmed by consistent similarities in brain imaging. If patients are categorised into discrete, pre-chosen illness entities and tested on a series of neuroimaging variables, differences between the groups might be erroneously seen to confirm the establishment of the pre-chosen boundaries, when either a continuum or other method of categorisation may be more appropriate. Large numbers of patients with a broad range of diagnoses, including those straddling the proposed boundaries, must be studied before the diagnostic utility of these tests can be fairly and objectively assessed.

An important future direction concerns understanding the numerous methodological and statistical limitations inherent in neuroimaging studies. Clinical variables may also significantly influence the outcome of neuroimaging investigations. Variables such as specific symptom profile, medication status, chronicity, severity of illness, level of arousal and the actual performance achieved on neurocognitive tasks undertaken during brain imaging are often satisfactorily controlled. A trend towards multimodal imaging (more than one measure on the same patient) will allow us to develop a more comprehensive picture of the brain in psychiatric disorders, than that provided by a one-off measure. When such results are viewed in conjunction, patterns of regional abnormality may emerge in a way which strengthens the case for the abnormality being a true pathophysiological finding rather than a statistical artefact. Thus, data from individual studies pointing to frontal lobe hypofunction in schizophrenia may be considerably strengthened by a multimodal imaging approach. The interrelationship among the different and possibly complimentary measures of brain function may also be determined. Future directions need to involve more sophisticated mathematical analysis that reflects the complexities of brain function during specific activation tasks.

However, we must recognise that many of our explorations in neuroimaging have been undertaken during an era when our conceptual understanding of the human brain function is still extremely rudimentary. Many of the excursions have been technology-led rather than hypothesis-led and it is sometimes difficult to interpret meaningfully both normal and abnormal results.

It seems inevitable that visualising colour images of the brain will be augmented by a greater critical analysis of what these measures of brain function actually mean. Ultimately brain imaging has a more imminent potential to contribute to an understanding of patterns of brain dysfunction in major psychiatric disorders, than it has to affect substantially the diagnostic confidence of the psychiatrist dealing with these diseases 'at the coal face' of clinical practice.

Further Reading

Andreasen N C, 'Brain Imaging: Applications in Psychiatry', *Science*, Vol 239, 1988, pp 1381–8.
Pfurtscheller G and Lopes de Silva F H, *Functional Brain Imaging*, Hans Huber Publishers, 1988.

Acknowledgments

Professor R A Meares, C Rennie, C Kraiuhin, J Anderson and Y Zurynski for technical and conceptual exchange of information concerning imaging brain dysfunction.

Chapter 22

Psychological Testing

A Gannoni

Background

The major developments that shaped contemporary psychological testing date back to the nineteenth century during which time there developed a growing concern for the welfare of the mentally retarded and insane. Physicians, Itard (1799) and Sequin (1866), for example, were interested in the remediation of mentally retarded children. With the establishment of special institutions for the care of mentally handicapped people in Europe and subsequently the United States of America, there came a need to develop uniform criteria for identifying and classifying individuals to meet admission standards. At the end of the nineteenth century, Galton, an English scientist interested in human heredity, devised statistical methods to measure individual physical traits such as muscular strength, reaction time, vision and hearing. The psychologist Cattell (1890) and the psychiatrist, Kraeplin (1895), experimented with sensory tasks as a means of measuring intellectual ability, but found little relationship between these and clinical estimates of intellectual ability.

An alternative approach was provided by Binet and his colleagues with the publication, in 1905, of the Binet-Simon Scale which forms the basis of intelligence testing as known today. The scale consisted of 30 tests arranged in ascending order of difficulty and were designed to cover a wide variety of cognitive functions, with special emphasis on judgement, comprehension, and reasoning. Sensory and perceptual tests were included. Greater proportion of verbal content was included in this scale than in most tests developed at that time. The Binet scale has been revised on several occasions, the most recent being in 1986. The second major individual test of intelligence, the Wechsler-Bellevue Intelligence Scale was published, in 1939, 35 years after the original Binet Scale appeared. Versions of the scale for adults, and pre-school and school aged children have been developed. Most intelligence tests were primarily measures of verbal ability and non-verbal (performance) skills such as handling symbolic and abstract relations. It became apparent in the early 1900s that these tests measured only a sample of an individual's abilities. As a result, specialised tests to supplement the information gained from intelligence scales were subsequently developed.

Nature and use of psychological tests

The goal of psychological assessment is to provide quantitative and qualitative data, obtained in a highly structured, controlled setting, through the use of carefully designed measurement procedures appropriate to the areas to be investigated (Sparrow et al, 1989).

The value of utilising appropriate standardised measurement instruments under well defined conditions include the elements of objectivity and constancy. The subjective judgement of the examiner is thereby minimised.

In considering whether a specific measuring instrument is useful, the validity and reliability of the test must be evaluated. Validity relates to the degree to which the test actually measures what it purports to measure and reliability refers to the consistency of scores obtained. For example, test re-test reliability refers to the consistency of scores obtained by the same individual over two separate occasions, and inter-rater reliability indicates the degree to which the individual obtains the same result on the same test administered or scored by two examiners.

To establish the reliability and validity of a psychological test, the instrument is pre-tested on a large representative sample of persons for whom it is designed. Test authors strive to make this sample reflect the population of interest on variables such as age, gender, geographical location, socio-economic class and race. This group, known as the standardisation sample, provides the data to establish norms or the average performance of the various age groups. It also provides a way of evaluating the different degrees of deviation above and below the average performance, thus permitting the comparison of an individual with reference to the standardisation sample. In addition, the difficulty of each item is considered and thus selection of items for inclusion in a test can be guided by the proportion of persons in the pre-test trials who pass each item. On the basis of this information items can be ordered in terms of their level of difficulty across age groups. Standardisation procedures also extend to the administration details for examiners such as the use of test materials, specific instructions given to examinees through to the scoring criteria of individuals' responses and interpretation of results.

Considering the plethora of tests available, only some are presented here. These were selected on the basis of coverage of several age categories, areas of assessment and frequency of test usage in Australia (Sharpley and Pain, 1988). Each test has its own limitations and strengths, and no single instrument can provide a comprehensive assessment of an individual's functioning. Furthermore, interpretation of results must take into account the individual's physical attributes, cultural background, the nature or task requirements of the test, the individual's test behaviour, and the interaction between the examinee and the psychologist. Only

psychologists who are trained in life span development and assessment procedures are qualified to administer standardised psychological tests. This requirement ensures the protection of examinees against improper administration and interpretation of tests.

Intelligence tests

Developmental tests

The scales for assessing the developmental status of infants in the main, cover several areas, for example, motor, speech and language, cognitive and adaptive functioning. These tests require individual administration with the primary care-giver providing information to supplement the assessment.

It has been found that developmental tests have more limited predictive power for infants who fall within the average and superior levels than those who present with significant developmental delay. Developmentally disabled infants are more likely to obtain low intelligence levels at later developmental stages (Brooks-Gunn and Lewis, 1983). It is recommended that infants showing developmental delay be assessed again when older to monitor their development rate as some may show rapid development at later stages. Intelligence tests developed for pre-schoolers have a higher predictive value than developmental tests, as the content focuses more on cognitive functioning. The Intelligent Quotient of any given child may change as much as 20 points from early childhood up to late adolescence (18 years of age), but for most children measured intelligence remains relatively stable after five years of age (Zigler et al, 1984).

There are many developmental tests such as Bayley, Gesell and Griffiths etc which can be used to assess children's psychomotor development.

Bayley Scales of Infant Development (Bayley, 1969)

The Bayley Scales developed in the United States of America measure the developmental status of children aged two months to two and a half years of age. It is comprised of three scales:

- mental scale, containing 163 items sampling functions such as perception, problem solving and vocalisation;
- motor scale, an 81 item scale covering gross and fine motor abilities such as sitting, standing, walking and manipulation of hands and fingers;
- infant behaviour record which is completed by the examiner following the administration of both the mental and motor scales. This is designed to assess behaviours related to task completion and social development.

The Bayley Scales take approximately 60 minutes to administer. Data on reliability and validity have been included in the test manual. The Bayley Scales principally provide measures of current infant developmental status and information regarding detection of deficit areas.

Intelligence tests

This limited sample of individually administered intelligence tests cover the range of early childhood through to adulthood.

Intelligence tests provide a summary score, for example, an Intelligence Quotient (IQ), which is an overall index of the individual's functioning or performance on the test in relation to others the same age. See Table 1.

Table 1. Classification ratings for Intelligence Quotients (Wechsler Scales)

Intelligence Quotients	Classification
130 and above	very superior
120–129	superior
110–119	high average
90–109	average
80–89	low average
70–79	borderline
69 and below	mentally deficient or retarded

Stanford–Binet Intelligence Scale: Fourth Edition (Thorndike, Hagen, and Sattler, 1986)

This scale covers the age range of two years through to the adult level. Some sub-tests are based on early versions of the Stanford–Binet and include tests such as vocabulary, comprehension, copying, memory for sentences, memory for digits and quantitative items. In total, the Fourth Edition of the Stanford–Binet comprises 15 sub-tests covering four major cognitive areas: verbal reasoning, abstract/visual reasoning, quantitative reasoning and short-term memory. In general, the complete battery includes from 8 to 13 tests. Of the 15 sub-tests, only six cover the entire age range. These are vocabulary, comprehension, picture analysis, quantitative, bead memory, and memory for sentences. The Stanford–Binet: Fourth Edition has only one timed sub-test and total administration time is dependent on the number of sub-tests selected, the age and performance speed of the examinee. However, it is estimated that the complete battery can take from 30 minutes to 90 minutes to administer. The Stanford–Binet: Fourth Edition has been shown to have good validity and high test–re-test reliability.

An Australian adaptation of the Stanford–Binet Intelligence Scale: Fourth Edition is now available.

McCarthy Scales of Children's Abilities (McCarthy, 1972)

The McCarthy Scales of Children's Abilities is a valid, well standardised measure of cognitive abilities for the age range two and a half to eight and a half years of age.

It is an individually administered test consisting of 18 tests, grouped into five scales: verbal, perceptual–performance, quantitative, memory and motor skills. The motor scale examines fine and gross motor abilities, and a laterality scale is included for children aged beyond five years to assess left-right awareness, hand, eye and leg dominance.

The McCarthy Scales, standardised on the American population, provide a measure of general intellectual functioning based on the sum of the verbal, perceptual–performance and quantitative scales. Furthermore, they yield a profile of abilities that may be valuable in evaluating young children.

Wechsler Intelligence Scales

The Wechsler Pre-school and Primary Scale of Intelligence (WPPSI: Wechsler 1967)[1]

The WPPSI published in 1967 in the United States of America was designed for use for children aged four to six and a half years of age. It is a downward extension of the scales developed by Wechsler for school children (WISC-R) and adults (WAIS-R).

The WPPSI contains 11 sub-tests, eight of which are also used in the WISC-R. These include information, vocabulary, arithmetic, similarities, comprehension, picture completion, maze and block design. The remaining sub-tests are sentences (a memory test), animal house (speed and accuracy copying test) and geometric design (copying drawings). Sub-tests form two scales, verbal and performance with the test providing verbal, performance and full-scale Intelligence Quotients. Ten of the sub-tests are used to calculate the Intelligence Quotients. In addition, test age equivalents (essentially mental age scores) are given. The WPPSI has excellent psychometric properties including standardisation, reliability and validity, and is a valuable tool for assessing children's intelligence.

Wechsler Intelligence Scale for Children: Revised (Wechsler, 1974)

The WISC-R, published in 1974, is a revised version of the WISC (1949) and was developed as a downward extension of the Wechsler-Bellevue Intelligence Scale, an adult intelligence test.

The WISC-R covering the age range of six years through to 16 years 11 months consists of 12 sub-tests, two of which are used as supplementary tests. Six tests form the verbal scale (information, similarities, arithmetic, vocabulary, comprehension and digit span) and six form the performance scale (picture completion, picture arrangement, block design, object assembly, coding and maze).

Three separate IQ levels, verbal, performance and full-scale are calculated based on 10 sub-tests.

The WISC-R has excellent standardisation, reliability and concurrent validity. It is a major contributor to the evaluation of intellectual functioning of children and adolescents.

Australian norms are not available but an Australian adaptation including substitute items appropriate for Australian use have been added.

Wechsler Adult Intelligence Scale: Revised (Wechsler, 1981)

In its original form, the WAIS-R was called the Wechsler-Bellevue Intelligence Scale (1939), being revised in 1949, and again, in 1955 (that is, Form One).

This current version covers the age range 16 years to 74 years 11 months, and contains 11 sub-tests grouped into two scales, verbal and performance. The six verbal sub-tests are information, digit span, vocabulary, arithmetic, comprehension and similarities; the five performance sub-tests are picture completion, picture arrangement, block design, object assembly and digit symbol (similar to coding on the WISC-R). Three IQ levels for verbal, performance and full-scales can be determined.

Similar to other Wechsler scales, the WAIS-R has good psychometric properties with high reliabilities, and excellent standardisation. Item substitutions for an Australian adaptation are included.

Assessment of academic achievement

The assessment of academic achievement is vital in the evaluation of individuals displaying learning disabilities, mental handicap, behavioural disorders and giftedness. Numerous tests covering reading, spelling, mathematics, written language, receptive vocabulary, and auditory comprehension have been developed.

Individually administered tests have been selected for presentation in this section although group administered tests are available for measuring academic achievement.

---

[1] The WPPSI-R published in 1989 in America was designed for children aged three to seven years and three months. It is a revised version of the WPPSI (1967) and is a downward extension of the scales developed by Wechsler for school children (WISC-R) and adults (WAIS-R).

Neale Analysis of Reading Ability: Revised (Neale, 1988)

The original Neale Analysis of Reading Ability, an individually administered test, published in the United Kingdom in the 1950s, was devised to assess the reading rate, accuracy and comprehension of children aged 6 to 13 years of age. The revision of the Neale Analysis of Reading Ability published in 1988 was standardised on an Australian sample of children drawn from Victoria and South Australia. The revised test includes more up to date stories, information on diagnosis and new norms and assesses the same components of reading as the original test. It has two parallel forms of six graded passages of prose, and is a continuous reading scale for children aged 6 to 12 years of age.

Wide Range Achievement Test (WRAT): Revised (Jastak and Wilkinson, 1984)

The WRAT was originally published in the United States of America in 1936 with the most recent revision occurring in 1984. The WRAT–R contains three sub-tests, reading, spelling, and arithmetic and is divided into two sections: level 1 for 5 to 11 years 11 months, and level 2 for ages 12 through 74 years and 11 months. The WRAT–R takes approximately 30 minutes to administer, and ought to be considered a screening tool. No Australian norms are available.

Woodcock-Johnson Psycho-Educational Battery (Woodcock, 1977)

The Woodcock–Johnson Psycho–Educational Battery standardised on an American sample, covers the age range of three years through to adulthood. It includes 27 tests assessing three areas: cognitive ability, achievement and interest.

The tests of cognitive ability cover, for example, vocabulary, spatial relations, memory and quantitative concepts. Achievement tests cover 10 areas including reading, spelling, capitalisation, punctuation and knowledge of subject areas such as science and social studies. The interest areas covers interest in reading, maths, language, physical activities and social activities. The complete battery can be administered in two hours. However, it is recommended that the cognitive ability tests not replace other standardised measures of intelligence (for example, the Wechsler Scales and the Stanford–Binet Intelligence Scale: Fourth Edition) as its construct validity is not satisfactory (Sattler, 1988). However, the achievement tests are useful for the assessment of the specific academic areas for which it was devised. No Australian norms are available.

Assessment of adaptive behaviour and behavioural problems

Adaptive behaviour refers to the individual's ability to meet the demands of the environment. Measurement instruments thus focus on the personal and social competence of the individual within the context of his developmental status.

Vineland Adaptive Behaviour Scales (Sparrow, Balla and Cicchetti, 1984)

Vineland Adaptive Behaviour Scales (VABS) is a revision of the Vineland Social Maturity Scale published by Doll in 1953. The VABS assesses social competence of handicapped and non-handicapped individuals from birth to 19 years of age. It is available in three forms: survey form, expanded form, and classroom edition.

The survey and expanded forms use a semi-structured interview technique, with information obtained from a parent or care-giver familiar with the individual's daily behaviour. The classroom edition is a questionnaire completed by a teacher and covers ages three years through to 12 years. In each version, adaptive behaviour is measured in four domains: communication, daily living skills, socialisation, and motor skills. The survey and expanded forms also include a maladaptive behaviour domain. Adjustment for standard scores for Australian children for the survey form are available (de Lemos 1989; ACER).

Child Behaviour Checklist (Achenbach and Edelbrock, 1983)

The Child Behaviour Checklist (CBCL) is a standardised questionnaire completed by parents or care-givers on behavioural problems and competencies of children 4 to 16 years. There are parallel forms of the questionnaire, completed by teachers, by direct observers and the children themselves, with separate forms for each sex at ages 4 to 5, 6 to 11, and 12 to 16 years. The checklist is also available for ages two to three years and covers both sexes. The CBCL is presented in two parts. First is a social competence section designed to measure positive adaptive functioning, with a second section describing a range of behavioural problems (see chapter 18). An Australian replication of the Achenbach and Edelbrock normative study has been carried out (Rae Hensley, 1988).

Personality assessment

Personality tests are self report measurement instruments of emotional, motivational, interpersonal and attitudinal characteristics and hence are principally used in clinical and counselling settings. The MMPI and HSPQ presented briefly in the following pages are examples.

Projective assessment techniques on the other hand are unstructured tasks with vague or ambiguous stimuli presented, giving the individual an opportunity to respond idiosyncratically. The underlying hypothesis is that the way in which the individual responds reflects fundamental aspects of psychological functioning. Projective assessment techniques include sentence completion, story-telling, and inkblot techniques, and drawing tasks.

The House-Tree-Person Test, a drawing test, and the Rorschach Inkblot Test are described. The majority of published studies on the validity of projective tests are inconclusive (Gittelman Klein, 1986; Krahn, 1985). Projective tests are regarded as supplementary qualitative interviewing aids in the hands of a skilled clinician (Anastasi, 1988).

Minnesota Multi-Phasic Personality Inventory (Hathaway and McKinley, 1983)

The MMPI is designed for adults from 16 years of age and upward and consists of 566 statements to which the examinee is required to indicate whether each is true, false or cannot say. The inventory provides information regarding psychiatric symptomatology and personality characteristics. The current basic profile form for the MMPI includes not only the 10 original clinical scales (hypochondriasis, depression, hysteria, psychopathic deviate, masculinity–femininity, paranoia, psychasthenia, schizophrenia, hypomania, social introversion) but also four of the newer scales (anxiety, repression, ego strength, and the McAndrew alcoholism scale). Shorter and simpler versions are available for screening purposes.

Eysenck Personality Questionnaire (Eysenck and Eysenck, 1975)

The EPQ is a self report inventory containing measures of neuroticism(N), extraversion(E), psychoticism(P), and a lie scale(L).

High School Personality Questionnaire (Cattell, Cattell and Johns, 1984)

The HSPQ developed by Cattell and his colleagues to identify primary personality traits was designed for the 12 to 18 year old group. It parallels the Sixteen Personality Factor Questionnaire for adults and gives scores on fourteen factors including warmth, intelligence, emotional stability, excitability, dominance, enthusiasm, conformity boldness, sensitivity, withdrawal, apprehension, self sufficiency, self discipline and tension.

Similar inventories have been developed for the 8 to 12 year old group (Children's Personality Questionnaire), and the 6 to 8 year olds (Early School Personality Questionnaire).

House-Tree-Person (Buck, 1981)

This test requires the examinee to draw free hand, a house, tree and a person. The subject is then asked to describe and interpret the drawings. The three drawings are then repeated, with the examinee using a set of coloured crayons. This is followed by a shorter interview about the drawings and scoring is based on quantitative and qualitative analyses considering, for example, proportion and perspective of each drawing. The reader is referred to a review by Glow (1986).

Rorschach Inkblot Test
(Rorschach, 1921, 1948)

The Rorschach Inkblot Test developed in 1921 is considered applicable to preschoolers through to adults. It uses 10 cards, on each of which is printed a symmetrical inkblot. The examinee is required to interpret what each represents thus indicating the underlying aspects, such as perception and motivation of the individual's personality. Extensive scoring systems have been developed.

Neuropsychological assessment

Between the 1940s and 1960s the emphasis of neuropsychological evaluations tended to be concerned with the diagnosis of brain damage. Increasingly, investigators and clinicians became aware of the variability in neuropsychological conditions and the need therefore to focus their attention on the psychological sequelae of organic brain conditions.

Beside the development of single tests aimed to measure specific functions (for example, Wechsler Memory Scales, Benton Visual Retention Test), batteries of neuropsychological tests have been developed to incorporate a comprehensive range of standardised tests. Two examples are the Halstead–Reitan Neuropsychological Test Battery and the Luria–Nebraska Neuropsychological Battery. The Halstead–Reitan Battery covers a range of sensory motor and perceptual tests and an aphasia test covering several sense modalities and response modes. The Luria Test, more recently developed, is designed to assess a broad range of neuropsychological functions, such as motor function, rhythm, tactile functions, speech and memory. Both the Halstead–Reitan, and Luria Batteries have developed a range of tests suitable for children.

This section has highlighted a limited sample of the psychological tests that are available. Other areas of psychology such as health occupational, and cross cultural psychology in which tests can play a vital role have not been included. Neither has mention been made of other testing methods such as group and computerised testing. Like individually administered psychological tests, the aim is to gain objective and standardised data to aid in the evaluation and management of individuals.

Further Reading

Gittelman Klein R, 'Questioning the Clinical Usefulness of Projective Psychological Tests for Children', *Developmental and Behavioural Paediatrics*, Vol 7 No 6, 1986, pp 378–82.

Glow R A, 'The House-Tree-Person in Clinical Use, Australian Council for Educational Research', *Bulletin for Psychologists*, Vol 40, 1986, pp 16–18.

Krahn G L, 'The Use of Projective Assessment Techniques in Paediatric Settings', *Journal of Paediatric Psychology*, Vol 10 No 2, 1985, pp 179–93.

Rae Hensley V, 'Australian Normative Study of the Achenbach Child Behaviour Checklist', *Australian Psychologist*, Vol 23 No 3, 1988, pp 371–82.

Sattler J M, *Assessment of Children*, 3rd ed, Jerome M Sattler, San Diego, 1988.

Sharpley C F and Pain M D, 'Psychological Test Usage in Australia', *Australian Psychologist*, Vol 23 No 3, 1988, pp 361–9.

Sparrow S S, Fletcher J M and Cicchetti D M, 'Psychological Assessment of Children', in *Psychiatry*, Vol 2 (ed Michels R), Lippincott, Philadelphia, 1989.

Zigler E, Balla D and Hodapp R, 'On the Definition and Classification of Mental Retardation', *American Journal of Mental Deficiency*, Vol 89, 1984, pp 215–30.

Part 5
Psychiatric Syndromes

Chapter 23

Disruptive Behaviour in Children and Adolescents

J M Rey and D Blyth

Disruptive and antisocial behaviour disorders are a heterogeneous group of conditions which are characterised by behaviour which is socially inappropriate and causes disruption or distress to others. It includes a variety of problems which may be limited to the child's home and family or which may affect the school or the wider community. The behaviours may or may not be delinquent, violent or altogether lacking in aggressiveness, and can occur within the context of a variety of interpersonal relationships. Therefore, it is not surprising that this group of disorders carries with it a good deal of argument and controversy about nature, diagnosis and treatment.

Case example

John was a 10 year old boy who was referred by the school counsellor because of his difficult behaviour at school. He was inattentive, overactive, noisy and disruptive in the classroom. John's teacher found him difficult to manage and a negative influence on the other children because he refused to follow her directions and often answered back. He had problems with his peers and regularly became involved in fights and quarrels. Mother reported that John was also difficult at home; he argued with his brother and sisters, did not do his jobs around the house, screamed and shouted with little reason and had temper tantrums when he couldn't get his own way.

Disruptive behaviour similar to that described in the above case vignette is one of the most common reasons for referral of a child or adolescent to a psychiatric clinic. This group of conditions can be subdivided into oppositional-defiant disorders, conduct disorders, and attention deficit-hyperactivity disorders (these are described in chapter 24).

Oppositional-defiant disorder

As a general characteristic, children with this disorder display a persistent pattern of negativistic, hostile behaviour. They are resentful of authority, have temper tantrums, are argumentative and appear to do things deliberately to annoy other people, particularly parents and or siblings. They are stubborn, angry and vindictive. However, they seldom carry out serious antisocial acts and their conduct can be normal in many situations, such as when they are seen in the clinician's office. These children tend to blame circumstances, parents or other people for their behaviour. Severe conflict with family members or suspension from school is not an uncommon occurrence and this may have significant negative consequences for the child. Between 2 per cent and 10 per cent of children in clinical samples are reported with these symptoms.

The causes of this problem are likely to be varied, with contributions from both the child's temperament and his relationship with parents. Oppositional behaviour may be the result of an unloving and overcontrolled upbringing. Children in these circumstances tend to express angry feelings in a passive-aggressive way.

Abnormal oppositional behaviour needs to be distinguished from developmentally appropriate oppositionality. Normally a child learns to resist and, if necessary, to oppose the will of others as part of his development. This is characteristic of those phases of development when the child, and the adolescent, try to break away from the strong parental influence. Oppositional behaviour and negativism may also be secondary symptoms in a variety of conditions such as depression or elective mutism.

Conduct disorder

Conduct disordered behaviour is a persistent pattern of conduct which is insensitive to others and in which age appropriate societal norms or rules are broken. Truancy from school, running away from home, lying, vandalism, cruelty to animals or other people, bullying and physical aggression are some of the behaviours displayed by conduct disordered children. Conduct disorder is not equivalent to juvenile delinquency which is a legal concept that implies the child has been unlawful.

Conduct disordered individuals are often reported as having low self-esteem and a negative self-image. They sometimes show symptoms of depression and/or anxiety. Almost always they underachieve at school. Specific developmental disorders in reading and spelling are present in about one third, and may add frustration to the list of problems experienced by the child. Drug and alcohol abuse, sexual assault and promiscuity (often leading to teenage pregnancy) are also common among adolescents. The symptoms first appear during primary school years and usually worsen during adolescence.

Conduct disordered behaviour has dimensions of *socialisation* (ability to relate and show loyalty to some peers) and *aggression* (such as stealing in which confrontation with a victim is involved). DSM–III–R classifies conduct disorder into three types: *group type*, *solitary-aggressive* and *undifferentiated*. In the group type, antisocial behaviour occurs mainly as a group activity, while in the solitary-aggressive type, conduct problems, particularly of an aggressive nature, occur mainly outside group activity.

As many as 9 per cent of males and 2 per cent of females under the age of 18 years can exhibit conduct disorder. Prevalences, however, vary considerably from country to country, and between urban and rural settings. It is generally reported that there are more conduct disordered young people in large cities. However, there may be considerable variations between suburbs in the same city or between schools in the same suburb.

The study of disorders of conduct has given rise to a large body of theorising. Psychoanalytic theory emphasises the personal meaning of the antisocial act. It is concerned with the social effects of personality development which may result in a defective super-ego or conscience. Such theories consider that, in some cases, antisocial activities are the external manifestation of intrapsychic conflicts (acting out).

Social theories stress the contribution of familial and social influences. Deviant behaviour is considered a result of a chaotic and hostile family and social environment. Other environmental theories note that antisocial behaviour may be learned through association with criminal subcultures. Coercive family processes may be present. These interchanges are prolonged, involve multiple family members and do not lead to resolution of conflict within the family. The lack of pleasurable family activities, frequent punishment and lack of praise provide in these families the atmosphere in which repetitive cycles of aggression and disruptive behaviour may occur.

Until recently there was little research on the biological aspects of conduct disorder. Although it seems implausible that young people with conduct disorder are biologically different from their peers, the results of adoption and twin studies suggest that there may be some biological features that characterise the most severe groups. These are likely to be an exaggeration of personality traits rather than qualitative differences.

Overall, there has been a move away from theories which attempted to identify a single causal process to those which emphasise multifactorial explanations. A good clinical history and a thorough exploration with the young person of their personal history and their feelings will often reveal many important aspects.

Case example

Alison was 15 years old when a family crisis for which she was the subject of much blame pushed her into close association with delinquent youth in her neighbourhood. At a time when her own identity was fragile, she learned to value the tough 'pecking order' of this group, Alison began to stay away from home overnight, played truant from school and became heavily involved in shoplifting and illegal graffiti. Within a period of 12 months, after little previous history of antisocial behaviour, Alison had run away from home 15 times and was on multiple charges for theft and vandalism. On occasions, she had broken into the family home and on other occasions had assaulted her mother.

The family history revealed several generations of psychiatric disorder and anti-social behaviour. Alison's developmental history disclosed several important personal losses, a congenital hearing defect with subsequent imposed comprehension and speech lag, and evidence of early maternal neglect.

Isolated acts of antisocial behaviour are common, particularly during adolescence, but these do not justify considering someone as being conduct disordered. The most important task during assessment is to rule out the existence of a treatable condition which may manifest itself by conduct problems such as an organic brain disorder, epilepsy, early onset schizophrenia or, more commonly, an af-fective disorder. In these cases onset of the symptoms tend to be more acute and the life long pattern of typical conduct disorder is lacking. Children who have attention deficit hyperactivity disorder may later show conduct disordered behaviour. Specific learning difficulties are not uncommon.

Milder forms of conduct disorder may improve with time. More severe forms can develop into serious adult psychopathology. Early onset and the presence of aggressive behaviours are thought to be bad prognosis and are more frequently associated with the development if antisocial personality disorder during adulthood.

Treatment of disruptive behaviour disorders

The literature available on this topic does not often distinguish between the various types of disruptive behaviour. Multifactorial explanations for disruptive behaviour have given rise to a variety of treatments, but no single treatment approach has produced consistently good results for all disruptive behaviours. Building rapport and trust with young people with these types of complaints is not always easy. This is because of the inevitable discomfort experienced by a child who may be attending unwillingly under the pressure of parents, school or the legal system. Such young people can be hostile to authority figures (including the clinician).

When disruptive behaviour is the result of poor adjustment to circumstances, the linking of the precipitant, such as a significant personal loss, to a period of disturbed conduct in a previously non-symptomatic child is essential. Exploring the meaning of the loss and the impact of the stressor (for example, moving house, transition to high school) upon all the family members provides the ground work in establishing a better understanding between parent, child and siblings. Once empathy has been achieved and trust re-established, simple behavioural directives to modify disruptive behaviour can be effective.

Case example

Nigel was a 13 year old boy referred for stealing at the local high school. The history revealed non-compliance at home and school, running away from home and stealing during the previous six months. This period of disruption occurred after the separation of his maternal grandparents, which involved the geographical re-location of his grandmother (who suffered from schizophrenia) and his 14 year old uncle whom he regarded as a brother. Unable to express feelings of loss and afraid that he would inherit his grandmother's psychiatric condition, Nigel released tension through clashes with his parents, teachers and acts of daring with peers.

In order to understand the meaning of this loss, Nigel, who had been suspended from school, was asked to spend time at home, drawing pictures about the family. At the next session these drawings were discussed with his parents who also explained their feelings of loss and distress. Once these issues were discussed, and reassurance given to Nigel that he was not 'crazy', attention was focussed on his 'answering back' when directed to do household tasks. His parents were requested to observe how they handled Nigel's argumentativeness.

By the next session the parents had arranged for Nigel to spend time with his maternal grandmother and uncle in recognition of the importance of their relationship. Nigel's mother had been alerted to her contribution in fuelling arguments, through her over-reacting to any sign of resistance. She voluntarily changed to more positive, persuasive requests. Nigel was also transferred to a new school to maximise the effects of a fresh start. On follow-up Nigel's mother and father reported good progress at home and school with no recurrence of the previous problems.

In treating oppositional behaviour, several matters need to be borne in mind. Firstly, the longstanding nature of the conflict usually means that the parents are unable to differentiate issues on which they should take a stand from issues which are trivial and are not worth the fuss. Such distinctions will need to be made by the clinician. A useful way to provide a rationale for this is by using the distinction between age-appropriate and age-inappropriate behaviours: this helps to avoid dead-end discussions of 'good versus bad' conduct. In the case of older children, the idea of adolescence as a preparation for adulthood is also helpful.

Secondly, the child's oppositional behaviour can arise from a combination of a stubborn temperament and parents' perception that the child's willfulness is very powerful. The parents may lose confidence in themselves as managers of the child. If that is the case, the clinician will need to encourage and support the parents.

Thirdly, the negative patterns of interaction between the parents and child may become very rigid and exclude other, more pleasurable interactions. The therapist will need to set up alternatives and open up areas of new interest for the parents and the child.

Case example

Lisa was a 16 year old girl who presented with an 18 month history of argumentativeness, disobedience and oppositional behaviour accompanied by emotional withdrawal and sullen silence at home. The main focus of conflict was between the single mother and daughter. The pattern reported was that mother came home from work exhausted, was resentful of her teenage children lazing around and became furious when Lisa had not done her household chores. She berated the children during the evening meal and often Lisa was the target. When this happened, an escalation would occur with the siblings joining mother against Lisa. The girl then stormed to her room, isolated herself and was unable to concentrate on homework. The next day she would perform badly at school, and came home in a worse mood.

The mother was given the choice of deferring her argument with Lisa until after dinner or to take her outside, away from the interference of her brother and sister, and to argue there. Lisa's desire to be seen to be grown up was accepted. However, it was pointed out to her that her strategy for being granted more freedom was working in reverse. Lisa was asked to think of a way in which she could express her appreciation of her mother as a surprise, the surprise to be in such a manner that no-one would know who had initiated it.

Two weeks later mother reported that her daughter had been 'cured'. No further arguments occurred at the dinner table. One afternoon in the preceding week a bunch of roses had mysteriously appeared for her. Lisa made no direct claim to their origin. This had touched the mother deeply and enabled a restoration of a positive feeling and physical closeness with her problem daughter. Other arguments had ceased and Lisa was working hard at school. This progress was reported as continuing at a six month follow-up.

The variety, severity and frequency of antisocial behaviour shown by children with conduct disorders at home, school or in the neighbourhood requires careful assessment. The establishment of an effective management plan depends on the information available about the child and his circumstances. It is essential that there is a thorough history taken from the child and the parents. Useful information can often be obtained from the school and from other agencies (for example, departments of community welfare). Since conduct disordered behaviour may be a result of psychiatric disturbances such as schizophrenia or depressive states, it is necessary that a mental state examination be undertaken in the assessment. A physical examination or investigations, such as an electroencephalogram or a computerised tomography of the brain, may provide revealing signs of medical or neurological conditions (for example, drug use, epilepsy, degenerative brain disease). Assessment of intellectual functions, of possible specific learning difficulties, educational achievements and neuropsychological deficits can be extremely helpful.

The question of how the behaviours compare with other children of a similar age, sex, cognitive ability and socio-economic background also needs consideration. It is important to obtain a clear description of the incident(s) which precipitate referral; where and when did these incidents occur? Who was involved? What were the precipitants and consequences of the incident? What was the young person's feeling, intending and choosing before, during and after the events. How does he feel about detection? It is also necessary to know how the young person has interacted with his family over these incidents. What attempts were made to deal with or conceal the anti-social behaviour? How was the crisis dealt with and what consequences were set?

Often behaviour disordered children show a cluster of behaviours that express themselves with different frequency, severity and in different contexts, so that treatment may need to address a package of deviant behaviours, in which parental cooperation and involve-

ment is crucial. In some occasions, this can be done while the child is at home but in others, because of the severity of the problems or because parents are unable to set limits on the child's behaviour, the youngster may need to be placed in a *residential* setting.

Case example

Darryl was 12 years of age when he entered high school. He had a history of difficult behaviour since fourth grade, both at school and at home. Teachers had found him very resistant to directions in the classroom. He verbally abused teachers, assaulted other children and destroyed his own classwork or classroom furniture when attempts were made to enforce compliance with basic rules. At home the picture was similar: refusal to do chores, deliberately destroying others' possessions, verbally abusing parents and siblings when frustrated. During the first year of high school this pattern was compounded by repetitive outbreaks of anti-social conduct: truancy from school, stealing from home and the neighbourhood, deliberate vandalism and, on occasions, fighting with peers using a sharp weapon.

Two factors seemed to have contributed to the development of his conduct disorder. Firstly, Darryl had difficulties with learning in English and maths which made his attitude to school negative and his attention to tasks in the classroom poor. The larger classes, more difficult school work and stricter discipline of the high school clashed repeatedly with Darryl's pattern of disruption. Secondly, Darryl had experienced violent physical abuse in his own childhood which ceased after his parents separated at the age of six years. His consequent trust of his stepfather was poor and deteriorated further during early adolescence as Darryl attempted to prove his masculine identity primarily through aggressive and defiant acts.

Initial treatment aimed at behaviour modification at home and revised classroom management was insufficient to prevent Darryl from being suspended repeatedly from school. Likewise, although at home his behaviour had improved, the level of support for Darryl by his mother, stepfather and siblings was fragile. Darryl was referred to a residential program which specialised in children with both educational deficits and conduct problems (see chapter 11). After 12 months, Darryl was successfully reintegrated to home and into mainstream high school.

Conclusion

Disorders of conduct are an important area of childhood and adolescent disturbance; because they are relatively common, they create an economic burden for society and cause pain to individuals and families. Clinical experience indicates that often the question of treatment is secondary to the primary task of helping an over-stressed and under-resourced environment to provide more adequate care and control. Thus, the interface between mental health services, the legal system and welfare services require sustained collaboration in this complex area.

Further Reading

Haley J, *Problem Solving Therapy*, Harper & Row, New York, 1976.

Kazdin A E, 'Treatment of Anti-social Behaviour in Children: Current Status and Future Directions', *Psychological Bulletin*, Vol 102, 1987, pp 187–203.

Kay R L and Kay J, 'Adolescent Conduct Disorders' in *Annual Review*, Vol 5 (ed Frances A J and Hales R E), American Psychiatric Press, Washington DC, 1986.

Levy D M, 'Oppositional Syndromes and Opositional Behaviour', in *Psychopathology of Childhood* (ed Hoch P and Zubin J), Grune and Stratton, New York, 1955.

Patterson G R, *Coercive Family Process*, Castalia, Oregon, 1982.

Rey J M, Bashir M R, Schwarz M, Richards I N, Plapp J M and Steward G W, 'Oppositional Disorder: Fact or Fiction?', *Journal of the American Academy of Child and Adolescent Psychiatry*, Vol 2, 1988, pp 157–62.

Robins L N, *Deviant Children Grown Up*, Williams and Wilkins, Baltimore, 1966.

Rutter M and Giller H, *Juvenile Delinquency*, Penguin, Middlesex, 1983.

Chapter 24

Attention Deficit Hyperactivity Disorder

F Levy

Attention Deficit Hyperactivity Disorder (ADHD) is a syndrome manifested by behaviour which is overactive and where the person seems unusually distractible. It can be mild, moderate or severe. Such a person is restless and fidgety, constantly moving in the seat or moving about the office or room. If asked to be still he feels uncomfortable and cannot resist moving. He is impulsive and speaks or acts in a manner which interrupts others. The central feature of this syndrome is the child's inability to sustain attention on tasks or to patiently complete them. Often the child will shift from one task to the other without completing anything effectively.

Teachers and parents complain that the child does not seem to listen, to follow instructions or to obey commands. The behaviour is disruptive in the classroom and home and others are often adversely affected by the interruptions and noise. Sometimes the activities are dangerous and the child seems to lack an awareness of danger to self or others.

Clinical features

The onset of ADHD occurs before seven years of age; many children with ADHD have been identified as overactive from infancy. Such children are said to have 'never walked but always ran'. At these early stages of motor and language development most children are active and have a relatively low attention span, but the vast majority respond well to good parental guidance. A small minority remain excessively active and unable to sustain their attention on tasks at pre-school. Parents and

pre-school teachers may need support in structuring the management of these children. The problem becomes even more evident when such children begin school. At school, the behaviour of attention-disordered children contrasts with that of their peers who are able to cope with the demands of a classroom setting such as sitting at a desk and paying attention to instructions. Such children are soon perceived by teachers as problematic because they disrupt the classroom. They will usually be brought into treatment at this time, unless their unmanageable pre-school behaviour or behaviour at home has already brought them into a treatment situation.

Diagnosis of ADHD in adolescence is more controversial than in childhood. Until the 1960s, most clinicians believed that the symptoms of attention deficiency and hyperactivity disappear in adolescence. More recent evidence suggests that some children with this condition may continue to experience attention and personality problems into adolescence and adulthood. There is however, considerable overlap with conduct disorders in the older age group. Because of this, and because of concerns about the potential for drug abuse among adolescents, most clinicians are conservative about diagnosing ADHD after the age of 15 years, unless there is a very well defined and clear history of attention deficit disorder, which has required treatment since childhood.

Prevalence

Prevalence rates of ADHD have varied from 5 to 20 per cent in the United States of

America to 0.1 per cent in a London borough. This is because of differences in classification criteria and diagnostic practices in various settings. The prevalence of ADHD in boys is higher than in girls (ratio of 4:1).

Causes

Despite extensive research, the aetiology remains unclear. Brain damage, perinatal trauma, minimal brain dysfunction, and genetic inheritance have all been investigated with no definitive findings. Various forms of brain damage can produce nearly all of the psychiatric syndromes of childhood. Soft neurological signs such as motor impersistance are more common in severely hyperactive children, but they are not valid as a sign of cerebral pathology, because of considerable uncertainty about what causes them.

Recent research using xenon 133 inhalation and emission tomography has shown low cerebral blood flow in dopaminergic striatal areas of the brain in ADHD children. This low striatal activity was partially reversed by methylphenidate, which increased blood flow to striatal and posterior periventricular areas, and tended to decrease flow to primary sensory regions, indicating an important direction for future research.

As far as genetic theories are concerned, siblings of hyperactive children are more likely to be affected than are half siblings, suggesting a genetic factor. Also hyperactive children have an increased incidence of sociopathy or alcoholism in first degree relatives. These findings are however, most applicable to children who have a conduct disorder with hyperactivity rather than hyperactivity alone; and could also be explained by family interactions leading to conduct disorder and alcohol abuse, as readily as by genetic inheritance.

Another group of theories relates to environmental chemical factors such as lead intoxication. Low lead levels in the body are associated with poor social circumstances, which could in turn themselves be associated with factors leading to behaviour disturbance.

Some have postulated that food colours and preservatives might be involved in the genesis of hyperactivity. This claim has provoked a number of studies. So far no single study has reported a consistent dietary effect on the symptoms of the hyperkinetic syndrome. The reported positive findings are generally the result of post-hoc analysis, are relatively sporadic, and are greatly out numbered by studies producing negative results. Any improvement due to dietary restriction of alleged contaminants seems most likely to be a placebo effect. Overall, analysis of the results of dietary modification indicate that it is not an effective intervention for hyperactivity.

Diagnosis

Most authorities have relied on the criteria of DSM–III–R or ICD-9 for a clinical diagnosis. However, a clinical diagnosis should be supported by psychometric testing. In addition, a number of workers have in recent years been using tests of attention or vigilance (for example, the Continuous Performance Test and Paired Associates Learning Test) to help support a clinical diagnosis. The use of these objective tests is a very important advance, but such tests must be validated in carefully selected clinical samples. However, non-invasive brain imaging techniques hold great promise for future understandings of the ADHD syndrome. The various complex aspects of attention such as sustained attention, selective attention and focussed attention, measured by laboratory tests, need to be clarified. There has been a recent move by some workers to study the classroom performance of children with ADHD and this approach should be welcomed.

Other conditions need to be considered. A pre-school child may be manifesting rebelliousness towards parents, or oppositional disorder, or may just be poorly managed by parents who are unsure of themselves. Children with a hearing disorder such as 'glue ear' may show apparently poor attention. Occasionally a pervasive developmental disorder such as autism may be diagnosed as hyperactive. School-aged children with conduct disorders may be mistaken for ADHD; specific developmental disorder in reading or mathematics can be associated with attentional problems; and the associated frustration in class sometimes mistaken for ADHD.

Treatment

Drugs which act as central nervous system (CNS) stimulants have been the commonest form of treatment since Bradley described their effects in 1937. While most clinicians are agreed on the benefits of short-term stimulant medications such as methyl-phenidate or dextro-amphetamine for some children with severe ADHD, there is con-siderable controversy about whether such medications should be used in pre-schoolers and also whether their use should be curtailed in adolescence. Most clinicians advocate a conservative dose range of 0.7 to 1.0 mg/kg/day of methylphenidate (the dosage is halved for dextro-amphetamine). A high dose range may impair cognitive per-formance. This claim has been disputed by some workers, but recent reports of tolerance effects with high dose regimes suggest that conservative dose ranges should be used, especially in adolescence.

The side effects of CNS stimulants are also controversial, but impairment of appetite and growth have been described, particularly on high dose regimes. In addition, chronic motor tic syndrome (Gilles de la Tourette's Syn-drome) can develop in predisposed children who are on long term stimulant medication.

Most treatment regimes have emphasised the importance of multi-modal treatment for children with ADHD. Such management would include behaviour therapy, remedial education, speech therapy, and family therapy where indicated.

Treatment programs should be tailored to the needs of each individual child. For example, a pre-school child may require a structured behaviour management program with considerable support for the mother and other family members affected by the continual demands of the child on the mother's attention. On the other hand, a school-aged child may require greater emphasis on the use of medication, and possibly a remedial reading program where learning disability is also involved in the problem. An adolescent with a long history of problems at school may require both educational support and careful guidance in relation to career selection.

In all cases the families of a child with ADHD need support and guidance. It is important that parents have an understanding of the special difficulties faced by their child in coping with school, peers, teachers and siblings. It is also important that clinicians have an understanding of the stresses which the families of ADHD children may experi-ence in coping with their child's behaviour, and its effect on peers, teachers and employers.

Outcome

There have been a number of outcome studies which suggest that while the symptoms may change, many or some hyperactive children continue to have problems with attention and personality into adolescence and adulthood. However the degree of associated conduct disorder is a better predictor of adult anti-social adjustment than hyperactivity per se. Where a hyperactive child has experienced rejection and failure, he may continue to manifest anti-social behaviour such as lying, stealing and sometimes alcohol or drug abuse. Despite this, the outcome can be positive. For example, one patient went to boarding school during his adolescence, became a member of the school rowing team, worked for a stockbroker at 17–18 years, hated office life, joined the local police force and is now a popular member of the local station's youth squad and rowing team.

Conclusion

Attention deficit hyperactivity disorder remains a controversial condition of unconfirmed known aetiology. In severe cases it can cause considerable behavioural disrup-tion, particularly in the classroom. Children with this disorder are best treated with multi-modal treatment regimes, consisting of CNS stimulant medications, behaviour modifi-cation, remedial education and family support.

Further Reading

Lou H C, Henrickson L, Bruhn P, Borner H and Bieber Neilsen J, 'Striatal Dysfunction in Attention Deficit and Hyperkinetic Disorder', *Archives of Neurology*, Vol 46, 1989, pp 48–52.

Lowe T L, Cohen D J, Detler H, Kremnitzer M W, and Shawitz B, 'Stimulant Medications Precipitate Tourette's Syndrome', *Journal of American Medical Association*, Vol 247, 1982, pp 1729–31.

Mattes J A and Gittelman R, 'Growth of Hyperactive Children on Maintenance Regimen of Methylphenidate', *Archives of General Psychiatry*, Vol 40, 1983, pp 317–21.

Weiss G and Trockenberg Hectman L, 'Hyperactive Children Grown Ups', *The Guildford Press*, New York, 1986.

Zametkin A J and Rapoport J L, 'Neurology of Attention Deficit Disorder with Hyperactivity: Where Have We Come in 50 Years?' *Journal of the American Academy of Child and Adolescent Psychiatry*, Vol 26, 1987, pp 676–86.

Chapter 25

Developmental Aspects of Emotional Disorder in Children and Adolescents

R Kosky

Emotions are generally regarded as heightened feelings or mood. Emotional disorders of childhood refer to a group of conditions which are characterised by persistent symptoms of predominently anxiety, depression or both. These conditions contrast with conduct (or disruptive behaviour) disorders where the child's behaviour is of concern to others, but the child does not appear to suffer emotional symptoms.

Both ICD-9 and DSM-III have a number of categories which are relevant to the emotional disorders in childhood. These include, in both cases, the major categories for anxiety disorders and depressive disorders which are applicable to adults, as well as categories of disturbances of emotion specific to, or first evident in, childhood and adolescence.

In the ICD-9 classification the latter categories include emotional disorders whose main features are anxiety and fearfulness (313.0),[1] misery and unhappiness (313.1), sensitivity, shyness and social withdrawal (313.2) and relationship problems (313.3). Similarly, in DSM-III there are categories for separation disorders (309.21), avoidant disorder (313.21) and over-anxious disorder (313.00).

These separate categories for emotional disorders specific to childhood and adolescence are an attempt to recognise that, in these early years of life, the clinical picture is often mixed and relatively undifferentiated. However, syndromes commonly seen in neurotic adults, such as phobic disorder, obsessive-compulsive disorder, and somatoform disorder (see chapters 30, 31 and 34), are also encountered in clinical practice, among children.

Prevalence

Symptoms of anxiety are generally found among about 5 to 10 per cent of school children. Girls and boys are equally affected. Depressive symptoms are rarely encountered among children less than six years old but increase in frequency as children get older. Overall, depressive symptoms are found in less than 5 per cent of the school aged population, but as many as 2 per cent report symptoms of major depressive illness.

Normally, a health professional is only consulted if the symptoms lead to obvious loss of efficiency at school or play or if the persistence and severity of the symptoms worry the child's parents. It is generally considered that about 10 per cent of children who experience symptoms of anxiety or depression are referred for specialist help.

In a survey of over six hundred children and adolescents who were referred to a child psychiatric service in Western Australia, Kosky and colleagues (1985) found that over 50 per cent of the patients had anxiety symptoms as a leading cause for referral. The symptoms included generalised anxiety and fearfulness, over-sensitivity, irritability,

---

[1]   This is a diagnostic code of ICD-9, usually cited at the beginning of a paragraph in the ICD-9 Manual.

negativism and sleep disturbances. In older children and adolescents, symptoms of depression, tearfulness and sadness, helplessness and hopelessness were prominent and among the 12 to 16 year old age groups suicidal ideas, threats or attempts were present in 20 per cent of the total referrals.

Developmental aspects of anxiety disorders

The problem for parents and clinicians alike is to distinguish between emotional states which are part of growing up and those whose persistence or severity mitigates against normal developmental progress.

In each child there is an intrinsic drive to proceed along a developmental pathway. Maturation is facilitated by environmental influences, in the first instance by the parents' care. This care not only has its physical aspects—food, shelter, comfort, etc, but also its emotional aspects. From this point of view, the care should encourage development while discouraging the persistence of inappropriate infantile needs and behaviours.

A child is 'born' into a world of meaning long before he is born into the real world. In other words, children can be wanted or unwanted, planned or 'a mistake', conceived in order to hold a marriage together or can be the cause of marital separation and so on. Such meanings need to be explored by the clinician, since they are often powerful determinants of the parents' emotional feelings towards the child. While in the majority of cases, the child's conception brings joy to parents, for some it seems to be a cause of great personal and social difficulty. The question of abortion may have been raised, with continued ambivalent feelings towards the pregnancy as it proceeded. The pregnancy itself may be unpleasant. Most women experience health and happiness while pregnant. A few suffer illness and anxiety (see chapters 2 and 3).

Some conceptions follow one or more miscarriages and in some cases there is still unresolved grief about these, which can be carried over to anxieties about the present baby. In other cases, persistent attempts to have children fail and parents enter in-vitro fertilisation programs with high expectations of success. Babies conceived after long periods of infertility may be invested with great emotion and anxiety and be perceived as very 'precious'. In other cases, parents opt for adoption and occasionally follow adoption by soon falling pregnant with a natural child. Such circumstances can produce strains on the parents' loyalties. All these issues can contribute to how the parents react to the child in the early years.

Disturbances in the emotional and social attachments between parents and infant can be produced by the birth experience itself. For many mothers, the experience can be a shock. Good antenatal care can prepare parents. Allowing fathers to be present at birth and giving them consideration can help cement the relationships between the parents and the newborn.

Early nursing experiences are also important in the establishment of adequate attachments. Parenting skills are not entirely innate. Most are learned and they come from one's own experience of being parented. People who themselves have had inadequate parenting cannot be expected to possess the confidence and knowledge needed to make nursing the infant easy and joyful. Such people can become very anxious, lose confidence in themselves and ultimately become resentful and angry towards the child. This is particularly likely if a mother is on her own and feeding regularly, so that her sleep is broken and she becomes more and more tired. Simple social support and nursing advice at this stage can be very helpful and save a lot of trouble later by giving the mother confidence in her ability to parent the child. Fathers should not be forgotten and should be helped to share the nursing with mothers.

At around six months of age the normally developing infant clearly differentiates his care-giving parents from strangers, to whom he now shows an anxiety response. The absence of this response and the persistent failure to be discriminating in approaching strangers may be an early sign of inadequate attachment between the infant and the parents. The clinician may notice this by the readiness of a pre-school aged child to go into the clinician's office without a backward glance at the parents. Most children of this age want their parents to accompany them.

On the other hand, parents who are very anxious about their child and who perceive many threats in the environment, often create an atmosphere where the child too, becomes anxious. Under normal circumstances, the child at about 12 months begins to become quite mobile and may walk. As he does so, he explores the environment. In doing this, he moves from the 'secure' base provided by contact with the parents, into the unfamiliar environment. Most children, especially if they lose sight of the parents, get anxious and move back to 'base'. An overly anxious parent may prevent this explorative behaviour, providing instead a tendency to overestimate the dangers. In these cases the child can grow up timid and shy and avoiding social interactions. In extreme cases, the child may cling to the parents and attempts at separation can produce tears and clinging behaviour. For the mother and child (occasionally father and child) who are locked into these mutual anxieties, separation for kindergarten and school can be a dreadful experience culminating in persistent school refusal (see chapter 26).

As the child's intellect develops and he acquires the ability to abstract and create and use symbols, he can develop anxieties about the night. He invests this shadowy world with potentially harmful figures—thieves, kidnappers. Such imaginary forms may cause the child to try to stay awake, or to seek refuge in the parents' bed. Parental comfort in these circumstances is usually sufficient to calm the child, although some children benefit by a night light. Persistence of these fears after six years of age is unusual and permanent nightmares and sleepwalking and talking may signal an underlying, more troublesome, anxiety disorder.

Children between ages five and nine years are particularly liable to allow their imagination to provide magical interpretations of nature. It is during these times that they can attribute animalistic spirits to such phenomena as lightning and thunder and can be frightened of them. Not understanding the nature of the cause and effect, they can often fail to distinguish between wishes and actions.

Thus, a child who has been jealous of a baby sister can blame himself if the infant gets sick. One aspect of this type of magical thinking which is relevant to clinician, is that a child who feels jealous of his father and who is angry towards him may subsequently feel himself to blame if the parents separate and the father leaves. Another common circumstance is that a child may blame parents if he suffers pain due to, say, appendicitis. The child reasons that the parents are there to protect him and the pain is evidence of their failure to do so. The child's angry response can bewilder parents if they are unaware of this type of thinking.

Many children aged between five and nine years have rituals as part of normal behaviour. Such rituals include touching fence posts, walking only on pavement cracks (or avoiding these), bedtime rituals and rituals relating to personal hygiene. In the majority of cases, these are fleeting and only rarely (in about 0.3 per cent of the population) do these develop into an obsessive–compulsive neurosis. Nevertheless, the psychological mechanisms seem to be similar. The child feels compelled to do the ritual otherwise some unspecified harm may occur; the anxiety is allayed by the ritual, but only temporarily. The ritual appears to temporarily resolve some hidden anxiety, but does not resolve it. When such a neurosis develops, it is frequently found when the parents are perfectionistic, relatively inflexible and have high expectations of 'good' behaviour from the child. It seems that, in these circumstances, there is a relatively oppressive home atmosphere and the children are unable to express anger or find acceptable channels for it. This causes anxiety to build up, a situation which favours the development and exacerbation of ritualistic behaviour.

The same can be said of involuntary movement disorders and spasms in children when these are not due to neurological causes. Many children develop facial tics such as winks, sniffs, nods and movements of hands and legs. These are usually fleeting and spontaneously disappear, but sometimes they persist or constantly return. In these persistent cases, high levels of tension are usually present in the relations between the family members and the family is under significant stress.

Occasionally, the tics involve speech and the characteristic syndrome of Gilles de la Tourette can occur where vocal utterances, often swear words, are made involuntarily. It is important for the clinician to distinguish between these functional disorders and involuntary movement disorders which are the results of brain disease, such as Huntington's chorea.

Parents can be caught up in the child's ritual behaviour, especially if they have a similar character, and indeed the whole family can become dysfunctional around the rituals. In one case, a boy developed a bedtime ritual which progressed into checking all the lights in the house, checking under all the beds and chairs and changing all the bed linen. His parents and siblings progressively became involved and spent many hours on this ritualised behaviour. As a result, they became more and more tired and irritable with each other.

In children, many of the signs and symptoms of anxiety are physical in nature. Among these are pallor and sweatiness, rapid heart beat, dry mouth, dizziness, headache, stomach ache and poor appetite are common. Anxious children may present to health professionals with headaches, stomach aches or pains in the limbs. Sometimes, they may present on many occasions, but their complaints always warrant a medical examination. Such children are not helped by analgesics such as paracetamol, although these are commonly given to them. In a few cases, these anxious children can become addicted to the common painkillers with serious long term effects on their health.

At times, parental anxiety may cause minor physical symptoms in the child to be invested with great drama. Thus, an anxious boy was presented to casualty at the hospital by his excitable parents. He had some mild indigestion but his parents believed he was having a heart attack and demanded that he be admitted to the Intensive Care Unit. Occasionally, a child may develop a symptom where he loses the use of some function—usually paralysis of a limb, but sometimes vision or speech and even memory may seem impaired. These 'hysterical' symptoms can be the cause for alarm and they require thorough physical examination in case they are due to a hidden physical disease. They seem to be explicable in psychodynamic terms as a maladaptive resolution to an otherwise apparently unresolvable personal conflict. For instance, an 11 year old girl was torn in the conflict between pleasing her father, who wanted her to be a champion athlete and her mother, who was extremely anxious about her, worried she would catch cold if she trained and basically wanted to baby her. After a hurdling race she became progressively 'paralysed'. She became a bed patient who could be 'mothered', while being an 'athletic casualty' and saving face with her father.

In such cases, it is essential to be confident in quickly rehabilitating the child back to normal activity, by treating her as normally physically capable, while encouraging the parents towards other interests and activities and so take the focus off the child. Occasionally, among children, symptoms such as fainting, panic or euphoria may spread rapidly among a group. Such a phenomenon is sometimes referred to as 'mass hysteria'. In these cases, it is again essential to remove the drama, emphasising normality and also to separate the affected children.

Intrinsic factors may also be important in both anxiety and depressive disorders. Genetic predisposition seems likely in both conditions because of the familial pattern in many of these cases. However, with exception of manic-depressive psychosis, where the familial tendency is strong, the contribution of genetic vulnerability in the other conditions is relatively unclear.

Some links have been made between special types of personalities and types of emotional reaction. The early temperament shown by a young child seems to remain relatively constant and is predictive of his later personality. Thus, timid infants may develop as shy children and retiring adolescents. In one study, the factors of 'high intensity of emotional expression' and 'poor adaptability to new situations', which were measured among two year old children, proved better predictors of behaviour problems when these children were aged three years, than did factors relating to the home environment (such as marital discord, maternal depression and family adversities).

Earlier studies have also linked particular body types with particular behaviours. For instance, delinquents are more likely to be of a muscular build. However, such general observations are rarely helpful in clinical practices, since it is commonly found that a wide range of emotional symptoms may develop in various personality and bodily types.

Developmental aspects of depressive disorders

Depressive symptoms are more frequent among post pubescent children than among pre-pubescent children. They increase in prevalence markedly after about age 12 years, in both sexes. It has been suggested that the hormonal changes of puberty are responsible for an increase in the rate of depressive symptoms. However, the significance of the biological contribution of puberty is in fact unclear. Kosky and colleagues (1988) divided children referred to child psychiatric services into age groups, genders, pre and post puberty categories and into those with and without suicidal ideas. They concluded that the increase in suicidal ideas found among the older children was directly a function of age rather than of the subjects' pubertal status. However, more studies are needed before the issue is resolved.

In children, as in adults, depression may follow the experience of loss. In children this may include the separation of their parents. In most cases when parents separate, children stay in the care of the mother. In Australian studies, in two thirds of cases of parental separation, the newly single mother and children move to a new residence and this often means breaks with friends and school. In United Kingdom studies, one fifth of post divorce children rarely see their father again. This loss seems particularly hard for boys, who may become depressed and difficult to handle. These issues are covered in more detail in chapter 28.

Even in quite young children, separation from parents, if prolonged or numerous, can have significant effects. Anger and despair have been observed in hospitalised children separated from their parents. In severe cases, the child may seem to become emotionally detached from his parents and instead, becomes indiscriminately friendly to his nurses. Because of observations like these and the potential for long term personality disturbances, modern clinical practice is aimed at maintaining parental attachments while the child is in hospital. In modern hospitals, mother–child units have been provided and accommodation for parents or families now exist at most Childrens' Hospitals.

One of the psychosocial tasks facing adolescents is to develop attachments to peers. They may form the basis for further social development and later family life. Psycho-analysic theory suggests that before these attachments can occur, some of the emotional energy contained in the primary parent–child attachments must be given up. In terms of this theory, adolescence represents a time of vulnerability to depression because this process involves the loss of the primary attachment. Other, more socially based theories, have emphasised the important social tasks of adolescence, in particular the move from primary to high school or from school to work. These tasks are difficult for many adolescents because of high rates of unemployment and many young people may not be satisfactorily able to achieve independence. Failure to obtain work is associated with the development of symptoms of depression, which may in turn lead to excessive use of alcohol, and risk-taking behaviour with drugs, sex and motor vehicles.

In addition to these personal development issues, chronic marital discord in the home may produce a tense, uncomfortable environment leading to feelings of depression. Lack of warmth, praise, acceptance or love from parents is bound to create feelings of worthlessness in their children. Constant carping and challenging can lead children to despair of ever pleasing parents or winning their love.

Illness, especially chronic illnesses like cystic fibrosis, asthma and diabetes, may lead to a sense of continually battling against overwhelming odds. Depression can compli-cate virus infections, especially infectious mononucleosis (glandular fever) and influenza. Some young people may seek to alleviate their depressed feeling by using alcohol, cocaine or other drugs which, while temporarily working, only lead to worse feelings as they wear off.

Depressed children and adolescents have feelings of misery, sadness, worthlessness, hopelessness and guilt. They also invariably suffer sleep disturbances and usually eat less or, alternatively, they may binge on food. They lose concentration, lose interest in previously enjoyed activities, such as sport or clubs and do not contact friends, instead, tending to avoid social contacts. They may become slow in their movements or, less commonly, agitated. Suicidal thoughts may occur. Sometimes the depressed youngster becomes delusional and convinced he is ugly and worthless and that people are humiliating him.

Children who are depressed may run away from home (which may be the source of their depression), drink alcohol, take drugs and commit antisocial acts. These children, some of whom are very angry, may become caught up in the welfare or justice systems and receive scant psychiatric attention. Kosky and colleagues (1990) in a study of adolescents in custody reported that about 40 per cent had symptoms of depression, compared with about 10 per cent of adolescents in school.

Depressed children however, are usually quiet, conscientious, and withdrawn. Because of this, their condition is not often noticed by teachers or even by parents. Friends sometimes become alerted by suicide threats. Occasionally, the depressed child's irritability becomes a concern at home or school and is the signal that something is wrong. One alert teacher identified a depressed child in her class. He was 11 years old. She wrote to the psychiatrist and her letter, which is reproduced below, captures the features of such children.

Robert (a pseudonym) transferred to us at the beginning of this year and has been a student in my year five class from this time.

Physically he is always well groomed and tidy. He has obvious social problems with children of his own age. Robert does not communicate easily with his classmates and avoids social situations, including class discussions (small group or whole group), eating lunch on his own and not participating in group activities. He does, however, interact well with adults on a one-to-one basis. He has a poor self concept and generally is unhappy at school. Robert is frequently involved in social conflicts with other children and always sees himself as the 'victim'. When questioned about incidents and conflicts he often displays aggressive and sullen behaviour; invariably he cries during these crisis times. His academic achievements are poor in relation to the work often produced by students at this year level. Although Robert reads quite capably and for enjoyment, he rarely produces written or artistic responses to his reading.

Robert is only able to concentrate on a task for extremely short periods of time and rarely completes any work. He has little motivation to work and to achieve success. He is extremely reluctant to participate in any discussions and seems to spend a lot of time 'day dreaming'.

Suicidal behaviour in children and adolescents

Suicidal behaviour is commonly associated with symptoms of depression. Suicidal ideas are more common among children after about 12 years of age. About a quarter of all adolescents with depressive symptoms also develop suicidal ideas. Of those who think about suicide, about a quarter go on to make a suicide attempt.

Suicide is rare under the age of 12 years but children as young as six years have attempted suicide. In recent years the rate of suicide among teenagers has increased in Australia. The suicide rate for males 15 to 24 years is now around 30 per 100,000. For females the rate is about 13 per 100,000. Suicide is a leading cause of death in this age group.

In the 15 to 19 year old age group, females are more likely than males to attempt suicide. The lower suicide rate among females may be because they usually choose to poison themselves, a method which is relatively uncertain in outcome and allows time for medical intervention which could save lives. Boys choose more lethal means such as hanging and shooting. Some motor vehicle accidents involving young drivers may be suicide, so the actual suicide rate may be higher than the official records show.

Not a lot is known about the nature of suicide in young people. Much has been inferred from interviews with survivors of suicide and from suicide attempters. The characteristic feelings of worthlessness, hope-lessness, self blame and self denigration which accompany depression are almost invariably found among young people who have seriously attempted suicide. Thus, depressive illness is one dimension of the suicidal behaviour complex.

The other dimension appears to be the family interactions experienced by suicidal youngsters. Studies comparing suicidal children with non-suicidal children show that the suicidal group tends to come from families where there has been chronic tension and hostile interactions. Commonly these young people have witnessed violence between their parents or they have been the target of parental violence themselves and have been beaten or injured by their parents. Incestuous behaviour may cause a young victim to become suicidal.

Such families have usually become dysfunctional because of factors outside their control. Compared to other families, they have high levels of illnesses amongst the family members, financial problems, suffer losses due to separations and deaths and have other circumstances which place the parents and children under considerable psycho-social stress. The parents may lack the skills to overcome these adverse circumstances and so the families are plunged into a vicious circle of stress and adversity. Such family difficulties may culminate in a child's attempts at suicide.

Alongside the two main parameters of depression and chronic family dysfunction, another factor which studies associate with suicide attempts in children and adolescents is the personal experience of losses. Social supports, particularly someone who is close and affirmative, protect against the development of depression. Loss of these supports can result in grief, which may, in turn, become pathological depression. Such losses are more common than might be

supposed. Death of grandparents occurs for many young people during their teenage years and it is from grandparents that some adolescents get support and unqualified love. Separation of parents is also not uncommon and affects up to one in nine of all children before age 15 years.

Suicide attempts in adolescents are also associated with a history of use of alcohol or other drugs. Possibly depressed youngsters are more prone to use drugs because of the temporary mood elevating effect or pain relieving effect that is produced. For many, though, the longer term effects simply compound their innate depressive state and serve to increase their anguish and despair making a frank suicide bid more likely.

Treatment of emotional disorders

The management of emotional disorders in childhood and adolescence is similar in outline to that of adults with the added factor of the family which provides the immediate social environment for the child. No treatment of these disorders in young people is complete without taking the family into consideration.

Among physical treatments it is important to look at simple things such as diet, sleep times, exercise, and to advise correcting deficiencies in these. Medications aimed at reducing anxiety or at relieving depression are fully discussed in chapters 27, 28, 56 and 57. Medications form a useful adjunct to treatment in many cases and may be life-saving in severe depressions with suicidal ideation.

Psychological treatments vary. Some are based on learning principles, others involve the dynamics of the family or a group and others involve the working through of past personal experiences on an individual level.

Systematic analysis of behaviour and the application of corrective learning, such as with desensitisation to a feared situation or object, is of value in dealing with some anxiety states, panic attacks, phobias and obsessive–compulsive disorders.

Family therapy can be the primary mode of treatment for many forms of childhood emotional disorders. Here the emphasis is removed from the child whose symptoms are, instead, regarded as a sign of family dysfunction. Various methods of allowing the family members to identify and address their difficulties have been described (see chapters 59 and 60). *Groups* of other children and of parents have been used to help young people and parents learn new ways of dealing with their problems. These are addressed as they arise in the groups and the members and group leader attempt to develop more appropriate new methods to tackle these problems. Groups are particularly useful for learning social skills which can then be generalised outside the group.

On a larger scale, *milieu therapy* has proved especially effective in dealing with emotional disorders in childhood and adolescence. The development of a milieu does, however, require a stable child psychiatric inpatient unit.

Psychodynamic treatments based on psychoanalytic methods have proved useful in many forms of emotional disorder. Techniques have been developed to apply these methods to quite young children using play and play materials. A good knowledge of normal and abnormal child development is needed by the clinician before applying these techniques, otherwise the material brought forth by the child is apt to be misconstrued. These various psychological techniques are described in more detail in chapter 58.

More often than not alterations in the *social environment* of the child and family prove useful. Greater access to activities with peers (such as in Guides or Scouts) may improve social skills. Tutoring and a special educational program or a different school environment may increase confidence. More social activities for parents can take the focus off the child's problems. A bedroom separate from siblings may create new opportunities for the child to develop his own private resources. Sometimes the parents will benefit from working with a social welfare professional or a marriage guidance counsellor.

A decision may have to be made about *hospitalisation*. In the case of suicidal ideation or attempts, admission to hospital is usually the first consideration. If young people are sufficiently depressed to require anti-depressant medication, hospitalisation ought to be considered.

In the case of neurotic conditions which are crippling the child's activities, for example, severe handwashing or severe school refusal, hospital based treatment may be necessary. Nursing staff play an essential and crucial role in the management of hospitalised young people—both in day to day nursing care and as models of effective management of social and personal skills. This is discussed more fully in chapter 63.

It is salutory to remind ourselves that depression in childhood was not widely acknowledged by health workers prior to 1970. We have come a long way since then in the early identification and treatment of emotional disorders in childhood. Child psychiatric and mental health services have undergone considerable development and recently such services have developed closer links with schools and the community in trying to effect early changes to help children and adolescents in distress. One example is the 'whole school approach' where mental health workers are associated with selected schools and work closely with the teachers and parents where distressed children are identified. Many of these initiatives are currently being evaluated, so it should be possible to pick out the most effective of them.

Preventive measures have not been subject to the same level of intense development as the treatment methodologies, partly because they seem so complex. Yet, on closer examination, this may not prove to be the case. The struggles of parents who are unable to cope with overwhelming psychosocial stress have usually been identified in social welfare terms and efforts directed towards providing them with social support, such as money or housing. However, it may be more effective to consider their difficulties in terms of particular deficits in their interpersonal skills (for example, how to handle anger), their social skills (for example, how to utilise social supports), or their parental skills (for example, how to feed and wash babies). It is widely assumed that skills such as these are innate. It is usually overlooked that, in fact they are mostly learned, usually from parents. Hence, families with these personal and social deficits can span generations. Ante- and post-natal classes for mothers are one example of an attempt to deal with learning maternal care. At present, fathers are rarely encouraged to attend such classes!

Conclusion

In children and adolescents it is sometimes difficult to differentiate anxiety disorders from normal developmentally based anxieties, like separation anxiety. Health professionals should be guided by the age appropriateness of the anxieties, and by their severity, as to whether or not clinical intervention is required. Depressive disorders were long overlooked among children and adolescents. Now, it is widely recognised that they occur, and can be severe, and have a major impact on the young person's life. In extreme cases suicide attempts can occur and suicide is now a leading cause of death in 15 to 19 year olds. For depressive and anxiety disorders, treatments are usually effective.

References

Kosky R, McAlpine I and Silburn S, 'A Survey of Child Psychiatry Outpatients', *Australian & New Zealand Journal of Psychiatry*, Vol 19, 1985, pp 158-66.
Kosky R and Sawyer M G, 'Adolescents in Custody: Hidden Psychological Morbidity', *Medical Journal of Australia*, Vol 153, 1990, pp 24-7.
Zubrick S, Kosky R and Silburn S, 'Is Suicidal Ideation Associated with Puberty?' *Australian & New Zealand Journal of Psychiatry*, Vol 21, 1987, pp 54-8.

Further Reading

Bowlby J, *Attachment and Loss*, Vols I-III, Hogarth Press, London, 1974-1980.
Freud A, *Normality and Pathology in Childhood*, Penguin Books Ltd, Middlesex, 1973.
Haim A, *Adolescent Suicide*, Tavistock Publishers, London, 1970.
Rutter M and Hersov L, *Child Psychiatry: Modern Approaches*, 2nd ed, Blackwell Scientific Publication, Edinburgh, 1985.
Winnicott D W, *The Maturational Processes and the Facilitating Environment*, Hogarth Press, London, 1976.

Chapter 26

School Refusal

S P Ward

Definition

School refusal is a child's repeatedly stated intention of not attending school or, a child's rejection of attempts to get him to school despite having the physical capacity to be at school.

Truancy is absence from school without the consent of parents or school authorities, an absence occurring despite the child's expressed intent to attend school. It is often associated with anti-social behaviour. *School phobia* is the excessive, persistent and irrational fear of some aspect of school, leading to avoidance of school. It thus can manifest as school refusal.

Clinical features

School refusal often first shows itself at the beginning, or changing school or after a period of absence, such as vacation or following a minor illness. The onset may be sudden but is more often gradual with absences building up over a few weeks. The child can appear to be exceedingly frightened with concomitant physiological signs of anxiety (such as trembling, sweating, clammy hands, dry mouth, light-headedness) and panic attacks may be observed. A slower onset may present with physical symptoms such as nausea, vomiting, abdominal pains or headaches all of which may mimic physical disease. Dawdling behaviour may predominate until an outright refusal supervenes.

The child may express concern about a particularly feared aspect of school describing a teacher who has been unpleasant to him or bullying. This may appear to be trivial to an onlooker but to the child it seems all-threatening.

Previous personality

The child's coping style before the onset of refusal is variable. Many have been quiet, passive and conforming children who have been achieving appropriately in their school work. Some, however, have been more exuberantly outgoing and some have had academic difficulties.

Background

Various workers have described a family pathology that they believe is significant in the aetiology of school refusal. They describe an anxious, perhaps depressed parent who has had an overly close relationship with the refusing child. This 'special' relationship may have developed because of illnesses experienced by the child or because it is seen as special, for example, a last-born child. In this family pattern the other parent may be a somewhat passive person or can be absent due to death or separation.

Stress may be present for the child at school. There may be an unsympathetic teacher, peer group conflict or inappropriate academic expectations being placed on the child by parents and/or school.

Prevalence

Severe school refusal is not a common presentation in child psychiatric clinics. Severe refusal occurs in less than 1 per 1000 children, aged 10 to 11 years. Minor forms are much more common. Because of its association with changes in the school experience the age peaks are at 4 to 6 years and at 10 to 13 years. There is no particular social class trend.

Assessment

If the child presents with physical symptoms, medical investigations should be performed as quickly as possible to exclude physical disease. The child and family should then be given a definite statement by the assessing doctor that physical disease has been excluded as far as possible and attention needs to be given to emotional aspects of the presentation. Some families will want to avoid this emotional exploration and may request further medical tests.

In examining the emotions involved in the situation note should be taken of the child's temperamental characteristics. These characteristics, which are demonstrated early in the child's life, remain relatively stable and interact with the personalities, the expectations and the child-rearing styles of the parents. Thus the quiet, placid child can cause the anxious parent to become more anxious and this in turn communicated to the child. The family should be interviewed to further discern possible interactions that may be aetiologically relevant to the school refusal presentation, for example, marital difficulties with the child being exposed to arguments and threatened or actual separation.

It is essential for the health professional assessing the situation to contact the child's school to gain a broader view of the child, both academically and socially. Particular concerns that teachers may have about the child and their observations of the child in his various relationships should be obtained. Whilst such exploration can be done with a phone call, visits to the school may be required to establish the school's sensitivity to the child and the resources that they may be able to mobilise as part of the therapeutic effort.

Management

A formulation is developed around the various causal factors that may be involved. School refusal is a situation where the various professionals involved, together with the child's parents and in some situations the child, may have to meet in a case conference in order that the interplay between the emotional and physical symptoms can be delineated. The various role responsibilities of the professionals involved should be defined in order that overlap, with a possibility of attendant confusion, if not conflict, can be avoided.

Family therapy may be required to challenge maladaptive patterns of family interaction that may be present, particularly in relation to the intensity of the bond between a parent and the child, marital conflicts or sibling rivalry. A disengaged father may be given the task of taking his child to school in order to circumvent the separation anxiety present between a mother and the child. The therapist may involve himself in taking the child to school or may involve school personnel in this role.

The child's fears may be addressed in individual psychotherapeutic work. Fears about maternal well being, family dysfunction or the child's own experiences may be explored. These issues may not be consciously recognised by the child and sometimes can be attributed, through a process of projection, to school and its perceived authority in, and over, the child's life.

A sudden confrontation to the feared school situation may be appropriate with the therapist instructing that there be a rapid return to school. A more gradual systematic desensitisation to the school experience may be advisable and as part of this it may be appropriate for the child to attend full-time or part-time a psycho-educational facility with a small group emphasis and for this then to be overlapped with part-time return to the normal school situation.

Home tuition should be resisted as it may compound the avoidance by the family of the dynamic issues at play and in any case does nothing to help the child's inadequate social skills. Instruction in relaxation techniques to help alleviate anxiety or pain experiences may be warranted.

A short acting anxiolytic may be indicated to deal with intense anxiety in the morning. In the presence of symptoms of depression, a tricyclic antidepressant, like Imipramine, may offer a benefit as part of the comprehensive management of the situation.

An active liaison is usually required with the child's school to further define their involvement in management of the school refusal and in particular their role in behavioural techniques being employed.

The amount of attention that the school gives to physical symptoms should be clarified by the doctor. Who makes decisions about withdrawal of the child from the classroom situation into a sickroom, or even return home, needs to be carefully formulated.

A difficult case

Joanne, aged 14, was referred by a general practitioner at the instigation of her school.

Joanne and her family had come to Australia four months previously from the United Kingdom. In the United Kingdom there had been multiple moves for the family as her parents pursued a series of successful business enterprises. *Joanne* had attended five schools in this process and with each change of school had shown an initial reluctance to attend, a reluctance that would settle after several weeks at the new school.

Her parents had decided to emigrate to Australia believing that it would open up further profitable opportunities.

After visiting various places they had decided where they wished to reside but remained unclear as to whether to live in a city or the country. In the interim they had enrolled *Joanne* into a school and she had begun complaining of headaches each morning. Whilst the headaches would settle with analgesics they would recur during the mornings at school and persist until her parents were contacted to fetch her home. Her headaches had been extensively investigated by a general practitioner and whilst *Joanne*'s parents had accepted that there was no demonstrable physical illness they were reluctant to further expose her to distress and she had not attended school for two weeks prior to her referral.

Both in individual assessment and family assessment *Joanne* was diffident in presenting her concerns. She was depressed and a history

was obtained of an initial insomnia and awakening during the night.

Discussion with *Joanne*'s parents revealed her father's need to be successful following his own school failure. Whilst he could accept that *Joanne*'s new school had appeared to be responsive to her needs, he shared his daughter's view that she was not readily accepted by her peers.

Joanne was diagnosed as having a depression and was commenced on the antidepressant Imipramine. With this her disturbed sleep pattern settled and she regained her appetite. However, in both individual sessions and family sessions, she remained shy and reserved. *Joanne* returned to school after a school vacation. She was compliant with the efforts to get her to school in the mornings but again began to complain of headaches at school. The headaches would persist in spite of reassurance and *Joanne* undertaking relaxation exercises. The school felt that they could no longer devote school resources to caring for *Joanne* and they were required to ring her parents. Her father would respond rapidly to the school's summoning of him and it was discovered that he was waiting outside the school gates after dropping *Joanne* in the morning in the belief that he would probably be summoned anyway.

Joanne's parents were confronted with the opinion that the family's mobile lifestyle was detrimental to *Joanne*'s psychological and educational needs. However, her father was of the view that he would eventually find employment for *Joanne* in the business he had yet to establish. *Joanne*'s mother, who was passive throughout, concurred with her husband's opinion.

In an attempt to further challenge the intransigence of the situation *Joanne* was referred to two psycho-educational facilities but her parents rejected their offers of assistance and independently arranged for *Joanne* to have home tuition.

Prognosis

Most milder presentations of school refusal usually result in a rapid return to school. However, ongoing work may be required to give attention to individual and family psychopathology. More severe presentations, especially those in older children with more pervasive personality difficulties, may go on to later significant psychiatric disorders, for example, chronic anxiety neurosis or an avoidant personality disorder. A proportion of women with agoraphobia give a history of school refusal in their childhood.

Awareness by school, educational authorities, and primary health care workers can facilitate early intervention into school refusal before it becomes chronic. Extensive and protracted investigation of physical symptoms, unless based on solid clinical indications, can impede a rapid intervention.

Further Reading

Atkinson L, Quarrington B and Cyr J J, 'School Refusal: The Heterogeneity of a Concept', *Amer J Orthopsychiatry*, Vol 55 No 1, 1985, pp 83-101.
Hersov L and Berg I, *Out of School: Modern Perspectives in Truancy and School Refusal*, John Wiley & Sons, Chichester, 1980.

Chapter 27

Anxiety Disorders

L Evans and F K Judd

Anxiety

Anxiety is a common and normal emotion, essential for effective functioning. It is generally experienced as unpleasant and has a subjective feeling of foreboding. Any situation which threatens well-being may produce anxiety. Examples include personal conflicts, any type of frustration, threats of physical harm, threats to self-esteem and pressure to perform beyond one's capabilities. In such situations, anxiety is often protective, resulting in adaptive behaviour, to overcome or avoid the threat.

Pathological anxiety is defined in terms that relate to these normal reactions. Generally, it is defined as complaints of anxiety which are more frequent, more severe or more persistent than the individual is accustomed to, or can tolerate. A distinction is frequently made between 'state anxiety' and 'trait anxiety'. *State* anxiety refers to anxiety at a particular time, for example, 'I feel anxious now', while *trait* anxiety is equated with personality (anxious personality), a habitual tendency to be anxious in a variety of circumstances, for example, 'I often feel anxious'.

Anxiety *symptoms* are commonly found among patients in clinical situations. When present, symptoms may be due to an anxiety disorder, or may be secondary features of a variety of other psychological disorders, or may be due to an organic illness. Depression is commonly accompanied by anxiety. Anxiety may be a prominent feature of schizophrenia, particularly early in the course of that illness. Physical causes of anxiety are shown in Table 1. When anxiety symptoms first occur in patients over 40 years old, a physical cause should be strongly suspected. Substance intoxication and substance withdrawal are not uncommon among patients in mental health clinics.

Table 1. Physical causes of anxiety

Substance intoxication	eg caffeine, amphetamine, ritalin, cocaine
Substance withdrawal	eg alcohol, barbiturates
Endocrine disorders	eg hyperthyroidism, phaeo-chromocytoma, hypoglycaemia
Neurological disorders	eg temporal lobe epilepsy, cerebral tumor
Cardiovascular disorders	eg paroxysmal tachycardia

Anxiety *disorders* are common among the general population. In a recent New Zealand study, lifetime prevalences were found to be 31 per cent for generalised anxiety disorder, 11 per cent for phobias, 2 per cent for panic and 2 per cent for obsessive compulsive disorder. It has been estimated that anxiety disorders account for 15 per cent of the workload of Australian psychiatrists. Although not often treated as inpatients, individuals with anxiety disorders are frequently severely disabled by the severity and chronicity of their symptoms.

Symptoms of anxiety

The symptoms of anxiety are predominantly physical and it is often for diagnosis and treatment of these physical symptoms that the patient presents to the general practitioner or other medical specialist. Severe anxiety may also be one of the causes of the quest for oblivion or artificial boosts to confidence that can lead to the development of alcoholism and drug dependence. Anxiety is a complex response which can produce changes across three channels:

1. Physiological or physical
2. Psychological and cognitive
3. Behavioural

Common changes in each channel are as follows:

Physical symptoms

Anxiety can produce symptoms in virtually any system of the body, although an individual will generally only experience these in one or a few systems which are usually the same each time for that individual. On assessment, the patient may not complain of anxiety but may appear strained with a set facial expression and some tremulousness of the fingers.

Common physical symptoms are:

1. Increases in heart beat and respiration rate (and even hyperventilation), dropped heart beats, chest pain, sighing, yawning and fainting.
2. Gastro-intestinal disturbances such as dry mouth, nausea, vomiting, difficulty swallowing, indigestion, abdominal pain, increased flatulence and diarrhoea.
3. Headaches, vertigo, blurring of vision and tinnitus.
4. Body temperature changes with increased sweating.
5. Increased muscle tension with trembling, muscle twitching, cramps, loss of energy and chronic muscle pain.
6. Paraesthesia and tingling sensations.
7. Loss of sexual enjoyment, erectile impotence and menstrual disturbances.

Psychological and cognitive symptoms

The familiar physical concomitants of anxiety may be largely overshadowed by the psychological components of tension. The main complaints will be of a constant sense of being wound up and on the edge and of responding in a startled and irritable manner to all unexpected stimuli, no matter how trivial; loud noises are intolerable. There may be a constant feeling that something dreadful is about to happen which is termed a 'fear of impending doom'. Decisions are increasingly difficult to make, even about mundane or trivial matters, and there is a loss of normal spontaneity. Difficulties in concentration make reading, or even following a television program difficult and as assimilation is patchy through inattention, recall is often faulty and incomplete, presenting as a functional deficiency of memory. In elderly subjects, suspicion of an early senile dementia may not be possible to dispel without a period of observation. Tolerance of frustration is decreased and minor setbacks may precipitate explosions of rage or anger which are out of character. This is called irritability. Initial insomnia is common, sleep may be restless, unsatisfying and punctuated by frightening nightmares.

Many anxiety disorder sufferers have recurrent negative cognitions or thoughts. These may include a general sense of foreboding, recurrent agonising over past mistakes, or an exaggerated fear of failure or misfortune. Particular sorts of cognitions are commonly associated with specific anxiety disorders. For example, social phobics tend to think a lot about being rejected or disapproved of by others. When anxiety has been continuously present for some time, depression will often occur and depressive symptoms are particularly prominent in the middle aged and elderly patients. Only a very few people enjoy the feeling of anxiety: for most, it is an unpleasant feeling. Derealisation and/or depersonalisation are common symptoms.

Behavioural symptoms

These changes predominantly are non-verbal behaviours and/or avoidance:

1. Wincing, tics, nervous gestures, avoidance.
2. Rigid symmetrical posture.
3. Verbal dysfluency, resembling a mild thought disorder.
4. Avoidance of anxiety producing stimuli.

It is important to note that individuals vary enormously in the extent to which they experience these various symptoms. It is also significant that these channels are asynchronous. That is, responses across channels are not strongly correlated. It is not unusual for a person to have a strong physiological response but little cognitive response when anxious, or vice versa, which complicates diagnosis.

A special mention of avoidance behaviours needs to be made as these have diagnostic implications. A persistent or recurrent, irrational fear of a particular object, place or situation accompanied by a compelling desire to *avoid* it is referred to as a phobia. One of the commonest forms of phobia is agraphobia, the fear of being in public places. Other phobias include social phobia in which the person is afraid of behaving in front of other people in a way that would be humiliating or embarrassing. The term simple phobia refers to a fear of a fairly narrowly circumscribed object or situation. Examples include heights (acrophobia), closed spaces (claustrophobia), specific animals or insects, plane travel and so on.

Aetiology

There have been many theories about anxiety development. Freud was very influential in the development of psychodynamic theory and proposed that anxiety disorders are an unsuccessful attempt to resolve unconscious emotional conflicts. Important features of this approach are an emphasis upon early traumatic childhood development, the symbolic rather than actual significance of the anxiety inducing stimuli and the role of the anxiety as an ego defence mechanism (see chapter 2).

Freud used the term neurosis in this context. Prior to Freud's work, these conditions had generally been considered to be physical illnesses and it was Freud who brought attention to the psychological aspects of their aetiology and presentation. He described three forms of anxiety which were free-floating anxiety, phobic anxiety and a spontaneous form of anxiety which we now term the panic attack.

An alternative viewpoint is the behavioural theory which views anxiety as learned behaviour. Anxiety is considered to be acquired, like all other behaviour via modelling and direct experience.

There is now evidence that some of the anxiety disorders, at least, have a genetic factor in their aetiology and hence possibly some biological or biochemical basis to them. This has been argued most strongly for panic disorder with and without agoraphobia and for obsessive–compulsive disorder. Other causative models are discussed under the specific anxiety syndromes.

Treatment

General

Most varieties of psychological and physical treatments have been applied to anxiety disorders in the past. The importance of psychological factors in the aetiology of the neuroses has led to a predominance of such approaches therapeutically. Drug therapy is of importance for symptomatic relief of anxiety symptoms, particularly as this relates to autonomic hyperactivity and the subjective feelings of anxiety, fear and depression. Such therapeutic intervention has a particularly important part to play in preventing the escalation of complex anxiety disorders. However, dangers of drug dependence, particularly in those disorders where anxiety is prominent, should be carefully considered by therapists.

The introduction in the 1950s and 1960s of specific behavioural approaches to the management of anxiety disorders caused a revision of traditional ideas, so that a combination of relaxation training and systematic desensitisation by imaginal procedures became widely used. Further, refinements of behavioural techniques in recent years have produced other effective procedures for controlling anxiety and changing the behaviour and cognitions of sufferers. The currently held view is that better results are obtained from treatment which combines the different approaches.

Fortunately nowadays, many sufferers from the more severe forms of anxiety disorders present early in the course of their illness, as a result of public awareness of these conditions and a decrease in the stigma attached to them. The initial interview is vitally important, as it is during this interview that the therapeutic alliance must be established. It is absolutely essential to develop a good therapeutic relationship in order to treat the patient effectively, as, for example, those who have become phobic will eventually be asked to do those things which they believe to be impossible and to do this, they must have absolute trust in the therapist. For such a relationship to develop, it is important to give the patient plenty of time to describe their symptoms which they often do in great detail. Sometimes they will recount some detail in a way which suggests that they believe themselves to be the only person to have ever experienced such a feeling.

Once the symptoms have been recounted and a full history taken with a mental state examination, the diagnosis can usually be made. A major role of the general practitioner or other medical specialist in the management of these conditions is to identify them correctly, early in their course, saving the patient from unnecessary and sometimes intensive and expensive investigation and also the distress and inconvenience that these investigations and the illness itself can cause.

The diagnosis of phobic conditions depends on the recognition of the features outlined above and the exclusion of other physical and psychiatric conditions. Rarely, anxiety disorders can occur secondarily to, or be mimicked by physical conditions, such as thyrotoxicosis, labyrinthitis, Meniere's disease, temporal lobe epilepsy, cardiovascular syncope and phaeochromocytoma. More commonly, substance abuse or withdrawal can be responsible for the symptoms. At this stage it is important to give the condition a name and to reassure the patient firmly, that they are not mad and that they do not have some serious physical illness and that others suffer from this relatively common condition. Explanation of the condition and further education about it (aided by the use of books or instructional pamphlets if desired) will give reassurance and increase compliance with an intended regime of treatment.

Patients who are likely to discontinue treatment because their symptoms prevent them from attending outpatient treatment need inpatient admission as do those who are physically dependent on drugs or alcohol. Those patients who are extremely disturbed by their condition are better referred for specialist psychiatric consultation as are those in whom there is some doubt about the diagnosis. Where the symptoms are thought to be secondary to some other psychiatric condition, it is probably wise to refer the patient for a fully psychiatric assessment.

Drug treatment

Benzodiazepines. The benzodiazepines are effective in treating anxiety and do give relief to sufferers. They lower the overall level of anxiety and can reduce anticipatory anxiety. However, underarousal, which can be produced by excessive use of anxiolytics can interfere as much as excessive anxiety with the learning required when behavioural therapies are used. A certain degree of anxiety is necessary for exposure techniques to be effective.

It is best to avoid the shorter-acting members of this group of drugs if they are to be used on a continuous basis, as they can produce symptoms of withdrawal resembling anxiety. Many agoraphobic patients who are on regular long term treatment with these drugs will experience such withdrawal symptoms and might even have panic attacks induced by them. Taking further doses of the drug will relieve the symptoms, but can reinforce habituation and dependence. For long term use, the longer acting compounds are better, as blood levels fall more gradually and do not trigger off anxiety. The shorter acting benzodiazepines are more useful when used on an infrequent basis or for a short term. In theory, it is easier to wean patients off the long acting than the short acting benzodiazepines.

Tricyclic antidepressants. These drugs are helpful in reducing anxiety, blocking panic attacks in patients whose attacks are spontaneous, and dealing with some of the symptoms of depression commonly associated with the anxiety disorders. Those tricyclic antidepressants with a preferential action on 5-Hydroxy tryptamine (5-HT) have been shown to be useful in the treatment of obsessive compulsive disorder.

Monoamine oxidase inhibitors. Early work with the monoamine oxidase inhibitors (MAOIs) showed that they were effective in the treatment of 'atypical' depression and in patients with reactive depression who showed anxiety, hysterical, 'anxiety hysterical' symptoms and severe phobic anxiety symptoms as prominent features in their illness. Since this time, there have been many studies which have shown a positive effect of MAOIs in the treatment of agoraphobia, presumably by their action on panic attacks. Despite their effectiveness, the MAOIs are not widely used and should probably only be initially prescribed by specialist psychiatrists.

Beta-blockers. There is evidence that these drugs are effective in the treatment of the somatic symptoms of anxiety. These drugs only block the somatic symptoms, (for example, increased heart beat) and not the psychic experience of anxiety. They do not assist in giving up avoidance behaviour.

Other drugs. The 5–HT reuptake blocking drugs have been shown to be effective in treating agoraphobia with panic attacks and obsessive compulsive disorder. This augers well for the introduction of newer drugs with similar activity on 5–HT and a number of which are becoming available.

Behaviour therapy

Most other techniques of behaviour treatment require specialist assistance to be used appropriately and effectively. However, there are a number of useful and less complicated behavioural techniques which are most effective and which can easily be taught to the patient by the general practitioner. These include relaxation, hyperventilation control, the use of distraction techniques, keeping a behavioural diary, instruction in cognitive restructuring and thought stopping. Other more complex behavioural techniques are the exposure or desensitisation techniques, both graduated and flooding, and response prevention used in the treatment of avoidance (ie phobic) and obsessive compulsive behaviour (see chapter 58).

Psychotherapy

Supportive psychotherapy and counselling are most important and can help the individual to look more objectively at their behaviour and at some of the problems responsible for this. Group therapy is of value and is also most effective when it is run using an eclectic psychoeducational model. Some patients require more intensive forms of psychotherapy, but these are not now considered by most to be the treatments of first choice for the majority of patients with anxiety disorders (see chapters 25, 26 and 27).

Other treatments

These include stress management, marital therapy, treatment of alcohol and drug dependence and are used as and when appropriate.

Conclusions

Anxiety and phobic disorders are common, chronic and they can be debilitating. Treatment is most successful when a variety of biological, psychological and social therapies are combined. While treatment should initially focus on target anxiety symptoms, personal, social and vocational issues must also be addressed if the significant morbidity, due to these disorders, is to be reduced.

Further Reading

Freud S, *Introductory Lectures on Psycho-analysis*, George Allen and Unwin Ltd, London, 1922.
Hawton K, Salkovskis P, Kirk J and Clark D M, *Cognitive Behaviour Therapy for Psychiatric Problems: A Practical Guide*, Oxford University Press, New York, 1989.
Judd F K, Norman T R and Burrows G D, 'Pharmacological Treatment of Panic Disorder', *International Clinical Psychopharmacology*, Vol 1, 1986, pp 3–16.
Klein D F, 'Anxiety Reconceptualised', *Comprehensive Psychiatry*, Vol 21, No 6, 1980, pp 411–27.
Klein D F and Rabkin J, *Anxiety, New Research and Changing Concepts*, Raven Press, New York, 1981.

Marks I M, *Fears, Phobias and Rituals, Panic, Anxiety and Their Disorders*, Oxford University Press, New York, 1987.

Matthews A M, Gelder M G and Johnston D W, *Agoraphobia: Nature and Treatment*, Guilford Press, New York, 1981.

Roth M, 'Agoraphobia, Panic Disorder and Generalised Anxiety Disorder: Some Implications of Recent Advances', *Psychiatric Development*, Vol 2, 1984, pp 31–52.

Chapter 28

Affective (Mood) Disorders

P R Joyce

Depression and mania are the psychiatric disorders combined under the term of mood or affective disorders, on the assumption that a disorder of mood is the primary underlying abnormality. Both depression and mania have been described since antiquity, and have long and fascinating histories. Today there is still debate as to whether depression and mania should be seen as diseases, or as deviations from normality, or as reactions to psychological stressors. These positions are not necessarily mutually incompatible and debates are likely to continue for some time. However, it is important to have an understanding of the range of human suffering caused by depression and mania, to have some diagnostic system for classifying abnormalities of mood, and to have some understanding of the aetiology and treatment of these disorders.

Depression as a term has a variety of meanings and can refer to the *mood* of depression (comparable terms are sad, 'blue', unhappy); to a syndrome (in which a person who feels sad also has associated symptoms such as inability to concentrate, lack of energy, loss of interest, reduced appetite and insomnia); or to a disorder of depression (in which the person has a depressive syndrome and it is assumed that this syndrome is a primary disorder in its own right).

Although it has always been recognised that most people will feel sad and depressed under certain circumstances, it has also long been recognised that some people become depressed to a degree out of keeping with their circumstances. Some traditional diagnostic systems attempted to classify

depressions on the basis of an assumed aetiological basis, and termed those depressions that occurred after an upsetting life event as 'reactive' and those depressions which occurred spontaneously as 'endogenous'. Although there may be some justification for this type of diagnostic system such as the American Psychiatric Association's Diagnostic and Statistical Manual of Mental Disorders (DSM-III) third revision have avoided assumptions about causality, and classify mood disorders on the basis of their symptoms. This is not to say that some day in the future when more is understood about the aetiology and pathophysiology of mood disorders, that an aetiological and/or pathophysiological classification system could not be developed, but at present this is not the case.

Clinical features

Although there is consensus as to the core features of severe depressive and manic syndromes, there is considerably more debate about the less severe syndromes and the optimal way of classifying mood disorders. It is therefore helpful to begin by knowing about the clinical features of the more severe depressions and manias, and then to contrast these with the less severe disorders. When we have an understanding of the varying clinical pictures, it is then appropriate to consider the classification of the mood disorders.

Mania

The central mood change is one of elation or euphoria, and the associate symptoms are increases in the sense of well-being, self-esteem, energy and sexual drive. In addition, thoughts race and there is a decreased need for sleep. When mania is mild (hypomania) the above symptoms may be pleasant and a person may become more productive, witty and creative. However, as the manic state increases in severity, the mood becomes increasingly irritable, subjectively distressing and unstable. With this increase in severity of the manic state the thought content becomes increasingly grandiose, overactivity becomes marked, speech becomes very rapid and social judgment is impaired leading to inappropriate sexual activity, spending sprees, or reckless driving. Delusions, hallucinations and thought disorder may also occur.

Typically, the delusions associated with mania are grandiose; examples are that one is the most beautiful person in the world, that one is God, that one has special powers or a special mission in life. However, it is not uncommon for delusions to be of a persecutory or paranoid nature. The content of hallucinations tends to reflect the grandiose ideas.

Usually, manic episodes develop over a matter of days or weeks, and if untreated may last several months. However, there can be marked variations on this general pattern, and episodes can develop over a matter of hours and last for just a few days or up to many months or, infrequently, years.

Major depression

The central mood change in melancholia or severe depression is a dysphoric, unpleasant or sad mood. However, some psychiatrists believe that the core of severe depression is the loss of interest and the loss of the ability to enjoy pleasurable events. Associated with dysphoric mood and the loss of interest and pleasure, is a loss of the sense of self worth, a tendency to blame oneself for real or imagined wrongs, a feeling that one should be punished, ruminating over misfortune, a feeling that life is not worth living, suicidal thoughts and actions, a change in appetite or weight (usually appetite and weight loss), a change in sleep (of special importance is the inability to stay asleep), a slowing of thought and actions (psychomotor retardation).

In severe depression the thought content can be delusional, and the most common depressive delusional themes are those of worthlessness, guilt and nihilism. However, hypochondriacal and paranoid delusions are also not uncommon. Similarly, auditory hallucinations which may occur usually have depressive content, such as hearing voices saying that the person is bad and would be better off dead. Thought disorder, if present, is usually related to a slowing of the thought processes and in the extreme a patient can be mute.

A severe depressive syndrome with all the above symptoms has been called by many names, including: endogeneous, melancholic, endogenomorphnic, vital, psychotic or retarded depression. There is no controversy about the existence of such a syndrome, the controversy is about the relationship between states and other depressive conditions which are less clearly abnormal.

Mixed mood states

Patients who experience both manic and depressive states (ie patients with bipolar affective disorder) may develop mixed mood states at various times. In these conditions the patient experiences simultaneous, or rapid alternation between, both manic and depressive states. The most common mixed mood state is that of a patient who is over-active and pressured in speech, yet has depressive thought content.

Other depressive states

Some patients who have depressive symptoms may have only a few symptoms of severe depression. It is likely that these depressive states reflect a variety of conditions, some of which are very akin to severe depression while others border upon normal states and may be more closely linked to a person's life situation and/or their personality.

One subgroup of these depressive states which is of interest is so-called 'atypical depression'. This term has been used in a variety of ways. One describes those depressions with reversed 'vegetative' symptoms (ie weight gain, over sleeping).

Another describes those depressions which are associated with marked anxiety symptoms. This latter group is of interest because of some evidence that they may respond preferentially to monoamine oxidase inhibitor antidepressant drugs.

Classification of mood disorders

In developing a system for classifying mood disorders it is first necessary to establish the presence of a mood syndrome and to know its duration and persistence. If a mood syndrome (whether depressive or manic) occurs as part of a physical disease then such a syndrome is termed an organic affective disorder.

Organic affective disorder

An example of an organic affective disorder is the depressive syndrome which so often accompanies Addison's disease, which is due to a deficiency of adrenal corticosteroids. However, a depressive syndrome which is not caused and sustained by the physical illness is not termed an organic affective disorder (for example, a patient who develops a depressive syndrome following a myocardial infarction is not considered to have an organic affective disorder).

Bipolar affective disorder

The next issue in classification is whether the patient has ever suffered from a manic episode. If the patient has ever had a manic episode then the patient has a *bipolar affective disorder*. When a patient has had a clear cut manic episode there is no difficulty in making this diagnosis. However, many patients who present mainly with depressive episodes also at some time experience mild manic episodes (*hypomania*) and there are other patients who only develop mania if treated with an anti-depressant. Although most diagnostic systems do not have explicit diagnostic criteria for such disorders, it is useful to note that the patient has an atypical bipolar disorder rather than to ignore the evidence of a bipolar tendency.

This disorder is most likely to first occur between the ages of 15 and 30 years, although it can begin earlier or later. It may begin abruptly with either a manic or a depressive episode, although for some patients the onset is more insidious and the person may have suffered from mild mood swings for some years, which may date back to childhood. Bipolar disorder is an illness with a high likelihood of recurrence, however most patients have times when they are completely well between episodes of disorder.

Depressive disorders

When we move to the non-organic, non-bipolar depressive disorders there is considerably more controversy as to the best method of classification.

There is general agreement that there is a *severe depressive disorder*. This disorder is characterised by the onset of a severely depressed mood accompanied by loss of interest in previously enjoyed activities and feelings of worthlessness, guilt, hopelessness and helplessness. There may be recurrent suicidal thoughts or impulses, and sometimes a suicide attempt. Physical symptoms are characteristic and include insomnia (or a continual urge to sleep), slowness of action or sometimes agitation, fatigue, pain, loss of appetite and usually weight loss. In ICD-9 this condition is referred to as manic-depressive psychosis, depressed type. In this classification system a similar depressive type of psychosis can occur apparently provoked by a saddening stress such as bereavement or severe disappointment. In DSM-III-R severe forms of this disorder are referred to as melancholia. In both cases delusion and hallucinations (characteristically gloomy, frightening and guilt ridden) may be present.

Major depression may have its onset at any age, but most commonly starts during early and mid adult life. Like bipolar affective disorder, it has a tendency to recur, although this is not as marked as with bipolar disorder. However, probably half of the people who suffer from one episode of major depression will at some stage have another episode.

A patient who does not meet the strict criteria in DSM-III-R for bipolar or major depressive disorder could still meet the criteria for cyclothymia or dysthymia. *Cyclothymia* is usually a mild form of bipolar disorder and represents a disorder with recurrent but mild manic and depressive mood changes. *Dysthymia* is a chronic (ie, minimum of two years' duration) depressive state of varying severity. Dysthymias are almost certainly heterogeneous, and some are chronic (and perhaps mild) variations of bipolar disorder or of major depression, while others are more akin to a depressive personality or arise secondary to some other psychiatric or medical disorder.

Epidemiology

In the course of a lifetime approximately 1 per cent of the population will suffer from a manic episode, and thus the lifetime prevalence of bipolar affective disorder is also about 1 per cent. Given the high tendency to recurrence in bipolar disorder, about 0.5 per cent of the population may experience an episode of this disorder within any year. Bipolar disorder occurs at much the same rate in men and women.

Major depression is considerably more common than bipolar disorder and has a life-time prevalence of 5 to 10 per cent in men, and of 10 to 20 per cent in women. The six month prevalence of major depression is approximately 2 to 4 per cent in men and 3 to 8 per cent in women. Traditionally it was believed that major depression was most common in middle and late adult life. However, there is currently considerable interest in the probability that the epidemiology of major depression is changing; it appears that major depression is becoming more prevalent, that the difference between females and males is decreasing and the depression is first occurring at a younger age.

Aetiology

Genetics

There is no doubt, based on twin, adoption and family studies that bipolar affective disorder is caused largely by genetic factors. Despite recent research using DNA markers the mechanism of inheritance is uncertain, but it is most likely that bipolar disorder is genetically heterogeneous. Furthermore,

genetic factors are aetiologically more important in the early onset rather than the late onset bipolar disorders, which further highlights the aetiological heterogeneity of bipolar disorder.

Genetic factors are almost certainly important in the aetiology of major depression, although the effect is less than in bipolar disorder, and the evidence is less convincing. As in bipolar disorder, genetic factors may be more important in those depressions which start early in life rather than later in life. Also of note is that while both bipolar disorder and major depression occur in excess in relatives of bipolar patients, only major depression occurs at a greater than chance rate in relatives of patients with major depression.

Childhood experiences
See chapters 4, 7, and 25.

The adult social environment

There has been considerable interest, especially among women, as to the role of lack of employment outside the house, the absence of a confidant, and the presence of three or more young children in the home, as risk factors for depression. Recent studies have not consistently found these three features to be risk factors for the development of depression, although all require further research. Another important issue is the quality of the relationship with one's spouse; even if the evidence that this is of aetiological importance is inadequate, a poor relationship with one's spouse seems to be clearly associated with a poor outcome if a patient becomes depressed.

Personality

While it is clear that most people who develop a bipolar affective disorder and many who develop a major depression had no marked abnormalities of personality prior to the onset of their affective disorder, it also seems that people of certain personality types may be at increased risk of depression. Thus people with antisocial, borderline, obsessive compulsive and dependent personality disorders seem to be at increased risk of suffering from major depression.

Although, in some instances personality disorders clearly predate the onset of a depressive episode, abnormal behaviour as a result of depression may mask the presence of a depressive disorder. It is also becoming apparent that in some patients a personality disturbance may follow from the affective disorder, especially if it is chronic or partially treated.

Recent life events

There is considerable evidence that adverse life events are associated with the onset of depressive episodes, and possibly with manic episodes. It is also clear however that the presence or absence of adverse life events before the onset of a depressive episode is not clearly associated with any particular symptom pattern, nor does it necessarily indicate that the depression will improve without antidepressant drugs, or that it is less likely to recur in the future.

Physiological factors

Although childbirth is a complicated bio-psycho-social event, rather than just a physiological process, it is a potent event for precipitating depressive and manic episodes in some people, and it now seems that the vast majority of post partum psychiatric disorders are of an affective nature. Important risk factors for the development of a post partum depressive episode are a family history or a past history of affective disorder. Patients with bipolar history are especially prone to post partum disorders, and perhaps a third of women with bipolar disorder will experience a post partum affective episode.

Since antiquity it has been noted that there may be a seasonal pattern to the onset of affective episodes in many patients, with an excess of depressive episodes commencing in autumn and spring, and an excess of manic episodes in spring–summer. Recent years have also witnessed the clarification of a syndrome called *seasonal affective disorder*, in which the most common pattern is for a depressive episode to occur during the winter and to lift in spring. This disorder is also of interest because of the evidence that it may be treated by exposing the patient to bright light, which via the retina and pineal gland may affect adrenergic function.

It is also important to note that certain drugs (especially some antihypertensive drugs such as reserpine, alpha-methyl dopa and beta-blockers), may precipitate depressive episodes in some people. Similarly, certain physical illnesses, such as viral infections and myocardial infarctions, may precipitate depressive episodes.

Neurobioligical aspects of mood disorders

As the more severe major depressive disorders and bipolar affective disorder can occur so clearly without any psycho-social precipitants, and because genetic factors are so clearly of aetiological importance, there has been considerable interest in the neurobiological changes which occur in depression (and in mania). Over twenty-five years ago it was postulated that depression was associated with a depletion of noradrenaline and/or serotonin in the brain. The evidence for this hypothesis came from two main sources: drugs such as reserpine which induce depression in some people deplete stores of noradrenaline and serotonin in brain synapses, while antidepressant drugs such as tricyclic antidepressants and monoamine oxidase inhibitors increase the availability of these amines at central synapses by promoting the reuptake of the amines or by blocking their breakdown. This co-called 'amine hypothesis is depression' has stimulated considerable research, but it seems increasingly that it is not correct in its simple form. Over recent years there has been less emphasis on absolute levels of the brain amines and more interest in changes in amine receptor activity. Again this has come about because of evidence that the more important drug action for anti-depressant effectiveness is not amine reuptake but changes in adrenergic receptor functioning.

Concurrently with the biochemical research on the amine hypothesis of depression, other researchers have been studying hormonal and sleep changes in depression. Ultimately, these may be linked to the biochemical changes which occur in the brain, and it already seems that noradrenaline and serotonin are implicated in the hormonal and sleep disturbances of depression. Many such abnormalities have been documented in major depression, with the most studied being the increased cortisol production which occurs in many patients with major depression. This cortisol hypersecretion may be indirectly assessed by the dexamethasone suppression test, although a number of factors preclude this test from wide clinical usage. The most consistent sleep electroencaphalogram abnormality which has been shown to occur in depression is a shortened REM (rapid eye movement) latency. This is the time it takes for a person to enter their first episode of REM sleep after falling asleep. Normally, this is about 90 minutes, but can be very much shorter in some depressed patients.

The clinical significance of these neuro-endocrine and sleep markers is still being studied, but it appears that the presence of either a shortened REM latency or of cortisol hypersecretion may indicate the presence of a depressive disorder which is unlikely to improve in the short term unless anti-depressant drugs or ECT (electroconvulsive therapy) are used. It also appears that if cortisol hypersecretion does not normalise even if the patient is feeling much improved with treatment, then the patient is unlikely to stay well. Cortisol hypersecretion may also be associated with an increased suicide risk.

Treatment and management of major depression

Recognition and diagnosis

One of the biggest challenges for the better treatment of major depression is to enable better recognition of this disorder. The majority of patients with major depression do not see psychiatrists but are treated in general medical practice or are seen by other health professionals. It is thus important for all medical practitioners and allied health professionals to be able to recognise it. It has been suggested that the most useful questions to ask to detect depression reliable in health care settings are: (i) Have you had low energy?

(ii) Have you had loss of interests? (iii) Have you lost confidence in yourself? (iv) Have you felt hopeless? If a patient answers yes to any of these, go on and ask: (v) Have you had difficulty concentrating? (vi) Have you lost weight due to poor appetite? (vii) Have you been waking early? (viii) Have you felt slowed up? (ix) Have you tended to feel worse in the morning? Patients who answer yes to two of these questions have a 50 per cent chance of having a clinically important depressive disorder, and for scores above this, the probability rises sharply. Note that none of these questions enquire about mood per se, and many patients when told they have a depressive disorder say, 'but I don't feel depressed', however, virtually all will admit to not being their normal selves.

A management plan

Once the diagnosis of major depression has been made the next issue is the management of the patient. The first point is to find out what the patient understands about depression and what is likely to be acceptable treatment for the patient. The second point is to assess where and by whom the patient should be treated; do they need to be hospitalised, do they need specialist psychiatrist care, or can they be well treated in general medical practice? Most depression can be adequately treated in general practice with psychiatrists being referered the severe, chronic, recurrent or complicated depressions and those at greatest risk of suicide. A number of factors determine this decision, including the severity of the depression, the adequacy of social support, the risk of suicide, and occasionally whether the patient is homicidal. The most common situation in which one needs to enquire about harm to others is in the case of a mother with young children, when homicidal thoughts towards the young children may be present.

The next issue to decide upon is whether the patient is likely to require psychotropic drugs, or electroconvulsive therapy (ECT), or whether it is likely that the patient could improve with psychosocial treatments alone. If the patient has a major depression of at least moderate severity, and especially if there are a number of melancholic symptoms, or a past or family history of clear response to antidepressants, then an anti-depressant drug should almost certainly be prescribed.

Another issue to decide is what type of psychological intervention is appropriate. Would the patient benefit from psychotherapy, or does the patient require personal support while waiting for the antidepressants to work? This issue does not have to be decided immediately, and often psychotherapeutic work takes on greater importance after there has been some improvement in the patient's mood as a result of medication.

Other issues relate to whether significant people in the patient's life should be involved, and if so, in what way? How often does the patient need to be seen over the first period of time? Should the patient's partner, friend or parent also be invited to contact the therapist if difficulties arise? Should the patient continue his normal living routine? All of these issues should be considered for all patients and are not mutually exclusive. Thus a decision to prescribe antidepressant drugs does not mean that psychotherapy or supportive measures should not be used.

Psychotropic drugs

The tricyclic antidepressants and related drugs are the mainstay of the treatment of major depression. The original tricyclic antidepressant drugs, amitriptyline and imipramine, have not been surpassed in terms of efficacy by the wide range of antidepressants now available. All available antidepressants have some side effects, but with proper explanation, most patients can tolerate them without too much difficulty. All the antidepressants require one to four weeks for them to be effective, and given that side effects will occur immediately, patients must be told about this delayed action.

It is now known that there are marked differences in the way individuals react to the tricyclic antidepressant drugs. Thus, it is difficult to talk of an average dose or of a dose that will be sufficient for everyone. With drugs such as amitriptyline and imipramine, effective dosages probably range from 75 mg to 350 mg per day, although lower dosages

will be appropriate in the elderly. Tricyclics can usually be prescribed on a once daily basis at night, and it is usually necessary to gradually increase the dosage over a number of days or weeks.

With depressed patients who have delusions the likelihood that the patient will response to an antidepressant drug alone is quite low, and the patient may require an antidepressant–antipsychotic drug combination or ECT.

If a first trial with an antidepressant fails to produce a marked effect by six weeks, after having reviewed the patient's history, there are then a further series of treatment options. It is reasonable to try a different tricyclic antidepressant. Another option is to change to a monoamine oxidase inhibitor. This may be especially indicated in 'atypical' depression when there are considerable accompanying anxiety symptoms. Another option is to add lithium to the antidepressant which the patient is already taking. If these options fail there is still ECT and other drug combinations including the addition of thryoxine, or combining a tricyclic and monoamine oxidase inhibitor (see chapters 56, 57).

Other physical therapies

In the very severe depressions, and especially if psychotic symptoms occur as part of the depression, or if antidepressants have failed to be effective, then ECT may be indicated. ECT is given as a series of treatments (usually two or three per week) over two to four weeks. This treatment involves the patient under anaesthesia receiving an electric current applied to the head with the objective of inducing a seizure. Despite controversy which at times surrounds ECT, it is still generally considered to be effective and safe treatment for some patients.

Very occasionally a depressed patient who has failed to respond to a variety of treatments, and yet who is still seriously depressed, may be considered for psychosurgery.

Other physical therapies which have been used with some success in some depressed patients include exposure to bright light (especially for those with seasonal affective disorder), and sleep deprivation.

Psychotherapies

There is now considerable evidence that for some people with major depression both inter-personal psychotherapy are effective treatments. Interpersonal psychotherapy focuses on the patient's thoughts and feelings about current important relationships, while cognitive therapy concentrates on the patient's way of thinking and particularly tries to alter negative thoughts. Antidepressant drugs probably work best on symptoms, while inter-personal psychotherapy may have a special role in preventing relapse. Combinations of antidepressant drugs and of psychotherapies are probably superior to either alone for many patients, and there is no evidence that combining treatments negates the effective-ness of the other.

Outcome and longer term management

Untreated, most but not all, major depressive episodes will spontaneously remit over a number of months. However, a proportion, even with optimal treatment, may run a chronic course. After recovery from an episode of major depression there is a high likelihood of relapse in the immediate aftermath, and it is usual to prevent early relapse. Even after sustained recovery major depression can recur, and probably about 50 per cent of patients who have one episode of major depression will at some stage of their life have another episode of depression. When a patient has had three or more episodes of depression, the likelihood of recurrence is very high and long term prophylactic medication may be necessary to prevent relapse. With each episode of major depression there is some risk that the depression will become chronic.

In both the short and in long term, the most alarming complication of an episode of major depression is suicide. Probably about one to two per cent of patients will die by suicide within the first year of having their depresssive episode, with more dying over the next few years. Over the first year hopelessness, loss of the ability to enjoy pleasurable events (anhedonia), anxiety, panic attacks, associated alcohol abuse and cortisol hypersecretion are probable risk factors for suicide.

Treatment and management of bipolar affective disorder

Diagnosis

Whereas the majority of patients with major depression are treated in general practice, the majority of patients with bipolar affective disorder are at some stage likely to be seen by psychiatrists. This is because of the more disruptive nature of manic, as opposed to depressive episodes. If the first presentation of a bipolar disorder is as a major depressive episode, the bipolar nature of the disorder may not be recognised, although in young depressed patients (under 25 years) with delusions, hypersomnia and retardation, or a loaded family history of affective disorder, the likelihood of a future manic episode is high. If the first presentation of a bipolar affective disorder is as a manic episode, the differential diagnosis of manic episodes is important, and it is now clear that many manic patients on first presentation were previously diagnosed as having schizophrenia, presumably because of the frequent presence of delusions, hallucinations and thought disorder in many manic patients. As always the possibility of an organic disorder needs to be excluded.

Management of acute mania

More often than depression, mania requires admission to hospital. This is because the patient often fails to recognise that he is unwell and there is a need to protect the patient from the consequences of poor judgements and hyperactivity. Often manic admissions must be involuntary. These factors thus necessitate the admitting ward to be sufficiently well staffed with nurses and/or have some security to prevent the patient from leaving. In hospital a person with mania should be in a low stimulus environment and may need to be kept away from excessive interactions with other patients. The nursing of patients with mania can be extremely demanding.

Anti-manic drugs

In severe manic states antipsychotic drugs such as haloperidol or chlorpromazine are usually the first line of treatment in the first instance. Lithium may be added to the anti-psychotic drug at quite an early stage if the patient is not improving. If the mania is not too severe then lithium may be used alone to treat a manic episode. Fortunately, over 70 per cent of manic episodes will settle over the course of a week or two with the above medication, however, some manic episodes settle very slowly. A number of alternatives to antipsychotic drugs and lithium are currently receiving attention.

The continuing management of bipolar affective disorder

As bipolar affective disorder is a recurrent disorder, and because considerable personal and social damage can occur in manic episodes, prophylactic treatment to prevent future episodes is usually required. If people have two affective episodes in three years, then, without prophylactic treatment, 50 per cent will have another episode within six months, 80 per cent within a year and 90 per cent within two years. Lithium, the mainstay of the continuing management of bipolar disorder, will decrease this recurrence rate by half. If lithium fails to prevent future episodes then carbamazepine is an established alternative. Carbamazepine may have a special place in patients who have a rapid cycling (defined as more than four episodes in a year) bipolar disorder. If lithium and carbamazepine alone and in combination fail, then alternatives may include sodium valproate, verapamil, clonidine and lecithin. All these alternative treatments for bipolar disorder require further evaluation as regards to their efficacy.

Outcome of bipolar affective disorder

As stated above, bipolar affective disorder is a recurrent illness, with a high likelihood of recurrence, especially if there have been two or more episodes in the previous past two or three years. As it is a recurrent illness and prophylactic medication is required, there is a considerable need for education and support for bipolar patients. Even with lithium many patients have multiple episodes and may require frequent hospital admissions. Thus, although bipolar disorder is at times thought of as having a favourable outcome with normal functioning between episodes, it can also be an extremely devastating disorder with considerable morbidity. Like major depression, patients with bipolar disorder are also prone to suicide, and in some cohorts of bipolar patients up to 5 per cent or more have died by suicide. Another complication of bipolar disorder is substance abuse.

Further Reading

Conte H R, Plutchilk R, Wild K V and Karasu T B, 'Combined Psychotherapy and Pharmacotherapy for Depression: A Systematic Analysis of the Evidence', *Archives of General Psychiatry*, Vol 43, 1986, pp 471–9.

Goldberg D, Bridges K, Duncan-Jones P and Grayson D, 'Detecting Anxiety and Depression in General Medical Settings', *British Medical Journal*, Vol 297, 1988, pp 897–9.

Jablensky A, 'Prediction of the Course and Outcome of Depression', *Pyschol Med*, Vol 17, 1987, pp 1–9.

Joyce P R and Paykel E S, 'Predictors of Drug Response in Depression', *Archives of General Psychiatry*, Vol 46, 1989, pp 89–99.

Keller M B, Klerman G L, Lavori P W, Coryell W, Endicott J and Taylor J, 'Long Term Outcome of Episodes of Major Depression, Clinical and Public Health Significance', *Journal of American Medical Association*, Vol 252, 1984, pp 788–92.

Kendell R E, 'The Diagnosis of Mania', *J Affect Disorders*, Vol 8, 1985, pp 207–13.

Klerman G L, 'The Current Age of Youth Melancholia: Evidence for an Increase in Depression Among Adolescents and Young Adults', *British Journal of Psychiatry*, Vol 152, 1988, pp 4–14.

Paykel E S, 'Handbook of Affective Disorders', *Churchill Livingstone*, 1982.

Quitkin F M, 'The Importance of Dosage in Prescribing Antidepressants', *British Journal of Psychiatry*, Vol 147, 1985, pp 593–7.

Chapter 29

Suicidal Behaviour

R D Goldney

Each year in Australia approximately two thousand people, the population of a small country town, commit suicide. An unknown number, but no less than 40,000 to 50,000, the population of a regional provincial city, attempt suicide. In addition, no less than 15 per cent of the general population at some time or another have a degree of suicidal ideation.

In developed countries suicide ranks among the top ten causes of death, and in those under the age of 25 it is either the second or third most common cause of death. Despite these figures, suicidal behaviour tends to be denied by society in general as it is difficult to come to terms with the fact that so many people feel that life is not worth living. It is easier to help worthy charities that address illness in young children or promote healthy lifestyles instead of examining one of public health's biggest problems.

Prevalence

Suicide rates vary from country to country, with figures below 10 suicides per 100,000 population reported from Ireland, Malta and Egypt to those greater than 25 per 100,000 from Finland, Austria, Czechoslovakia and Hungary. The rates for males are invariably higher than those for females, and there is a general consistency of suicide rates in any given country over a period of time.

In Australia the suicide rate for males in 1985 was 18.2 per 100,000; a figure virtually identical to that of 18.9 per 100,000 for 1901. For females there was a small increase from

4.3 to 5.1 per 100,000 in the same time period. This consistency tends to obscure the fact that there have been variations in rate over the years, with the male rate peaking at 24 per 100,000 at the height of the Great Depression in 1930, and the female rate peaking at 10.8 per 100,000 in 1965. The latter peak may well have been related to the massive post-war influx of migrants to Australia and the ready availability of relatively lethal tranquillisers and sedative drugs.

In addition to the fluctuations by sex there have been changes in age-specific rates, with a reduction in the rate of the elderly and an increase in childhood and adolescence. Despite these changes, the elderly remain the group with the highest risk of suicide, and the young, notwithstanding frequent sensational media reporting, still represent only a small proportion of the total number of those who suicide.

Official statistics of suicidal behaviour have been questioned and it is almost certain that suicide is under-reported. Estimates of under-reporting between 1.2 and 3.8 times have been given, and it is reasonable to assume that at least half as many again as the official statistics do in fact commit suicide in our society.

The reasons for this under-reporting are several. There is a reluctance to conclude that death has been caused by suicide for fear of causing distress to the surviving family, because of the general religious proscription of suicide and because many life insurance policies are void when death has been self-intentioned. Furthermore, the medical profession itself has been tardy in acknow-ledging that adolescents and even young children can have severe depressive illness with intense suicidal ideation. In the absence of medical acknowledgment of these conditions it is not unexpected that coroners would be reluctant to find verdicts of suicide.

Classification

Suicide and attempted suicide have tradition-ally been considered separately although there has always been the acknowledgment that there is a degree of overlap. The World Health Organisation has defined suicidal behaviour as 'self injury with varying degrees of lethal intent' and suicide itself as 'a suicidal act with a fatal outcome'.

Just as there have been problems in the delineation of suicide per se, so authorities have also debated the definition of attempted suicide. This has largely revolved around issues of motivation of the distressed subject in terms of their suicidal intent and the medical lethality of their suicidal actions. It is important to note that few suicidal subjects definitely want to end their lives, and the majority have mixed feelings about living and dying. The dilemma remains that any risk to life is significant, and subjects may not be aware of the lethality of the method of suicidal behaviour which they are employing.

As a result of these questions about suicidal motivations a number of synonyms for attempted suicide have arisen. These have included 'pseudocide', 'self-poisoning', 'para-suicide', 'acute poisoning', 'deliberate self-injury', 'self-injury', non-fatal deliberate self-harm', and even 'propetia', meaning rushing head-long into harm. Fortunately these terms do not obscure the fact that clinicians appear to be relatively consistent in what constitutes the behaviour necessary for inclusion in these categories and there is probably no advantage in any of these terms over and above the long used 'attempted suicide'.

Notwithstanding these questions, it is important to note that many of the issues underlying suicide, attempted suicide, and, indeed, suicidal ideation share common characteristics and there are reasonable grounds for considering them together.

Causes

Suicidal behaviour is an area in which the application of the biopsychosocial model is particularly important. Many disciplines have contributed to our understanding, as will be evident from the diverse theories presented below.

Genetic factors

Twin and adoption studies indicate that there is probably a genetic factor in suicide. Danish–American research has demonstrated that of those who suicided more of their biological relatives had suicided than had their adopted control relatives. It is thought that the genetic factor could be related to transmission of schizophrenia, alcoholism or manic depressive illness and there has also been a suggestion that there could be genetic factor related to impulsivity and aggression which is sometimes observed in persons who commit suicide.

Biochemical factors

Biochemical abnormalities in the brain, particularly in the serotonin system, have been implicated, and these appear to be related to impulsivity and aggression rather than any specific psychiatric diagnosis. People who commit suicide by the more impulsive and violent methods such as hanging, shooting and jumping from a height are more likely to have decreased 5–hydroxyindoleacetic acid, a metabolite of serotonin, in their cerebro-spinal fluid. Furthermore, follow-up studies of persons who have low 5–hydroxyindoleacetic acid in their cerebro-spinal fluid and who have attempted suicide in a violent manner are more likely to commit suicide subsequently than similar subjects with normal quantities of this substance in their cerebro-spinal fluid.

The peak seasonal incidence of suicide in spring and autumn has raised hypotheses about the relationship of mood disturbances to changes in the hours of sunlight. These may mediated biochemically by the pineal gland.

Other studies have examined cortisol secretion which appears to be increased from the adrenal gland and the relative reduction in electrodermal responsivity in patients who

have made suicide attempts. The latter finding
may be related to the observation that those
who cut themselves usually state that they do
not feel pain at the time.

Peri-natal factors

Although classical psychoanalytic theory has
always postulated that early life events are
of importance in psychiatric illness, there has
been little empirical data to support that view
in the context of suicide. However, a recent
Scandinavian study suggests that there is an
association between events at birth, such as
mechanical birth trauma and a predilection
for a violent lifestyle in adult life. These
provocative findings are explained on the
basis that there could be an 'imprinting'
process at birth which leads to adult self-
destructive behaviour. Although somewhat
speculative, this hypothesis has heuristic value
which will undoubtedly lead to more research
in this area.

Physical illness

Physical illness is thought to be associated
with approximately half of all suicides. Thus
epilepsy, multiple sclerosis, Huntington's
chorea, Cushing's syndrome, peptic ulcer and
cirrhosis have all been reported to be
associated with suicide, and more recently
acquired immune deficiency syndrome
(AIDS) has been implicated. Occult cancer
can also contribute to mood disturbances
which may lead to suicide.

Psychiatric illness

Patients with psychiatric illness have about
a ten times greater risk of suicide than the
general population. The degree of this risk
depends on the nature of the illness, its severity
and the extent of hospitalisation. Thus severe
illnesses with tormenting delusions and
hallucinations lead to greater hospitalisation
with concomitant feelings of hopelessness and
a greater risk of suicide.

Depression is the illness which is most
commonly associated with suicide, with two-
thirds of those who suicide being afflicted with
a major affective disorder. It is important to
note that a major affective disorder does have

an appreciable mortality as well as ongoing
morbidity and as many as one in six (15 per
cent) of those with this condition will die by
committing suicide. Suicide is more frequent
either at the beginning or at the resolution
of a depressive illness and the paradox of the
latter suicides is that these patients feel not
only that they now have the energy to commit
suicide, but they do not wish to risk the
possibility of ever becoming so profoundly
depressed again, and the only way to prevent
that is by committing suicide (see chapters
25, 28).

Schizophrenia also has a high rate of suicide
with up to 10 per cent of subjects dying in
this manner. Suicide in this case is not often
a consequence of responding to hallucinations
or delusions. More frequently it is related to
the fact that the schizophrenic process
appreciably disrupts a young person's employment and interpersonal adjustment, such that
they not only have a severe psychiatric illness,
but also fewer emotional and community
supports (see chapters 32, 38).

Alcoholism is the third major psychiatric
condition which may lead to suicide and
approximately 15 per cent of those who are
alcohol dependent die in this way. As with
patients with schizophrenic illness, those who
are alcohol dependent tend to lose their social
and interpersonal supportive networks in
addition to being particularly susceptible to
secondary depressive disorders. Furthermore,
suicide in response to psychotic phenomena
when acutely intoxicated or when undergoing
withdrawal symptoms is not uncommon (see
chapter 42).

Those who have personality disorders or
who are drug dependent are also more likely
to commit suicide. These persons are more
likely to have impaired social and interpersonal relationships and they are prone to
becoming acutely depressed. When this is
combined with their impulsivity and the ready
availability of a method of suicide, it is not
unexpected that suicide frequently results (see
chapters 14, 43).

Social factors

Social factors are of considerable importance
in contributing to suicidal behaviour. The very

fact that there is such a wide diversity of rates of suicide in different countries points to this. The first to delineate clearly the importance of social factors in suicide was Durkheim who examined European demographic and social data. He postulated three broad types of suicide: the egoistic which occurred when a person was deprived of his close personal and social relationships; the anomic which occurred when an individual felt as if he had lost the usual social norms of functioning, such as might occur during war or a significant economic depression; and the altruistic, which resulted from an excessive sense of duty to society such that the individual would take his life rather than risk disintegration of their society. Examples of the latter are the suttee of Indian widows and the Hari Kiri of certain sections of Japanese society.

Whilst Durkheim's work has been extremely influential in the field of suicidal research, more recent sociological work has tended to focus on less all-embracing theories. It is now generally accepted that the rate of suicide is positively correlated with a wide variety of social factors such as loneliness, isolation, alcoholism, urban rather than rural residence, upper socio-economic status and being an older single, widowed, separated or divorced male.

Those who *attempt* suicide are more likely to be younger women, more often separated and/or divorced, in the lower social economic groups, and living in a crowded urban setting. They are more angry and depressed with personality disturbances and often alcohol will have been used in association with a recent interpersonal conflict.

It is important to appreciate that conclusions drawn from populations studied in urban Australia or the United States may have little relevance to people in less developed societies. Furthermore, even within one particular country, clusters of suicide dependent on age can influence sociological surveys. Thus older persons who have retired to a seaside resort and who may be widowed and depressed with physical illness are different to younger subjects who have moved to a city and who may have emerging psychotic illnesses or severe personality disorders. Cognizance of these factors is required in assessing individual studies.

Migration is frequently considered to be a predisposing factor to suicidal behaviour. This has been borne out by studies in the United States and Australia where there were massive influxes of migrants after World War II. It is difficult to delineate the exact factors which may predispose such persons to increases in suicidal behaviour, as these persons have frequently been subjected to considerable disruption in their lives in their country of origin, with forcible separation from family and friends and loss of economic security, all factors which can lead to an increase in suicidal behaviour even in the non-migrant.

In Australia there have been studies which have shown that migrants who have come from European countries with a high rate of suicide tend to have a higher rate of suicide in Australia than Australian born subjects. Similarly, subjects from those European countries which have traditionally had a lower suicide rate have had a lower rate than Australian born. Other work has demonstrated that the children of migrants have suicide rates approximating those of other native born Australians, rather than that of their parents' original country (see chapters 3, 47).

Unemployment has been associated with an increase in both those who attempt and commit suicide. However, it is difficult to determine whether this is cause or effect, as it is reasonable to assume that those who are coping less well psychologically are more likely to be unemployed, and hence a self-fulfilling prophecy of an increased number of unemployed in those who engage in suicidal behaviour will inevitably emerge. There is no doubt that for some individual subjects unemployment is a potent factor in their final suicidal act, but it is more likely that other intervening variables such as depression or the reaction to their unemployment of a significant other in that person's life has been of more significance. Thus the issue of whether or not unemployment per se contributes to suicidal behaviour remains unresolved.

Imitation or 'copy-cat' suicide has been considered in the last decade as a potent contributing factor, particularly in the young.

There have been a number of studies which have demonstrated that there is an increase in suicide, particularly of an imitative kind, after extensive media exposure. This raises a number of issues including those related to the freedom of the media and the wish of the general public to be made aware of dramatic events such as suicide. The dilemma remains that available evidence suggests that the reporting of suicide does seem to be followed by further imitative suicide and restraint by the media is clearly appropriate.

Availability of method

The availability of the means of suicide influences the proportion of suicides by a particular method, but it is doubtful whether it influences the overall rate. Suicide is predominantly by firearms in North America, whereas in Europe it is by hanging and in Britain by drug overdose. The use of domestic gas used to be a prominent means of suicide in Britain and it was argued that the conversion from coal gas to natural gas was responsible for a reduction in suicide, but a similar reduction was not noted in The Netherlands. However, the majority of subjects who suicide in The Netherlands do so by hanging and therefore any reduction by the elimination of the coal gas method of suicide would not make an impact on their figures. When Australian domestic gas was changed from coal to naturally derived gas there was an increase in suicide by carbon monoxide poisoning from motor vehicle exhausts, and this appeared to be in proportion to the decrease in suicide from domestic gas. This suggested that Australians substituted one form of gas poisoning for another when the previous form became unavailable.

It is possible that changes in prescribing habits may have an effect on suicide rates. The change from the relatively lethal barbiturate hypnotics and sedatives in the 1950s and 1960s to the much safer benzo-diazepine drugs in subsequent years may well have contributed to a decrease in suicide, as could have the blister packaging of drugs which interferes with the impulsive taking of large quantities of medication. Whilst variations in availability of method appear to

be of significance in the short term, their importance is probably only related to the extent to which any one method is used, rather than influencing the overall incidence of suicide as a whole in any given population.

Interpersonal events

The interpersonal environment is very important as a final precipitant to suicidal behaviour. Suicidal subjects experience a greater number of stressful life events than those with psychiatric illness alone or those in the general population. Precipitants are usually related to arguments with a significant other person, or to the breakdown in relationships. Chronic social problems such as marital difficulties, unemployment, poor accommodation, poverty and antisocial behaviour are also more likely to be associated with suicidal behaviour than is a more stable family environment.

Intra-psychic factors

Although all the above factors are of undoubted importance, suicidal behaviour ultimately is a uniquely personal phenomenon. Every individual who is suicidal has his own idiosyncratic view of the world. Frequently that view becomes quite constricted and alternatives to suicide appear remote. The final act is often precipitated by the experience of loss of an interpersonal relationship and fantasies of retribution or retaliation are frequently present. These feelings are undoubtedly aggressive in nature, but rather than being appropriately projected out into the environment they are turned in upon the self, so much so that suicide has been referred to as 'murder in the 180th degree'. Coupled with feelings of retaliation and retribution there is a sense of omnipotence that suicide is not only the solution of one's own problems, but it is the ultimate method of making others feel sorry for their actual or imagined acts against the suicidal subject. At times of intense suicidal ideation fantasies of being reunited with significant others who may have died in the past are particularly important danger signs, especially if the person who has previously died has also commited suicide.

The important issue of suicidal behaviour in children and adolescents is discussed in chapter 25.

The prediction of suicide

Although suicide is a significant cause of death in our society, it is still an uncommon occurrence and in a general sense it is impossible to predict. Suicide has a low base rate and for events with such a low base rate statistical methods of prediction are very weak. The usual predictors are increasing age, severe psychiatric illness with prolonged hospitalisation, previous suicide attempts and use of psychotropic drugs in groups at high risk, such as those attending a psychiatric hospital. However, the number of false positives predicted in the course of delineating those who will suicide is so great that prediction is of little practical value. Whilst such statistical information could be taken as grounds for nihilism in one's management of suicidal subjects, it really is only an indication that specific checklists or questionnaire approaches to the management of suicidal behaviour, when taken in isolation from the clinical context, are unlikely to be of value. Thus we have to rely on our clinical assessment of individual patients who present either with suicidal ideation or having already attempted suicide.

The risk factors for suicide are summarised in Table 1.

Management of suicidal behaviour

The management of suicidal behaviour can be divided into the areas of prevention, the management of those who have already demonstrated their suicidal disposition and, finally, the care of those who may be bereaved by suicide.

Prevention

It is unrealistic to expect suicidal ideation can be prevented. Humans are introspective and will continue to ponder the meaning of existence and, as such, it is inevitable that the question of one's own mortality will arise. Such existential musings merge imperceptibly into significant suicidal ideation. The provision of the optimum peri-natal and early childhood experiences lead to a greater sense of security with a resultant enhancement of self-esteem and a minimisation of psychiatric and interpersonal problems, although it is probable that the more severe mental illnesses will continue to emerge unremittingly. Only prompt recognition and treatment of these offers hope in reducing their considerable morbidity.

There have been a number of self-help organisations, such as the Samaritans and Crisis Care counselling services, which have allowed suicidal subjects the opportunity of talking about their problems in an anonymous and non-threatening manner. The role of these services and other preventative measures are discussed more fully in chapter 68.

A number of studies have indicated that those who both commit suicide and attempt suicide are likely to have consulted a medical practitioner in the few days before their act. It is therefore important to ensure that a full assessment of the overall situation is made as, with adequate management of psychiatric illness and its concomitant distress, suicidal acts are potentially preventable.

Assessment and management

Assessment of suicidal subjects is essentially similar to the assessment of any other patients. A full history should be taken, a diagnosis formulated and, with the patient's co-operation, a plan of management instituted. The initial establishment of rapport and a therapeutic alliance is particularly important. Comfortable surroundings with privacy should be used, and the therapist, if unknown to the patient, should introduce himself, and indicate that a certain amount of time has been set aside for the initial interview before discussing what treatment can be offered.

Challenging or direct questions which could be interpreted as critical will rarely help. Comments such as 'things seem to have got on top of you' or 'you must have been pretty upset' are often sufficient to allow patients to talk about their difficulties, and the open-ended question 'Can you tell me more about it?' is particularly useful. Some patients may

Table 1. Evaluation of unjustified suicide risk

Variable	High risk	Low risk
Demographic and social profile		
Age	Over 45 years	Below 45 years
Sex	Male	Female
Marital status	Divorced or widowed	Married
Employment	Unemployed	Employed
Interpersonal relationship	Conflictual	Stable
Family background	Chaotic or conflictual	Stable
Health		
Physical	Chronic illness	Good health
	Hypochondriac	Feels healthy
	Excess drug intake	Low drug use
Mental	Severe depression	Mild depression
	Psychosis	Neurosis
	Severe personality disorder	Normal personality
	Alchoholism or drug abuse	Social drinker
	Hopelessness	Optimism
Suicidal activity		
Suicidal ideation	Frequent, intense, prolonged	Infrequent, low intensity, transient
Suicide attempt	Multiple attempts	First attempt
	Planned	Impulsive
	Rescue unlikely	Rescue inevitable
	Unambiguous wish to die	Primary wish for change
	Communication internalised (self-blame)	Communication externalised (anger)
	Method lethal and available	Method of low lethality or not readily available
Resources		
Personal	Poor achievement	Good achievement
	Poor insight	Insightful
	Affect unavailable or poorly controlled	Affect available and appropriately controlled
Social	Poor rapport	Good rapport
	Socially isolated	Socially integrated
	Unresponsive family	Concerned family

Source: Adam K, 'Attempted Suicide', *Psychiatric Clinics of North America*, Vol 8, 1985, p 183, with permission.

remain resistant, but by stressing that it is important to try and understand what has happened, and by the use of silence, which further indicates a willingness to listen, most will respond and rapport can be gained. More direct questions may be necessary in order to elucidate the sequence of events leading to suicidal behaviour, and the role of significant others should be sought. This may require a systematic enquiry of relationships with family members and friends.

Suicidal intent can be determined on the basis of the degree of planning, the knowledge of the lethality of the method, and the presence and content of suicide notes. If patients are asked an open-ended question such as 'What were your feelings about living and dying?' or, 'I guess you had mixed feelings about living and dying' at the time of the attempt, rather than 'Did you really want to live or die?', they are usually able to verbalise their ambivalence and motivations.

The elucidation of symptoms of both psychological and physical illness should be pursued carefully. Depression, schizophrenia alcohol and other drug dependence are the most common psychiatric illnesses and concomitant physical illness, and the use of prescribed drugs which may have contributed to depression, should be delineated. The risk factors noted before should be carefully evaluated and after having established these, decisions about specific treatment must be made. *Hospitalisation* may be necessary unless it is quite clear that there is no risk to life and a plan of management has been agreed upon. It is mandatory if there is a high degree of suicidal intent. Difficulties can arise when there is a discrepancy between expressed suicidal intent and that objectively assessed, and compulsory detention in a psychiatric inpatient unit may be required. If so, it should be emphasised to patients and their relatives that it is done out of concern for the immediate future rather than as punishment for suicidal behaviour.

Irrespective of psychiatric diagnosis, successful management requires the establishment of a *trusting relationship* as it is usually the disruption of such a relationship that has precipitated the suicidal crisis. Thus a therapist must be willing to accept the demands that these patients may make. Such demands are not met unconditionally or in an open-ended manner, but with tact in pointing out the patient's own responsibilities for his actions. It is useful to insist on the patient clearly describing what options they have, beside suicidal behaviour, should they find themselves in a similar crisis in the future.

Not all patients require or accept ongoing therapy. In the absence of psychiatric illness and when suicidal behaviour has resulted in a re-orientation of interpersonal dynamics, further contact may be more limited. Such support should focus on specific interpersonal difficulties, and it is usually beneficial to involve significant others. The presence of a neutral therapist allows the verbalisation of aggressive and jealous feelings between

couples in a controlled manner, whereas such feelings may have been acted out in the past by using suicidal threats and actions.

For patients with clearly defined psychiatric illness standard treatments should be followed. Because the majority of those who attempt suicide use psychotropic drugs, some have suggested that drugs should never be used for these patients. Such an attitude unnecessarily limits one's options, especially in relation to depression, which may specifically require antidepressant therapy, even in the younger age groups. It is reasonable to consider the short-term use of minor tranquillisers for patients with prominent symptoms of anxiety, and major tranquillisers for those with extreme hostility or poor impulse control, and, of course, for those with a schizophrenic illness.

Although clinicians should keep an open mind about the use of psychotropic medication in the management of those who attempt suicide, the majority of patients can be assisted by non-pharmacological means.

Recent work has demonstrated that specialised social work or community nurse follow-up for patients without psychiatric illness may be as effective in terms of prevention of further suicide attempts as conventional medical care, but more effective in producing better social adjustment. This indicates that it is not sufficient for medical practitioners simply to feel confident in their own assessment and management of individual suicidal patients, but that cooperation with social workers and community nurses is required if as full an impact as possible is to be made on the morbidity associated with suicidal behaviour.

Those bereaved by suicide

Although suicide is potentially preventable, it will never be eliminated entirely. An important component of the overall management in this area is providing solace for those who have been bereaved by suicide. Just as it is difficult for many people to acknowledge that death has occurred even as a result of natural illness, so it is particularly difficult for some of those who have been bereaved by suicide to acknowledge that their relative or friend could have taken his own life. Suicide is not only an indication of one's own hopelessness, but it also emphasises the impotence of both the helping professions and others in the life of the deceased. Such impotence is difficult to accept and frequently blame is attributed elsewhere by those who find it difficult to concede that suicide may have actually occurred. Sometimes community attitudes towards the survivors are seen as unhelpful, as blame may be attributed to them, and there is usually a distancing of others from those so bereaved, a distancing which is almost invariably perceived as outright rejection.

An acceptance that not only has suicide occured, but that it has occurred as a result of a person having a psychiatric illness which has proved difficult to treat can sometimes provide comfort to survivors. Many wish to know if genetic factors are of importance and one can be comforting in noting that although there may well be such a factor, any such genetic linkage is not strong. Many of those bereaved find some comfort either by drawing an analogy between suicide following severe psychiatric illness and death from physical illness, or by accepting the certainty of death rather than having to tolerate the uncertainty of the chronically suicidal subject with erratic impulsive behaviour.

Support groups have been established for those bereaved in this manner and many report a considerable sense of relief at being able to share their thoughts and feelings in the presence of others who have been similarly bereaved.

Conclusion

Suicidal behaviour has been present throughout man's history and is likely to remain so. It has a fascination for many and challenges our sense of autonomy. In a sense it is our one great freedom, the freedom of choice of our own life or death. However, in acknowledging that freedom there is the need to pursue our understanding of why some who have suicidal ideation then go on actually to commit suicide. In the pursuit of this understanding there have arisen moral, sociological and medical theories, none of which by itself has proven to be sufficient to explain all aspects of suicidal behaviour. Despite the inadequacies of our present knowledge, medical and other health professionals are uniquely placed to alleviate some of the morbidity associated with suicidal behaviour, and to influence the actual suicide rate.

Further Reading

Black D W, 'Suicide and Parasuicide', *Current Opinion in Psychiatry*, Vol 2, 1989, pp 225-9.

Goldney R D and Burvill P V, 'Trends in Suicidal Behaviour and its Management', *Australian and New Zealand Journal of Psychiatry*, Vol 14, 1980, pp 1-15.

Hassan R and Tan G, 'Suicide Trends in Australia 1901-1985', *Suicide and Life-Threatening Behaviour*, Vol 19, 1989, pp 362-80.

Kosky R, 'Childhood Suicidal Behaviour', *Journal of Child Psychology and Psychiatry*, Vol 24, 1983, pp 457-68.

O'Carroll P W, 'A Consideration of the Validity and Reliability of Suicide Mortality Data', *Suicide and Life-Threatening Behaviour*, Vol 19, 1989, pp 1-16.

Roy A, 'Suicide', in *Comprehensive Textbook of Psychiatry*, 5th edn (ed Kaplan H I and Sadock B J), Williams and Wilkins, Baltimore, 1989, pp 1414-27.

Chapter 30

Obsessive Compulsive Disorders 1: Children

F Levy

Definition

Obsessive compulsive disorder (OCD) is characterised by recurrent ideas, thoughts and impulses, which are persistent and experienced as senseless, uncomfortable and intrusive into the normal thought stream and consciousness. They may try to ignore or suppress these invasive obsessions or to distract themselves from acting on them. When they do yield to obsessional impulses, the behaviour is repetitive, intentional and stereotyped (ie a compulsion). Although the behaviour seems to be designed to alleviate the intrusive obsession, it in fact has only a temporary comforting effect and the impulse returns, so the behaviour is repeated. Ultimately such obsessions and compulsions cause personal distress, aggravate others and become socially crippling.

Prevalence

The disorder is reported as presenting rarely in clinical populations of children. The incidence is 1 per cent in child psychiatric inpatients and 0.2 per cent in child populations. However, recent data indicates that the disorder may be more common. Flament et al (1985) studied over 5000 unselected adolescents in the State of New Jersey, and found an incidence of about 0.33 of the total population, with suggestions that this was a minimal figure because many children are secretive about the disorder.

Aetiology

In the past, psychodynamic explanations linked obsessional traits with concern about toilet training during child-rearing, but no evidence has been shown for this theory. More recently family factors have been considered important in modelling rigidity and obsessive behaviour.

Serotonin re-uptake inhibitors such as clomipramine have been found to have a relatively specific effect in treating the systems of obsessive compulsive disorder. This had led to a 'serotonin hypothesis' which has been discussed by Rapoport (1986) and Zak et al (1988). Both authors conclude that while there is some evidence that a serotonergic defect is associated with OCD, there is no direct evidence of a causal relationship. Rapoport (1986) also reports some suggestions of soft neurological associations such as increased ventricular brain ratios on CT scans, but these await further evidence from brain imaging techniques such as positron emission tomography or xenon inhalation. It is possible that ritual-like behaviours will be traced to specific parts of the brain. For example, studies of basal ganglia lesions in squirrel monkeys suggest that the globus pallidus may mediate some ritual-like behaviours.

Diagnosis

The diagnosis of this disorder is made clinically, based on a history of obsessional thoughts and compulsive actions, which interfere with social and educational adaptation. In adults symptoms more usually form part of a related personality structure, but in children symptoms may occur in isolation, or coupled with other symptoms and personality traits. The most commonly reported symptom associations are with Tourettes' Syndrome (a chronic motor and vocal tic syndrome) and with neurological conditions. For example, obsessive phenomena have been recognised in association with temporal lobe epilepsy.

Differential diagnosis

Obsessive compulsive disorder can appear as an isolated condition or it may be associated with other entities such as depressive disorders, schizophrenia, or Tourette's Disorder. In such conditions, the primary diagnosis should be made first, but an associated diagnosis of OCD may also be made.

Treatment

OCD in children, as with adults, generally resists psychodynamic treatment. However, behavioural treatments such as response prevention with relaxation have been shown to have an important role in the treatment of compulsive behaviour (see chapter 61).

Recent interest has focused on the development of promising psychopharmacological treatments using serotonin re-uptake inhibitors. Flament et al (1985) reported significant improvements in a group of 19 adolescents after five weeks on clomipramine (mean dose 141 mg/day). The effect appeared independent of an antidepressant action, and has been replicated in a number of double-blind studies in adults. According to Zak (1988) serotonine in re-uptake inhibitors are more effective for obsessive thoughts than compulsive rituals, which may require exposure and response prevention.

Outcome

Obsessive compulsive symptoms have been notoriously resistant to treatment in the past, with the best results obtained from behavioural treatments. The advent of specific pharmacological agents is too recent for assessment of long term outcome, but provides a very useful addition to the treatment of this distressing condition.

Conclusion

Childhood and adolescent OCD has been gaining increasing attention from child psychiatrists, with suggestions that the condition is under-recognised and under-referred. In addition, interesting pharmacological and neurological findings, as well as possible associations with Tourette's Disorder, make this a very interesting condition.

Further Reading

Bear D and Fedio P, 'Quantitative Analysis of Interictal Behaviour in Temporal Lobe Epilepsy', *Archives of Neurology*, Vol 34, 1977, pp 454–67.

Flament, M, Rapoport J, Berg C, et al, 'Clomipramine Treatment of Childhood Obsessive Compulsive Disorders', *Archives of General Psychiatry*, Vol 34, 1985, pp 977–83.

Hollingsworth C, Tanguay P, Grossman L and Pabst P, 'Long Term Outcome of Obsessive Compulsive Disorder in Childhood', *Journal of the American Academy of Child Psychiatry*, Vol 19, 1980, pp 134–44.

Judd T, 'Obsessive Compulsive Neurosis in Children', *Archives of General Psychiatry*, Vol 12, 1961, pp 126–44.

Rapoport J, 'Childhood Obsessive Compulsive Disorder', *Journal of Child Psychiatry and Psychology*, Vol 27, No 3, 1986, pp 289–94.

Zak J P, Miller J A, Sheehan D V, et al, 'The Potential Role of Serotonin Re-uptake Inhibitors in the Treatment of Obsessive Compulsive Disorder', *The Journal of Clinical Psychiatry*, Vol 49 (supplement), 1988, pp 23–8.

Chapter 31

Obsessive Compulsive Disorders 2: Adults

N McConaghy

Patients with obsessive compulsive disorder (OCD) are distressed by recurrent obsessive thoughts or images, or compulsions to carry out certain acts. Diagnostic criteria for this disorder are outlined in the chapter, 'Obsessive Compulsive Disorders: Children' (see chapter 30).

Clinical features

A useful distinction is made by some workers between obsessions and ruminations in adults. *Obsessions* are fears that the subjects will harm someone, usually themselves or a loved one, or doubts that they have done so. The harm might be thought to be through physical violence but more commonly by contamination with dirt, chemicals, glass fragments or germs. It can be magical, for example, by failure to perform a ritual, such as carrying out all acts in three or perhaps, seven stages or, it can be by leaving electric switches on or taps dripping.

Ruminations are repetitive thoughts not concerned with an act, but they cause the patient to feel guilty (for example, sexual or blasphemous thoughts). Patients can develop phobias of situations or stimuli connected with their obsessions. For example, they may avoid touching objects, going into areas which they think are contaminated or to heights from which they fear they may throw themselves, or into situations like public transport in which they fear experiencing sexual thoughts concerning other passengers. People with sexual ruminations may report an apparently hallucinatory experience of seeing the genitals of a fully dressed person sitting opposite them. Patients report that they feel compelled to perform compulsions to help prevent them carrying out obsessive thoughts or to check that they haven't carried it out. For example, after touching an object which they feel is contaminated, they must wash their hands many times. Fearing they may have driven over someone, they must drive back over the road and check that they have not done so.

Research findings suggest that the apparent senselessness of obsessions and compulsions is recognised by about half the patients with the symptoms. Carrying out a compulsion is usually, but not always followed by reduction in tension.

Obsessions and compulsions are present in about 70 per cent of patients with OCD, and obsessions or ruminations in about 25 per cent. Compulsive behaviours alone are rare.

Patients with OCD commonly report feelings of anxiety or episodes of depression, which may be severe. Up to 25 per cent report phobias and/or compulsions before the age of 14 years. The illness commences in over half the patients before the age of 24 years. When the illness commences in adolescence, it frequently improves significantly after about 12 to 18 months, but can return in adulthood in a more chronic form, often fluctuating in severity.

Prior to the introduction of behavioural treatment, OCD was considered to respond poorly to treatment and commonly persisted for the patient's lifetime. However, about half the patients, even with severe symptoms, continue working at some level.

The DSM-III-R description states that complications include abuse of alcohol and anxiolytics. In my experience most patients dislike the feeling of loss of control which drugs produce and are quite resistant to taking either prescribed or non-prescribed drugs. Also in patients with OCD, suicide appears to be rare.

Prevalence

Prevalence surveys of American city populations have reported rates of 3 per cent in women and 1.9 per cent in men, being highest in the 18 to 44 year old age group. Two-thirds had symptoms in the previous six months, indicating the chronicity of OCD. These surveys were carried out by lay investigators using structured interviews. Attempts to validate the diagnoses reached in such surveys, by using independent psychiatric interviews, indicate that the prevalence of OCD reported in them seems to be significantly exaggerated. A recent New Zealand survey using psychiatric interview found no cases of OCD in a sample of 314 women.

Causes

Obsessional symptoms are common in the relatives of OCD patients although the research has not yet been carried out to determine to what extent this is indicative of genetic or environmental transmission. A genetic relationship between the OCD and some forms of involuntary recurrent disorders which include tics has been postulated.

OCD has been noted to occur more commonly following neurological damage such as found in encephalitis and head injury. Recent studies have reported abnormalities in the caudate nucleus and putamen areas of the brain. The apparent specifity of response of OCD symptoms to tricyclic antidepressants, which block serotonin reuptake in the brain has led to the hypothesis that alterations in the secretion of serotonin and compensatory changes in brain serotonin receptors are of significance in the development of OCD.

Diagnosis

Currently in research studies preference tends to be given to the use of structured interviews for diagnosis. One such interview is the Composite International Diagnostic Interview (CIDI).

Defined diagnostic criteria, such as those of the DSM-III-R, are applied to the CIDI responses. Significance is attached to the obsessive compulsive symptoms only if they have persisted for several weeks, or in the case of obsessions, only if the patient tried to resist the thoughts.

Operational diagnoses reached by the use of a structured questionnaire such as this are highly reliable. They exclude the influence of the clinician's subjective diagnostic ability. However, it is not clear if the response patterns validly capture the clinical entity of OCD. Clinicians rely in practice on their diagnostic judgment following a history and examination, utilising cues which they may not be able to describe easily.

Another problem with operational diagnoses is that many patients present with symptoms which do not completely fit criteria for the operational diagnosis. In a research study such patients can be excluded. In clinical practice of course they cannot. Subjective judgment is necessary in understanding these cases.

In the author's experience it is as important, when making diagnosis of OCD, to pay attention to the content of the symptoms, as much as to their form. That is to say, if the content is of guilt concerning harm or other unethical, immoral or sacrilegious acts, as outlined under clinical features, this has as much clinical significance as whether the ideas are experienced as intrusive and senseless and are resisted.

When the onset of OCD is recent, ie within a year and the patient is over 35, a likely underlying diagnosis is depressive disorder. Enquiry concerning loss of interest, appetite, weight and sleep disturbance, reveal these symptoms which are characteristic of depression.

In patients over 55 years presenting with OCD of recent onset, early dementia needs to be considered.

Treatment

When OCD is of recent origin (ie within the last 6 to 12 months), and there are indications in the patient's history of stress or conflicting emotions, discussion of these with explanations of ways they might be alleviated or resolved may be adequate to resolve the condition. If the resolution requires that the patient becomes more assertive or socially adequate, social skills training might be helpful. For the patient with considerable anxiety, relaxation training, combined with systematic desensitisation to stress situations may be indicated. Depending on their orientation, some psychiatrists treat such patients with insight oriented psychotherapy.

If stress or conflict situations are not apparent and, if, as will be more likely in patients over 30 to 35 years of age, signs of depression are present, antidepressants in adequate doses should be given a trial of at least six weeks. Probably most psychiatrists would currently use clomipramine because of its apparently specific anti-OCD action, but patients whose symptoms appear part of a depressive disorder possibly respond as well to any of the antidepressants.

When compulsions have been present for months or years, response prevention therapy may be instituted. Response prevention is most effective if it can be administered on an outpatient basis. Patients are asked to select some situations which provoke their compulsions only mildly and are instructed to expose themselves to these situations, but not to carry out their compulsion following the exposure. In order to monitor progress and to encourage the patients to tolerate the increase in anxiety which often results, they need to be seen at least weekly initially. They should be on full doses of clomipramine (150 mg nocte) during this period beginning with smaller doses. Occasional patients who cannot carry out response prevention as outpatients will respond to its supervised administration if they are admitted to a hospital. Such patients require dedicated nursing to encourage them to expose themselves to the situations provoking the compulsions while resisting the need to perform them. Following discharge they are likely to relapse unless they return as outpatients for further supervised sessions, or have domiciliary visits from staff to supervise their behaviour in their homes. Patients should show early improvement with response prevention, so excessive perseverance with this treatment is not warranted.

Some psychiatrists have treated established OCD with clomipramine alone and they report complete or near complete remission of symptoms in a number of patients. However, it appears most of their patients relapse if the medication is ceased. In the author's experience virtually all patients who respond to 'response prevention' combined with clomipramine are eventually able to cease medication. Patients commonly respond to response prevention treatment who have compulsions which are entrenched and take up hours of their day, but who nevertheless, are able to carry out their work and daily activities satisfactorily. Response prevention is rarely effective for those patients who report that their whole waking time is taken up by their OCD symptoms. Even if they are admitted to hospital and show improvement in response to the intense supervision and attention of nursing staff, they commonly relapse following discharge. Such patients usually give a life-long history of inability to cope with stressful situations—examinations at school, difficulties at work and in their emotional life—so that they usually describe poor school and work records and give a history of dependant or unstable personal relationships. In older classifications, such people were considered to have inadequate personalities. They best fit the DSM–III–R categories of avoidant or dependent personality disorder.

OCD patients with passive-aggressive, paranoid or schizoid personality features commonly resist response prevention. They may consider some of their rituals rational and necessary or become hostile and aggressive if strongly encouraged not to carry out the rituals. Such patients therefore respond poorly. The symptoms of passive-aggressive people may control their families. If the families cannot be encouraged to prevent this, change is unlikely. Those patients with OCD who also have compulsive personalities so that they control their aggression and are perfectionistic, often cooperate extremely well with response prevention. They can be ideal subjects for treatment, if they are able to enjoy the normal aspects of their lives and feel their symptoms limit this enjoyment. A useful question to ask such people is: 'How would your life be different if you didn't have these symptoms?' Patients who list all the things they would like to do but are hampered by their symptoms are likely to do well. Those who say they would feel much more comfortable but do not seem to wish to change their actual behaviours are not.

The less common group of patients with obsessions or ruminations which have persisted for months or years without compulsions are best treated by clomipramine combined with aversive therapy. With aversive therapy, unpleasant, but not painful electric shocks are administered to the patients' fingers, after they read phrases describing their obsessions or ruminations.

A few patients with severe disabling OCD who have failed to respond to drug treatment, behaviour modification or psychotherapy may be considered suitable for some form of psychosurgery. Psychosurgery for OCD usually involves severing neuronal connections of the limbic system of the frontal lobe of the brain. Some, whose symptoms persist following leucotomy, then show a response to behaviour therapy, though prior to the operation they did not. The issue of brain surgery for OCD is however, controversial.

Further Reading

Anthony J C, Folstein M, Romanoski A J, et al, 'Comparison of the Lay Diagnostic Interview Schedule and a Standardised Psychiatric Diagnosis', *Archives of General Psychiatry*, Vol 42, 1985, pp 667-75.

Catts S and McConaghy N, 'Ritual Prevention in the Treatment of Obsessive-Compulsive Neurosis', *Australian and New Zealand Journal of Psychiatry*, Vol 9, 1975, pp 37-41.

Emmelkamp P M G, Van Linden Van Den Heuvell C, Ruphan M and Sanderman R, 'Home-based Treatment of Obsessive-Compulsive Patients: Intersession Interval and Therapist Involvement', *Behaviour Research and Therapy*, Vol 27, 1989, pp 89-93.

Grayson J B, Foa E B and Steketee G, 'Obsessive-Compulsive Neurosis', in *Handbook of Clinical Behavior Therapy with Adults*, (ed Hersen M and Bellack A S), Plenum Press, New York, 1985.

Quality Assurance Project, 'Treatment Outlines for the Management of Obsessive-Compulsive Disorders', *Australian and New Zealand Journal of Psychiatry*, Vol 19, 1985, pp 240-53.

Chapter 32

Psychoses in Adolescence

R Kosky and B Waters

Psychosis implies severe mental disorder in which the patient has no or poor insight in his mental condition, and his concept of and contact with reality is impaired. It is usually associated with disorder of thoughts, perception, affection, behaviour, and relationship with the external world.

Psychotic disorders tend to be diagnosed among adolescents later than should be the case. This is because ideas about normal behaviour during adolescence tend to be confused. It is widely believed that adolescence is a time of storm and stress and that young people are prone to instability, moodiness, rebellion and sometimes bizarre ideas. However, studies of the prevalence of emotional and behavioural symptoms among adolescents in the general population suggest that only a minority at any one time (between 5 and 10 per cent) report symptoms. A survey of high school students in Adelaide, using a self report questionnaire, indicated that about 10 per cent scored in the region that might indicate some clinical relevance to their symptoms. Long term studies of adolescents growing into adults, such as that undertaken by Grinker and his colleagues, also fail to support the notion that adolescents are an especially disturbed group or that adolescence is a particularly vulnerable time for psychiatric illness. In short, adolescents are mostly physically and emotionally healthy and severe or persistent deviations from the normal emotional and behavioural expectations should be taken seriously.

It should also be noted that psychoses in adolescence can be overlooked because the young person's behaviour brings them into contact with the juvenile justice system. Young persons who are in custody on remand report higher prevalence of symptoms than those in the general population and there is reason to suppose that children identified as young offenders may receive inadequate psychiatric care or assessment. Because of the rate of suicidal behaviour among young people in custody, particularly aboriginals, this matter has become of public concern.

There are four main psychotic conditions dominating the psychiatric conditions found in adolescence. These are schizophrenia (once called dementia praecox), affective illness, drug induced psychosis and disintegrative psychosis. These will be considered in turn.

Schizophrenia

Schizophrenia commonly manifests itself for the first time during adolescence. When this happens, it seems particularly tragic, as very often there are no tell-tale signs of abnormality before the first psychotic episode and a young person's life seems to be rudely destroyed. It is a frightening and bewildering experience for the child, the family and others who know the young person. It is, for them, hard to take in or to understand what has happened. The tendency for the parents is to blame themselves and to go back over how they treated their son or daughter, trying to find reasons for the breakdown. Previous theories of 'schizophrenogenic parents' who caused the illnesses in their children, have no scientific support although, of course, parents with high expectations of their child, or who carp and criticise their actions, can add to stress, which may trigger the first episode. Similarly, social expectations and tasks and school pressures all may contribute, although these circumstances are faced by many young people without breakdown.

Clinically there appears to be two main forms which schizophrenia can take in adolescence. The first is dominated by an acute onset and very disturbed features. In this form, there is marked thought disorder and very loose associations of ideas, so that conversation is often incomprehensible. Such young people usually experience delusions and hallucinations. Distressingly, their delusions may include their parents, who they believe may try to harm them or be possessed by devils, etc. In a large number of cases in the acute stages of the illness, emotions are unpredictable, change rapidly, and are often incongruous with laughing or crying at inappropriate times or the person is seemingly confused. Because of this affective reaction, it is sometimes difficult to differentiate these acute attacks of schizophrenia from mania.

Case example

An 11 year old boy went to the cinema with his brother to see a horror film. When he came out, he fell to his knees in the street, praying. It was not clear what he was saying, but later it became apparent that he was praying in order to avoid thinking about his parents, who he believed would be killed by his thoughts. He said he was accompanied by the Devil, with whom he conversed. He tried to stab his mother and then himself. Previously, he had been an excellent student and athlete. There had been no obvious reason for his breakdown. He never fully recovered.

The other clinical form of schizophrenia in adolescence is of an illness with much slower onset, a gradual loss of interest, activity, social contacts, and a general blunting of personality in all its aspects. These young people, particularly hard to diagnose because of the slow course of the illness, may have no obvious thought disorder (although they show poverty of thought) and rarely have hallucinations or delusions, although they may be very suspicious of others. They may also develop bizarre philosophical beliefs. Parents can become exasperated with such adolescents and see them as rebellious, negativistic and unaffectionate. Sometimes the parents find them unbearable to live with and the young person finds himself on the streets or in a flat where he may fail to look after himself adequately. Some end up in gaol.

Case example

A 14 year old girl was adopted at an early age by upper middle class parents. She gradually seemed to turn against her parents, although she had been an excellent student and talented musician. Finally, she had taken to living in the garage, the inside of which, including the window, she painted black. She defaecated into plastic bags which she threw into the lane next door. Finally, she set the furniture on fire. By this time the parents had lost any sympathy for her, and when she recovered from this stage of her illness they refused to have her back home.

In a large number of cases the acute symptoms can be managed at home. Adolescents in the early stages of the illness respond particularly effectively to antipsychotic drugs (see chapters 56, 57) and these can often be supervised by parents, general medical practitioners and visiting nurses with frequent outpatient visits for psychiatric care. Teenagers are particularly sensitive about taking psychotropic drugs and these need to be carefully explained to them. Support from the family is very important at this and later stages.

If there is a reason to suspect that the young persons may harm themselves or others, it will be necessary to provide them with specialised care in hospital. In many cases this will be a psychiatric unit of a general hospital. However, in some States there are specialised psychiatric units for adolescents, which will accept psychotic teenagers. These may be preferable to adult units, since the treatment and rehabilitative aspects are geared to the particular social and emotional needs of young people and can provide special programs for school work.

In rare cases where treatment is refused the young person, with the parents' consent, may have to be admitted to a psychiatric hospital. Most doctors are hesitant about doing this, but the need to get the psychosis under control is imperative. Where parents refuse consent, application can be made to the Minister for Community Welfare or to Guardianship Boards for treatment permission. In all these cases, it is essential to try to maintain the support and cooperation of the parents, who are usually under severe stress and often the subject of critical comment from friends and relatives who deny the child's illness.

The family of the schizophrenic teenager living at home usually requires support from the beginning of treatment. They and the young person should be well informed about the diagnosis and the prognosis. The parents should also be informed about the patient's need to take medications and about possible side effects. However, it is preferable for the teenagers to take as much charge of their own medications as is possible and is safe. They should return to school or work as soon as possible. This may need to be done gradually, starting on a part-time basis, initially, in the least stressful situation. The patients also need counselling. They need to talk about how to let their peers know about what happened to them in a way which will not expose them to ostracism. Sometimes a small group of other young people with similar problems can usefully share these experiences.

The medication may affect learning abilities. Neuroleptics affect concentration and also may make the young person sleepy. The dose or the type of drug may need to be changed if this becomes a problem.

Parents and other family members may also need counselling to help them deal with the impact of the disorder. They may be frightened, depressed, and, if one of the parents has a family history of schizophrenia, they may feel they have passed it on to the child. As well, parents may need help to deal with the desire most adolescents have to be left alone. Parents often try to over-protect psychotic adolescents. However, if the adolescent has been quite suspicious or withdrawn, they may perceive the parents' protective urges as very intrusive and a build up of antagonism may even precipitate a worsening of their condition. Parents need to be counselled about how to maintain a 'safe' distance from their child which balances care against being over-protective.

A single episode of schizophrenia in a previously well adjusted adolescent may be followed by complete or almost complete recovery. Good predictors include an acute onset, clear stressful precipitants, and a good premorbid personality. Overall, the younger the age of onset, the worse the prognosis. Adolescents have not usually established adult levels of social skills and vocational capabilities. These developments are interrupted by the illness. Rehabilitation of adolescents may be more difficult than adults because they lack these basic skills. It is essential that education and social development is maintained as far as possible, and it is for this reason that adolescents should return to school or work as soon as possible. If they cannot return to their previous level of functioning, their highest level of functioning should be ascertained and pursued. Encouragement should be given to maintain peer and other social relationships.

There is a high risk of suicide associated with schizophrenia in adolescence. Intelligent adolescents seem to be at a somewhat higher risk, possibly because they are able to understand that they have something wrong with their brain function and they become very depressed about this.

Affective psychoses

Symptoms of depression occur in about 5 to 10 per cent of adolescents in general population surveys. Major depressive illness is much less common, occurring in about 1–2 per cent. When severe features of depressive illness occur the illness is similar to that in adults. There is a morbid depressed mood, accompanied by feelings of worthlessness, helplessness and hopelessness. Ideas of reference (people talking about one), feelings of ugliness and inferiority occur, and may reach delusional intensity. Usually the patient is slowed up in thinking and actions but occasionally the depressive illness in adolescents is accompanied by agitation. These features are associated with poor sleep, loss of appetite, loss of interest, difficulty concentrating and irritability.

While this picture is unmistakable to the trained eye, it is often overlooked by parents, teachers and friends, because the sufferer usually becomes quiet and withdrawn. If depressed young people are agitated, their behaviour can be mistaken for 'naughtiness'. For these reasons, seriously depressed adolescents are often delayed in their referral to specialist medical help and their condition may be taken seriously only if they threaten or attempt suicide. This is particularly unfortunate since their condition readily responds to antidepressant medication, appropriate nursing, rehabilitative care and psychotherapeutic assistance.

Depressive psychosis, sometimes with marked delusions, often paranoia, can result from steroid and other medications. This needs to be considered, especially in young people with chronic medical conditions such as steroid dependent asthma.

Case example

A 15 year old boy tried to kill himself. He left a long, rambling, depressed and paranoid letter. He was asthmatic and on numerous medications including quite high doses of steroids. Several months earlier his best friend had suicided and he had brooded over this. He recovered in hospital with good nursing care, psychotherapy, antidepressant medication and a very much lower daily steroid dose.

Mania is less common than depressive psychosis in adolescence, but very much more dramatic. Euphoric mood, singing, joking and overt sexualisation is characteristic, accompanied by pressure of thoughts and speech. The patient may seem incoherent and unable to respond to reason. Manic adolescents are extremely disorganised and may even be violent. Delusions and hallucinations are common. It is often difficult to differentiate this picture from acute onset schizophrenia and mania should be considered in every adolescent first diagnosed with schizophrenia.

Mania in adolescents usually responds rapidly to antipsychotic drugs, but lithium

should be considered at an early stage. If the symptoms are not too severe, and the family feel they can cope, treatment at home with close supervision may be possible. However, severely depressed or manic adolescents need hospitalisation especially if they are reckless or suicidal.

As with schizophrenia, family counselling is necessary to help deal not only with the impact of the disorder, but also the parents' grief and then their natural sense of guilt. Once again, it is unlikely that any parental action has caused the illnesses directly although nonspecific stress may be present in the family. For both depressive psychoses and manic-depressive psychoses (bi-polar affective disorders) strong inherited tendencies exist, so it is likely that a parent or other close relative had a similar condition.

Early rehabilitation is essential, with return to school or work as soon as possible being the goal. Social skills groups and step by step rehabilitation in the hands of skilled health professionals, particularly nurses and occupational therapists, working to an individual management plan (either on an inpatient or outpatient basis) is the basis of early rehabilitation.

Maintenance of preventive medications is necessary. Even if the young person is well, they should continue on their antidepressants, neuroleptics or lithium for several months or a more prolonged time, since relapse can follow the too-early cessation of medication. It is often difficult for young people or their parents to understand this and in many cases, there is a strong impulse to stop taking the medication. Relapse will often follow the cessation of medication. Good medical counselling about the biochemical basis of these illnesses and the action of the medications (and their side effects) as well as a trusting relationship with a general medical practitioner or visiting nurse, can be a helpful support.

With adequate medication, both maintenance and preventive, the outcome is good. Most respond well but a minority do have relapses which do not seem to be adequately controlled by drugs. Such relapses can have devastating social effects, particularly manic attacks. It is important that appropriate medical and nursing care is instituted early in relapses.

Suicide is a serious risk in both depressive and manic psychosis. About a quarter of all adolescents with depressive symptoms get suicidal ideas. These intensify in more severe depressive states. Mania may lead to reckless behaviour especially drinking and driving which can lead to injury and death.

Drug induced psychosis

While drug induced psychosis is rare amongst adolescents generally, it is a common form of acute presentation of adolescents to psychiatric services, especially in big city hospitals. The psychosis may be a direct result of intoxication or of a hallucinogen (like LSD), or it may be due to withdrawal from drugs, or to brain damage from excessive drug use.

In most cases the acute presentation is of a delirium (see chapters 41 and 43) with clouding of consciousness and this distinguishes this form of psychosis from acute schizophrenia. In practice the differentiation is not so easy, especially in an extremely disorganised patient. There are also changes in perception, memory problems, incoherence, sleep–wake disturbances and disorientation in time, person and space.

Alcohol is by far the most commonly used drug among adolescents. Its intoxicating effects are well known but, in particular, judgment is impaired, behaviour disinhibited and sometimes aggressive. Opiates produce euphoria and then sedation. Accidental overdose and use of needles contaminated with HIV virus present dangers to those who inject these and other drugs. LSD produces hallucinations and amphetamine-like drugs (cocaine) produce aggression and psychosis (see chapter 43).

In treating these intoxications in adolescents it is necessary to try to identify the drug. Blood tests may help. In extremely disturbed persons, antipsychotic tranquillisers may be useful, but the general rule should be to avoid further chemical insult to the brain. Rest in a well lit room, good nursing care, quiet talk and reassurance are usually sufficient to allow the time necessary for the body to excrete the drug. In some cases,

especially with LSD and amphetamines, more persistent psychoses occur including 'flashbacks'.

Later, it is important to establish whether the patient is dependent on the drug, in which case appropriate treatment may be instituted (see chapter 43).

Disintegrative psychoses

These psychoses are the result of brain disease and are extremely rare. Nevertheless they do occur, tragically, in childhood and adolescence. Males are more often affected than females. They are due to neurological disorders, including brain infection (such as cerebral measles, or amoebic infection), disorders of brain metabolism and enzyme systems, Huntington's disease, chronic poisoning (for example, by lead), cancers of the brain and Acquired Immune Deficiency Syndrome (AIDS).

The clinical picture is usually of a normal child who develops changes in their personality or behaviour. These may include cognitive problems—trouble with maths or reading, problems with memory. They also include behavioural changes, irritability, aggressiveness and impulsiveness which create difficulties in relationships with parents, siblings and friends. Speech, language and comprehension deteriorate and there is deterioration in school and work performance. Several months may pass before it is apparent that there is brain function deterioration and often these young people are mistakenly thought to be suffering an emotional crisis. As deterioration continues neurological signs appear including movement problems. Blindness can occur in some conditions. Neurological investigations (see chapters 20, 21) reveal the underlying brain disease.

In non-progressive conditions the deterioration may stop. In others it continues until death.

It is rarely possible to reverse the underlying disorder. Psychotic disturbances may be ameliorated by antipsychotic drugs. It may be necessary to control epilepsy with anticonvulsants.

Early neurological investigations and a neuro-psychological assessment may be helpful in establishing a baseline of intellectual functioning from which progress can be monitored. A multidisciplinary rehabilitation team is always necessary in these cases in order to re-establish the patient to any appropriate level of functioning.

With progressive disorders particularly, the parents and family need much counselling and support. The illness and, if likely, the death of these young people is usually especially distressing and the physical changes that occur are very hard for parents to cope with. Even in cases of non-progressive illness the circumstances can be overwhelming to parents.

Case example

Brad was a 17 year old, only son, of a single mother. He went swimming one hot afternoon in the local pool. Later he became feverish and then unconscious. He had amoebic meningitis and was treated with high doses of antibiotics. He survived but was left with little memory of the past and was unable to recognise his mother. Despite remedial teaching he learnt little. His mother, grief stricken, left him in the children's home and went interstate.

Summary

Psychoses in adolescence create extraordinary disruptions in the lives of the patients and their families. Schizophrenia and disintegrative psychosis represent overwhelming tragedies for most families and for the young sufferers, while depressive and manic illnesses, often in young people, can lead to death by suicide and reckless behaviour. Psychosis in adolescence requires coordinated medical nursing and rehabilitative treatments which are complicated by the developmental level of the young person and by the need to help them achieve adulthood as adequately as possible.

Further Reading

Grinker R R Snr, Crinker R R Jnr and Timberlake J, 'Mentally Healthy Young Males', *Homoclites, Archives of General Psychiatry*, Vol 6, 1962, pp 405–53.

Evans J, *Pre-adolescent and Adolescent Psychiatry,* Academic Press, London, 1982.

Masterton J F, *Treatment of the Borderline Adolescent, a Developmental Approach*, John Wiley & Sons, New York, 1972.

Stein B A, Elliott K C, McKeough M J, 'Trends in Adolescent Psychopathology', *Canadian Journal of Psychiatry*, Vol 27, June 1982, pp 301–6.

Chapter 33

Schizophrenia

V Carr

Schizophrenia is one of the most puzzling conditions in the field of mental health. It is difficult to define, descriptions seem incomplete and our understanding is quite rudimentary. Just as our comprehension of the condition is insufficient, so our capacity to appreciate the personal experience of the sufferer is also limited. We all know sadness, fear and elation, for example, and so we can readily empathise with depressed, anxious or manic individuals. The fragmentation of experience, disorganisation of behaviour and the bizarre beliefs occurring in schizophrenia are not so familiar to us, or so we think, and hence the schizophrenic experience seems quite foreign. This is unfortunate, as it probably serves to alienate further those in our community who most need acceptance and human warmth.

Schizophrenia may not be a single disorder, it may have one or more of several possible causes and its development may proceed along more than one path. It is therefore preferable to use the term 'schizophrenic syndrome' which, while treating the disorder as a single entity for the sake of convenience, leaves open these possibilities.

The syndrome occurs basically in two forms: an 'active' or acute form, and a 'chronic' or residual form. The acute form is characterised predominantly by delusion, hallucinations and disturbances in affect and in the flow of thinking (thought disorder). These symptoms are often referred to as 'positive' or 'productive' symptoms. The residual form is marked by loss of initiative, social withdrawal, apathy, impaired emotional expression (blunted affect) and slowing of thoughts and actions. These features are referred to as 'negative' or 'deficit' symptoms. There is often overlap between the two forms with symptoms of one form co-existing with those of the other. However, the distinction is a useful one as each has somewhat different implications for treatment.

Epidemiology

Difficulties in defining schizophrenia have led to different approaches to diagnosis. This variability has, in turn, made estimates of incidence and prevalence of schizophrenia problematic. Hence, figures vary depending on the criteria used for diagnosis as well as the populations studied. Figures given for annual incidence of schizophrenia vary between 0.1 and 1.0 per 1000 population. British and European studies tend to report figures at the lower end of this range while North American studies tend to yield the higher estimates. These discrepancies are probably not real population differences but reflect variations in diagnostic criteria.

The prevalence of schizophrenia is taken to be in the vicinity of 2.5 to 5.0 per 1000 of population and the lifetime risk is generally given as 1 per cent.

Although the prevalence of schizophrenia in males and females does not differ, the syndrome is likely to make its first appearance earlier in males (15–25 years) than in females (25–35 years). Childhood schizophrenia is rare as is the onset of new cases after the age of 50. With few exceptions the rates of schizophrenia do not vary significantly from region to region or from one country to another.

The above figures do little, however, to convey the impact that schizophrenia has on the community. For instance, it has been estimated that the direct and indirect yearly costs of schizophrenia now amount to about $1.5 billion in Australia. More hospital beds are taken up by people with schizophrenia than any other illness and about 50 per cent of all psychiatric hospital beds are occupied by schizophrenic persons.

Clinical features

Prodromal phase

In the early or prodromal phase of schizophrenia, a variety of symptoms may occur which change in type and severity over time. These are generally non-specific manifestations of the disorder but they may persist for many months before the emergence of the acute form of the syndrome. These early features may include vague unease or listlessness. Symptoms of mild anxiety or depression together with inexplicable pains or reports of weakness may emerge. There may be a loss of concentration and a deterioration in the quality of school work or occupational skills. A growing tendency to avoid people may take friends by surprise and an attitude of remoteness or indifference may offend them. Uncharacteristic moodiness and irritability may surface leading to tension in the home. This is a very frustrating time in which the affected person appears to have changed in a puzzling way that is difficult to define. Medical or psychiatric consultation at this time is often unproductive as a diagnosis of schizophrenia cannot be made on the basis of these features alone. Hence, appropriate treatment cannot be undertaken unless clear evidence for schizophrenia emerges by way of the acute form of the syndrome.

Acute form

Characteristic features of acute schizophrenia include delusions and hallucinations. The former are defined as relatively fixed, false beliefs, not shared by other members of the patient's socio-cultural background. They tend to be held firmly in spite of an absence of objective evidence to support them and may play a part in governing the person's behaviour. For example, persecutory delusions, which are very common in this condition, once caused a male patient to complain to the police that certain people were piping poisonous gas into his flat and he had tried unsuccessfully to thwart their supposed malevolent intentions by blocking the air-conditioning ducts with rags. Other types of delusions include delusions of reference, and of control. Special diagnostic significance is placed on delusions of the possession of thoughts. These include the belief that thoughts are inserted into, withdrawn or even broadcasted to others from the person's mind against their will.

Hallucinations are sensory perceptions occurring in the absence of the appropriate external stimulation of the sense organs. In schizophrenia they are typically auditory in type but hallucinations in other modalities (visual, olfactory, etc), while relatively uncommon, are not unknown. Again, special diagnostic significance is placed on auditory hallucinations in which the individual hears his own thoughts spoken aloud and voices discussing or commenting about the patient in the third person.

Disturbance in the form of thinking is another important sign that may be present in acute forms of schizophrenia. The stream of thought becomes disrupted by shifts from one idea to another that is unrelated or only obliquely related to the preceding idea. The patient tends to be unaware of the lack of connection between the ideas. As a result, the patient's speech may be difficult to follow (loose association) or, in severe cases, quite incoherent.

Other symptoms of acute schizophrenia include emotional expression that is discordant with the content of the person's thinking (incongruous affect). This often takes the form of inappropriate smiling, laughing, and/or crying. Non-specific symptoms which may accompany the acute phase include anxiety, depression, agitation, impulsiveness, poor judgment, impaired concentration and unusual, stylised or stilted movements.

Patients often lack insight into the nature of their predicament and tend to deny that they are ill. This can make it difficult for them to accept the need for treatment.

Residual form

When the acute phase has subsided, the clinical picture that emerges is often marked by loss of drive and initiative. The person tends to be apathetic, and social withdrawal together with long periods of inactivity may be prominent. Levels of functioning at work, school or at home often decline and there may be self-neglect with inattention to personal hygiene and grooming. Typically, affect is blunted. Speech may become vague and circumstantial in form or, alternatively, reduced in rate and amount. The patient may display odd beliefs and eccentricities of behaviour.

Diagnosis

Diagnosis is made on the basis of the presence of symptoms of the acute syndrome and an overall duration of illness of at least six months. The duration criterion may include a period consisting solely of symptoms of the residual form, provided that acute symptoms have been present for at least some of the time. In addition, evidence of a decline in functioning in areas such as work, social relationships, home duties and self-care must be present before the diagnosis can be made. Some have criticised the latter requirement as it serves to delineate a condition based partly on disability criteria rather than on the direct manifestations of the disorder. It is thus inclined to bias the diagnosis in favour of including persons who are likely to have a poor outcome. That is, the use of disability as a diagnostic criterion identifies a group of patients with a poor prognosis by definition. The extent to which this undermines hopefulness and therapeutic effort is open to speculation. However, schizophrenia, variously defined, is known to have a good outcome (normal or near normal functioning) in 20–30 per cent of cases with a further 20–30 per cent having moderate degrees of impairment, but associated with a reasonable

quality of life. Generally speaking, if the follow-up period is sufficiently long (for example, 20–40 years) the outcome is significantly better than would be expected on the basis of a much shorter follow-up period. It is important therefore not to prejudice outcome by the simple act of making the diagnosis.

When symptoms of the acute syndrome are present, unassociated with lasting disability and the overall duration of illness is less than six months, then the diagnosis of schizophreniform disorder is made. Understandably, since the disability criterion for schizophrenia is not met in this case, the condition tends to have a relatively good prognosis. Similar illnesses of even shorter duration and associated with considerable emotional turmoil are referred to as brief reactive psychoses. These are thought not to be forms of schizophrenia. If the acute symptoms of schizophrenia occur concurrently with those of mania or major depression then the condition is often referred to as schizo-affective disorder. This is often regarded as a diagnosis of indecision on the part of the clinician concerned since, with the passage of time, such cases tend to become more clearly distinguishable as either schizophrenia of affective disorder.

Differential diagnosis should include manic illness, schizo-affective illness, psychotic depression and a number of organic conditions which can mimic schizophrenia, including induced psychosis (especially amphetamine and LSD), temporal lobe epilepsy and delerium.

Subtypes

Three of the traditional schizophrenia subtypes continue to be distinguished even though none, with the possible exception of paranoid schizophrenia, have any implications with respect to aetiology, pathogenesis, treatment or outcome. *Paranoid* schizophrenia is characterised by relatively well organised delusions with a persecutory and/or grandiose theme. Thought disorder, affective disturbance and bizarre or disorganised behaviour are absent in this subtype. The features of *catatonic* schizophrenia include marked lack of responsiveness to the environment and reduced spontaneous activity (stupor); mutism; inexplicable resistance to instructions or attempts to be moved (negativism); the maintenance of rigid, often bizarre postures which may be associated with 'waxy flexibility'; and occasionally, excited, apparently purposeless motor activity. In *hebephrenic* (disorganised) schizophrenia, the clinical picture is dominated by thought disorder; incongruous affect which may be shallow or 'silly' with inappropriate giggling; disorganised, sometimes childish behaviour; and delusions that are changeable and poorly organised.

To these traditional subtypes have been added *undifferentiated* schizophrenia and *residual* schizophrenia. The former identifies a group in which there are generally features of more than one of the traditional three subtypes so that the disorder cannot definitely be subtyped along traditional lines. Residual schizophrenia refers to the residual form of the syndrome described previously in which delusions, hallucinations or thought disorder are not apparent.

Aetiology and pathogenesis

The cause of schizophrenia is not known. In approaching this subject it is helpful to keep in mind a model for integrating information from among predisposing, precipitating and perpetuating factors. A useful stress–diathesis model put forward by Joseph Zubin is presented here in modified form (Figure 1). This model postulates a basic vulnerability (diathesis) or predisposition for developing schizophrenia which is, in principle at least, measurable in terms of cumulative risk factors. Just as predisposition to a heart attack may be measurable by means of such risk factors as family history, obesity, tobacco smoking, blood cholesterol and other factors, so it is proposed that predisposition to develop schizophrenia may be quantifiable in an analogous way. The second component of the model, conceived as being orthogonal to the first, is stress. Stressors may vary in type and severity, are usually thought of in terms of environmental events or physical conditions, and are regarded as precipitating factors which act on an individual's profile of vulnerability to cause the symptoms of schizophrenia to appear. Whether an episode of illness occurs is said to depend on the nature and severity of the stressors, the degree of individual vulnerability and the interactions between each of these sets of factors. A third concept in the model is that of protective versus perpetuating factors. These help to determine the outcome of the interaction

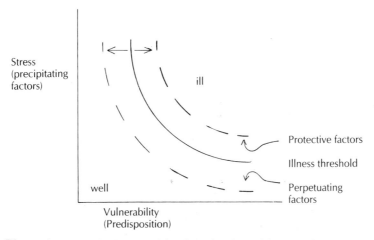

Figure 1. *Stress-diathesis model. Adapted with modifications from Zubin J and Steinhauer S, 'How to Break the Logjam in Schizophrenia: A Look Beyond Genetics', J Nerv Ment Dis Vol 169, 1981, pp 477–92 © by Williams & Wilkins, 1981.*

between stressors and individual vulnerability by altering a hypothetical illness threshold. Below this threshold no illness is said to occur as a result of the stress–vulnerability interaction but above it the illness will become apparent. Protective factors serve to raise the illness threshold and thus help to protect the individual from the occurrence of episodes of the illness. Examples of protective factors include coping skills and social support. Perpetuating factors are those which lower the illness threshold and thus increase the likelihood that the patient will suffer an episode of the illness.

Finally, we need to consider what are termed mediating mechanisms. This term refers to the abnormal biopsychological processes by which interactions between stress, vulnerability, protective and perpetuating factors are believed to mediate in the emergence of schizophrenic symptoms.

Predisposing factors

1. Genetic

There is a large body of evidence from family, adoption and twin research to suggest that genetic factors are important in the cause of schizophrenia. The risk of developing this syndrome in first degree relatives of schizophrenic patients is about 10–15 per cent. If both parents suffer from schizophrenia then the risk of their offspring becoming ill is between 35 per cent and 40 per cent. In monozygotic twins the concordance rate for schizophrenia is approximately 50 per cent while in dizygotic twins this figure drops to 10–15 per cent. Thus, while it can be stated that genetic factors appear to play a role in the aetiology of schizophrenia, heredity cannot be taken as the sole basis for explanation of the syndrome. Indeed, most schizophrenic patients do not have a family history of schizophrenia. Clearly, then, environmental factors must also be regarded as having some importance in causing schizophrenia. Exactly what is inherited and how it is inherited are the questions that now need to be addressed. It is hoped that research in molecular genetics may yield answers to these questions.

2. Environmental

It has been proposed that there may be a causal role for physical factors impinging on the individual during the prenatal and perinatal periods. For example, obstetric complications of different kinds may cause injury to neural tissue and thus compromise subsequent neurological development in some crucial respect. The fact that more schizophrenic patients tend to be born in winter months has been interpreted by some authorities as indirect evidence for the causal role of viral infection of the brain in schizophrenia. In any event, a wide range of subtle neurological abnormalities have been reported in schizophrenic patients. These vary from clinical anomalies ('soft signs'), through cerebral atrophy, enlargement of the cerebral ventricles and thickening of the corpus callosum to microscopic changes in neural tissue. The fact that a number of patients with temporal lobe epilepsy may sometimes display schizophrenic symptoms lends credence to the argument for the role of neurological abnormalities in the aetiology of schizophrenia.

The non-physical (ie social) environment has been examined repeatedly to identify factors which may predispose individuals to develop schizophrenia. There appears to be no significant effect of socio-economic status or culture on the predisposition to schizophrenia. The family may have a part to play but the evidence presented so far has either been refuted or failed confirmatory tests. The concept of the 'schizophrenogenic' mother has been discarded and there is no evidence that certain 'abnormal' patterns of family relationships contribute to schizophrenic vulnerability. Disordered patterns of communication in families have been described but on close scrutiny substantial doubt has been thrown on their role as predisposing factors. In all of the family work it has been difficult to determine whether the various factors identified pre-date the onset of schizophrenia or represent a reaction to the schizophrenic member of the family.

Attempts to seek vulnerability markers have led to the identification of personality characteristics thought to predispose to schizophrenia. Schizoid personality traits provide one example, but their specificity in relation to schizophrenia remains in doubt. In studies of children thought to be at high risk for schizophrenia several biological variables have been investigated but the results so far are inconclusive.

Precipitating factors

The evidence for physical factors as precipitants is difficult to tease out. It is possible that a variety of physical disorders, including the effects of head injury, may trigger an episode of schizophrenia but insufficient evidence has accumulated in favour of this hypothesis so far. Certainly it is the view of many clinicians that some drugs may precipitate schizophrenia or schizophrenia-like illness. Examples include drugs such as amphetamines, cocaine, marijuana and the hallucinogens (for example, LSD, psilocybin and phencyclidine (PCP)).

Psychosocial stressors have also been regarded by clinicians as precipitants of schizophrenic episodes. It has been reported that schizophrenic patients experience a number of stressful life events in the period shortly before an acute episode of their illness. Loss of a job, failure in school, accidents, death of a relative are all examples of the kinds of stressors sometimes reported in the weeks preceding the onset of acute symptoms. The difficulty in evaluating the causal role of life events lies in determining to what extent they are independent of schizophrenia as opposed to being merely the effects of the prodromal or early stages of the illness. Studies that have striven to distinguish these two kinds of life events tend to confirm that independent events appear to play an important role in precipitating acute symptoms.

Perpetuating factors

These factors need to be divided into two categories: those that lower the illness threshold for acute symptoms and those that perpetuate the residual form of the syndrome by worsening negative symptoms and increasing disability.

Of the former, a large amount of face-to-face contact between patients and families who display high levels of 'expressed emotion' (EE) has been widely reported to increase the likelihood of relapse of acute symptoms. The concept of EE embraces the phenomena of hostility, critical comments and emotional overinvolvement. To what extent these characteristics are independent of schizophrenia or represent a reaction to the presence of a schizophrenic family member is open to debate. High EE can be regarded as a particular form of continuous psychosocial overstimulation which increases the likelihood of acute symptoms.

Factors which perpetuate negative symptoms and worsen disability tend to be just the opposite—understimulating. Impoverished social environments (for example, social isolation in the form of solitary living circumstances), barren institutional life, lack of opportunities for activity or productive work and the consequences of poverty all contribute to clinical deterioration in the form of increased apathy, blunted affect, inactivity, loss of social competence and self-neglect.

Protective factors

It is a reflection of the narrow biomedical orientation which emphasises abnormality and disability that hardly anything is known of the factors which protect the patient from symptomatic relapse and disability by raising the individual's illness threshold.

Extrapolating from other areas of psychiatric research, it is possible to speculate that a wide range of coping techniques, personal resourcefulness and flexibility, problem-solving skills, 'ego strengths' and social supports may act as protective factors in relation to schizophrenia. This is an under-researched area to which attention will hopefully be directed in the future.

Mediating mechanisms

1. Neurochemical

The dominant theory in this area is known as the 'dopamine hypothesis'. This holds that schizophrenia is related to an overactivity of dopamine-mediated neurotransmission in certain neural pathways in the brain, particularly the meso-limbic system. Indirect evidence for this hypothesis is derived from a knowledge of the actions of amphetamine (which can cause schizophrenia-like symptoms) and antipsychotic drugs (which block dopamine receptors and ameliorate acute schizophrenic symptoms). This is supported by post-mortem studies and certain brain imaging techniques both of which enable quantification of dopamine receptors.

2. *Psychophysiological*

The numerous studies of autonomic 'arousal' (readiness of the nervous system to respond to stimuli) indicate that there may be some abnormality in its control or modulation in schizophrenia. Some patients seem abnormally unresponsive whereas others are overresponsive. Level of arousal is thought to affect attention and the way in which individuals handle information input. Studies of attention and information processing in schizophrenia are numerous and difficult to interpret. However, they suggest that there may be some abnormality in the early ('preattentive') stage of information processing in schizophrenia with consequent overloading of, and interference with the serial processing stage. Since environmental factors (for example, psychosocial stressors and high EE families) influence arousal levels, and abnormalities in attention and information processing are reported in schizophrenia, it is possible that the phenomenon of arousal may mediate the effect of environmental stressors in precipitating acute schizophrenia symptoms.

Attempts to understand information processing abnormalities in schizophrenia in terms of brain functioning provide the rationale for the numerous studies involving Event Related Potentials (ERP). These techniques are capable of mapping the electrical activity of the brain in the hundredths of a second following stimulus inputs. Research in this field has yet to identify the neural basis for information processing dysfunction in schizophrenia.

Numerous research efforts involving various techniques have sought to identify the nature of the alterations of brain function in schizophrenia. Studies of regional cerebral metabolism and blood flow, together with computed electroencephalographic studies and neuropsychological tests often yield conflicting results. However, evidence from these studies suggest abnormalities in the functioning of the left cerebral hemisphere and the frontal lobes in schizophrenia. At this stage it is not possible to be any more precise than this and certainly no definite conclusions can be drawn from this line of research.

Treatment

The cornerstone of treatment is the establishment of a firm and lasting relationship between the patient and a committed therapist who is willing to be responsible for planning and co-ordinating the patient's treatment. The therapist has a pivotal role to play in integrating the various components of treatment and should be prepared for an undertaking that will continue for years. A long term commitment is very important as schizophrenia is a condition generally characterised by repeated relapses, levels of disability that require continuing rehabilitative efforts and, typically, small gains are made gradually but accumulate over many years. Consequently, treatment and rehabilitation is undermined if the therapist changes every six months or so.

Hospitalisation

Treatment in a psychiatric inpatient facility is useful early in the course of the illness for diagnostic purposes. Many conditions can mimic schizophrenia and a thorough diagnostic assessment to rule out these conditions, together with an evaluation of the patient's deficits and assets, need to take place in a well-resourced hospital. Inpatient care is also very useful if the patient is unable to take care of his basic needs and in cases where there is a danger to the health, safety and well being of either the patient or others. In the latter instances, the patient may have to be detained in an approved hospital against his will. The laws that govern procedures for this purpose vary from one State to another.

Hospitalisation for a patient's care and protection is preferably brief with an active treatment program aimed at controlling symptoms and maximising levels of function, thus enabling early return to the community. Hospitalisation should also provide optimal levels of support and reassurance with an important element being to instil hopefulness for recovery and resumption of a normal or near normal life. Practical issues that need attention usually include accommodation, employment, welfare, social support and self-care which includes matters of hygiene, nutrition and budgeting. An important function of hospitalisation is to help the patient link up with the various aftercare resources that may be required.

Medication

The introduction of antipsychotic drugs in the 1950s revolutionised the treatment of schizophrenia. The common property of these drugs is their ability to block dopamine receptors in the brain. At least part of their therapeutic action may be related to their ability to reduce arousal. Their effects can be considered three-fold:

1. Immediate or non-specific effects

In the very short term these drugs have a rapid calming or *tranquillising* effect. Agitation, restlessness, overactivity, severe anxiety, irritability and impulsiveness, unpredictable behaviours tend to settle fairly quickly after administration of the drugs. Also, a restful, quiet atmosphere can assist this action and enable smaller doses to be effective than would otherwise be the case in an overstimulating environment. This tranquillising action may require from some minutes to several hours to begin but takes effect more quickly if given by injection. Non-specific tranquillisation caused by the drugs must be distinguished from their specific antipsychotic effects.

2. Delayed or specific effects

When given in appropriate doses over a longer period of time, these drugs exert specific *antipsychotic* actions. That is, they help to counteract delusions, hallucinations and thought disorder. This process usually takes two to four weeks but sometimes longer. It cannot be hurried.

3. Long-term effects

When given in amounts that are usually less than those required for the immediate and delayed effects, antipsychotic drugs have a very important role to play in preventing relapse of acute symptoms. This can be referred to as their *prophylactic* effect. Continuing use of maintenance doses of these drugs is very useful in preventing readmission to hospital and thus helping to maintain the individual patient living in the community.

It should be kept in mind that antipsychotic drugs represent merely one component of treatment, albeit a very important component. As such they are complementary to, but do not replace, high quality psychosocial treatments.

Since all of the antipsychotic drugs are effective in controlling the acute symptoms of schizophrenia, there is little basis to choose between the different varieties available other than their profile of side-effects. Broadly speaking, the so-called 'low-potency' drugs (for example, chlorpromazine, thioridazine) are more likely to be associated with the side-effects of sedation, postural hypotension and anticholinergic actions (for example, dry mouth, blurred vision, constipation). On the other hand, high potency drugs (for example, haloperidol, fluphenazine, trifluoperazine) are more likely to produce neuromusclar side-effects (for example, Parkinsonism, akathisia, acute dystonia). A more detailed discussion of the actions, side-effects and complications of these drugs can be found in chapters 56, 57. There is no therapeutic advantage in taking more than one antipsychotic drug concurrently.

For practical purposes, most acute episodes of schizophrenia will respond to 200–800 mg per day of chlorpromazine and 5–20 mg per day of haloperidol. The daily dose for maintenance therapy is usually between 20 to 50 per cent of these levels. Maintenance drug therapy should be continued for several years on the lowest effective dose possible. It is difficult to determine whether and when these drugs can be safely discontinued. Even patients who have been well while taking medication for several years may relapse within months of discontinuing the drugs.

Whether this represents true relapse of the illness or merely a drug withdrawal reaction is not known. The best strategy is to enlist the active participation of the patient in managing his own drug therapy in consultation with the therapist. This entails the patient developing a good understanding of the effects of varying drug dosage in his own particular case and an awareness of the early signs of relapse so that treatment can be reinstituted or the dosage increased rapidly when necessary in order to forestall a recurrence of acute symptoms. This is the basis for the 'intermittent' treatment strategy which may be very useful for insightful patients. The collaborative strategy described above is also useful in helping to avoid chronic overdosage which may not only lead to severe side-effects and certain complications such as tardive dyskinesia but may also exacerbate the negative symptoms of the residual form of schizophrenia.

Other medical treatments such as lithium or benzodiazepines may be useful adjuncts to antipsychotic drugs for some patients. Electro-convulsive therapy (ECT) is rarely effective except in life-threatening catatonic schizophrenia or severe depression which has supervened.

Psychosocial therapies

These need to be thoughtfully integrated with the other therapeutic modalities and carefully tailored to meet the unique needs of individual patients.

1. *Individual psychotherapy*

In the first instance this needs to be supportive in its orientation with emphasis in the early stages on the establishment of a trusting relationship with the therapist. In this context, an educative focus can help patients learn about their illness and methods of coping with it. They can also be taught useful information about medication, its therapeutic and adverse effects. The individual therapeutic relationship can act as a vehicle by which ego strengths can be supported and consolidated. The ego function of reality testing is a particularly crucial example in

schizophrenia. Advice, reassurance and explanation are also important components of psychotherapy in schizophrenic patients. Further psychotherapeutic work may appear indicated but the nature and goals of this work very closely depend on the type of psychological or interpersonal difficulties the individual patient is experiencing along with their illness. It is important that the therapy be problem-focused and not overstimulating or too demanding for the patient's psychological resources.

2. *Family therapy*

In the beginning, families should be given as much information about schizophrenia (symptoms, treatment and outcome) as they need to understand the patient and assist with his management. This can go a long way towards relieving the family of feelings of guilt or self-blame for the patient's condition. Counselling and advice should then be problem-focused and opportunity given to allow families to have their questions answered satisfactorily. Specific counselling methods for reducing levels of 'expressed emotion' have been devised and these can play an important part in preventing relapse. These tend to incorporate ways of improving the family's problem-solving skills which, by reducing conflict, have the effect of ameliorating their propensity to get angry with or criticise the patient.

3. *Group therapy*

In the residual phase of schizophrenia group therapeutic approaches can sometimes be useful provided they are supportive and accepting rather than uncovering or confrontational in their orientation and provided also that the focus is on practical tasks and solving problems of everyday living. A specific example can be found in social skills training groups. These need to be well-structured in their mode of functioning. Their goals are to enhance social competence so that survival in the community may be improved and quality of life increased through the development and maintenance of social relationships.

4. Behaviour therapy

The principles of learning theory can be applied in a variety of settings and in several ways (for example, token economies) to improve functioning. Techniques incorporating a system of rewards contingent upon the occurrence or disappearance of certain target behaviours can be effective in reducing a range of disabilities associated with schizophrenia. This mode of therapy can lead to improvements in the areas of social skills, self-care, independence and communication while also reducing socially inappropriate or maladapative behaviours. Unfortunately, many patients relapse when discharged from this kind of therapeutic environment. That is, the acquired behaviours fail to generalise when the systematic application of reinforcers is withdrawn (see chapter 61).

Rehabilitation

The task of minimising or overcoming the handicaps associated with schizophrenia is essentially one of rehabilitation. This illness may adversely affect human functioning in many areas. Examples include occupational functioning, academic performance, household chores, parenting tasks, recreational activities, budgeting, nutrition, hygiene, grooming, social competence and other activities of daily living. Rehabilitation in each of these areas needs to be targeted at specific deficits identified through careful assessment of each individual by a multidisciplinary team. The latter may comprise occupational therapists, clinical psychologists, social workers, vocational guidance officers, psychiatric nurses, teachers and the therapist primarily responsible for the patient.

Rehabilitation often requires special facilities such as day hospital centres, industrial therapy units, community health centres, employment training programs, community 'drop-in' facilities and client-run businesses. A realistic series of achievable goals need to be set and the rehabilitation program individually tailored to the needs of the particular patient. Suitable accommodation is mandatory but often difficult to find. Well-supervised hostels oriented towards

rehabilitation can be very useful in promoting independent living and socialisation.

Outcome

When patients recover from an acute episode of schizophrenia they may struggle to integrate the experience, to accept and make sense of what happened by trying to grasp the meaning of the illness in the context of their own lives. This mode of recovering treats the illness experience as an important, albeit unwelcome, learning opportunity. Another mode of recovery involves trying to suppress all memories of the event, to treat the illness as an alien event that has no personal relevance or significance to the individual— the 'less said about it, the better' style of recovery. In either case, patients often emerge from an acute episode of schizophrenia with their self-confidence and self-esteem severely injured. This may take a long time to recover and can be associated with profound feelings of hopelessness and depression.

It is in the months after recovery from the acute illness that suicide is most likely to occur. Approximately 10 per cent of schizophrenic patients commit suicide and about half of all cases make a suicide attempt at some time. The patient most likely to commit suicide is a young male who has suffered a series of relapses and has found himself failing to live up to the high expectations of himself and his family. A severe disappointment with subsequent despair and hopelessness may be the final event that triggers the suicide.

The long-term outcome of schizophrenia has not changed significantly since the advent of antipsychotic drugs. A good outcome occurs early in 20 to 30 per cent of cases and many of the remainder show moderate degrees of impairment but with a satisfactory quality of life if followed for a long time.

It is impossible to predict the outcome accurately in individual cases. However, good prognostic signs include sudden onset, brief acute episodes with prominent affective symptoms, older age of onset and good premorbid functioning in terms of work, social relationships and psychosexual adjustment.

Schizophrenia is one of the most disabling psychiatric disorders. There are effective treatments but they need to be administered in a multidisciplinary framework. A good outcome is possible with the aid of time, patience and a caring environment.

Further Reading

Bleuler E, *Dementia Praecox or the Group of Schizophrenias*, International Universities Press, New York, 1950.

Cutting J, *The Psychology of Schizophrenia*, Churchill Livingstone, Edinburgh, 1985.

Rollin H R, *Coping with Schizophrenia*, The National Schizophrenia Fellowship, Burnett Books, London, 1980.

Strauss J S and Carpenter W T, Jr, *Schizophrenia*, Plenum Medical Book Co, New York, 1981.

Chapter 34

Pain: Psychiatric Aspects

I Pilowsky

Virtually any psychiatric condition can present with pain as the main symptom, but this is especially the case in anxiety, depressive and somatoform disorders. This obviously means that such presentations are very common amongst people attending general practitioners and a variety of medical specialists. It is important, therefore, that a proper diagnosis be made as early as possible, so as to avoid unnecessary investigations and treatments.

Pain is not easy to define, however the International Association for the Study of Pain has agreed on the following definition: 'Pain is an unpleasant sensory and emotional experience associated with actual or potential tissue damages or described in terms of such damage'. The important aspect of this definition is that it emphasises the fact that pain is an *experience* of a particular type and, therefore, to fully understand someone's pain, we have to take their feelings and thoughts into consideration. This means that we need to know whether they are anxious, depressed or angry, and what they think has caused the pain and what the future holds in store for them. All this is apart from making a thorough appraisal of any physical factors or inputs to the pain experience, which helps to clarify the nociceptive[1] aspects of the pain experience.

Although, as stated above, any psychiatric syndrome can present with the complaint of pain, there is a group of conditions in which

pain is a particularly prominent feature of the syndrome. These syndromes are referred to as somatoform disorders in the Diagnostic and Statistical manual of the American Psychiatric Association, 3rd Edition, Revised (DSM-III-R). Somatoform disorders consist essentially of conditions in which the patient has somatic complaints and disabilities for which an adequate somatic cause cannot be found. It is assumed that these patients are suffering from emotional and psychological distress, which is expressed in somatic rather than psychological terms. What allows one to be more confident that this is happening, is the finding that the patient rejects the idea he has personal problems or that any emotional distress exists, and is offended by the suggestion, even when such stresses are obvious to any objective observer. We can deduce from this attitude that it is more comfortable for the patient to conceptualise and communicate his problems in somatic rather than psychologic terms. This form of defensive coping is described as somatisation or somatising behaviour.

The four main forms of somatoform disorder are: somatising disorder, hypochondriasis, conversion disorder and somatoform pain disorder. Pain may be present in all these conditions, but it is the main complaint in somatoform pain disorders.

All these somatoform disorders are forms of abnormal illness behaviour, which is defined as:

> an inappropriate or maladaptive mode of experiencing, perceiving, evaluating or responding to one's own state of health which persists despite the fact that a doctor (or other

---

[1] Nociception refers to the body's response to a stimulus which is noxious or would become noxious if prolonged.

appropriate social agent) has offered an accurate and reasonably lucid explanation of the nature of the person's health status and the appropriate course of management (if any), with provision of adequate opportunity for discussion, clarification and negotiation based on a thorough examination of all parameters of functioning (psychological, social and biological), and taking into account the individual's age, sex, education and sociocultural background.

This has to be borne in mind when assessing patients. Particular attention should be paid to providing the patient with a proper explanation of their health status, or at least ensuring that it has been done by someone in a position to do so, preferably in the presence of the person who will continue management. If the explanation has not been given, or is deemed to be incomplete, the diagnosis of a form of abnormal illness behaviour should be recorded as 'provisional'.

The somatoform disorders will each be described briefly, after which we will focus on the meanings and significance of pain.

Somatisation disorder

This is not a common condition. It is a chronic disorder, characterised by a tendency to regard oneself as 'sickly' with frequent presentation of focal conversion symptoms of a neurological nature. Such patients appear to find comfort in the care of doctors and tend to agree passively to active treatments including operations. The developmental history may reveal a childhood experience of medical treatments and possibly hospitalisation, against a background of a severely deprived family life.

Conversion disorders

These disorders involve a loss or alteration of function which suggests a physical disorder, but without objective evidence for a pathological process which should be associated with such a disorder. Examples would be symptoms such as blindness or a paralysed limb. What is also important is the way the person thinks and feels about the disability. In the classic case, the patient reports a lack of preoccupation with the cause or significance of the symptom, although there is an awareness of discomfort and disability.

Psychosocial stresses which may be linked to the symptom are denied, even when they are obvious to most people who take an objective view of the patient's situation. The patient's overt affect may be serene ('la belle indifference') and anxiety or depression strenuously denied. On the other hand, such uncomfortable affects may be acknowledged, but attributed entirely to the disability and suffering caused by the physical symptom.

Hypochondriasis

Hypochondriasis differs from conversion disorders in that the patient is preoccupied with concerns about their health and overly aware of bodily symptoms. The preoccupation may take the form of a phobia, with fears of death due to a stroke, heart attack, etc, or it may be a firm conviction of the presence of disease, such as cancer. However, this conviction may not be sufficiently firm to be considered a delusion, but rather a morbid preoccupation which, in a typical case, is present more often than not, ie more than 50 per cent of the time. Hypochondriasis may be primary or secondary. When it is secondary, the condition considered primary is usually a depressive illness, but may also be an anxiety disorder and occasionally schizophrenia (especially in the very early stages). In primary hypochondriasis anxiety and depression are minimal—the patient is concerned and preoccupied with the fear of having a serious disease. This concern is based on the way the person interprets their bodily sensations and on the various signs present in their body, which they believe indicate the presence of the illness. It is characteristic of this disorder that despite medical reassurance, and any number of examinations and tests, the belief persists and continues to preoccupy the person. In this case, the belief does not reach a delusional intensity, ie the person can accept that the belief is unfounded yet they are unable to shake off the fear.

It is interesting to note that the two systematic studies carried out to establish the validity of the diagnosis of hypochondriasis as an independent entity, differed in their findings; with Kenyon concluding that hypochondriasis was always secondary, usually to a depressive illness, and Pilowsky finding that hypochondriasis could be regarded as primary—as indeed DSM-III-R does. The difference between the two studies may be accounted for by the fact that Kenyon studied the casenotes of patients referred to a psychiatric hospital while Pilowsky personally studied outpatients, inpatients and day patients referred to the University Psychiatric Unit of a general hospital. The important point to be drawn from this, is that patients with hypochondriasis or any other somatoform disorder do not readily seek treatment from psychiatrists. They are usually seen by a variety of specialists and general practitioners and regard this as appropriate; indeed, they will usually resist referral to a psychiatrist, although they are more likely to accept psychiatric help in a general hospital where the psychiatrist can be regarded as a member of multidisciplinary team, such as a pain clinic. They will also be more accepting if the referring physician emphasises a continued interest in seeing the patient.

Somatoform pain disorder

This consists of a preoccupation with feelings of pain either in a situation where the appropriate medical evaluation fails to reveal any organic pathology or physiological mechanism to account for the pain, or where the complaints of pain are grossly in excess of what would be expected from the physical findings.

The psychological significance of pain

Somatoform pain disorders cannot be adequately managed unless there is some understanding of the meanings which the pain may have for the patient and the ways in which the patient may be predisposed or vulnerable to the development of a somatoform pain disorder. These issues have been dealt with in a classic paper by George Engel. Based on his clinical contact with a series of patients suffering from chronic pain, in the absence of somatic pathology adequate to account for the type and intensity of the pain, nor the associated impairment of function, he was able to describe the meanings of pain and personality patterns associated with what he termed 'psychogenic pain'. He found that

apart from the obvious association between pain and the idea of bodily harm, pain was also associated with ideas of guilt, loss, with aggression and punishment, with reconciliation and care-giving and, at times, with sexual arousal and pleasure (masochism). Engel also encountered certain developmental patterns in these patients, ie childhood experiences which might predispose to chronic pain as part of an unconscious adaptive strategy. For example, some patients had experienced a great deal of physical punishment as children often followed by 'making up' when they were given the only positive regard they received from their parents. Other patients give a history of having one dominant aggressive parent and the other a submissive one. These and other similar experiencs may lead to a personality type (described as 'pain-prone' by Engel) in which pain is utilised unconsciously as a way of assuaging real or fantasied guilt, and also as a state which reunites them with someone upon whom they can depend for love and support.

Management of chronic non-malignant pain (including somatoform pain disorders)

General principles

There is a tendency for some patients whose pain is largely a consequence of psychosocial problems, to resist the suggestion that there is any point in considering their suffering from a psychosocial perspective. This is the case, of course, when a crucial psychological function of the pain experience is to achieve subjective emotional equilibrium by avoiding the need to face up to personal problems. It is important, therefore, to help the patient realise that the pain should be approached from a multidimensional point of view, ie with proper attention to somatic, psychological and social factors which are somehow associated with the pain or perhaps a consequence of it. It may be asserted with reasonable confidence, based on clinical experience and theoretical considerations, that provided the clinician shows unambiguous acceptance of the patient's pain experience and suffering, it is invariably possible to shift the focus to the psychosocial domain, from a diagnostic and management point of view.

Thus, pain of this sort calls for a multimodal approach and this may require a collaborative, multidisciplinary team, such as exists in Pain Clincs which are associated with most major teaching hospitals—certainly in the case of Australia and New Zealand.

The approaches available for the management of chronic pain include:
1. psychopharmacological
2. psychotherapeutic
3. cognitive–behavioural
4. relaxation and biofeedback
5. group and marital therapy.

1. Psychopharmacological approaches

Those which have been found effective in chronic pain involve chiefly the use of antidepressants (in particular tricyclics). Amitriptyline has been most commonly used and is effective in doses lower than those used for the treatment of depressive disorders, unless, of course, the pain is associated with a depressive illness. The rationale for using such drugs is based on the fact that the endogenous pain suppression system is dependent on serotonergic and, to some extent, adrenergic activity.

2. Psychotherapeutic approaches

Supportive psychotherapy is always a keystone in the management of chronic pain. Allowing the patient time to speak freely about somatic and psychosocial problems, so that these can be clarified and emotions ventilated is a basic approach to any condition. Judicious advice, where appropriate, and support for the patient's own coping strategies with praise and reinforcement will help boost a usually low self-esteem. Such support at four to six weekly intervals may be necessary over long periods of time.

Individual psychotherapy on a weekly basis over 10 to 20 weeks may be used in some patients who require greater insight into the nature of the pain experience, the part it plays in their interpersonal relationships and their ways of coping. Patients more suited to this type of treatment have less severe pain which

is not continuous, and they tend to accept the role of psychosocial factors. They are younger and tend to have head and neck pain. It is not unusual for a patient to report satisfaction with the effects of such treatment on their quality of life and ability to cope, even though they may consider the pain itself to be unchanged or to have worsened in some ways. Individual psychotherapy combined with a tricyclic tends to be an effective combination, with advantages over psychotherapy alone (see chapter 58).

3. Cognitive–behavioural therapy

This is used most often for patients who are clearly disabled by the pain and spend much of the time sitting or reclining. There are a number of inpatient units for such treatment which usually lasts three to six weeks. The program is highly structured with regular graded exercises playing an important part. Patients are advised not to seek sympathy and care from others because of pain, and their relatives are similarly advised. However, improvements in functioning are reinforced with praise and attention. It is particularly important that the patients keep a regular record of the amount of pain on a scale from 0–10, as well as a record of their activities and exercises, and that these be presented in a graphic and visual form.

The cognitive part of the treatment involved helping the patient to find ways of modifying the way he thinks about the pain and what it might mean in terms of somatic damage. For example, it is important to explain that pain after exercise does not necessarily indicate tissue damage. Help is also given to develop ways of distracting attention from pain and other health preoccupations onto thoughts and activities which reduce anxiety (see chapters 58, 61 and 63).

4. Relaxation and biofeedback

These refer to exercises aimed at reducing muscle tension and thus pain. Such techniques can form a part of any pain management program. Biofeedback involves presenting the patient with an auditory or visual signal indicating the amount of tension in a group of muscles, thus giving feedback as to the amount of relaxation achieved. This form of muscle biofeedback works especially well in patients with head and neck pain.

5. *Marital and family therapy*

This is important where obvious conflicts exist, but also where close ones are reinforcing invalidism by their over-protective attitudes. Group therapy is usually a part of any structured inpatient programs and allows patients the opportunity to learn from each others' experiences and provide mutual support.

Prognosis

It is difficult to make general statements about prognosis for patients with somatoform pain disorders because, thus far, reports have come from relatively disparate contexts, involving heterogeneous populations. However, there appears to be a consensus emerging that, given a rational, structured approach to chronic pain problems, one may, at the very least, save the patient from unnecessary, time-consuming, expensive and, in some cases, potentially dangerous, investigations and treatments. Actual percentages improving range from 40 to 70 per cent.

Furthermore, as mentioned earlier, a great deal may be done to improve a patient's functioning and attitudes without necessarily removing the pain. Indeed, most patients will agree at the outset that total pain removal is not a realistic objective. Some patients may go so far as to say that they simply want to know that there is no further medical or surgical intervention available for their disorder, and are content to 'live with the pain', while making the best adaptation they can achieve. Gains of this sort are highly desirable for patients who might otherwise be destined for a life dominated by pain, invalidism and constant involvement with the health care system.

References

Engel G, 'Psychogenic Pain and the Pain-prone Patient', *American Journal of Medicine*, Vol 26, 1959, pp 899–918.

Kenyon F E 'Hypochondriasis: A Clinical Study', *British Journal of Psychiatry*, Vol 110, 1964, pp 478–88.

Pilowsky I, 'Primary and Secondary Hypochondriasis', *Acta Psychiatrica Scandinavica*, Vol 46, 1970, pp 273–85.

Further Reading

Bellisimo A and Tunks E, *Chronic Pain. The Psychotherapeutic Spectrum*, Praeger, New York, 1984.

Merskey H and Spear R, *Pain: Psychological and Psychiatric Aspects*, Bailliere, Tindall and Cassell, London, 1967.

Pilowsky I, 'Abnormal Illness Behaviour', *British Journal of Medical Psychology*, Vol 42, 1969, pp 347–51.

Pilowsky I, 'The Psychiatrist and the Pain Clinic', *American Journal of Psychiatry*, Vol 133, 1976, pp 752–6.

Pilowsky I, 'A General Classification of Abnormal Illness Behaviours', *British Journal of Medical Psychology*, Vol 51, 1978, pp 131–7.

Pilowsky I and Barrow C G, 'A Controlled Study of Psychotherapy and Amitriptyline Used Individually and in Combination in the Treatment of Chronic Intractable "Psychogenic" Pain', *Pain*, Vol 40, 1990, pp 3–19.

Chapter 35

Post-traumatic Stress Disorder

A C McFarlane

Since the time of the American civil war, psychiatrists have recognised that extremely distressing events cause considerable emotional distress and psychological malfunction. During and after both the First and Second World Wars there was much discussion about whether servicemen developed a unique pattern of symptoms or whether the large numbers of psychiatric casualties suffering from depressive and anxiety neuroses were similar to those seen in the civilian population. In the last 15 years, the impact of the Vietnam war on a generation of veterans has led to a much greater awareness of the long-term psychological sequelae. This increased knowledge led to the definition of post-traumatic stress disorder (PTSD) in the third edition of DSM-III. However, the chronicles of history document that this disorder has affected people throughout recorded time. Samuel Pepys, in his famous diary gave a graphic account of his own post-traumatic symptoms following the fire that devastated London in 1666.

Events which can precipitate post-traumatic stress disorders are those which are outside the range of usual human experience and that would be markedly distressing to almost everyone. These stressors include any serious threat to a person's life or physical integrity (for example, rape, motor vehicle accident or violent assault), destruction of a person's home or community (for example, in a natural disaster or house fire), or seeing another person who is mutilated, dying or dead. It is important, however, not to be too rigid in the definition of a traumatic event because people's perception of the danger-

ousness or threat posed by an event depends on range of factors, such as their past experience. Also, the personal meaning of the trauma determines the degree of distress and whether or not aspects of the experience continue to haunt the victim. For example, a man who had been brutally tortured was not most preoccupied by these assaults which caused excruciating pain or the times where he thought he might die, rather he was haunted by the memory of hallucinations he had experienced during an episode of delirium caused by sleep deprivation, starvation and physical pain which challenged his most basic sense of self control.

Clinical features

The diagnostic criteria for post-traumatic stress disorder include three sets of phenomena. The first is characterised by *re-experiencing the trauma* in a variety of ways. The sufferer may complain of recurrent and intrusive recollections of the trauma which may dominate his mind for many hours. There may be recurring dreams of the event and these focus on general themes of death, injury or personal safety. Less commonly, there are intense flashbacks to the traumatic event which feel as though the event were actually recurring. Alternatively, the patient may experience intense physiological distress when confronted with a symbolic reminder or events that resemble the trauma. For example, the unexpected smell of smoke may be sufficient to make the victim of a bushfire disaster vomit. Such re-experiencing phenomena tend to become less frequent with time but they are often triggered by reminders. They are more intense and pervasive forms of the normal distress response that can affect any person who has, for example, come close to death.

Patients tend to complain about another set of phenomena which relate to *disorders of attention and arousal*. They have difficulty falling and/or staying asleep and they are more irritable than usual. War veterans particularly have outbursts of anger that can sometimes lead to assaulting others. Difficulty concentrating disrupts day to day functioning and is reflected in increased forgetfulness and problems completing tasks. Great sensitivity is manifested by the person watching for danger or threat and by their feeling of increased vulnerability. Patients show an exaggerated startle response, reflecting their distractibility and their arousal. They may become intensely anxious if exposed to a real or symbolic reminder of the trauma. For example, a boy who witnessed a savage attack by a German Shepherd dog on a friend, became panicky when a change of weather occurred because the attack occurred at approximately the time a cool change had arrived.

The third set of phenomena represent attempts by the person to *control* his emotional lability and arousal and by a continuing preoccupation with the trauma. This is perceived to be irrational because of the intensity of feeling. Such patients attempt to shut out the recurring thoughts and feelings of the trauma and avoid any activity which reminds them of the trauma. Places or situations which are associated with the event may be actively avoided. This avoidant behaviour may even include loss of memory for important aspects of the experience.

The distress associated with the emotional lability of post-traumatic stress disorder may also involve psychic or emotional numbing. This mechanism leads to feelings of detachment or estrangement from other people and loss of interest in activities which the individual previously enjoyed. This can reach the point where the person loses the ability to feel emotions of any type, particularly intimacy and tenderness. This disturbance can be very distressing for a spouse who may also have endured the impact of the trauma.

In children, re-experiencing phenomena may be manifested in their play which focuses in a recurring way on the general theme of the trauma. A child's withdrawal and emotional numbing can be misinterpreted as 'good' behaviour because the child becomes quiet and conforming. Adolescents can show a marked change in their orientation to the future, for example they might avoid any commitment to a career or stable relationships because they now see no guarantee of a stable future.

Onset and prevalence

Symptoms usually begin soon after the trauma. In the weeks immediately after the event it is often difficult to distinguish post-traumatic stress disorder from a more normal distress response which is also characterised by re-experiencing phenomena. Sleep disturbance and high levels of anxiety, at this early stage, are markers of a higher risk of developing clinically significant symptoms later. In a minority of sufferers (10 per cent) PTSD may not develop for months or even years after the trauma.

The prevalence of PTSD depends on the severity of the trauma and the duration and intensity of exposure. This will vary widely within the victims of the same event or type of event. Studies of disasters, including the Bhopal chemical disaster in India, the eruption of Mt St Helens Volcano in Seattle and the Ash Wednesday bushfire disaster in South Australia showed that between 15 and 40 per cent of victims developed symptoms of PTSD.

Few longitudinal post disaster studies have been conducted which means that little is known about the natural history of post-traumatic stress disorder. However, the disorder appears to have a chronic course in the majority of people. Most continue to have symptoms for more than one year after the trauma.

Aetiology

No theory of psychopathology can fully explain all the features of PTSD. There has been an ongoing debate about the relative importance of predisposing factors in its aetiology. However, the way people respond to trauma is inevitably moulded by their individual perception of the event. This is influenced by the individual's past experiences, individual personality traits and his perceptions of other people's characteristic ways of reacting to him. While the trauma becomes the focal determinant of an individual's initial reaction, these other characteristics colour his longer-term adjustment. The fact that PTSD is not an inevitable consequence of severe trauma emphasises the involvement of a range of factors which modify individual responses. The resilience of the majority of the victims to the impact of traumatic stress is a notable demonstration of people's adaptability to adversity.

There are no predisposing factors which inevitably lead to PTSD. However variables such as a personal or family history of psychiatric disorder, a tendency to use avoidance as a normal defence, the personal characteristic of being particularly reactive to environmental stimuli (neuroticism) and the experience of other adverse life events in close proximity to the trauma are thought to be important vulnerability factors. In fact, people become unusually sensitive to distressing life events experienced in the aftermath of a trauma. Similarly the effects of the trauma on other family members such as nightmares and flashbacks can act as a constant reminder of the horror of the trauma. If a third party is being sued for having caused the triggering event, the adversarial nature of the legal system can maintain a sense of victimisation and perpetuate symptoms in PTSD.

At a physiological level, PTSD may involve a disturbance in the catecholaminergic systems of the brain and in the function of the locus coeruleus, a small nucleus in the midbrain which controls the attention to environmental stimuli and the modulation of an individual's state of arousal. The repeated exposure of rats to inescapable electric shocks leads to a depletion of their brain noradrenaline. This is the neurotransmittor of the locus coeruleus and this effect demonstrates how an environmental event can lead to a biological change in brain functioning.

Psychological mechanisms are also involved in the symptom patterns seen in PTSD. The content of a patient's traumatic ruminations are often influenced by previous life experiences and conflicts. For example, an elderly farmer who found his dead workmate's body after a disaster was preoccupied by an intense sense of guilt about his own survival. This death had reactivated his guilt about a wartime experience. As a pilot in the airforce he had changed places with a colleague flying a particular mission. The plane he was to have flown crashed with the death of all the crew. The disaster which happened many years later triggered intense ruminations about this wartime tragedy.

Events which symbolise the trauma (for example, the touching of a light switch for a person who has been electrocuted); and real reminders (for example, travelling in a car for a motor accident victim) may trigger a conditioned response of intense anxiety. Furthermore, avoidance of the reminders serves to perpetuate the individual's traumatic fear and leads to a generalisation of the anxiety. A cognitive processing model focuses on the cognitive mediation of the stress response and the affect generated by a traumatic event arises from the discrepancy between the degree of threat and the coping resources available to deal with it. The working through of the event involves the integration of the experience with the person's previous inner models of the world.

Assessment of PTSD

The process of assessment can have a potentially beneficial effect in its own right. Often the assessment interview will be the first setting where people can confide the real nature of their personal trauma. The simple process of unburdening the distress with another person can play an important role by evoking a sense of hope. This contrasts with the demoralisation and feelings of isolation that are part of the aftermath of trauma. An excessive enthusiasm on the part of the health professional for patients to disclose the full affective quality of their experience should be avoided because it will more often cause withdrawal from treatment, rather than lead to a rapid improvement. The successful assessment interview is characterised by only brief moments of intense affect which the patient is encouraged to control.

PTSD is associated with another psychiatric disorder in more than 50 per cent of patients. People will often focus on symptoms of depression and panic attacks rather than speak of recurring and intrusive thoughts which they will even actually avoid telling the interviewer. For this reason, PTSD can be easily overlooked. Somatic symptoms (for example, chest pains, headaches and shortness of breath) are a frequent focus of complaint and can be the primary reason for seeking medical attention. They need to be thoroughly assessed medically. Alcohol abuse occurs in approximately 30 per cent of patients who have PTSD. Often successful treatment of PTSD is difficult because of the perpetuating role of an underlying anxiety or depressive disorders. When the patient is describing the event, it is important to explore the perceptions of his experience and thoughts during and immediately after the trauma, in addition to discussing the reality of the experience. For example, a woman who was trapped in her upturned car was terrified that the petrol dripping from the tank would ignite. Her fear was particularly vivid because she had worked as a nurse in the burns unit of a teaching hospital. The content of the patients' post-traumatic imagery should be examined in relation to the aspects of the traumatic experience which are particularly remembered (for example, a police officer who had to take the wedding ring off the corpse of a woman was intensely preoccupied by this experience as his wife had died one month earlier and he had also removed her ring). People's perception of threat often has little to do with their actual experience of trauma, but has more to do with the individual meaning of the traumatic experience.

Management

There are three separate sets of problems in post-traumatic stress disorder that require attention in treatment. What works for one set of symptoms will not necessarily be useful for another. A psychotherapeutic approach is the central treatment of the intrusive memories. Catharsis alone has little role to play except in rare circumstances where the patient is amnesic in relation to the trauma. Specific behavioural strategies are useful in overcoming avoidance and should focus on exposure to real and symbolic triggers of the patient's anxiety symptoms.

Control of the patient's disturbed attention and arousal is often critical to the success of the treatment of post-traumatic stress disorder. Relief of these symptoms plays an important role in ensuring a patient's commitment to the treatment process. Once these distressing and disabling symptoms are decreased, people often find it much easier to focus on and think through their traumatic memories. Medication, used as a short-term adjunct to psychotherapy can be particularly useful in this regard. Tricyclic antidepressants and monoamine oxidase inhibitors are the most effective and commonly used medications. The reasons for prescribing these drugs need to be explained in detail and the possible side effcts also should be discussed. The need to remain on medication requires regular review. There is little role for sedatives (for example, benzodiazepines).

Numbing and withdrawal require a specific focus in their own right as they do not necessarily respond to the psychological techniques aimed at the intrusive memories or the anxiety.

In an acute disorder, the social and interpersonal problems are still evolving and are therefore more amenable to treatment, because they are not yet entrenched. In long-standing post-traumatic stress disorder, the underlying disturbances of attention and arousal may be less of a problem than the constructed affect and emotional estrangement in relationships. Family and group therapy is often required to allow a focus on the interpersonal and social dimensions of the effects on the family and other people.

Conclusion

Many uncertainties remain about the aetiology and treatment of post-traumatic stress disorder. The effects of traumatic stress are frequently missed and can lead to a chronic disability. While patterns of response to severe trauma can be described, it is important not to over-generalise about the nature. There are many ways that people respond to disaster. Their reactions are moulded by their individual perception of the event, which in turn is influenced by the victim's past experiences, personality traits and expectations of other people.

Thus, careful assessment of these issues and attention to the individual preoccupations of each patient are central to the adequate treatment of post-traumatic stress disorder. Similarly, a treatment program will often use a number of therapeutic methods concurrently, emphasising the need for a multi-dimensional approach of this disorder.

Further Reading

Ettedgui E and Bridges M, 'Post-traumatic Stress Disorder'. *Psychiatric Clinics of North America* , Vol 8, 1985 pp 89–103.

Figley C R, *Trauma and its Wake: the Study and Treatment of Post-traumatic Stress Disorder,* New York, Brunner/Mazel , 1985, Vol 1 and 1986, Vol 2.

McFarlane A C, 'The Treatment of Post-traumatic Stress Disorder', *British Journal of Medical Psychology,* Vol 62,1989, pp 81–90.

Chapter 36

Eating Disorders

A Hall

Eating disorders are characterised by overconcern about weight and body fatness and by self imposed abnormalities of eating and dietary intake sufficient to impair physical and mental health. Ninety five per cent of sufferers are female and the majority are aged between 15–25 years.

The most clearly defined syndromes are anorexia nervosa which was described as a medical condition in the nineteenth century and bulimia nervosa which has only been described in the last 20 years.

Anorexia nervosa

The four features of anorexia nervosa are extreme thinness, an overriding fear of putting on weight and becoming fat, a disturbed perception of the body and, in females, amenorrhoea.

Clinical features

Typically anorexia nervosa begins in a teenage female who has lost some weight by dieting. Less commonly it may begin when weight is lost through illness. The patient is unable to stop dieting because she becomes overwhelmingly concerned about getting fat and this concern intensifies as more weight is lost. The weight loss is usually rapid, and the full syndrome commonly develops within a few months.

For the diagnosis to be made, the patient should weigh less than 85 per cent of the population average weight for age, height and sex or, have a Body Mass Index (BMI = $\frac{wt(kg)}{ht(m)^2}$) of under 18. Body Mass Index is a measure of weight related to height increasingly used in medicine as an index of obesity. The normal range of the BMI in women is 20–25. In patients less than 15 years of age paediatric growth charts are used to estimate the degree of underweight.

The thinness may be hidden by loose clothing, but some patients exhibit their extreme thinness apparently oblivious to the effect of their emaciated appearance on others. Typically even extremely thin patients are characteristically alert and physically active. All the physical changes can be explained by starvation which results in lowered metabolism, marked loss of body fat and alteration of hormones. The pulse and blood pressure are low and the circulation is poor so that the patient feels cold and is liable to fungal infection of the nail beds.

Growth stops, sexual feelings are reduced and menstrual periods are absent unless the patient is on a contraceptive pill. Anaemia is unusual although the number of white blood cells is often reduced. Demineralisation of bones may develop after three to four years of low weight and amenorrhoea.

Fats and sugars are avoided. Meat, eggs and full-cream dairy products are often not eaten at all because of their fat content. Complex carbohydrates (cereals and vegetables) which are currently popular diet foods tend to be favoured. Daily intake become progressively more restricted and will often be reduced to a few apples, raw vegetables, and a little cottage cheese or lean chicken or fish. Patients deny that their intake is inadequate for them to remain active and healthy.

Eating behaviour varies considerably. Some nibble small quantities of food throughout the day while others may eat nothing all day but have an apparently adequate meal in the evening. They avoid eating with other people if they can, but, on the other hand, are extremely interested in food and take a great interest in other peoples' eating.

As starvation progresses, patients may break their rigid dietary rules and eat small quantities of 'forbidden' food and then counteract this by self induced vomiting, laxative taking, increased exercise or even more rigid restrictions. When patients are required to eat adequately they may hide food, lie about their intake, or secretly purge the food.

Some patients become compulsive about exercise. They may feel compelled to go for a long run every day irrespective of the weather, the social convenience or, the state of their health and, if exercise is prohibited they may exercise secretly in the middle of the night or in the shower.

Psychopathology

The starvation state causes impaired concentration and greatly diminishes the ability to think flexibly. People with anorexia nervosa are constantly preoccupied with thoughts of food and this subject may take up much of their conversation. Their intense fear of gaining weight and becoming fat differentiates them from naturally thin people or people who have lost weight for other reasons. Fear of becoming fat is the motivating force in the patient's life, and other concerns become secondary. It is important to recognise that sufferers value continuing weight loss, because this proves fat is not being deposited. Long hours are spent at school work in order to control thoughts of food, and social occasions may be avoided because they may involve being required to eat. Family members or friends may be regarded as enemies because of their wish to fatten the patient.

Patients develop abnormal beliefs about their weight and shape. They can perceive other peoples' weight and shape realistically but are unable to do this for themselves. They will believe for example that loose folds of skin caused by rapid weight loss are 'rolls of fat' or that a one kilogram weight gain 'will make me like an elephant'.

Prevalence

Anorexia nervosa is predominantly a disorder of young women with only five to ten per cent of cases occurring in males. A disproportionate number of cases come from upper socio-economic status families.

Studies in Sweden and the United Kingdom have found a prevalence of about one in two hundred 15–18 year old school girls. The mean age of onset in most referred patients is 17–18 (±3) years. It can occur in children as young as eight and in older women.

New patients with anorexia nervosa have been found to present to specialist services in America, Great Britain and New Zealand at the rate of approximately 5 per 100,000 population per year.

Causes

There is no single cause for anorexia nervosa. In individual, biological and personality factors, family factors and sociocultural factors are likely to contribute to the onset and perpetuation of the disorder.

The findings of a recent combined twin and family study suggest that there may be a genetic predisposition to anorexia nervosa. Fifty-six per cent of 25 female identical twins and only 5 per cent of female non identical twins were concordant for anorexia nervosa. A family history among first degree relatives was found in 5 per cent of cases. People with anorexia nervosa are likely to have more perfectionist and obsessional personalities than average. In many patients the anorexia nervosa comes on after a period of personal and family stress. In some patients the onset of anorexia nervosa appears to be precipitated by fear of developing adult sexuality. However, one study found that at the time of onset, the sexual experiences of anorexia nervosa patients were no different from those of others of their age and social class. Controlled studies have shown that the families of people with anorexia nervosa have difficulty in solving conflicts and tend to avoid discussing negative feelings. While stresses in the family may vary from extreme to mild, a common situation is an apparently well functioning family who cope with problems by denying that they are much affected by them. An increased family incidence of depressive illness has been found in anorexia nervosa.

Eating disorders are relatively common in cultures which are food rich but value slimness in women and have a high prevalence of restrictive dieting. Recent studies in the United Kingdom, America and New Zealand suggest that classical anorexia nervosa may not be increasing in incidence although bulimia is increasing. Cultural pressure to be slim does not seem to be a sufficient cause for the development of anorexia nervosa and individual and/or family vulnerability factors need to be present as well.

Management

The management of anorexia nervosa involves persuading patients to normalise their diet and weight and assisting them to increase their self confidence and recognise and deal with personal and family stress. Treatment is difficult because the behaviour and thinking are a way of life which patients are frightened to give up.

It is essential to first take a detailed history from the patient not only to make the diagnosis but to establish rapport which is necessary for subsequent treatment over the next year or so. The history should include a lifetime weight history, a menstrual and sexual history and a detailed history of dietary intake including specific enquiry about bulimic feelings and practices, vomiting and laxative taking, exercise patterns and the person's attitude towards normalising weight.

It is important to obtain a full understanding of the family relationships, as well as the patient's relationships with friends and the extent of social activities. The history should include enquiry about obesity and eating disorders in other family members and friends.

Physical examination should include recording the patient's height and weight, resting pulse and blood pressure, and estimation of dehydration and loss of subcutaneous fat. It may be necessary to obtain a full blood picture and estimation of electrolytes as well as other laboratory investigations such as thyroid, liver and renal function tests. Assessment also should include interview with the parents to assess the parents' personalities and the family stresses. Similarly, an older patient's partner should be seen. Whenever possible, the family should be seen together to enlist their help in improving the patient's eating, and to clarify the family dynamics and the need for family therapy.

In considering differential diagnosis, the distinguishing features of anorexia nervosa is the preoccupation with fears of weight gain and fatness. Weight loss from other causes does not lead to this preoccupation. Weight loss from physical illness can be accompanied by difficulty in eating adequately and undue feelings of fullness after eating. Weight loss can occur in many physical diseases especially in cancer, thyroid and liver diseases. Vomiting as a result of anxiety can lead to marked weight loss but the characteristic eating disorder psychopathology is absent.

Even with expert treatment, recovery takes a minimum of one to two years and is rarely steady. The aims of treatment are to prevent death, to gain weight and improve the chances of full recovery by attention to personality and relationship factors. The methods used will depend on the results of the assessment and the facilities available, but for all patients it is essential to:

1. Establish and maintain a positive relationship with the patient by recognising their overriding fear of fatness and understanding their history and life situation.

2. Identify stressors in the family and at school or work.

3. Prescribe an adequate diet aimed at preventing further weight loss.

4. Educate the patient about energy balance and the physical and psychological effects of starvation.

5. Educate and support the family, particularly to improve parental confidence.

In specialist eating disorder clinics this multidimensional therapy is tailored to the individual's needs by a team of mental health professionals providing individual and family therapy, nutritional expertise, and outpatient and inpatient weight restoration programs.

Hospital admission may be necessary as a life-saving measure in patients with rapid weight loss. It also may be necessary if the patient fails to improve with outpatient treatment or, to relieve family stress. The aim of the admission and the treatment needs to be made clear to the patient, to the family and to the nursing and other staff of the hospital involved.

Achieving positive energy balance requires time consuming nursing care to persuade the patient to eat regular balanced meals and prevent food disposal and excessive exercise. This can take up to six to eight hours daily of experienced nursing staff time. Very rarely tube feeding may be necessary. Throughout hospital admission, it is essential that the patient is recognised as a unique individual with their own particular problems and life situation and not as 'an anorexic', and that staff work with the family. A recent study showed family therapy, which was begun after weight gain in hospital, had a better one year outcome than individual therapy for young patients with anorexia nervosa. In any case, the parents and family need education, support and encouragement to work together to ensure improvement in the patient's health, both by helping with the patient's eating and by learning to recognise and deal with family stress.

Individual psychotherapy is usually necessary in most patients and takes the form of longterm supportive relationship/ educational therapy aimed at improving the patient's understanding of the physiological and psychological effects of starvation and improving their self confidence and their ability to cope with their feelings and personal relationships.

Anti-anxiety medication before meals may be useful if the patient will agree to take this. Antidepressants and major tranquillisers such as thioridazine are commonly used although scientific studies of their efficacy are lacking.

Prognosis

All long term studies have shown that about a quarter of patients referred to specialist care with anorexia nervosa remain under weight and chronically anorexic while about a quarter to a third fully recover. The rest recover weight and menstruation but have eating disorders ranging from mild overconcern about diet and weight, to severe bulimia nervosa. Death in the first few years of illness with anorexia nervosa has become rare with the availability of modern refeeding programs but a 20 year follow-up study showed a death rate of 16 per cent—ie most chronic patients eventually die of the disorder.

Bulimia nervosa

The features of bulimia nervosa are an overwhelming urge to eat huge quantities of food, with binges occurring at least twice weekly, behaviour aimed at controlling the fattening effect of the binges (such as vomiting, laxative or diuretic taking and very strict dieting or exercising), and preoccupation with weight, body shape and dieting.

Clinical features

Bulimia nervosa typically starts in young women who have been chronic dieters for years and often follows an episode of weight loss. Once bingeing has occurred the potential patient becomes excessively fearful of weight gain and the syndrome becomes established by ongoing attempts at restrictive dieting and vomiting or purging after binges.

Most patients are of normal weight (unless they are also suffering from anorexia nervosa) but weight may fluctuate by as much as 7–10 kg between bouts of bingeing and bouts of food restriction.

In patients with frequent vomiting, salivary glands may be enlarged, there may be calluses on the knuckles (grazed by the teeth when inducing vomiting) and dental enamel may be eroded. Low potassium is a particularly dangerous consequence of purging behaviour, and death from cardiac arrest has been described in bulimic patients.

Hormone levels are usually normal and menstrual periods are rarely absent. Despite normal weight, bulimic patients spend most of their time eating very little and have been shown to suffer from the effects of chronic starvation.

The characteristic feature is episodes of eating large quantities of food in secret while restricting eating publicly. The binges may be planned or unplanned. Patients will eat anything they can find in the kitchen, or will buy food for bingeing and eat it in secret at home. They eat food regarded as 'forbidden' for restrictive dieters such as hamburgers, fish and chips, biscuits, chocolates and sweets. Patients may spend a large proportion of their income on food. Most patients plan to vomit after binges and drink large quantities of fluid to help this. The urge to binge characteristically occurs after eating following restricting food for days. In severe cases, patients will have days on end of binge eating and vomiting several times a day interspersed with days of semi-starvation.

Most patients have taught themselves to vomit by thrusting their fingers down their throats, and vomit repeatedly to make sure that all the binge food is eliminated. Some patients take huge quantities of laxatives to produce diarrhoea in the mistaken belief that this will prevent absorption of food.

Like anorexia nervosa patients, bulimia nervosa patients are constantly preoccupied with thoughts of food and weight although the fear of fatness is of a lesser degree unless anorexia nervosa coexists.

Most patients start the day with a resolve to stick to a strict diet and avoid the hated and feared bingeing. Following bingeing and purging the patient may feel shame, guilt and depression.

Prevalence

Bulimia nervosa is more common than anorexia nervosa. In New Zealand, bulimia nervosa has a prevalence of 3 per cent among women aged between 18 and 24 years but is less common in other age groups. Approximately 5 per cent of patients are male.

Causes

All restrictive dieters have some bulimic urges but the bulimia nervosa patient, once they have given in to these and found themselves bingeing, becomes terrified of weight gain, and diets even more strictly, which in turn increases the bulimic urges. It is not known why bulimia nervosa develops in some chronic dieters and not in others, but life-long markedly low self-esteem is characteristic of bulimia patients despite many of them leading apparently successful lives. Bulimia often starts during a time of stress, and preoccupation with control of bingeing and weight then takes precedence over dealing with these problems. The bingeing itself results in self-loathing and self esteem becomes even more impaired. There are some reports that bulimia patients have experienced a high rate of sexual abuse in childhood. Alcohol abuse and compulsive thieving occur in a small percentage of patients and are part of a pattern of difficulty with impulse control in these patients.

Management

The principles of management and the assessment of the patient are the same as those for the anorexia nervosa patient.

Patients need to be persuaded to stop restrictive dieting and eat regular normal meals and accept their own healthy weight. It can help reduce the guilt and shame if patients understand that constant dieting causes physiological changes which reinforce the binge urges. Symptoms are often greatly improved when the patient tells their family or their friends about their secret behaviour and enlists their help to achieve normal eating and prevention of the opportunities to binge. Group treatment can be very effective for well-motivated patients and includes education, encouragement of behavioural change and increasing social skills to improve self-esteem.

Equally effective is individual cognitive/behavioural and/or relationship therapy. Patients may be asked to keep a diary of eating behaviour, of their moods, and of their life events, and to discuss these in individual therapy sessions. Treatment may need to be intensive (once or twice weekly) for several months. Some patients are greatly helped by antidepressant medication, for example imipramine. Hospital admission is only indicated for underweight patients with life-threatening disturbances in fluid and electrolyte balance.

Prognosis

The long term outcome of bulimia nervosa is not reliably known as there have been insufficient follow-up studies. Short term follow-up or intensive treatment shows very considerable improvement in a majority of patients who complete the various programs.

Further Reading

Beumont P J V, Burrows G D and Capser R C, *Handbook of Eating Disorders*, Pt 1, Elsevier Science Publications, Amsterdam, 1987.

Duker M and Slade R, *Anorexia and Bulimia*, Open University Press, Milton Keynes, 1988.

Garner D M and Garfinkel P E, *Handbook of Psychotherapy for Anorexia Nervosa and Bulimia*, Guilford Press, New York, 1985.

Huon G F, Brown L B, *Fighting with Food: Overcoming Bulimia Nervosa*, New South Wales University Press, Sydney, 1988.

Pirke K M, Vandereycken W and Ploog D, *The Psychobiology of Bulimia Nervosa*, Springer-Verlag, Berlin, 1988.

Chapter 37

Obesity

A Hall

Western cultures have a demonstrably negative social attitude towards obesity. The National Institute of Health statement on the health implications of obesity states that: 'Obesity creates an enormous psychological burden. In fact, in terms of suffering, this burden may be the greatest adverse effect on obesity.'

Negative social attitudes are learnt early and children have been shown to prefer leanness to chubbiness and even children with diabetes would not choose to exchange their chronic illness for obesity. In other studies of children's attitudes, silhouettes of obese children are attributed unfavourable traits such as cheating, dirtiness, laziness, sloppiness, meanness and stupidity. Obese people have been discriminated against in educational and vocational settings.

Mental health professionals are not immune to such cultural attitudes. In a recent study 120 mental health professionals were asked to evaluate a case history accompanied by a photograph of the patient. While all other information remained constant the level of obesity as observed in the photograph was altered. The patient when shown as obese was attributed significantly more negative symptoms than the same patient not appearing obese.

Obesity and illness

There is a significant positive relationship between degree of overweight and the development of cardiovascular disease, diabetes and certain types of cancer, although the mechanisms of the associations are poorly understood.

The distribution of body fat has been found in recent research to be important in that abdominal obesity is more closely associated with coronary artery disease and diabetes than fat on the buttocks and thighs. The waist to hip ratio is obtained by measuring the waist at the level of the umbilicus and the hips at the level of the greatest protrusion of the buttocks. The ratio is usually less than 1 in women. The higher the ratio the greater the risk of obesity related disease.

A genetic basis for obesity?

While dietary habits and life style have long been known to influence obesity there is now powerful evidence that weight has a major genetic component. In a study of 540 adult Danish adoptees there was a strong correlation between the adult weight of the adoptees and that of their biological parents, but no correlation between their adult weight and that of their adoptive parents. This relationship was true for a whole range of body weight from very thin to very fat.

This study provides the best evidence to date for the hypothesis that inheritance is more important than childhood environment in determining adult body weight. The Ten State Nutrition Survey in the United States of America examined 40,000 people. It showed that the children of lean parents were leanest, the children of obese parents were the most overweight, and parents with intermediate weights produced children of intermediate weight. These findings could be explained by either environmental or genetic influences or both.

Evidence in favour of a genetic basis has

been found by comparing twins. In one study of 40 identical and 61 non-identical same sex twins of school age, one or both of whom was overweight the identical twins were much more alike in measurements of skin fat and weight than the non-identical twins. The Swedish twin registry, which has observed 14,000 same sex adult twins, also showed much greater concordance for obesity in identical than non-identical twins. A longitudinal study of 514 pairs of American white male twin veterans, over a period of 20 years, showed evidence of significant concordance in weight. The largest twin study to date, of 1974 identical and 2097 non-identical male twins showed that concordance for different degrees of overweight was twice as high in the identical as in the non-identical twins. The inherited mechanism may be a low rate of energy expenditure.

There is a growing body of research confirming that there are large differences between individuals in food intake and amount of exercise while maintaining the same relative weight.

Management of obesity

Although a recent Australian study showed that obesity is at least as common in men as in women, well over 90 per cent of all persons under treatment for obesity are female. The majority of them have buttock and thigh obesity which is less of a health hazard that abdominal obesity. If reduction of obesity related disease were the aim of treatment men with abdominal obesity would form the majority of people being treated and adolescent males would be the most appropriate targets for preventive programs.

The management of established obesity requires assessment of the person's degree and type of obesity, their medical and family history and life style. Mild obesity is often defined as BMI 26 – 30, moderate as 31 – 40 and severe as above 40 (BMI = Body Mass Index $\frac{wt(kg)}{ht(M)^2}$). Mildly obese persons

with medical risk factors and all moderately and severely obese people may benefit medically from weight reduction. However, no current program of weight reduction reliably produces long term stabilisation of weight at 'normal' level in people with established obesity. The best results are from behavioural programs which aim at a permanent change in life style with reduction in total energy intake from food, particularly lower fat intake and increase in energy output from exercise. The modest permanent decreases in weight (approximately ten per cent) produced in obese people by this regime are beneficial to health even if the cosmetic effect is not as great as the person might like. There is growing evidence that short term dieting with rapid weight loss is harmful to health in that much of the weight loss is loss of protein rather than fatty tissue. Repeated weight loss–gain cycles result in an increase in the proportion of body fat.

Surgery is the one treatment which can profoundly reduce body weight in patients with very severe obesity. It is only appropriately considered for the 0.5 per cent of obese persons who are over twice their ideal body weight. At least 50 per cent of patients treated this way have a major reduction in body weight (greater than 40 kg) on a long term basis and their psychosocial functioning and state of mind are usually substantially improved. However, most become chronically tired and suffer from vitamin and other nutritional deficiencies.

Summary

Prejudice against the obese is the greatest handicap of obesity. Recent research has shown that genetic makeup is a major contributor to obesity and that abdominal obesity (measured by the waist to hip ratio) is a better measure of the health risk of obesity than weight per se. Weight reduction programs should be aimed at improving total health by permanent change in life style and eating habits.

Further Reading

Hall A, 'Obesity: Time for Sanity and Humanity', *New Zealand Medical Journal*, Vol 102, 1989, pp 134-6.

'National Institute of Health Consensus Development Panel on the Health Implications of Obesity', *Annual International Medicine*, Vol 103, 1986, pp 1073-77.

Trusswell A S, 'Epidemiology of Obesity', in *Eating Disorders: Prevalence and Treatment*, (ed Touyz S W and Beumont P J V), Williams & Wilkins, Sydney, 1985, pp 83-94.

Trusswell A S and Wahlquist M I, 'International Symposium on Nutrition and Obesity', *Medical Journal of Australia*, Special Supplement, Vol 142, No 7, 1985.

Young L M and Powell B, 'The Effects of Obesity on the Clinical Judgments of Mental Health Professionals', *Journal of Health and Social Behaviour*, Vol 26, 1985, pp 233-46.

Chapter 38

Problems of Psycho-sexual Development and Function

B Boman

Human sexuality is a complex phenomenon, and while biological forces determine whether an individual has either male or female anatomy and physiology, sexual behaviour is primarily determined by upbringing and culture.

Chromosomes are the basic building blocks of sexuality, a female having two x chromosomes and a male one x chromosome and one masculinising y chromosome. During the third to fourth months of foetal development, the 'y' chromosome induces the formation of testicular tissue which manufactures the male sex hormone, androgen, and this then causes the foetus to develop as a morphological male. In the absence of exposure to such an in-utero androgen flux, and irrespective of the underlying chromosomal sex, a foetus will develop female anatomical characteristics.

In mammals other than humans, androgen also causes the development of a centre in the pre-optic nucleus of the hypothalamus responsible for male sexual behaviour, while in its absence, centres for female sexual behaviour will develop in the ventromedial and anterior hypothalamic nuclei.

In humans, while similar hypothalamic centres are induced, their effect on later sexual behaviour is much reduced and the sex one is recognised as being at birth (ie the sex of assignment) and subsequent patterns of rearing are much more powerful determinants of sexual behaviour. Thus, girls whose mothers were administered progesterone (a medication with androgenic activity) during pregnancy to prevent miscarriage, were found to be aggressive and tomboyish and, as adults, to be self-assertive and to have masculine interests, but still to be securely feminine in their sexual orientation. Likewise, in the androgen insensitivity syndrome, where the tissues of a chromosomally male foetus are unable to respond to normally produced in-utero androgen, the child is born with female external genitalia, raised as a female and develops a fully female identity. Controversy still exists as to whether other aspects of behaviour can be primed by foetal androgen exposure. Thus there is some evidence that male aggression and the acquisition of visuospatial skills are enhanced by its presence and the acquisition of verbal skills by its absence.

Theories

Probably the most influential theory of psychosexual development has been that of Freud, who suggested that a child's sexuality began to emerge at about four or five years of age. In the boy, this generates an intense oedipal rivalry between him and his father for the mother's affection, which is resolved only by the fear of retribution from the father. In the girl, Freud described a similar rivalrous triangle between her and her mother for the father, which is resolved when the little girl, envious of the genital appendages of brothers and male playmates, but realising she has no way of altering her own 'inferior' genital endowment, turns in disappointment from father. Freud considered such forces to be less capable of leading to a successful resolution of the oedipal triangle than the fear of retribution in the boy and that hence female sexuality was more insecure and prone to disruption. In both sexes, the resolution of this oedipal triangle leads to the identification of the child with the parent of the same sex (see chapters 2 and 58).

Erik Erikson, another influential psychoanalytic theorist, expanded on the importance of a child learning appropriate sex specific behaviours from identifying with and imitating the same sexed parent. He emphasised the part culture plays in determining the different expectations placed on boys and girls in such things as dress, play, aggression and manual dexterity.

Now that it is realised that a child's sense of maleness or femaleness (ie gender identity) begins to crystallise out by eighteen months, and is firmly developed by three years, more emphasis is placed on earlier experiential influences. For example, it is appreciated that parents begin to sex stereotype their offspring right from birth and react in quite different ways to male and female babies. It is also apparent that, in contrast to what Freud postulated, masculinity rather than femininity is the more precarious state and that gender identity disturbances like transsexualism are considerably more common among males. Modern psycho-analytic writers like Stoller have hypothesised that gender development is more straightforward for girls, for all they have to do to attain a female orientation, is to identify with their mothers, the first person to whom they have bonded. Boys, on the other hand, have first to separate from their mothers before they can begin the process of developing their masculinity. An excessive intimacy between mother and son can impair this process of emancipation and make it more difficult for the boy to attain a masculine identification. Such an emancipation is assisted by the presence of a warm, non-threatening father and impeded by one who is a poor role model because of either his passive ineptitude or his hostility towards and devaluation of his son.

Gender identity disturbances

The essential feature of these conditions is the conviction that one's gender identity is the opposite to one's anatomical sex. They occur more often among males.

During childhood

Gender identity disorder of childhood has at its core the strongly and persistently stated insistence by the child that he belongs to the opposite sex. Such beliefs are accompanied by a repudiation by the child of the appropriateness of his genitals and by cross-gender behaviours. Such features are often observed to begin by the second or third years of life. An example of a gender identity disturbance would be a little boy who experiences persistent distress about being male, has an intense desire to be a girl, spontaneously dresses in his mother's or sister's clothes, jewellery and make up, takes part in girls' games and fantasises about growing up to be an attractive and elegantly dressed woman. These interests and his associated feminine mannerisms, so unlike boys of his age, often lead to him being teased and rejected, and he can easily then go on to develop secondary emotional disturbances. Many boys with gender identity disturbance tend to lose their more overtly feminine traits around eleven or twelve, but while achieving a masculine gender identity, very often develop a same sex preference. However, a small number will retain their firm sense of femaleness into adult life and actively pursue methods to change their sexual morphology by both hormonal and surgical means.

Transsexualism

This is an adult condition in which individuals after puberty are quite convinced that they are inhabiting a body whose gender is the opposite of their true sexual identity and have a sense of repugnance about their genitalia. Gender reassignment surgery long term follow-up studies are not optimistic and suggest that, at best, such procedures only modestly improve levels of psychosocial functioning and should be considered only for those who have successfully lived as a member of the opposite sex for at least two years and who are generally well adjusted personally and socially. The prevalence of this relatively rare condition is about four times more common among males than females.

It has been suggested that an overly symbiotic and excessively intimate relationship between a boy and his mother, and having a father who is remote, critical or hostile can so impair the development of a boy's masculine gender identity that transsexualism may result, though, of course, such parental behaviours may just be secondary responses towards an innately feminine boy.

Homosexuality

While homosexuality is no longer considered a psychiatric disorder, it may still be a source of distress to the affected individual. Homosexuality is considerably more common among males and probably varies little in prevalence across social and cultural boundaries. Some one third of males have a homosexual experience leading to orgasm (usually in adolescence) and, at a conservative estimate, four per cent of males are exclusively homosexual.

Homosexuals do not have a sense of repugnance towards their genitals and have a gender identity congruent with their appearance. While abnormalities of in-utero androgen secretion or function may have a minor priming role for adult homosexual behaviour, more aetiological emphasis is given to early experiential influences.

The bulk of evidence suggests that homosexuality, per se, is not associated with an increased risk of psychiatric disorder.

Paraphilias

The paraphilias, or sexual deviations, have as their essential component the need for abnormal fantasies or behaviours to achieve sexual arousal and satisfaction. They are considerably more common among males and while they are uncommonly encountered in clinical settings, the fact that a wide market exists for magazines, videos and equipment

catering for such activities suggests that they are not rare.

A common theme running through these conditions is of a male who feels inadequate and insecure in his masculinity, who tends to be inept and timorous in his sexual encounters and who lacks self-esteem, assertiveness and self confidence. Such men find women threatening and sexual relations with them a potential source of humiliation, failure and embarrassment. Not infrequently, they are prone to anxieties about their sexual performance and this often causes problems with sexual arousal. The paraphilias, then, can be considered to be a defence against such fears and insecurities by humiliating, demeaning or shocking the woman involved (exhibitionism and sexual sadism), by engaging in sexual activities with children (paedophilia), inanimate objects (fetishism), or animals (zoophilia) which are viewed as less threatening, by seeking sexual arousal in an anonymous encounter (frotteurism and voyeurism) or by allowing the woman to humiliate via bondage and discipline (sexual masochism). These conditions almost always emerge around puberty and their first appearance after 40 would strongly suggest either an organic mental disorder such as Alzheimer's disease or an affective disorder (either depression or hypomania).

Exhibitionism, paedophilia and sexual sadism are clinically important because of their legal and human consequences. Fetishism and sexual masochism tend to be regarded by the community with greater tolerance and health professionals would probably direct their attention with these latter conditions towards helping the person come to terms with their sexuality rather than embarking on the generally fruitless course of 'normalising' it.

Exhibitionism

This is a recurrent, intense and often distressing urge to expose one's genitals to strangers with the intent of inducing shock and surprise and is definitely not an invitation to mutual sexual activity. Adolescent girls are the usual targets. Such acts seldom are a prelude to either sexual assault or violence.

The exposure and associated masturbation (either during or later) only temporarily relieves the impulse. Another feature of the condition is the conscious or unconscious wish for apprehension and punishment, manifesting itself in the considerable risks of apprehension such people take. Most young men appearing before courts on their first exposure charge will not reoffend. However, a second or third charge strongly suggests a recidivistic course. Social skills and assertiveness training and behavioural techniques like orgasmic conditioning (where the person is instructed to masturbate and switch his fantasy from a deviant to a more conventional one at the point of orgasm), in conjunction with supportive counselling, usually produce positive results. Aversive conditioning, where sexual arousal engendered by the deviant stimulus is followed by an electric shock, is now much less widely advocated.

Paedophilia

Adult sexual activity with pre-pubertal children, or paedophilia, can either be heterosexual or homosexual. The former is significantly more common, often involves an adult well known to the child (frequently in a position of trust or authority) and usually consists of the adult looking at or fondling the unclothed child or having the child manipulate the adult's genitals. On the other hand, homosexual paedophiles often indulge in oral and, or anal sex and tend to have relationships with a larger number of boys, usually with whom there has been no earlier involvement. Heterosexual paedophiles are often married and their behaviour frequently follows a period of life stress, while in the case of homosexual paedophiles sexual activity with pre-pubertal boys is the usual and preferred sexual behaviour. Paedophiles often have immature, *Peter Pan* like qualities, tend to identify with and indulge the children with whom they become involved, and, not infrequently, have been victims of child sexual abuse during their own childhoods. However, because paedophilia has at its core the dynamic of arousal stimulated by dominance and power over a helpless victim, there always remains the risk, albeit not great, of assault and possibly homicide.

Sexual sadism

Sexual sadism involves the infliction of physical and/or psychological pain to achieve sexual excitement. The partner may be consenting or non consenting. The need for total control and power over a passive and intimidated victim eloquently highlights the underlying feelings of sexual inadequacy to which such people are prone. While most cases of this type of sexual behaviour take place with a consenting partner and little injury is inflicted, some men need to progressively increase the intensity of their sadistic activities to attain sexual arousal and, in these instances, there is the very real potential for serious injury. The need for dominance and power over a helpless victim is also a common dynamic in men who participate in rape.

Apart from first conviction exhibitionism, the prognosis for the paraphilias are not good. Behavioural modification using aversive conditioning, anti-androgen drugs like cyproterone acetate, individual and group psychotherapy, assertiveness and social skills training have all been advocated but with only limited success.

Disorders of sexual arousal

These are among the most common sexual disorders that health professionals are likely to encounter. Pioneering work by Masters and Johnson delineated the basic physiology of the human sexual response. The first or appetitive stage, consists of sexual fantasies and a desire for sexual activity. The second, or excitement stage, leads on to a subjective sense of arousal accompanied by physiological changes. In the male, these consist of penile tumescence and erection and the appearance of lubricating secretions from Cowpers' glands. In the female, there is pelvic vasocongestion, vaginal lubrication, clitoral retraction, swelling of the external genitalia, formation of the orgasmic platform by vasocongestion and increased muscle tension of the outer third of the vagina. The third or orgasm stage is associated with rhythmic contractions of the perineal muscles and reproductive organs. In the male, the sensation of ejaculatory inevitability is followed by contractions of the vas, seminal vesicles, prostate and urethra and the emission of semen. In the female, there are rhythmic contractions of the outer third of the vagina and proximal labia minoria. The final or resolution stage is accompanied by general relaxation and well-being, during which males are refractory to further erection and orgasm, but women may respond to additional stimulation and have the potential for multiple orgasms.

Aetiology

The aetiology of disorders of sexual arousal can be divided into immediate, triggering factors and more remote, predisposing ones. The immediate ones include a lack of knowledge about proper technique, anxiety, an excessive need to please the other partner or unrealistic and intimidating demands for performance. These issues often occur against a background of marital discord where the sexual dysfunction can be used as a way of getting back at the other partner. People also bring into a relationship insecurities and vulnerabilities from adverse childhood experiences such as being raised in a puritanical atmosphere where sex is regarded as sinful or being exposed to repeated incestuous experiences, which can also predispose to sexual dysfunction in adulthood.

Most common disorders

The two common disorders of sexual functioning in males are *erectile dysfunction* and *premature ejaculation*. Erectile dysfunction is relatively uncommon in men under 35, but increases in frequency with age. Premature ejaculation, in contrast, is more common in younger males, because they generally respond more readily and more intensely to sexual stimuli. Before erectile dysfunction is put down to a psychological cause it is important to exclude other factors such as medications acting on either the central or autonomic nervous systems (for example, anti-hypertensives).

In women there are three relatively common disorders. Sexual arousal disorder consists of the failure to achieve or maintain either the lubrication and swelling responses or the subjective feeling of sexual excitement during sexual activity. Inhibited orgasm refers to a marked delay or absence of orgasm following the arousal phase of sexual activity. The sexual pain disorders in females are twofold. Dyspareunia refers to genital pain experienced during sexual intercourse despite the presence of adequate lubrication and muscle relaxation. Vaginismus is a painful condition in which involuntary spasms of the muscles around the vagina interferes with sexual intercourse. Provided physical disease can be ruled out as a causal factor, in most instances a combination of psychological and physiological processes seem to be operating to produce these dysfunctions.

Treatment

If no medical conditions have emerged to explain the sexual arousal difficulties, most clinicians would adopt a treatment program of relatively short duration encompassing educational, psychotherapeutic and behavioural components. A core tenet is that, because the disorder of sexual arousal reflects difficulties in the couple's relationship, both partners must be involved. In this regard, the use of joint male and female therapists can facilitate effective communication between the partners and can interpret material from both a female and male perspective in a relaxed and unembarrassed fashion.

The simple educative process of explaining normal sexual functioning and of clarifying any misconceptions the couple may have can, of itself, relieve much anxiety. Thus, many couples are unaware of the crucial role of clitoral stimulation in the female sexual response or that men experience a refractory period after orgasm. The psychotherapeutic strand of treatment will centre around the reestablishment of communication between partners so that, for example, resentment is expressed directly rather than indirectly through the medium of the sexual dysfunction.

The basic behavioural technique used is that of desensitisation, which aims to reduce the performance anxiety associated with sexual failure which has been built up over time. This is achieved by proscribing any genital contact and then teaching the couple exercises where

254

they can learn to give and receive pleasure from non-genital contact, a technique called *sensate focusing*. Initially, this might involve the touching and massaging of non-genital areas, with each partner describing to the other their responses. Gradually, stimulation of an increasingly genital erotic nature is allowed, but only as each earlier exercise can be performed free of anxiety. Initially, genital stimulation is permitted only with the goal of arousal. When this can be achieved without anxiety, orgasm (initially non-coital but then coital) is permitted.

Aspects of the program will vary with the kind of disorder, for example, with premature ejaculation, the female partner manually stimulates the man to erection and impending orgasm, but then stops and squeezes the coronal ridge of the penis for a few seconds until the sensation of ejaculatory inevitability abates. In vaginismus, the involuntary nature of the spasm is demonstrated to both partners by a pelvic examination. Systematic exercises to relax the pelvic musculature are then taught in conjunction with the technique of inserting progressively larger vaginal dilators. With anorgasmia, the woman is given exercises in masturbation, where alone and in a relaxed atmosphere, she learns to enjoy the sensual feelings that otherwise would be submerged in the tensions of coitus.

The outcome of such techniques is generally quite favourable, especially when the sexual dysfunction is not associated with significant psychopathology. Masters and Johnson, for example, reported success rates in the order of 70 per cent for erectile dysfunction, 80 per cent for premature ejaculation and 98 per cent for vaginismus.

Summary

While chromosome complement and the presence or absence of an in-utero androgen flux determines external sexual morphology, human sexual behaviour is primarily dependent on upbringing and culture. The spectrum of disturbance of gender identity, is more common among males, reflecting the more complicated biological and psychological processes involved in the development of masculinity. In adulthood, gender identity is resistant to change but, on the other hand, sex reassignment surgery for transsexualism seldom produces better than modest improvement in psychological adjustment.

The paraphilias are also more common among males and often reflect feelings of sexual inadequacy and low self-esteem. In addition, exhibitionism and paedophilia are criminal offences, the latter being more serious because of the greater danger of physical and emotional damage to the victim.

The physiology of sexual arousal with its appetitive, excitement, orgasm and resolution phases can often be impaired by psychological or medical factors. Erectile dysfunction and premature ejaculation in men and anorgasmia and vaginismus in women are relatively common, but in the absence of underlying physical illness, often respond to a program of anxiety reduction, marital counselling and instruction in proper sexual technique.

Further Reading

Bell A P and Weinberg M S, *Homosexualities: A Study of Diversities Among Men and Women*, Simon & Schuster, New York, 1978.

Gadpaille W J, 'Research into the Physiology of Maleness and Femaleness', *Archives of General Psychiatry*, Vol 26, 1972, pp 193–205.

Masters W H and Johnson V E, *Human Sexual Inadequacy*, Little Brown & Co, Boston, 1970.

Stoller R J, 'The Impact of New Advances in Sex Research on Psychoanalytic Theory', *American Journal of Psychiatry*, Vol 130, 1973, pp 241–51.

Chapter 39

The Psychiatry of Late Life

S Ticehurst

The elderly present their illnesses in ways that are often different from younger adults. The assessment and management of their problems often have different means and goals.

The psychiatry of the elderly deals with people who are both elderly and suffer from mental disorders. It does not deal solely with people who have dementia. Various services will have different criteria of 'elderly', but the age of 65 is a convenient starting point.

Demographic trends

The populations of most Western countries are becoming 'greyer'. This is because of increased life expectancy and lower birth rates. The post war 'baby boomers' will compound this effect when they reach their senior years early next century.

In Australia, those over 65 have risen from 8 per cent of the population in 1947 to 10.5 per cent in 1986, and will increase still further to near 12 per cent in the year 2000. This means that the 'old old' (those aged over 75) have become a significant sector of the population this century, whereas they were only ever a hardy elite for most of human history. They are the heaviest users of health services and the most liable to contract age-linked disorders such as dementia.

Despite this, it is important to remember that the majority of elderly people in Australia are both physically and mentally well.

Mental disorders in the elderly

The most serious mental disorder found among old people is *dementia*. This condition is the major reason for hospitalisation and nursing home care. Dementia is fully discussed in chapter 40.

Depression is relatively common in the elderly and severe cases may be mistaken for dementia. In essence, its presentation is similar to that described in chapter 28. However, failure to eat or drink properly may have more serious consequences for the elderly than for younger adults and, in particular, dehydration may be a problem. *Suicidal behaviour* among the elderly is not common but the lethality of suicidal acts increases with age, so that the elderly are more likely to succeed than younger people.

Treatment for depression in older people follows that described for younger adults in chapter 28. However, caution needs to be taken when prescribing antidepressant medication to old people, as they are more prone to experience side effects, the consequences of which may be quite serious, for example, for a frail person, a fall in blood pressure on standing due to medication may result in dizziness, collapse and a serious injury. Electroconvulsive therapy may be useful for some seriously depressed people.

Mania is uncommon in the elderly and when it occurs has the features described in chapter 28 for younger people viz elation, grandiosity, overactivity and unreality. However, such behaviour may be an unexpected result of medication. Hospitalisation is almost always necessary.

Schizophrenia rarely develops for the first time in old age. Some aging people with schizophrenia develop a dementia-like syndrome, others retain intellectual clarity accompanied by their fixed bizarre beliefs and disturbed thought patterns and behaviour. Some evidence is found in the former group for brain shrinkage. Drugs need to be carefully monitored in the elderly person with chronic schizophrenia.

Delerium is not uncommon in the elderly. The clouding of the sensorium characteristic of this condition may be due to many causes which need careful elucidation and urgent treatment (see chapter 41).

While schizophrenia is uncommon as a new condition in old age, paranoid states are not. *Paranoid disorders* are characterised by prominent false fixed beliefs (delusions) of a persecutory or grandiose type. Many diseases can present as paranoia. Dementia, delirium and depression can all present with delusions concerning theft, slight, jealousy, or strangers in the house etc. Many physical illnesses can present with paranoid symptoms. These include overmedication and circulatory problems. Paranoia may also be made worse by social isolation and deafness. It is always important to consider the many possible causes of paranoid symptoms. A full medical and psychiatric assessment is necessary before assuming that the patient is suffering simply from a late onset primary psychiatric disorder.

Once a diagnosis is made of late onset paranoid disorder, it is essential for some member of the health care team to establish trust with the patient so that treatment will be complied with successfully.

The aim of treatment should be to protect the patient from the harm they may suffer as a result of their beliefs. This may involve protecting them from irate neighbours and inappropriate police intervention.

The long term outcome in these rare psychiatric disorders is somewhat uncertain. Nevertheless, in the short term at least, they can respond well to treatment. Antipsychotic medication in small doses usually dampens the paranoid symptoms to the point where the patient can continue their life in relative peace.

Alcohol related problems decline with age as people either moderate their habits or suffer the consequences of illness and death. Nevertheless, alcohol problems remain the third most common mental disorder in elderly

men. A smaller, but clinically important group of 'late onset' alcohol abusers may present atypical ways. These can be women who have suffered recent bereavement and may present to general medical or geriatric services with falls, confusion or lack of self care. Treatment in the elderly is similar to that in earlier years. However, more emphasis on home assessment and follow up, thorough medical examination and awareness of cognitive deficits caused by alcohol is necessary. Many of the 'late onset' drinkers may respond favourably if underlying precipitants such as grief, loneliness or depression are correctly identified and properly managed.

Benzodiazepine abuse has supplanted barbiturate and bromide use in the elderly as the availability of these drugs has changed. The addictive potential of benzodiazepine tranquillisers is now well publicised. Elderly patients can suffer from a withdrawal reaction after as little as four weeks' use. Rebound anxiety and insomnia in withdrawal can give way to delirium that may last longer than alcohol withdrawal (see chapters 42, 43).

Some *personality disorders* may present in old age as the 'senile recluse syndrome'. Such elderly people live in squalor by choice and resist attempts to make themselves more presentable. These patients may have personalities of the introverted or paranoid type. However, it must be stressed that such a presentation can occur with many psychiatric disorders.

Perhaps more common in Australian society is the 'personality' problem that becomes apparent when people unsuited to institutional life are admitted to nursing home or hostel accommodation. Previously independent assertive individuals can cause great problems in the routine-dominated atmosphere of an institution. Similarly, people with a dependent personality can place enormous demands on staff who often have not the time to spend with such needy patients. One such example is the patient with multiple physical complaints who seems to the staff to be needing attention and concern rather than treatment. Another problem for institutional staff is the 'manipulative' patient. Such a person may be able to split staff into opposing camps and then play one off against the other in a destructive way. Many of these patients would never come to a psychiatrist's attention if they had remained at home. Usually an extended interview will clarify the problem, and relatives may supply examples of previous similar behaviour in other social settings. Treatment may involve psychotherapy for the patient and support for the staff to deal with the disruption by enhancing their understanding of the underlying problem.

It must be kept in mind that personality change in late life is often the precursor of brain disease. Previous personality traits may be accentuated by a dementing illness. Depression can present as introversion, dependency or hypochondriasis (see chapter 14).

Many elderly people are understandably anxious about developing physical illness and fear becoming dependent. However, there is evidence that patients with marked anxiety tend to lose their symptoms to some degree as they age. A housebound person may be one form of presentation. If a patient does have a phobic disorder in old age that is not caused by an other illness, then that person is likely to have been anxious all their life (see chapter 27).

Sleep disorders are not uncommon in the elderly, however elderly people tend to require less sleep. Their sleep patterns may be disturbed by the need to go to the toilet more frequently, breathlessness or pain. It is important in the elderly that sedatives not be the immediate response to complaints of insomnia. Anxiety, depression, alcohol and tranquillizer abuse, dementia, delirium and adjustment to stresses such as bereavement can all be associated with sleep disturbance. Sleep apnoea may also be an unrecognised cause of insomnia in the elderly. Symptoms that may point to this disorder include snoring and daytime tiredness.

A full medical and psychological evaluation to rule out these causes should be followed by a non pharmacological treatment plan involving the development of a regular routine and other behavioural techniques. If sedatives are used, they should be restricted to a maximum of two to three weeks, because of the rapidly developing problems of tolerance, dependence and loss of efficacy.

'Normal' experiences of ageing with mental health implications

Grief

Losing one's closest emotional partners becomes increasingly common with age. Widowhood is almost universal among elderly women due to a life expectancy greater than men. Losing a life partner may be a particularly damaging event and the process of grief has been well documented. When the loss is not accepted, possible consequences include depression, alcohol abuse and physical illness. Bereavement is linked to a higher mortality rate, especially among widowers. In some cases, the grief may become prolonged and fail to be resolved. Such abnormal grief reactions may cause the sufferer to become socially isolated and incapacitated as his life becomes fixated on the loss or handicapped by its denial. There is now evidence that timely intervention can prevent abnormal grief reactions. An empathic listener can help facilitate the grief process. The ability of such a listener to tolerate the sufferer's shock, denial, anger and sadness are vital parts of this process. Those particularly at risk have had ambivalent feelings about the lost person. That is, their feelings include many negative ones which have not been resolved during life. Bereaved persons who have few effective social supports are also at risk.

Retirement

Retirement is a life change that requires psychological and social adjustment to adapt to new roles and priorities. Most people make this transition with little distress and enjoy their retirement. In contrast, the poor, the sick and those retrenched early seem at risk of psychological consequences. People failing to adapt may become anxious, depressed or begin to abuse alcohol or other drugs. Retirement programs aimed at smoothing the transition are becoming widespread. Perhaps an even more important preventive intervention would be to ensure an adequate standard of living for all retirees.

Assessment and management of the elderly

All aspects of assessment and management should be guided by an appreciation of the psychological, biological and social determinants of a person's condition. Any intervention should be calculated to cause the least disruption to the person and to ensure no disability is added as a result of the intervention. People should be assessed both to make a clinical diagnosis as well as an assessment of their potential level of functioning.

The home visit has been adopted in pychogeriatric practice to provide invaluable information concerning the patient's abilities and needs. The elderly patient should be approached with respect. Surnames should be used unless permission is given otherwise. The approach to taking a history should be unhurried and courteous.

The most important part of assessment is a careful and detailed history. Relatives, neighbours, local doctors and many other sources may need to be approached before the entire picture is revealed. This is particularly so when the patient is confused and cannot give a reliable history himself. Physical examination and appropriate laboratory tests reveal previously undiagnosed conditions more commonly in the aged.

Psychological tests

In the elderly, psychological tests are most often used to measure aspects of cognitive functioning such as memory, abstraction, calculation, attention and concentration. Screening tests looking for evidence of physical impairment of the brain are becoming very widely used in the elderly. Perhaps the best of these is the Mini Mental State Examination (MMSE). This test is scored out of 30 and compares very favourably with many other questionnaires available, because it covers a broad range of cognitive functioning. The MMSE will still miss cases of dementia, especially early ones, and it will falsely identify as demented some patients who are depressed or who have language difficulties. People who have difficulty concentrating because of anxiety, depression or schizophrenia, and those who are poorly educated or developmentally delayed may also falsely score as if they were demented. Amongst those who are identified by the MMSE as impaired, there may be those suffering from dementia, delirium, amnestic syndromes or depressive pseudodementia. Further testing using more complex instruments may be carried out by a psychologist. The results of such testing can quantify strengths and deficits in different areas of functioning, aid in diagnosis and provides baselines against which future improvement or deteriorations can be measured.

Although very valuable tools, the results of psychological tests should always be interpreted in the overall clinical context and they are always dependent on the circumstance of their administration.

Medical tests

Many physical illnesses can mimic psychiatric illness especially in the elderly. Common examples include hypothyroidism presenting as depression and hyperthyroidism as anxiety. Delirium is basically a psychological presentation of underlying physical illnesses. Dementia may be caused by a number of potentially reversible diseases. More commonly, sudden exacerbations of behavioural disturbances may be caused by a physical illness in a dementing person. The elderly do not present with the typical symptoms of medical illnesses as often as younger adults. For example, myocardial infarction may present as confusion without chest pain. Pneumonia can present as confusion without a temperature. Many of the treatments used in psychiatry of the elderly may adversely affect mental state and their doses may need to be altered.

For all of these reasons, the use of diagnostic tests are often necessary to complement the history and clinical examination. Such tests include full blood count, serum biochemistry, kidney and liver function tests, thyroid function tests, vitamin B 12 and folate estimations, syphilis screening, urine examination, chest X-ray and electrocardiogram. Just how many of these laboratory investigations are required depends on clinical judgments. Cranial computerised tomography (CT scans) provide an invaluable demonstration of brain structure whereas the electroencephalogram (EEG) measures aspects of brain function. The former is becoming more important in the investigation of brain pathology in the elderly, whereas the latter is becoming less important (see chapters 19, 21).

Service provision—the multi disciplinary team

Psychogeriatric services may be part of geriatric or of general psychiatry services. Ideally, they can provide short and long stay treatment centres, inpatient assessments and community programs. It is generally accepted that optimal care will be delivered by a team with skills in all these areas of management. This requires a multidisciplinary approach. The potential problems caused by delay in assessment are important; service delayed is often service denied. Overzealous treatment may be as damaging as lack of treatment. Inappropriate institutionalisation should be avoided. A well functioning team will be flexible and responsive with well established cooperation with other facilities and agencies who deal with the elderly. These will include Government Welfare, Housing, Health and Veteran Affairs departments as well as general practitioners, hostel and nursing home owners.

Institutions

Less than one in ten elderly people in Australia are in institutional care. Despite this, institutionalisation remains a source of anxiety among the elderly. They realise that being in a nursing home may imply loss of personal freedom and increased dependence on others. Nursing homes and psychogeriatric units vary in their capacity to maintain the dignity of their residents. An important factor in this variability is the attitude of the staff. All institutions impose rules and routines on residents. Unwillingness to comply with such routines may be labelled as deviant behaviour and 'psychiatric' labelling can occur.

Dementia is the most common single reason for nursing home care. A dementing person may be confused concerning showering, toiletting and other routines if the purpose of the routine cannot be communicated. A non demented resident may resent being told what to do by staff many years his junior. Even the most enlightened and flexible institution has to struggle to overcome the sense of loss of purpose, frustration, boredom and apathy that may follow institutionalisation. One of the most difficult problems is that of those who wander away. For them locked facilities may be necessary. Again these vary in quality.

Community treatment and the burden of caring

Caring for a person with dementia exacts a toll. This toll is physical, social, financial and psychological. The majority of unpaid carers, relatives and friends of the elderly person draw on a long-standing knowledge and love of the 'healthy' person now dementing. Most of these carers rely on support from paid and unpaid, skilled and 'unskilled' helpers. The health and welfare systems remain at the periphery of care, most of which is conducted by families. As thinking swings away from institutional care, more and more resources need to be channelled into community care. Nevertheless, community based services are unlikely to supplant the care provided by relatives, friends and neighbours. The family is likely to remain the cornerstone of community care. Consequently, the future may well see more distress amongst carers, rather than less, unless better supports are provided for them.

Caring for ageing patients with psychiatric disorders can be especially stressful. Families can also benefit from practical financial and emotional support from the government and non government agencies for the dementing elderly (see chapters 44, 63, 64).

Drugs

One of the major advances of geriatric medicine has been to spread the message that the elderly are particularly susceptible to the side effects and interactions of prescription drugs. This is no less the case in geriatric psychiatry. Many consultations sought from psychogeriatric services are at least partially due to the results of medication, particularly psychotropic drugs.

Confusional states are the most common modes of presentation, but many drugs can cause depression, anxiety, delusions and hallucinations. For example, any of the drugs used in treating Parkinson's Disease can cause visual hallucinations and delirium. Likewise, drugs used to treat high blood pressure have been linked with depression.

The drugs that psychiatrists use in the elderly also cause similar problems. The antipsychotic drugs such as haloperidol and thioridazine can cause a condition almost identical to Parkinsons' Disease which may interfere drastically with the function of an elderly person. They also can cause a severe form of restlessness called akathisia which can be very distressing. Acute dystonic reactions where muscle spasm in awkward positions are less common in the elderly but still occur. Sedation, sudden drops in blood pressure on standing and confusion can occur with all these drugs. A late complication of antipsychotic drug use is tardive dyskinesia. This usually involves a chewing, rolling motion of the muscles around the mouth which comes on after some months' exposure. If not detected early and the drug ceased it is usually irreversible.

Lithium is a very effective drug in preventing the swings of bipolar mood disorder. It has also been used to prevent recurrent depressive illnesses and in the treatment of resistant depression. Owing to declining kidney function with age, doses of lithium should be a fraction of usual adult doses. The toxic effects of lithium are particularly likely to occur in the elderly if they become dehydrated (see chapter 57).

Psychotherapy

The elderly can benefit from psychotherapy. Listening to an elderly person's worries and troubles with respect, being empathic when they are distressed and helping them to clarify things in their own minds are all parts of supportive psychotherapy. More sophisticated forms of psychotherapy have been adapted

for elderly patients. Therapist–patient issues are often focused differently, for example, by the patient relating to the therapist as if he were his child. The goal of psychotherapy in late life is usually to support and comfort rather than change the person's defences or coping style. This is probably owing to ideas about cost effectiveness rather than any documented lack of response by elderly patients to more ambitious therapy. Particular modes of therapy have been proposed. Reminiscence therapy involves an elderly person going back over life events. It is similar to the 'life review' where developmental tasks of other life stages may be reworked. (see chapter 58).

Social work

The complexity of social security health and welfare legislation is often very difficult for the elderly patient to understand. Health care professionals often fail to recognise the particular needs of the elderly patient. Complex intergenerational dynamics come into play as society changes often rapidly. Women are now part of the paid work force, people are retiring earlier. Such social stresses highlight the need for a social work service that can act as the patient's advocate when in contact with all these other systems (see chapter 64).

Behavioural approaches

The idea that reinforcement shapes human behaviour is still as relevant in old age as in youth. Positive reward to increase desired behaviour can be used in many health care settings. Many institutional programs aim at change through behavioural techniques. A particular 'problem' behaviour can be analysed with respect to what leads to it, what is associated with it, what reinforces it and what does not reinforce it. Points of intervention can be identified and the frequency of the behaviours before and after treatment can be noted. This may mean that a regular nurse is assigned with a regime of step by step explanation. If this approach reduces the behaviour then the approach can be further modified to enhance its successful components. Reality orientation in which a disoriented patient is gently reminded of their whereabouts is an example of how repetition and reinforcement can be used to obtain a particular goal even in dementing patients (see chapter 61).

Occupational therapy

Occupational therapists can add an important extra dimension to the assessment and management of the elderly patient. Often the behaviour of the patient cannot be modified, but the living environment may be. With increasing stratification of levels of care for elderly patients and an increased emphasis on home care, an occupational therapist can provide invaluable information about appropriate placement and management (see chapter 65).

Diversional therapy

Many diversional programs have became standard in day centres, nursing homes and other institutional settings. The aim is to enrich the lives of those involved. Many elderly psychiatric patients may benefit from these approaches. However, the critical question is one of the correct degree of stimulation. Too much stimulation can overwhelm an elderly patient who has cognitive impairment. Too little stimulation can lead to apathy and boredom with regression in behaviour. Each patient has a different threshold, and a skilled therapist will take this into account. Music groups where participation in age appropriate music is encouraged but not enforced allow an opportunity in which patients may find their own level. Many people seem to retain their capacity to enjoy music well after they have lost even basic language skills.

The problem of morale

Elderly patients with psychiatric illness are doubly stigmatised. They are often at the bottom of the pile when it comes to resource allocation. Such patients often confront health professionals with their own mortality and a sense of helplessness when they do not respond quickly to treatment. This is compounded by the youth oriented values of our society. Nevertheless, such patients have to be cared for and the emotional reactions of anger, frustration and depression dealt with. Not everyone is suited for caring for these people, and forcing people to do so can have disastrous consequences. Staff often need a break and capacity to transfer temporarily to other duties with different rewards is highly desirable in any system dealing with elderly psychiatric patients.

The actual care of patients who regress in the process of their illness is often very demanding physically as well as mentally. Faecal and urinary incontinence, disinhibited sexual behaviour, aggression and repetitive demands without appeasement all place a unique blend of emotional and physical demands upon carers. This requires flexibility and acceptance combined with a great deal of patience. At best, carers under such distress may begin to see themselves as an elite group dealing with problems that no-one is prepared to handle. Support and understanding from staff who do not participate in direct patient care is essential. At worst, carers can become immensely dispirited and deliver poor care or even become aggressive and frustrated themselves. Indirect signs of increasing difficulties include demands for the patient to be moved, increased requests for medication, increasing anger directed at outsiders or fellow carers and increased sick leave.

The elderly patient from a different ethnic background

Such a person can be one of the most isolated that a health care worker may meet. Many aged people who migrated in their earlier years have been dislocated by forces of war and political upheaval. They may have no family network and feel lost in an alien world. If they begin to suffer from dementia, their English as a later acquired language is lost first. If institutionalised, it may be in a setting where they can no longer eat the food of their own culture or practice their religion. Even the most basic of human exchanges can be lost and assumptions made on the basis of inadequate knowledge or stereotypes. A first step is to engage an interpreter, preferably from a trained health service. Questions of confidentiality can become a major problem when the only interpreters available are relatives, neighbours or friends. A skilled interpreter can translate as well as enlighten the health professional as to cultural norms and expectations. This is particularly important in relation to the understanding of unusual behaviour. Multicultural psychiatric centres have recently been established in Melbourne and Perth, which adopt an approach which attempts to consider the patient in their cultural context and to identify the behaviour within that context (see chapter 47).

Self help groups

Sufferers and carers have formed numerous groups. The Alzheimer's Disease And Related Disorders Society (ADARDS) is probably the one of most relevance in the field of dementia. These groups allow for carers of patients with dementia to meet and exchange their practical help as well as allowing for the group processes of expression of feelings. There is little evidence available to say whether this function of the groups is beneficial or not. Some relatives find them a great help, others do not. There is no doubt however, that they can act as a powerful advocacy group for a relatively neglected group of people. They also act as a focus for information and education.

Ethical and legal issues

'Rights versus risks'

One common dilemma in psychiatry of the elderly occurs when a patient is deemed by others in the community to be at risk of harming themselves either directly or indirectly. However, at which point a person's rights should be overridden is a complex issue. It is usually a question of degree. At one end, for example, is the patient who sets fire to his house or wanders on to the road and is run over by a car. At the other is a man who will not wash or shave, but who otherwise manages to look after himself. Of vital importance is whether the patient has a mental disorder which is impairing his function. If

none is present, then most would say that rights outweigh risk. However, if the patient has a severe mental illness and particularly if this is potentially treatable, Mental Health legislation usually allows for compulsory treatment of the underlying mental disorder.

Difficulties often arise when a patient is becoming demented and yet retains some capacities. A person who is able to survive alone at home in every respect, but who wanders off and needs to be returned home by the police or neighbours is a good example. Such people often lock themselves out and need to have the locks replaced regularly. At some stage they may be referred to a mental health facility and the admitting doctor is requested to admit the patient to solve the problem. To admit to hospital in this situation, the doctor may be doing the patient a disservice. Dislocation from the community and subjection to the possible adverse effects of hospital management may have consequences.

People who leave the gas on or misuse electric heaters and other appliances may cause fires and burn themselves or their houses. At some point the threshold for hospitalisation is crossed as the disease progresses. The threshold largely depends on the presence or absence of support structures, the degree of impairment, the circumstances of the referral and the degree of acceptance of the offered services.

Every health worker should become aware of the legislation regarding compulsory treatment for mental illness and guardianship.

Informed consent

Central to any debate on rights versus risk and involuntary treatment in the elderly is the question of informed consent. In mentally ill and dementing patients, this capacity is often impaired. Again it is a question of degree with no absolute dividing line between the mentally competent and incompetent person. A person giving informed consent must be able to understand what treatment is being offered, what the treatment is for and the possible consequences of both having the treatment and not having it. If a person is incapable of informed consent, then their refusal of treatment must be viewed with caution. In these instances, we look at the legislation to provide reflections of what is acceptable to the community in terms of rights versus risks. A person with advanced dementia is very unlikely to be able to give informed consent, whereas a person with Huntington's Chorea may need a sophisticated assessment over some time before an opinion can be offered (see chapter 50).

Euthanasia

This controversial issue often arises in clinical practice with the elderly. The relatives of patients with dementia often test the water with statements such as 'If I was like that I know what I'd want you to do'. Others are more blunt. Society is struggling to deal with this problem. A distinction has been drawn between passive and active euthanasia. Passive euthanasia in the sense of allowing elderly people with terminal dementing illnesses to die in comfort is no doubt widely practised.

People with dementia are rarely capable of making a rational judgment concerning euthanasia. Relatives do not have the legal power to speak for the patient. Active euthanasia in a dementing person implies that another person both takes responsibility for the act and physically performs it. This is such a dangerous precedent that it has been widely repudiated.

One danger needs to be emphasised. It is not uncommon for severely depressed patients to develop delusional beliefs about having cancer, or that their spouse is suffering so much that they need to be put out of their misery. Likewise, paranoid patients may feel that others are persecuting them or suffering persecution. When such beliefs lead to someone's death, as they may occasionally do, it may be seen to be a form of euthanasia. Care in interpreting such events is necessary. Similarly, carers may become so stressed that they resort to desperate measures. Lessening the burden prior to this stage is infinitely preferable.

Restraint—physical, chemical, architectural

Physical restraint may be used where patients are disruptive and risk harming themselves or others. Such restraint can take the form of posy belts, chair tops that can be fastened, gloves and bed rails. Mechanical restraints of this kind have been associated with an increased mortality rate. This does not mean that restraint causes death. At least equally likely is the hypothesis that the agitation leading to restraint is caused by some undiagnosed medical condition which proves to be fatal. Every nursing home and psychogeriatric unit should have an acceptable policy on restraint.

Many patients who are demented and restrained will actually become more agitated and the method is often counterproductive. The concept of physical restraint can also include action of staff who have to deter patients from leaving or who encourage them to perform such routines as bathing and toiletting.

Between a quarter and a half of dementing patients in nursing home settings receive some form of sedation. There is no doubt that in some cases the patient benefits from such prescriptions. In others, however, it is the institutions which benefit by having quieter, compliant patients. Many patients on such medications have unpleasant side effects.

Architecture designed to cater for wandering patients is an important aspect of modern nursing home and psychogeriatric setting. Nursing homes have been slow to adapt to the increasing numbers of poorly functioning patients. They have often not been encouraged by government support. Fire regulations and concern over being sued for imprisonment whilst attempting to preserve the rights of non demented patients have often deterred nursing homes from taking in demented people. Yet, architecture is beginning to come to terms with providing appropriate secure environments for ambulant confused patients. Purpose built units have been provided, either free standing or as part of other complexes. The old Swanbourne Hospital in Perth was replaced with modern villa-style units based on an eight bed self contained module. Landscaping and fences provided security for people likely to wander off. Private homes may be modified to minimise the distress of carers who live with confused patients.

Property management

Each Australian State has its own legislation to deal with looking after the financial affairs of patients who are either temporarily or permanently incompetent owing to mental illness. A manager can be appointed to ensure that the patient's interest are safeguarded. When public trusteeship is proposed, there must be clear evidence that the patient has impairment in reasoning, judgement or memory such that they can no longer manage their affairs.

Conclusion

A knowledge of the biological and psychosocial aspects of ageing will aid health professionals in their contacts with elderly people. Although there are continuities in presentation throughout the life cycle, age brings specific problems that affect presentation and management. Knowledge of these issues allows a more rational approach to the elderly patient. It is likely that this area will be one of marked growth and changing ideas in the coming years as the number of elderly increase in the Australasian communities.

Further Reading

Kay David W K and Burrows G D, *Handbook of Studies on Psychiatry and Old Age*, Elsevier, Amsterdam, 1984.

Kendig H L, *Ageing and Families*, Allen and Unwin, Sydney, 1986.

Levy R and Post F, *The Psychiatry of Late Life*, Blackwell Scientific Publications, Oxford, 1982.

Mace N L and Rabins P V, *The 36 Hour Day*, Johns Hopkins University Press, Baltimore, 1981.

Murphy E, *Affective Disorders in the Elderly*, Churchill Livingstone, Edinburgh, 1986.

Chapter 40

Dementia

S Ticehurst

Dementia is a serious disorder affecting mental functioning. Its prevalence increases with age. It is now assuming greater importance as the number of elderly persons grows relatively larger in our community

Definition and clinical features

Dementia is a syndrome rather than one disease. This means that 'dementia' implies a clustering of symptoms and signs that is fairly consistent despite different underlying diseases causing the syndrome.

In dementia, there is usually an overall change in personality. In particular there is evidence of impairment in short and long term memory. Impairment in short term memory (inability to learn new information) may be indicated by inability to remember three objects after five minutes. Long term memory impairment (inability to remember information that was known in the past) may be indicated by inability to remember past personal information or facts of common knowledge.

In addition, dementia is often characterised by an impairment in abstract thinking which can manifest itself by an inability to recognise relationships between concepts. There is also often an impairment in social judgment. The patient may commit embarrassing social gaffes, swear inappropriately or, for instance, urinate publicly.

Other disturbances of higher brain functioning may also be apparent. These include aphasia (disorder of language), apraxia (inability to carry out motor activities despite intact comprehension and motor function), agnosia (failure to recognise or identify objects despite intact sensory function) and 'constructional difficulty' (inability to copy three dimensional figures).

There is often evidence of a specific organic cause or else it is not possible to account for the disturbance by the presence of depression or another psychiatric condition.

Typically, there is a gradual onset over at least several months and steady downward progression over years. A mental state examination reveals widespread impairment of intellect in the absence of an altered level of consciousness. This means that the patient, despite being alert and able to concentrate, has a diminished capacity to perform mental tasks.

The advanced stages of dementia may bring physical symptoms such as muscular rigidity and a shuffling gait. Patients may eventually become unable to walk.

The behavioural symptoms of dementia that cause most concern to carers are repetitive demanding behaviour, disturbed sleep, wandering, aggression and incontinence. Delusions can occur in 10-30 per cent of cases. These are usually beliefs that someone is entering the house or stealing misplaced belongings. Such beliefs rarely become elaborated into the systematised delusions seen in schizophrenia or the paranoid disorders. Hallucinations are less common but can occur. They are almost always visual and rarely as frightening as the hallucinations in delirium. Depression may occur in patients who also have dementia. Other patients will have incontinence. Tearfulness may occur whenever an emotional subject is raised. Anxiety and tearfulness can be provoked in dementing patients, when their grasp on reality is unsure. One such situation occurs when questions concerning memory and orientation are asked. This requires sensitivity of the clinician to the anxiety of the patient and a willingness to have a more neutral, less taxing conversation.

Epidemiology

At the age of 65, approximately one per cent of Australians will have dementia whilst at age 80, between 20 and 30 per cent will suffer from the disorder. Dementia is the most common reason for long term institutional care in Australia. At least as many people with dementia are cared for at home as reside in nursing homes.

At the present time, Australia is experiencing a rapid increase in the number of elderly citizens. This will continue into the next century as the adults of the 'baby boom' become old. Because age is the most important risk factor for dementia, the number of people with dementia will virtually double between the 1980s and the first decade of the next century.

Causes

The most common causes of dementia in Australia are Alzheimer's disease (50 per cent), cerebral circulation (multi infarct) dementia (20 per cent), a mixture of the first two, and alcohol (less than 10 per cent).

Multi infarct dementia probably includes a group of disorders which have the end result of reducing blood flow to the brain until the nerve cells are damaged. When this damage becomes great enough, the reserve capacity of the brain is overcome and the patient shows signs of dementia. The most common cause of this disorder is atherosclerosis. The strokes that accumulate to cause this disorder are usually small and numerous. Occasionally, several large strokes can also produce dementia.

Multi infarct dementia can often be differentiated from dementia of the Alzheimer's type on clinical grounds. The patient with multi-infarct dementia often has a history of high blood pressure, step-wise rather than gradual progression, focal neurological signs, evidence of generalised blood vessel disease, relative preservation of personality, relatively focal nature of cognitive deficits and a greater amount of emotional lability and depression. Making this distinction is at present of limited usefulness, because the outlook for the two diseases processes is very similar.

The underlying cause of Alzheimer's disease is unknown. There have been many theories put forward, but none as yet has been firmly established. Deficiency in aluminium, a viral infection, toxins, a genetic disorder and an acceleration of the normal ageing process have all been proposed. Widespread damage and cell death are seen in cortical areas of the brain. The fluid filled ventricles within the brain are widened and the brain takes on a shrunken appearance.

Alcohol related dementia is the end result of heavy alcohol use, usually over many years and in large quantities. The damage in this type of dementia is usually in structures at the base of the brain and in the frontal lobe. It may be due to thiamine deficiency or to a direct neurotoxic effect of alcohol.

There are many other causes of dementia which are much rarer. Some of these are potentially reversible. As the age of onset of dementia increases, the chances of dementia being reversible decreases. At the age of 65, as many as one in ten cases of dementia are caused by potentially reversible diseases. By the time the age of onset has risen to 80, the change of dementia being reversible has fallen to less than one in 100. Some of these causes include; normal pressure hydrocephalus, meningioma, subdural haematoma, syphilis, vitamin deficiency and endocrine disorders, including thyroid disease. Neurological disorders that may be associated with dementia including Parkinson's disease, AIDS and Huntington's chorea.

Risk factors

Advancing age is the most important risk factor for the development of dementia. Alzheimer's disease has a familial tendency.

In general, a positive family history increases only slightly a relative's chance of developing dementia. However, there are some families in which a strong genetic component exists, particularly for early onset Alzheimer's. A past history of head injury or thyroid disease are other factors said to increase the risk of Alzheimer's disease.

Hypertension, smoking, diabetes and poor diet may all be factors in the dementia caused by atherosclerosis. Alcohol can cause dementia when taken in excess over a prolonged period of time, especially if this is accompanied by a poor diet and lacking in thiamine.

Assessment and diagnosis

The diagnosis of dementia rests on a thorough assessment. The history of development of symptoms is the most crucial aspect in this process. It is essential to gain such a history from both the patient and a source who has known the patient well. Concrete examples of symptoms should be sought rather than accepting generalisations. For example, a relative's opinion that the patient is 'vague' or 'confused' should be backed up with examples to illustrate their point.

The history should be followed by a mental state examination to determine the extent of clinical features mentioned above. Physical examination and laboratory investigations are directed primarily at revealing the underlying cause of the syndrome and any other illnesses that may increase the level of confusion or behavioural disturbance. A list of investigations is included in the 'Medical Tests' section of the chapter 'The Psychiatry of Late Life' (see chapter 39).

Social assessment includes an estimate of the resources available to the patient. The availability, skills, health and attitudes of carers are probably the most important factors in maintaining a dementing person in the community. Such caring places immense strains on the physical and mental health of those providing it. Financial concerns and social isolation among the carers are also very important. A home visit can prove invaluable in gaining information on living conditions, social support and evidence of failing abilities and cleanliness. A dementing patient often feels more secure in a familiar environment and it may provide a more realistic appraisal of which abilities are preserved and which are lost.

Differential diagnosis

There are several conditions that can present in a similar fashion to dementia. This is particularly the case when a patient is being seen for the first time and is unable to give an adequate history.

Widespread cognitive impairment also occurs in *delirium*. However, it differs from dementia, in that it has an altered level of consciousness, is usually sudden in onset over hours or days, perceptual disorders are often prominent and there is usually a disturbed sleep wake cycle. A delirious person may have marked autonomic arousal and may be quite ill from the underlying physical cause of the delirium. The importance of excluding delirium lies in the fact that delirium is best regarded as a sign of underlying medical illness which must be treated (see chapter 41).

Depression may mimic dementia in a way that has been described as 'pseudodementia'. Such a depressed patient may have become increasingly despondent over a period of weeks or months and no longer takes an interest in life. As a result, they perform poorly in everyday tasks and at cognitive testing. The history is usually shorter than dementia, being over weeks or a few months. There may be a past or family history of depressive disorder and the patient often looks depressed. They may have sleep and appetite disturbances and their thoughts are full of gloom, pessimism and guilt. Their physical activity is often retarded as well as their thinking. Occasionally, a trial of antidepressant treatment is required to clarify the diagnosis (see chapter 28).

Schizophrenia in its advanced state can mimic dementia, especially in a mute patient who has been in an institution for a long time. *Amnestic syndromes* associated with alcohol use may be misdiagnosed as a global dementia. Such syndromes usually only involve memory and are not progressive once the original cause (alcohol) is no longer in evidence. Focal brain lesions such as *tumours*, *haematomas* and *strokes* may cause cognitive impairment that mimics dementia. More usually, the patient has focal neurological signs and areas of preservation of intellect. *Mental retardation* or developmental disability can be mistaken for dementia if an adequate history is not available (see chapter 38).

Clinical course and prognosis

Dementia typically progresses over time, causing increased impairment of mental functioning. The severity of dementia has been divided into mild, moderate and severe. In mild dementia, work and social activities are impaired. However, the capacity for independent living remains, with adequate personal hygiene and relatively intact judgment. In the moderate stages, independent living is hazardous and some degree of supervision is necessary. As the disease moves into the severe stage, activities of daily living are so impaired that continual supervision is required to maintain such things as personal hygiene. The patient is largely incoherent or mute. This whole process is gradual with one stage merging into the next and with much individual variation in progression.

Few patients survive ten years. Most patients succumb to pneumonia or other common causes of death. Survival seems to be increasing and this seems to be due mainly to a higher quality of nursing care.

Management

Many of the principles underlying the management of the patient with dementia are included in chapter 39 on 'The Psychiatry of Late Life'.

In most cases of dementia, there is no reversible cause or curative treatment. Treatment is based on reducing symptoms and ameliorating the distress of the patient and the carers. A full biological, psychological and social assessment provides the basis for administering comprehensive treatment strategies. An individualised treatment plan can be formulated with the information gathered in the assessment.

What general interventions are available?

The aim of intervention is to optimise current functioning and limit increased disability due to reversible physical, social and psychological factors.

In the early stages of dementia, 'reality orientation' can be used to gently remind the confused person of his surroundings. As dementia increases, this approach tends to produce increased anxiety. As this occurs, many therapists switch to 'validation therapy'. In this, the patient's internal world and thought processes are accepted without confrontation. A guiding principle for psychological intervention is to utilise the abilities which have been retained.

Social interventions are numerous and provide real opportunity to aid the dementing person and their carers. Education and training courses and self help groups such as Alzheimer's Disease and Related Disorders Society (ADARDS) can be invaluable in supporting carers. Home help, respite care, day care, community options, home nursing, meals on wheels, day and night sitters, mobilisation of informal support networks and other innovations provide valuable practical assistance to carers.

Residential care

As many as 50 per cent of persons with dementia will be placed in nursing care or hospital at some stage of their illness. There are no rigid rules as to when placement is desirable. Placement decisions should only be made after a comprehensive assessment of the available resources, the patient's present and anticipated problems, the caring network capabilities and the wishes of both the patient and their caregivers. At present, the major difficulties in placement arise with the patient, who does not yet fit criteria/admission to nursing home, but who has exhausted the resources of their carers.

Psychotropic drugs in dementia

Psychotropic drugs are in widespread use for the control of behavioural complications of dementia. This is particularly the case in nursing homes and hostel settings, where prescription rates vary markedly. Between 20–70 per cent of institutionalised dementing patients are receiving psychotropic medications. Haloperidol and thioridazine are the two drugs used most commonly. They may be effective in 30 per cent of cases, but the evidence of their usefulness is otherwise limited. Up to 90 per cent of patients will suffer side effects from such medication. Thus, medication can never be seen as the sole answer to problems such as wandering, aggression and agitation in dementing patients. The best use of such drugs is for short periods at low dosages in particularly disturbed patients (see chapter 57).

Behavioural problems

When a patient with dementia presents with behavioural problems, several questions should be asked.

1. Is there a physical illness making this behaviour worse? A sudden change in the behaviour of a person suffering from dementia should demand review of their medical status. Usually, such a change is linked with a physical illness. The patient is unable to describe symptoms because of his impairments. Delirium may be present. Common causes include prescribed drugs, alcohol, infections in the urine, chest or skin, faecal impaction, pain, strokes, heart attacks and sensory impairment.

2. Is there a psychiatric disease making the behaviour worse? This is less common than a physical cause of deterioration in a dementing patient. However, a depressive, paranoid or manic illness may be superimposed on dementia. Evidence for this includes a past or family history of such a disorder. The mental state examination reveals the characteristic changes seen in those illnesses.

3. Is there a social factor making the behaviour worse? The burden of caring for dementia may lead to, or become intermingled with, marital discord, depression, chronic tiredness, poverty and chronic ill health in the carers. When such problems increase, they can be responsible for the carers being unable to cope with behaviour that they previously could tolerate. Dementing patients are more able to pick up non verbal language than verbal communication. Thus, an exasperated or angry carer can provoke a similar reaction in the patient. This may lead to an escalating cycle of discontent. Very occasionally, the elderly dementing patient is subject to abuse and exploitation.

The pre existing relationship with carers is also most important. If the relationship was strained before the onset of dementia, it is less likely to remain health in the years of decline. A sudden dislocation in the caring network such as sickness or holidays may lead to behavioural difficulties. Institutional routines and practices which require a dementing person to wash, eat and sleep to the regime of another, can also precipitate behavioural disturbances.

After the questions above concerning reversible factors have been addressed, many patients will still show behavioural problems for at least some part of their illness. Two of the most difficult behaviours are wandering and aggression.

The 'wandering' patient

The architecture of the accommodation for dementing patients is all important. It must be safe and familiar. It can be made secure by a combination of fences, locks, gates, landscaping, double handles, mirrors on doors and exit planning. Identification strategies including bracelets, can be linked with alarm systems. In the community, neighbour awareness, spare keys in strategic places, local police involvement and schemes to develop contact points with informal networks, can all aid in the management of wandering and confused people. Staffing strategies in institutions include adequate staff to follow and redirect wandering patients. Drugs are of limited usefulness and should never replace constructive environmental changes. Physical restraint tends to increase agitation and only compound the problem.

The 'aggressive' patient

The most common form of hitting out in patients with dementia is reactive aggression. This occurs when a carer is trying to help a patient who does not understand or appreciate the need for such assistance.

Sometimes pain can accentuate this problem. Carers presented with this problem should attempt to see the incident from the position of the dementing person. It must seem odd to have a stranger come into your house, try to undress you and put you in a shower when you have not formed the idea that you wanted a shower in the first place. Many elderly people have conservative attitudes to nakedness and the need for bathing, which are totally different from the carers, who are attempting to provide such a service. Strategies for minimising this problem include an explanation of the procedure every time, a warm gentle approach with the flexibility to be able to leave and come back later if necessary. Having enough time is very important. Unfortunately, many professional carers have too little of this valuable commodity. Staffing levels must be adequate when such procedures are attempted. Strength in numbers ensures safety for not only the staff but also for the patient.

Unpredictable aggression is rarer, but presents major problems when it does occur. The importance of physical illness in precipitating sudden aggression must not be overlooked. The previous personality of the patient may provide clues as to reasons for aggression. Architectural solutions which provide such patients with space to move, are usually most successful in reducing unpredictable outbursts. A behavioural analysis of the events leading up to and reinforcing aggressive outburst, may identify points at which preventive interventions could occur. Dealing with the reactions of those who suffer as a result of such aggression is important. Adequate staff levels, training and support from administration and medical staff are needed to maintain morale in carers dealing with the few patients who manifest continued aggressive behaviour (see chapter 48).

The legal mechanisms for intervention

The care of dementing patients has been increasingly 'legalised' as concerns for human rights has increased. This often creates anxiety in professional carers. Each State has its own legal framework for decisions regarding the care of dementing patients. These may take the form of guardianship or mental health laws or be covered by 'duty of care'. Each carer who deals with dementing patients should become aware of the legislation that covers their work (see chapter 50).

Conclusion

Dementia is one of the largest health problems facing our community. Over the next generation, it will assume greater importance. The effects spread out from the sufferer and involve carers, families, health and welfare professionals, housing and welfare authorities. There is no cure for the disorders that cause the majority of cases of dementia, but much can be done to alleviate the burden of caring and improve the comfort of those who are afflicted. This can only be achieved if sufficient resources are allocated to the task. Health professionals can aid in this by expanding their knowledge of dementia and by becoming skilled in the interventions which can be utilised.

Further Reading

Bernlef J, *Out of Mind*, Faber, London, 1988.
Cummings J L and Benson D F, *Dementia: A Clinical Approach*, Butterworths, Boston, 1983.
Mace N L and Rabins P V, *The 36 Hour Day*, Johns Hopkins University Press, Baltimore, 1981.
Pitt B, *Dementia*, Churchill Livingstone, Edinburgh, 1987.
Reisberg B, *Alzheimer's Disease*, The Free Press, New York, 1983.

Chapter 41

Delirium

S Ticehurst

Definition

Delirium is a syndrome and not a disease in itself. It is a collection of signs and symptoms that represent the brain's response to illness. Delirium is a transient organic mental syndrome characterised by a global disorder of cognition and consciousness. Delirium is often missed clinically because of the transitory fluctuating nature of symptoms and their lack of recognition amongst health care personnel. It has been described under many names, including acute brain failure, acute confusional state, acute organic brain syndrome and encephalopathy.

Clinical features

Delirium is characterised by impairment of the ability to maintain attention to the environment or on a logical stream of thought. As a result the patient exhibits disorganised thought patterns and rambling incoherent speech. They may misinterpret environmental stimuli and experience illusions and hallucinations. They are disorientated in time and place. They become confused about their environment and themselves. Their memory is impaired. They have marked sleep disorders with disturbed sleep–wake cycles.

Such symptoms in delirium develop rapidly over the course of a few hours or days. The level of impairment often fluctuates.

An impaired level of consciousness may be difficult to detect and this often requires considerable clinical experience. It can present as drowsiness or as 'hyperalertness', where sounds and touches can cause an exaggerated startle reaction. Attention and concentration are impaired and include difficulty in maintaining the thread of a conversation, often wandering off the topic. Poor concentration can be tested clinically by asking the patient to name the months of the year backwards or by other memory tests. Wakefulness at night, and daytime sleepiness is the usual pattern of sleep–wake disturbance. In the period before the onset of delirium, patients will often describe dreams of increased vividness. In the more severe forms, patients suffer from perceptual disturbances such as illusions (the misinterpretation of external stimuli) and hallucinations. Illusions are more prominent in half light where the patient may interpret folds in the bed clothes as people or animals. Hallucinations are usually visual and can include animals, insects, people and monsters. They are often vivid and brightly coloured and may be accompanied by intense fear. Hallucinations involving smell, touch and hearing may also occur. Patients trying to remove insects from their skin or bed clothes can become extremely distressed. Perceptual disturbances have been reported in up to 50 per cent of elderly patients with delirium. Frightening paranoid delusions may develop, which are usually transitory and ill defined. A patient may believe that hospital staff are trying to poison him. Such beliefs can lead to uncooperativeness and in some cases, suicidal behaviour.

Since the symptoms fluctuate markedly during a 24 hour period, they may be missed if only a single interview is performed. The patient may misidentify staff as friends or family. New information is very difficult to retain and the patient may remember some things and not others.

The patient may show signs of autonomic arousal, including sweating, a rapid pulse, raised blood pressure and dilated pupils.

A less obvious presentation of delirium is that of the so called 'quiet' delirium. This form is usually not as well detected because the patients sits or lies in a hospital ward quietly confused with little obvious behavioural disturbance.

Epidemiology

Patients suffering from delirium are often in hospitals and nursing homes because of the relationship between the disorder, physical illness and age. Between 15 and 25 per cent of the patients, especially elderly people in a general hospital, will suffer a delirium during their stay. As many as 90 per cent of these *may not* be diagnosed as having a delirium. This is partly because of the transitory nature of the disorder. Another reason for the poor level of detection is the failure of staff to pick up the signs and symptoms. Patients with delirium stay in hospital longer than non delirious patients and they have an increased risk of dying in hospital.

Risk factors

Delirium is more common at the extremes of age. The maturing brain of the child and the ageing brain have decreased capacities to deal with disturbances to their functioning. The higher prevalence of delirium amongst the elderly is also related to the increase in physical illness that occurs with age. Another factor is the prescription of drugs to older people and the diminished capacity of the elderly body to deal with these, especially when several are used simultaneously. Patients with dementia and cerebrovascular disease are at increased risk of delirium.

Patients who abuse alcohol and the benzodiazepines may also be more likely to suffer from delirium. Sleep loss, sensory deprivation or overload, bereavement or relocation may be precipitating factors in some patients with delirium.

Aetiology

Delirium is the final common pathway of illnesses which cause a disturbance in the metabolism of the brain. The electrical activity of the brain is altered without any permanent destruction of brain tissue. The exact mechanism by which delirium is produced is unclear. One theory is that the area affected in the brain is responsible for arousal and alertness. This area is at the base of the brain and the effects of disturbed metabolism in this area spreads to have an influence on the functioning of the brain as a whole.

At any age life threatening illness, severe infections, drug intoxication or withdrawal and head injuries may be complicated by delirium. Alcohol is a particularly common cause of delirium in the general population. It can do so through intoxication and withdrawal as well as through associated causes such as subdural haematoma as a result of falls in intoxicated patients.

Young children often become delirious when they suffer fever from any cause. In the elderly, the cause is often prescribed medications, especially psychotropic drugs such as tranquillisers, sedatives and antidepressants. Other common causes at all ages include infection in the chest, urine, skin or elsewhere, congestive cardiac failure, faecal impaction, a recent stroke and dehydration. Delirium is particularly likely to develop after anaesthesia and surgery. The number of physical illnesses that can cause delirium is too large to list here, but pneumonia is a common cause among both the young and the old.

Differential diagnosis

Like dementia, delirium involves a widespread impairment of mental function. However, it differs from dementia, in that dementia is of chronic onset and does not have the level of disturbed consciousness seen in delirium. Perceptual disturbances and autonomic arousal are much less common in dementia.

Depression, mania, paranoid psychoses and schizophrenia may all be present with disorganised behaviour, irrational thinking and psychotic phenomena. In these conditions, the level of consciousness is not usually altered and the electroencephalogram is usually normal. An adequate history and physical examination may establish a longer time course of events and the absence of an underlying physical illness.

Clinical course and prognosis

Most episodes of delirium are brief. The usual outcome is complete recovery which parallels treatment of the underlying disorder. However, in 20–30 per cent of patients, the underlying disease process leads to death. In a few patients, delirium can continue for days and even weeks if the illness causing the disorder is not recognised or does not respond to treatment.

Diagnosis

The history of recent onset is very important. A reliable corroborative source of information should be sought to gain an adequate history. Relatives and carers should be questioned about fluctuations in the degree of symptoms over time. They can also provide valuable information concerning medical illnesses which may be responsible. A careful mental state examination is necessary. It may be that repeated examinations during the course of the day will provide the best picture of the periodic fluctuation which is part of the syndrome. Close observations in hospital can provide confirmation of the presence and degree of symptoms. A physical examination may reveal signs of autonomic arousal and previously unrecognised signs of underlying physical illness. There is no definitive test to prove the presence of delirium. Electroencephalographs (EEG) showing generalised slowing of the brain wave patterns may be helpful, especially when repeated recordings are taken which show change over time, in line with the clinical picture. However, they may be difficult to administer in an agitated patient.

Management

A patient diagnosed as having a delirium needs to be in a safe environment and have a comprehensive medical assessment as soon as possible. Treatment is directed at finding and remedying the underlying physical cause.

Careful observation is required both to aid in the diagnosis and to prevent the patient from coming to harm or inadvertently harming others. Appropriate laboratory investigations to help identify the illness responsible should be undertaken urgently.

Several early management strategies are useful. The confused patient responds best to an environment where the sensory input is moderate. Too little stimuli can predispose the patient to illusions and hallucinations. Too much stimuli can increase confusion.

A separate, well lit area with no dangerous objects or open windows is preferred. Orientation devices such as a clock and calendar may help. Approaches by staff should be gentle and reassuring, with as much explanation and repetition as possible. Having regular staff and encouraging visits by relatives and familiar friends can aid the delirious patient. Sensory deprivation in the form of eye patches and no hearing aids should be avoided. Attention to adequate fluid intake is necessary. A wandering patient may benefit from identification bracelets.

Medication can be used to settle a very agitated patient, especially if psychotic features are prominent. However, minimising sedation is a general rule as medication may increase confusion and disguise valuable clinical signs. Haloperidol has been seen by many as the best drug to use in such situations, because it causes minimal hypotension and has little in the way of anticholinergic effects that may cause delirium. However, it may produce neuro-muscular rigidity and should not be used in delirious patients at high doses or for prolonged periods (see chapter 57).

Conclusion

Delirium is an under diagnosed and poorly researched syndrome. Its diagnosis should herald urgent medical investigation to diagnose and treat the underlying illness. Health care professionals in acute medical settings must become skilled at recognising delirium.

Further Reading

Lipowski Z J, *Delirium: Acute Brain Failure in Man*, Springfield, Illinois, Charles C Thomas, 1980.

Lipowski Z J, 'Delirium in the Elderly Patient', *The New England Journal of Medicine*, Vol 320 No 9, 578–82.

Chapter 42

Alcohol Dependence and Related Problems

R G Pols

Australians and New Zealanders are among the heaviest drinkers in the English speaking world and rank high in the world as a whole. As such, alcohol dependence and related problems are very common, on their own or in association with other psychiatric illness. In fact, alcohol related psychiatric illness is the most common psychiatric illness in general population surveys.

Definition

The standard dictionary definitions of alcoholism usually refer to the compulsive, excessive consumption of alcohol. In common usage, the term also includes withdrawal symptoms. However, the term 'alcoholism' is subject to varying definitions and interpretations. For our purposes, it can be described as a chronic, progressive, relapsing syndrome characterised by increasing alcohol consumption, dependence, withdrawal symptoms and the development of a wide range of social, physical and psychological problems with progressive personal decline.

Causes of alcoholism

The aetiology of alcoholism is a relatively elusive problem. Many factors have been implicated:

1. Strong statistical evidence has been found for a *genetic factor* in alcoholism. Reviews of adoptees have shown a correlation of alcoholism (both primary and secondary to other illnesses) with an alcoholic history in the biological parents.

2. However, other family studies have shown that alcoholism is more likely to be transmitted to children when the behaviour of the alcoholic parent is disruptive of family routines and rituals. The *family pattern* of handling of severe alcohol problems is an important factor and suggests the need to consider family systems in management.

3. Among *physiological factors* are the observations that there may be disturbed metabolism or reduced levels of neuro-transmitters in alcoholics (similar to the findings in affective disorders). This may explain the frequent association of alcohol with depressive symptoms.

4. Psycho-analytic theories have suggested that drug addictions are due to a fixation at an early stage of development. This results in strong dependency needs, an inability to tolerate frustration and fears of sexual impotency. These characteristics are established by over-indulgent and over-protective parents. Other psycho-dynamic theories also emphasise the alcoholics' longings for warmth and comfort, feelings which are released by alcohol, which is a substitute for the mother's milk.

5. However, the development of patterns of problem drinking may also be due to *learned behaviour*. For an anxious or otherwise predisposed individual, the pleasurable effects may be highly rewarding and a habit may become quickly established. For many workers, this is the simplest way of viewing the cause of alcoholism. For others, it is a simplistic explanation.

6. Alcoholics have more *sexual problems* than non alcoholic persons in the general population, but the role of sexual maladjustment in the development of alcoholism is uncertain.

7. *Occupation* plays an important part and alcoholism appears to be an occupational hazard among people who conduct their daily business over beer and spirits. Alcoholism may become a greater risk for people as they get promoted in work and acquire greater responsibilities and have more social engagements. *Pressure from peers* can be a major factor in increasing drinking patterns and in nourishing them. This may be particularly the case in subgroups of the population, for example, among undergraduate students, some ethnic groups and among socially deprived and unemployed people.

8. Alcoholism can arise secondary to psychiatric illness, particularly depression and anxiety where the use of alcohol may initially have blunted the anxious and depressed feelings.

Classification

The *responsible use* of alcohol can lead to the well-known beneficial effects; employment for many people, excise revenue to governments and pleasure for many.

Conversely, the excessive use of alcohol results directly in physical, social and psychiatric problems for the individuals who use it. Indirectly, excessive alcohol use affects many others and imposes a huge cost burden to our community. This high level of excessive use of alcohol in Australia led the National Health and Medical Research Council (NH & MRC) to indicate that alcohol should be used responsibly. Their recommendations are summarised in Tables 1 and 2.

Acute alcohol intoxication

This is responsible for most of the deaths associated with alcohol use. It is characterised by recent consumption of sufficient alcohol to cause intoxication in most people. This produces maladaptive behavioural changes such as disinhibition of sexual or aggressive impulses, lability of moods with euphoria or

Table 1. NH & MRC guidelines for responsible drinking

Men

NO MORE THAN 4 standard drinks (40 gm) on any one day and no more than 28 drinks in any one week

Women

NO MORE THAN 2 standard drinks (20 gm) on any one day and no more than 14 drinks in any one week

ABSTINENCE IS DESIRABLE IN PREGNANCY

ABSTINENCE WHEN PERFORMING HAZARDOUS ACTIVITIES (eg driving)

ABSTINENCE WHEN IN HAZARDOUS ENVIRONMENTS (eg water sports)

Source: Pols R G and Hawks D, *Is There a Safe Level of Alcohol Consumption?*, NH & MRC, Canberra, 1987.

Table 2. Responsible drinking in social situations

- Plan your drinking behaviour
- Drink slowly. Your body can handle only about one drink per hour
- Alternate alcoholic and non alcoholic drinks
- Count your drinks
- Dilute your drinks with mixers
- Fill your own glass
- Eat whilst drinking
- Take non alcoholic drinks
- First drink should be non alcoholic
- Use small glasses
- Stick with one beverage
- Say 'no thank you'
- Serve yourself
- Avoid rounds
- Seek help if you find drinking hard to control

Source: Pols R G and Hawks D, *Is There a Safe Level of Alcohol Consumption?*, NH & MRC, Canberra, 1987.

depression, impaired judgment, social and occupational functioning. It is accompanied by at least one of the following: slurred speech, uncoordination, unsteady gait, nystagmus and a flushed face. There should be no evidence of any other psychiatric disorder which could account for these symptoms.

When people have been drinking (even at

0.05 mg per cent or as little as 2–3 standard drinks), the ability to react quickly to more than one thing at a time is seriously impaired. Studies show a dramatic increase in the number of mistakes made driving under the influence of increasing levels of alcohol intoxication.

There are a number of factors which need to be taken into account when considering alcohol intoxication. First, the *amount of alcohol consumed*. Standard glasses for alcoholic beverages contain approximately 8–10 gms of alcohol or 1 unit. Each such unit will raise a person's blood alcohol level (BAL) by between 0.005 to 0.015 mg per cent on a breathalyser. The concentration of alcohol also varies enormously amongst alcoholic beverages as beer ranges from 1.8 per cent to 5.8 per cent, wine 9.2 per cent to 16 per cent, fortified wines 22 per cent to 28 per cent and spirits 35 per cent or more alcohol by volume. Thus, standard glasses are of different volumes so that a nip of spirits (30 mls) contains approximately the same amount of alcohol as a 115 ml glass of table wine, ie approximately 10 gms of alcohol.

The second factor is the *size of the person who is drinking*. When alcohol is absorbed it disperses to every part of the body. If a person is small, there is only a small distribution volume. For example, in a 50 kg man, one standard drink may well raise his BAL by 0.015 per cent. The same standard drink may raise a 100 kg man's BAL by only 0.005 per cent, a threefold difference. The smaller the person, the higher the BAL will be for any given drink.

The third factor is the *rate of metabolism of alcohol by the body*. This depends on the size of the person's liver and whether or not the liver has developed the capacity to metabolise alcohol at an increased rate. The more people drink, the more the liver responds by increasing the rate of breakdown of alcohol. This is due to enzyme induction. Heavy drinkers may have a very much increased rate of alcohol breakdown.

The fourth factor is *gender*. Women are on average of a smaller build than men. This results in them having a smaller distribution volume than men. Proportionally, women also have a larger amount of fatty tissue and

although alcohol distributes throughout the whole body, it predominantly stays in the non fatty tissue. Their smaller body also means that they have a smaller liver and therefore a reduced metabolic capacity in comparison to males as well. This accounts for the lower drinking limits for women than men recommended by the NH & MRC. In the examples above, a 50 kg woman may have reached a BAL of 0.02 per cent with one standard drink and a 100 kg woman a level of 0.01 per cent.

The last factor is the *absorption of alcohol from the stomach*. On an empty stomach BAL rises very rapidly. Drinking with meals leads to a slower and steadier rise of BAL.

On average the body will be able to cope with about one standard drink per hour, otherwise alcohol accumulates and progressively increasing intoxication develops. The effects of alcohol on cognitive function are also more severe when the blood level is rising than when it is falling.

Idiosyncratic intoxication

Rarely some people respond in an unusual way to intoxication with alcohol. This idiosyncratic response consists of maladaptive behavioural changes, such as aggressive or assaultive behaviour which occurs within minutes of ingesting an amount of alcohol insufficient to induce intoxication in most people.

These people should be advised to abstain from alcohol. Sometimes they have some evidence of underlying minimal brain dysfunction and they should be fully assessed medically for evidence of this.

Alcohol abuse

Alcohol use can lead to four groups of problems: socio-economic, physical, psychiatric and alcohol dependence. Alcohol use can cause any one or more of these types of problems. For example, people can develop dependence without any other problems. However, when problems result from the use of alcohol, alcohol itself may be used as a way of trying to cope with them. For example, a man who gets drunk repeatedly at weekends may find that his wife complains or even threatens to leave him. He may become depressed or annoyed about his wife's reactions, storm out of the house and go to the pub and 'drown his sorrows'. This type of problem drinking is called 'alcohol abuse'. It is defined by a maladaptive pattern of alcohol use indicated by continued use despite the person's knowledge that he has a persistent problem which is caused or exacerbated by alcohol and by the recurrent use of alcohol in situations in which its use is physically hazardous, for example driving while intoxicated.

Thus, alcohol use which leads to any problems, without there being dependence, is classed as alcohol abuse. Alcohol abuse is very common and evident among drinking drivers. People die and many are injured daily in Australia and New Zealand because of driving while under the influence of alcohol. The intoxicated driver and his passengers contribute to this problem if he drives, or they allow themselves to be driven, in this way.

Alcohol dependence

One of the important effects of alcohol is the phenomenon of *tolerance*. People who drink heavily gradually learn to talk without slurring, or without much evidence of poor coordination. The body also adapts to the effects of alcohol. The cell membranes of nerve and muscle, particularly, learn to work efficiently even in the presence of the sedating influence of alcohol. Alcohol depresses the activity of nerve cells, so these cells increase their activity to adapt to alcohol when it is present frequently. Finally, the body adapts by increasing the rate at which the liver metabolises or breaks down alcohol.

Normally the body can cope with about 10 mg of alcohol (1 standard drink) per hour but in seriously dependent drinkers this level can increase substantially. This whole process of accommodation to alcohol is called the development of tolerance.

Tolerance involves cellular or *neuro-adaptation*. When neuro-adaptation has developed, the person can only function normally when alcohol is present. When the blood alcohol level drops, these people start to show signs of alcohol withdrawal. *Dependence* refers to the phenomenon whereby a certain amount of alcohol in the body is required for normal functioning and is identified clinically by the phenomena of tolerance, withdrawal and awareness by the person that his control over drinking is impaired.

Alcohol dependence can be said to be present when at least three of the following characteristics are present:

1. Alcohol is taken in larger amounts or over a longer period than the person intends.

2. Unsuccessful efforts to cut down or control alcohol use.

3. A considerable time is spend in activities necessary to obtain and consume alcohol (for example, pub time) or recovering from the effects of intoxication.

4. Frequent intoxication or withdrawal symptoms interfere with work or home life, or alcohol use is dangerous (for example, driving when intoxicated).

5. Important social, occupational or recreational activities are given up or restricted because of alcohol use.

6. Continued alcohol use despite knowledge of having a persistent or recurrent problem that is caused or exacerbated by the use of alcohol.

7. Marked tolerance to the effects of alcohol and increasing consumption is necessary in order to achieve intoxication or desired effect.

8. Development of characteristic withdrawal symptoms.

9. Alcohol is used to relieve or avoid withdrawal symptoms.

10. There is a compulsion to drink alcohol.

The severity of alcohol dependence can be categorised as:

(a) *mild:* symptoms result in only mild impairment in occupational functioning, social activities or relationships with others;

(b) *moderate:* the functional impairment, while serious, is not yet completely incapacitating;

(c) *severe:* there are many or all of the above characteristics. The symptoms interfere substantially with work, social activities or relationships with others.

Alcohol withdrawal

This condition is associated with alcohol dependence. It occurs when the person's usual intake of alcohol is reduced or stopped altogether. The sedating effects of alcohol are absent and there is increased activity of the nerve and muscle cells which have become used to the alcohol effects. This leads to many signs of neural over activity. There are several degrees of severity of alcohol withdrawal. The most common and the mildest is the hangover. The nausea and tremulousness that people feel are mainly due to alcohol withdrawal. A more severe form of withdrawal is defined as *uncomplicated alcohol withdrawal*. It is manifested by coarse tremor of hands, tongue or eyelids and nausea or vomiting, malaise or weakness, autonomic hyperactivity (for example, tachycardia, sweating, elevated blood pressure), anxiety, depressed mood or irritability, transient hallucinations or illusions, headache and insomnia.

These symptoms and signs of uncomplicated withdrawal usually only occur in people who have been drinking very heavily for quite a long time, but they can occur after a binge drinking. There is a continuum of adaptation to the effects of alcohol which ranges from no tolerance to extreme dependence where people are able to drink amounts which would kill others. High levels of tolerance are in fact quite common. Some people, although severely impaired by alcohol intoxication, can still drive at blood levels of 0.15 per cent (ie 10–15 drinks in 1 hour!). Non tolerant people would be too intoxicated at these levels to even walk to their car. It must be remembered that people who are tolerant to high blood alcohol levels are in fact, very dangerous on the road because their neuro-motor skills are seriously impaired at these levels. The fact that their judgment is also impaired makes them even more dangerous. Such drinking leads to the most common alcohol related casualties, namely alcohol-related motor vehicle accidents.

Alcohol withdrawal delirium

The most severe form of alcohol withdrawal is *alcohol withdrawal* or *delirium tremens*. It is characterised by a reduced ability to attend to the external environment (for example, questions must be repeated because attention wanders) and difficulties shifting attention to new stimuli (for example, repeating the answer to a previous question when asked about something new), cognitive impairment, as indicated by rambling, irrelevant or incoherent speech. Delirium is also characterised by a reduced level of consciousness, (for example, difficulty keeping awake during examination), perceptual disturbances (misinterpretations and hallucinations), disturbance of sleep–wake cycle with insomnia or day time sleepiness, increased or decreased psychomotor activity, disorientation to time, place or person, and memory impairment.

The delirium develops over a short period of time after drinking has stopped and tends to fluctuate over the course of a day. It is accompanied by marked autonomic hyperactivity, for example, tachycardia, sweating, increased temperature and blood pressure and respiratory rate.

The progression of symptoms starts as simple alcohol withdrawal but instead of settling the excitement and agitation progressively worsens. Autonomic overactivity causes an increased temperature, heart-rate, sweating and tremor. Mentally, the senses are overstimulated and sensory misinterpretation or illusions occur. These progress into hallucinations, usually of a tactile type 'like ants crawling on the skin'. Visual and auditory hallucinations are also common. Disorientation in time, place and person may develop and persecutory delusions are common.

The syndrome usually occurs between 24 and 72 hours after the person has stopped drinking. These persons are seriously ill and should be treated in hospital. Convulsions can occur in 10–30 per cent of cases. Death can occur in 10 per cent of cases and may be due to infection, epilepsy, cardiac failure, metabolic problems or suicide.

The management of alcohol withdrawal delirium consists of:
1. Nursing in a well lighted, peaceful, calm, quiet, comfortable environment which is safe.
2. Consistent staff taking a supportive, reassuring approach.

3. Monitoring physical observations.

4. Fluid and electrolyte replacement.

5. Vitamins, especially thiamine, before the withdrawal starts (as soon as the patient is seen).

6. Sedation with appropriate drugs is mandatory. Patients may need 40 mg or more of diazepam over 24 hours. Sometimes antipsychotic medication is required, such as haloperidol up to 40 mg per day, in addition.

The most important principle in the treatment of alcohol withdrawal is the early recognition that it is occurring. Because of this, some hospitals routinely observe patients who have a history of moderate alcohol consumption for signs of withdrawal.

Some hospitals also use a simple screening questionnaire called the 'CAGE'. Four questions are asked in admission:

c   Have you ever felt you ought to cut down on your drinking?
    Yes/No

A   Have people ever annoyed you by criticising your drinking?
    Yes/No

G   Have you ever felt bad or guilty about your drinking?
    Yes/No

E   Have you ever had a drink first thing in the morning to steady your nerves or get rid of a hangover (an eye-opener)?
    Yes/No

If a person answers YES to two or more, then some degree of alcohol dependence can be expected. Such patients should be fully assessed to see if other alcohol related problems are present. They should all receive simple information and advice about the responsible use of alcohol.

Polysubstance dependence

It is also not at all uncommon for patients who use alcohol excessively or are dependent, to use other psychotropic substances. These are most commonly the benzodiazepines. Withdrawal from these substances is likely to occur. This presents a more dangerous situation as there is tolerance to two or more different types of drugs and withdrawal is usually much more severe. Convulsions are very common in addition to the delirium.

Alcohol hallucinosis

This is an unusual disorder, the cause of which is uncertain. However, severe alcohol dependence, poor nutrition, vitamin deficiency and absolute or relative alcohol withdrawal are often implicated (see chapter 45). The patient experiences auditory hallucinations in a setting of clear consciousness, there is not evidence of any delirium. It is characterised by vivid and persistent hallucinations (auditory or visual) which develop shortly after cessation of alcohol use.

The hallucinations are frequently self-denigrating in nature. Sometimes there can be a risk of the patient acting upon the hallucination and trying to kill himself. This is most likely when patients are still intoxicated and they live in depressing circumstances.

This psychotic illness requires hospitalisation and subsequent management of the alcohol withdrawal syndrome. Antipsychotic medication is usually required (haloperidol) and suicidal ideation and risk need careful assessment and observation.

Alcohol amnestic syndrome

This condition is also called the Wernicke-Korsakoff syndrome after the two men who described the acute and chronic pictures respectively. The main cause is an acute lack of thiamine (vitamin B_1). The body only stores reserves of water soluble thiamine for several days. Metabolising alcohol uses up thiamine and when patients are drinking very heavily they do not get hungry due to inflammation of the stomach (gastritis) and fail to replenish thiamine from the diet.

The lack of thiamine has important effects on brain structures. The mamillary bodies and peri-aqueductal grey matter around the third ventricle show congestion, with small haemorrhages. Similar lesions are sometimes also present in the floor of the fourth ventricle. The amnestic syndrome is identified by impairment in both short and long term memory. Impairment in short term memory is shown by an inability to learn new information (inability to remember three objects after five minutes). Long term memory impairment is shown by inability to remember information that was known in the past. For example, a person may not know what happened to them yesterday, their birth place or their occupation. They may have forgotten facts such as past Prime Ministers or well known dates.

The amnestic syndrome is not due to delirium. It is also different from dementia in that there is no impairment in abstract thinking, judgment, or other disturbances of higher cortical function and there is no evident personality change.

Symptoms emerge during an extended period of heavy drinking. Patients have double vision, vomiting and nystagmus associated with inability to remember new information, delirium, peripheral neuropathy and uncoordinated gait.

This situation is an acute medical emergency which requires the giving of thiamine (200 mg), and vitamin B complex intravenously (IV). If treatment is early enough, full clinical recovery can occur. Otherwise, due to irreversible structural lesion of some part of brain, recovery does not occur.

However, in many cases, a chronic amnestic syndrome remains (Korsakoff psychosis). The patient is unable to remember new information and fills in the gaps with remnants of old, retained information or makes up answers to questions. This is called confabulation. This condition responds only very slowly to methods of memory retraining and usually patients are severely handicapped by this condition, often requiring hostel or other supervised care for the rest of their lives.

Australia has about 20 times the rate of alcohol amnestic syndrome compared to the United States of America or many European countries. Although it is uncertain why this is so, there is some evidence which points to the fact that in those countries thiamine is added to flour and food. Adding thiamine to beer is a preventative measure which has only recently been considered in Australia.

Dementia associated with alcoholism

It is thought that repeated episodes of low levels of thiamine deficiency may cause a global dementia in patients with chronic alcohol dependence. In this condition there is evidence of impairment in short and long term memory. There is also impairment in abstract thinking, as indicated by inability to find similarities and differences between related words, difficulty in defining words and concepts and other similar tasks.

Impaired judgment, as indicated by inability to make reasonable plans to deal with interpersonal, family and job related problems and issues is also present and other disturbances of higher cortical function, such as 'constructional difficulty' (for example, inability to copy three dimensional figures, assemble blocks or arrange sticks in specific designs) may occur. Personality change, alteration or accentuation of pre-morbid traits is a common finding. These disturbances interfere significantly with work, social activities or relationships with others. All other causes of dementia have to be excluded for the diagnosis alcoholic dementia to be made (see chapter 40).

Other psychological conditions associated with alcoholism

Morbid jealousy

Although not exclusively found amongst patients who are dependent upon alcohol, it is more common among alcoholics. Patients develop persistent and relatively refractory delusions of infidelity in respect of their spouse or partner.

The setting for this illness usually has three elements; excessive drinking which impairs sexual potency or pleasure, chronic marital conflict and the use of the mental mechanism of projection by the patient. These elements reinforce the development of delusional thinking. The sexual relationship of the patient and his partner is frequently very poor, both due to the effects of intoxication and marital conflict. This heightens the alcohol dependent person's suspicions that the partner could, or must be obtaining sexual satisfaction with someone else. Projection allows attribution of the fantasied infidelity to the partner. This then provides an explanation for the problem the subject is facing. This protects the person from having to resolve the problem by ceasing drinking and the solutions seems to lie solely with the partner.

This illness can be very difficult to treat because it is so difficult to establish a treatment alliance. Occasionally also, it leads to domestic violence and even homicide. It requires treatment with antipsychotic medication, abstinence from alcohol and marital counselling.

Major depression

Patients who have alcohol dependence may experience considerable downward social mobility. These losses may result in grief and shame and such patients have a much greater risk of suicide than the rest of the population. In one research study over an eight year period, some 9 per cent of a cohort of patients with alcohol dependence suicided.

Some patients who suffer from depression may use alcohol as a way of trying to cope with their feelings. Alcohol can act as a depression relieving agent in the short term. Patients who use alcohol in this way may have a family history of affective disorder. After such people are withdrawn from alcohol, they can become very depressed and be at significant risk for suicide (see chapter 28).

Anxiety disorders

A significant percentage (5–15 per cent) of patients who develop alcohol dependence start drinking to cope with anxiety. In these situations a history of drinking *before* going out of the house or entering a social situation and relief of anxiety 'after a couple of drinks' will be found. Such people are often unaware of their high levels of anxiety, especially if they have social anxiety, while they may be frightened of mixing with people and they find themselves 'the life of the party' once they have had some alcohol. In these cases the anxiety disorder needs treatment in its own right (see chapter 27).

Personality disorder

Many patients who develop alcohol dependence or abuse show a personality disorder. Thus it is not uncommon for patients with antisocial or borderline personalities to drink heavily and irresponsibly (see chapter 14).

Schizophrenia

In a sequential survey of casualty patients at a psychiatric hospital, 23 per cent of patients who were suffering from schizophrenia had a significant blood alcohol level when they presented for treatment. It seemed that some patients with this disorder were using alcohol as a form of self medication for their illness.

Such patients and their families require education and information about their drinking behaviour. A review of their antipsychotic medication is also indicated because alcohol may be being used by patients to deal with troublesome hallucinations. Phenothiazines or haloperidol are far more effective if this is the case (see chapter 38).

Management of alcohol dependency

The key to the development of a treatment plan is thorough assessment. There is good evidence in the case of alcohol related disorders that thorough assessment is therapeutic in its own right. There are three levels of intervention in these problems.

Primary prevention

This is really a nationwide strategy. For example, compulsory breath testing and compulsory seat belt use is aimed at reducing deaths and injury on the roads. Adding thiamine to flour or alcoholic beverages may prevent the high rate of the Wernicke-Korsakoff Syndrome in Australia.

Other legislative interventions have been shown to be important in the prevention of alcohol related disorders. It has been suggested that the rate of alcohol related problems within a given community is related to the average amount of absolute alcohol consumed by each person. If the level of drinking is reduced by a small amount, then the level of alcohol related problems will decline by a much greater amount. In Australia, where per capita consumption of alcohol has fallen by about 8 per cent since 1981, alcohol related deaths have fallen by about 16 per cent. Increasing the cost of alcoholic beverages by taxation may reduce alcohol consumption. Restriction of the number of liquor licence outlets or the age at which people are allowed to drink, also reduces overall consumption and the incidence of alcohol related problems in a community.

People have also started to take individual action when there has been a high level of alcohol related problems. For example, some aboriginal communities have declared themselves 'dry areas'. Other community groups have lodged complaints about drunkenness, noise, fighting and other social disturbances suffered by neighbours of licensed outlets. In some instances licences have been modified and restricted. Some groups have also tackled specific problems such as Mothers Against Drunk Drivers (MADD) and they have had considerable influence in the United States. Health workers should be aware of these possibilities and consider being involved in social actions.

Secondary prevention

Individual patients are assessed and a program of management is negotiated with them and carried out. All intervention should occur as early as possible so that the most effective outcome can result (see chapter 68).

Assessment

The information required from a person when an alcohol related problem presents is as follows:

1. *Consumption.* How much alcohol has been consumed by this person over the last week? This can be assessed accurately by asking patients to keep a diary of drinking.

2. *Dependence.* What degree of tolerance or dependence does this person have? An estimate should be made to see if dependence is mild, moderate or severe.

3. *Problems.* How many and what variety of problems are associated with this person's drinking? Physical ill health may be a problem. Finances, arguments or work related problems may occur. Drink driving, domestic violence or assault may be the issues. A full list of problems should be determined and written down.

4. It is also helpful to learn about:
   - the family drinking pattern
   - drinking cues, ie are there particular

situations (people, places, mood states, etc) which precipitate drinking or drinking which is out of control?
- the historical development of the present drinking pattern
- previous treatment, ie what may or may not have been helpful before? What has led to relapse previously?

Once all this information is available, the person should have a medical examination to assess their physical health. All people who drink heavily should have investigations done to assess the functions of their liver and red blood cells.

An agreement then needs to be reached with the patient to cooperate in treatment. The first step is reviewing the role of alcohol in the creation of problems found. Patients need to be motivated to focus upon alcohol consumption as a problem. This is often very difficult because the norms used in Australasian society are of excessive consumption. Confrontation about the problem, persuasion towards change and cooperation for specific behavioural changes will be required.

Minimal intervention

Evidence is accumulating that the provision of detailed assessment, followed by specific advice about cutting down on consumption, is very effective for persons who are in trouble with alcohol use.

Controlled drinking

The aim is to achieve the responsible, controlled use of alcohol which carries no adverse consequences. This means that patients need to agree to drink no more than a responsible limit and adopt responsible patterns of alcohol use. Some patients lose control of their drinking in specific social or drinking situations. If this is so, the agreement with the patient should include a strategy to deal with those situations, so that the relapse is prevented.

Controlled, responsible drinking is a goal which can be achieved by many patients. If there is severe dependence on alcohol, however, controlled drinking strategies are progressively less likely to be successful.

Abstinence

Dependent patients may find great difficulty achieving controlled drinking. The achievement of a period of abstinence for six months leads to a favourable outcome after four years. Hence, the first phase of treatment of a patient with moderate alcohol dependence should be that of detoxification followed by abstinence. This may be assisted at times with the use of *disulphiram* which blocks the breakdown of alcohol from acetaldehyde to acetate. If patients taking these substances drink alcohol, they become quite ill, vomit and develop a flushed face, bounding pulse and a drop in blood pressure. They then learn that they cannot drink and use these drugs at the same time. These substances can be a useful adjunct to treatment for some patients as they need to stop taking the medication for four days before they can drink alcohol without such ill effects.

Alcoholics Anonymous (AA) can also be an important source of support for some patients to strengthen their resolve. AA was founded in America by R H Smith and W William in 1935 who became abstinent after many alcohol related problems. They found that they could help and support each other to maintain their sobriety. AA is a self help group which embodies an essentially religious and spiritual approach emphasising the need for new and different values. Members know each other by first name and go to meetings as often as they feel it is necessary to sustain their sobriety. At the meetings, members share their life story. AA is not acceptable for every patient, but if the approach is acceptable, it can be extremely helpful.

Alanon developed from the needs of the partners of AA members, who formed themselves into a support group. It has developed a parallel format of sharing and support. One of the very useful features of Alanon is that it provides the opportunity for the partner of an alcohol dependent person to learn strategies to disengage from taking responsibility for controlling their partner's drinking. *Alateen* was formed as a support group for the children of patients with alcohol dependence.

Women for Sobriety was formed in the United States in 1972. It is an approach which uses a format not unlike that of AA. It provides a forum specifically to examine drug and alcohol dependency from a woman's perspective. There are only very few Women for Sobriety groups in Australasia.

During the period of abstinence, or controlled drinking, many issues usually need to be addressed. These involve problems in relationships, work, health and legal issues. The patient has to learn how to live with a dramatically reduced alcohol intake or without any alcohol at all and this means a different lifestyle for many. During this time, patients may relapse and it may be necessary to *start again*, taking particular care to plan strategies to prevent relapse. A success rate of 20 per cent abstinence at 12 months can be expected even for quite severely deteriorated patients. Less seriously dependent patients usually do better than this, especially if they are followed up regularly for 12 months.

Some patients show other psychiatric illness when they stop drinking. In these cases, that illness requires treatment in its own right.

Summary

Alcohol consumption may have severe physical, psychological, financial and social consequences. It is important for *all* clinicians to be aware that alcohol related problems are extremely common and that effective treatments are available. Early intervention with advice to achieve controlled, responsible alcohol use should be the first goal and this can be achieved by most patients. If dependence is severe, abstinence may be the only way in which control over drinking can be achieved.

Further Reading

Alcohol and Liquor Advisory Council, *Action on Alcohol Kit*, ALAC, New Zealand, 1985.
Edwards, Griffith, *The Treatment of Drinking Problems*, 2nd ed, Blackwell, Oxford, 1987.

Pols R G and Hawks D, *Is There a Safe Level of Daily Alcohol Consumption?*, NH & MRC, AGPS, Canberra, 1987 (reprinted 1989).

Robins L N, Helzer J E, Weisman M M, Orvaschel H, Gruenserg E, Burke J D and Regier D A, 'Lifetime Prevalence of Specific Psychiatric Disorders in Three Sites', *Archives of General Psychiatry*, Vol 41, 1984, pp 949-58.

Royal College of Physicians, *A Great and Growing Evil*, A Report on the Medical Consequences of Alcohol Abuse, Tavistock, London, 1987.

Royal College of Psychiatrists, *Alcohol: Our Favourite Drug*, Tavistock, London, 1986.

Chapter 43

Other Substances Abuse

R G Pols

Australia was described as 'a medicated society' by the Senate Standing Committee on Social Welfare in 1981. That statement indicates an aspect of the way in which Australians use chemical substances other than alcohol. However, it is difficult to know what is meant by 'drug problem','drug abuse' or 'substance abuse', and completely satisfactory definitions have not really been agreed upon. In this chapter 'drug use' refers to the use of psycho-active substances taken to achieve a subjective effect. This usually means the use of illegal drugs such as heroin, cocaine, amphetamines, LSD, as well as the illegal use of legal chemicals such as glue and petrol or the deliberate misuse of prescribed medications.

Drug use and drug problems

The reasons people use chemical substances which are dangerous to themselves, are not well understood. The habit of using chemical substances as a part of everyday life may be part of our culture because the use of a wide variety of drugs is actually sanctioned and taught through modelling by parents and society from early in life.

In a recent South Australian survey of children and adolescents in Year 11 at school (15 and 16 years old), it was found that 30 per cent of girls and 24 per cent of boys smoked tobacco, 40 per cent took analgesics and 40 per cent drank alcohol on a once a week basis or more frequently. At least 30 per cent had used illegal drugs at some time.

Substance abuse affects about 12 per cent of adult men and 5 per cent of women, mainly young people, yet unfortunately, it has not been a high priority area for many mental health professionals.

When mortality is examined, alcohol causes 16 per cent of deaths and prescribed medication and illegal drugs account for less than 2 per cent of deaths.

Alcohol and illegal drugs lead to premature death and therefore the years of life lost are probably a better indicator of the relative seriousness of these problems. While tobacco causes 52 per cent of total years of life loss, alcohol causes 37 per cent and opiates and other drugs 11 per cent.

A model of drug dependence

There are many predisposing factors within individuals, their families and society that contribute to the likelihood of a person using a particular substance. Parents are models for their children, and a parent who has frequent headaches and commonly uses analgesics tends to convey the message to their children that it is a good, useful and normal thing to take medication. A particularly traumatic childhood, leaving a person very insecure, anxious and seeking approval from others may lead towards experiments with heroin under the influence of pressure from peers. The effects of heroin can powerfully reinforce the continued use of the drug by providing an insecure person with a sense of calmness.

There can be immediately antecedent factors which lead to episodes of drug use. These include social factors such as a drug using peer group or individual factors such as anxiety, insecurity and wish to please.

The experience of the drug taking itself may be rewarding. For example, a 10 year old boy mixing with a group of 14 year olds who are smoking cigarettes may be encouraged to smoke. He may be persuaded to use three or four cigarettes, but becomes extremely nauseated owing to the toxic effects of nicotine. This may be socially humiliating and physically unpleasant. Such circumstances may make it less likely for him to use cigarettes again (ie avoidance learning). On the other hand, he may find that the cigarettes are pleasant and he is given praise by his friends. He is likely then to use the cigarettes again (ie approach learning).

With some chemicals however, there is another phenomenon which is the most powerful reinforcer of all. This is the development of addiction.

The development of addiction

There are overlapping concepts which need to be understood: tolerance, neuro-adaptation and dependence. *Tolerance* refers to the fact that in response to acute and chronic drug use, the person and body respond by needing more of the drug to achieve the same effect.

People learn to be able to carry out tasks while they are intoxicated, for example they may drive a car more slowly. The metabolism of the drug is speeded up by means of enzyme induction so that after the continuous use of, say, barbiturates over three to four weeks, the rate of breakdown will increase two fold. Moreover, physiological functions change. In the case of opiates such as heroin, there are two ways in which cells adapt to the presence of the drug. They become more active to combat the depressant effect of the drug and they develop more receptors. Thus, a higher dose of drug will be needed to block receptors and to overcome increased cell activity.

When the cell is adapted to work in presence of the drug, this is called neuro-adaptation. When the drug is withdrawn the cells respond and produce the symptoms of physiological withdrawal, which are usually characteristic for a particular drug.

Dependence includes neuro-adaptation and tolerance. It involves in addition an awareness of the person of a craving for the drug. The subjective sense of loss of control has important learning components, the association of the situational, personal and physiological circumstances of drug use. For example, a person who has been opiate free for months, may suddenly experience craving and symptoms of withdrawal when presented with needles used in drug taking. Similarly, people can experience a 'high' when they think they are taking an active substance when they are actually using a substance which has no psychoactive pharmacological effect.

Thus, a typical life story of a heroin user might include:
1. The psychological rewards of a relief of chronic insecurity and anxiety.
2. The effect of heroin to give a sense of euphoria or optimism.
3. Adaptation to heroin, becoming less sensitive to its effects so that doses need to be increased.
4. The sense of belonging to and approval by a peer group, further rewarding drug taking behaviour.

The mode by which a drug is taken has an important influence on the effects of the drug. In the case of opiates, the intravenous (IV) route produces a very powerful euphoria, described by users as 'the rush'. This is a strong, reinforcing effect for people, because it is immediate and intense. It is an important reason for opiates being so addictive. In the same way cocaine, which is 'smoked' and inhaled, also causes a similar immediate, acute euphoria.

'Addiction' can be said to be established when there is tolerance, dependence, neuro-adaptation and when the person continues to use the drug in spite of having significantly harmful consequences. Because 'addiction' is a term which is very difficult to define without making value judgments, classificatory systems have chosen dependence as the more useful term.

Psycho-active substance dependence is characterised by at least three of the following characteristics:
1. The substance is taken in larger amounts, or over a longer period than the person intended.
2. Efforts are made to cut down or control substance use but fail.

3. Much time spent in activities necessary to get the substance (for example theft), taking the substance (for example chain smoking), or recovering from its effects.

4. Frequent intoxication or withdrawal symptoms when expected to fulfil major role obligations at work, school, or home.

5. Important social, occupational, or recreational activities are given up or reduced because of substance use.

6. Continued use of the substance, despite knowledge of its harmful effects.

7. The need for markedly increased amounts of the substance.

8. The development of withdrawal symptoms.

Opiate dependence

These drugs include opium, morphine, heroin and pethidine. They are extremely addicting because of their effects (euphoria and sedation) and because the body rapidly develops tolerance. Over the past decade, many naturally occurring peptides with opiate-like actions have been identified in nervous tissues. These are called endorphins. They produce an effect by interacting with opiate receptors formed in nervous tissue. The exact physiological purposes and the tissue targets of the endorphins are still unclear. However, it is thought that they may play a role in the experience of pain and in a number of psychiatric disorders, including depression and schizophrenia. Their role in drug addiction is unclear.

Opiate intoxication is characterised by initial euphoria followed by apathy, mood swings, psychomotor retardation, impaired judgment and impaired social or occupational functioning. In addition, physical effects of the drug are present on examination, including pupillary constriction, drowsiness, slurred speech and impairment in attention or memory.

Opiate withdrawal

The opiate withdrawal syndrome is characterised by a history of cessation after prolonged (several weeks or more) use of an opiate or reduction in the amount of opiate used, followed by craving for the drug, nausea or vomiting, abdominal cramps and diarrhoea, muscle aches, lacrimation and rhinorrhea, pupillary dilation, piloerection (gooseflesh or 'cold turkey'), or sweating, yawning, shivering, fever and insomnia. In addition, signs of anxiety and agitation occur with increased blood pressure and heart rate.

Consequences of intravenous drug use

Heroin is the drug which is most often used intravenously (IV). Problems include the consequences of the use of non sterile equipment. This can lead to infections. Infected equipment which is shared can also spread infection from person to person. Of particular importance is Hepatitis B and HIV (AIDS). In a Sydney study, syringes collected at a needle exchange program contained as many as six blood groups. Thus, needle sharing can be a major public health problem. The important issue of needle sharing and AIDS infection is dealt with in chapters 53, 54.

Treatment of heroin use

One of the major problems for drug users who are seriously dependent upon heroin is the fact that their lives revolve completely around obtaining and using the drug. Heroin becomes the first priority in their lives. The only effective way for people who are in such an existential dilemma to stop drug using, is for them to deliberately choose to stop. Ultimately, people will weigh the costs and benefits of the habit. With drug dependent people, the major role for health professionals is to try to minimise the harm resulting from drug use and to maximise the opportunities for them to cease drug use.

Drug users frequently come into contact with health professionals through physical illness, overdoses, or antisocial activities. Frequently, they lose drug using peers by accidental overdoses, suicides or illnesses. In a British cohort, over a 10 year period, 18 per cent of IV drug users died.

It is at critical times when the costs of continued drug use confront users that they are more likely to be engaged in a therapeutic relationship. If such good supportive relationships can be established, it can lead to a positive outcome in many cases over a period of three to five years. A number of specific approaches will be briefly discussed.

Diversionary programs are especially useful for drug users who have got into trouble with the law as they are offered alternatives to prison. There are also a number of programs in prisons. Of particular interest are predischarge programs for those likely to relapse after leaving prison.

Detoxification programs are where drug users are withdrawn from the drugs under supervision. Up to 50 per cent of detoxified patients are reported to remain drug free after six months.

Drug maintenance programs are currently confined to opiate dependence. Methadone, a long acting opiate, is given to substitute for street heroin. The aim is to help patients to stabilise their lives and move away from drug taking as a full time activity, which is the case when people are part of the 'drug scene'. This aim is often only slowly realised over a period of three to five years.

Initially, drug substitution reduces the need to obtain drugs as it blocks the drug withdrawal syndrome without giving the patients the acute euphoria resulting from IV heroin use. In practice, patients gradually reduce their use of street drugs in addition to the methadone, although some sporadic use is common.

Some patients do not commit themselves to more change than this, but the overall cost of their drug use is less. In such patients, the maintenance is a harm reduction strategy because such patients expose themselves to less risk from adulterated street heroin, infected needles, crime and prostitution. However, amongst this group there are also some who persist in needle sharing and street drug use, usually with one or several confidants. This continues to be of grave concern and currently new educational programs are being developed for such patients, so that the spread of HIV infection can be reduced.

Many patients do respond to the increased stability which a methadone maintenance program can give and go on to commit themselves to moving away from drug use over time.

Therapeutic communities allow people to choose to live in a group situation away from drug involving life for a period of several months. They can review their priorities and the way in which they deal with people. If patients complete these programs, they usually do very well in the long term. Success rates vary from 20–80 per cent in different programs, but many patients relapse a number of times on the road to recovery.

Narcotics Anonymous (NA) is a program based upon the Alcoholics Anonymous model (see chapter 42). It is a very useful program for patients who are willing to accept such a philosophy. Often it is used as a complimentary program to therapeutic community activities and assists patients in maintaining a drug free lifestyle. The support network offered by NA members to patients in trying to give up a drug using lifestyle is very helpful.

Women for Sobriety is for women and is derived from the Alcoholics Anonymous model. It however, focuses upon the specific needs and aspirations of women. *Naranon* is an independent group loosely related to NA which meets for the purpose of supporting relatives of drug dependent people.

Assessment, support, information and good health care are the most basic of interventions but are always the core of any good and effective treatment programs. Most people in trouble as a result of drug use have multiple health and social problems. Assessment, support, advice and treatment for any illness will be required, often repeatedly before individuals are ready to make the decision to alter their lifestyle.

Education and information are needed by all drug users. This should include matters about drug use and its effects, drug problems, treatment options and services which are available to help them. In particular, information needs to be given to them about the dangers of the use of dirty equipment in the spread of Hepatitis B and HIV (AIDS) infections.

Needle exchange programs have been established so that dirty needles can be exchanged for clean ones cheaply or for no cost, in locations where users can access them readily. These programs appear to have had limited, but definite success in some areas. Most drug exchange centres also provide condoms and education literature on AIDS for drug users.

Experimental drug substitution programs have also been used by some very experienced specialists in this area. Prescription of IV heroin, methadone and other drugs have been used at times to attract some of this group into a therapeutic relationship, often the first step to a graduate process of change.

Stimulant dependence

Stimulants include substances such as cocaine and amphetamines.

Cocaine is mostly used recreationally by middle and upper class people. Most people experiment only once or twice, but unfortunately, cocaine is extremely addictive. This is especially so in the form known as 'crack' which can be smoked. This gives an immediate, extremely intense euphoria which is the main addiction-producing effect.

Amphetamines are also frequently used by intravenous injection for recreational purposes. They are also used by some people who need to stay awake for long periods, for example, truck drivers and students. Unfortunately there is also an increasing number of young people who use amphetamines in combination with alcohol to continue partying without sleep from Friday to Sunday. Other amphetamine derivatives are prescribed to women as appetite suppressants or to children for hyperactivity. In these situations, people can become dependent.

These substances release chemicals from nerve cells which produce euphoria (adrenalin, non-adrenalin, dopamine and 5-hydroxytryptamine). When stimulation becomes excessive they can precipitate rage and violence and distortions of perception, including paranoia or delirium. Such disturbances are a form of organic psychosis.

Stimulant withdrawal leads to a severe clinical syndrome, the most important feature of which is severe depression. It is believed to be related to depletion of the neurotransmitters, noradrenaline and 5-hydroxytrypt-amine. It is also characterised by severe craving. These factors can lead to suicide attempts.

Sedative dependence

Sedatives include barbiturates, alcohol and benzodiazepines. Barbiturates and alcohol cause similar pictures of dependence and withdrawal. In the case of barbiturates there is a greater danger of epileptic seizures. Death, as a result of epilepsy, is a possibility and should be guarded against during barbiturate withdrawal. Seizures in the case of barbiturate withdrawal should be treated with a barbiturate rather than other anticonvulsants.

Benzodiazepine dependence is more common in Australia and New Zealand than was previously realised. It presents a characteristic picture of increased tolerance to high doses of medication and with a typical withdrawal syndrome as shown in Table 1.

Table 1. Symptoms of benzodiazepine withdrawal

Features include:
Sleep disturbance
Hand tremor
Profuse sweating
Poor concentration
Dry retching
Nausea
Weight loss
Palpitations
Muscular pains
Epileptic fits
Psychosis

Mood changes include:
Irritability
Tension and anxiety
Panic attacks
Malaise
Depression

Perceptual changes include:
Depersonalisation
Intolerance to noise, light and touch
Numbness
Paraesthesia
Unsteadiness and a feeling of motion
Strange smells
Metallic taste

The withdrawal syndrome lasts for several days.

Many people become dependent on benzodiazepines as a way of coping with the stresses of life. These sedatives should never be prescribed continuously for anxiety for more than eight weeks and a course of treatment for anxiety lasting only 10–14 days is preferred.

Treatment of dependency involves withdrawal of diazepam, reducing the dose by about 10 per cent per day. Other ways of dealing with the patient's stress or anxiety need to be found and the patient treated accordingly (see chapter 27).

Hallucinogens

A wide variety of classes of drugs can produce hallucinations. Lysergic acid diethylamide (LSD) disturbs dopamine pathways; the plant 'Angel's Trumpet' (Datura) and certain fungi ('magic mushrooms') contain psylocin and psylocybin which have atropine-like effects. Benzene and other volatile solvents have direct intoxicant effects. Cannabis (delta-9-tetra-hydro-cannabinol, or 'THC') has a variety of effects. All can cause disturbance in perception.

The most common clinical condition is one of organic psychosis. The clinical picture is of gross perceptual distortion including visual, auditory and tactile hallucinations and paranoid or grandiose delusional misinter-pretations. Mood is disturbed with agitation, anxiety and/or elation or depression. The person may or may not be delirious.

Some of these drugs, such as LSD and the atropine-like drugs, produce a psychosis frequently and some such as cannabis do so very rarely. However, all can cause hallu-cinations and delusions, depending on the dose of the drug taken, the vulnerability of the individual and the setting in which the drug is taken.

Any drug related delirium or psychosis is a medical emergency which may require good nursing management and quiet reassuring atmosphere and possibly, antipsychotic medication.

The major danger of these drugs is the quite bizarre behaviour when people have been intoxicated. This has sometimes led to violence, including homicide and suicide. These substances are therefore, generally speaking, dangerous.

In the case of volatile solvents, the main danger is that they can produce sudden cardiac arrhythmias and death.

Should drugs be decriminalised?

It has been argued that most of the problems related to drug abuse are due to the fact that drugs are illegal. If drugs were legalised then the large profits from the criminal supply and distribution networks would disappear. Drugs could then be supplied at low cost, of known potency and sterile for intravenous use. Against this view is the considerable data suggesting that increased availability of any drugs results, inevitably, in an increased incidence and prevalence of problems related to that drug. For example, in Western Australia, the introduction of Sunday trading in alcohol was associated with a 38 per cent increase in fatalities and admissions to hospitals due to motor vehicle accidents.

However, answers depend greatly on the ways the problems are defined. While legalising drugs could remove all the criminal problems, policy makers are uncertain about how many people would experiment with drugs, if the legal sanctions were removed. They are concerned that we might become a population which uses heroin, cocaine and marijuana in situations of minimal stress. Some argue that this would be particularly likely amongst the deprived, poor unemployed who are in any case, marginalised people in our society. Nevertheless, the concern about the spread of AIDS is such that the option of legal distribution of drugs does need serious consideration.

Should health and welfare workers take a more active public health approach?

Health workers have been amongst the most active in the changes which have occurred in tobacco use. Some people are taking an active role in the reduction of alcohol related problems. In a Western Australian community a disco, which had some 3000 patrons every week, had its liquor license due for review. Because of alcohol related problems such as noise, public nuisance, trespass, property damage, offensive drunken behaviour and illegal parking on private property, citizen action forced restrictions to this license.

More directly, health and welfare professionals need to be more aware and attentive to drug use and its consequences so that early intervention is possible. Early in the progression of drug use, it is relatively easy for the habits of individuals to be modified. Assessment and advice is effective if it is supported by simple, relevant educational literature.

Summary

Various forms of drug use are very common in Australia, but with the exception of tobacco, addiction affects only a small group. Dependence, tolerance, neuro-adaptation and withdrawal are all powerful reinforcers for continued drug use. Dependent drug use has many adverse consequences which usually lead to progressive social, physical, psychological, financial and personal decline. Drug dependent people often seem to have little in life to live for and a great deal of persuasion is necessary to enable them to achieve a drug free lifestyle.

Management needs to be directed at good assessment and treatment of ill health, harm reduction strategies, the foundation of a supportive treatment relationship and the continual encouragement to patients to move towards achieving an exit from a drug using lifestyle.

Further Reading

Brown V A, Manderson D, O'Callaghan M and Thompson R, *Our Daily Fix: Drugs in Australia*, Australian National University Press, 1986.
Commonwealth Department of Community Services and Health, *Statistics on Drug Abuse in Australia, 1987*, AGPS, 1987.
Gossop M, 'Addiction and After', *British Journal of Psychiatry*, Vol 152, 1988, pp 307-9.
Petursson H and Lader M H, 'Benzodiazepine Dependence', *British Journal of Addiction*, Vol 76, 1981, pp 138-45.
Pols R G and Henry-Edwards S, *The Role of General Health Workers in Detection and Early Intervention for Alcohol and Other Drug Problems*, National Health & Medical Research Centre, 1988.
Royal College of Psychiatrists, *Drug Scenes*, Alden Press, Oxford, 1987.
World Health Organisation, 'Nomenclature and Classification of Drug and Alcohol Related Problems: A WHO Memorandum', *Bulletin of the World Health Organisation*, Vol 59 No 2, 1981, pp 225-42.

Part 6
Community

Chapter 44

Community Psychiatry

G Smith and M Harries

The term 'community psychiatry' has been used by some writers descriptively and others prescriptively, that is, as describing services provided in certain ways and in certain places, or as an ideal in the light of which services are to be judged and developed. While some see it as a specialist field in its own right, with its own theoretical and practice base, others see it simply as the good practice of psychiatry carried out where the majority of mentally ill people spend the major part of their lives—in the community.

It was in its recognition of the dynamic nature of the relationship between the individual and his social environment, that community psychiatry began to diverge from institutional psychiatry, which had characterised practice during the preceding 150 years. It developed as a philosophy and practice model, in part, as a reaction to institutionally based care and in part, as a response to changing values and attitudes within the mental health professions and the broader community, during a period in which strong emphasis was being placed on individual rights and on the modification of the environment as the primary avenue of social changes.

It is the theoretical orientation, rather than any specific treatment technique or activity, which differentiates community psychiatry from other models of mental health care. Community psychiatry is informed by a 'systems' approach which recognises the dynamic nature of the relationship which exists between an individual displaying mental disturbance and the individual's family and broader social environment. This is shown on Figure 1. It is recognised that factors in the family (for example, bereavement) or in the broader social environment (for example, natural disasters) can lead to mental disturbance in individuals. As a corollary, factors in the individual's biological or psychological state lead to mental disturbance and this will produce reactions in the family and in the broader social environment. It is the recognition of this interaction which defines the focus for, and characteristics of, community psychiatry.

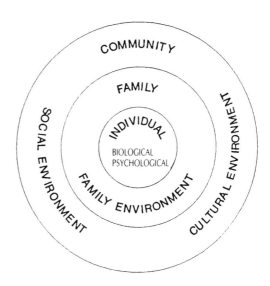

Figure 1. *Bio-psycho-social system.*

Two other key elements of community psychiatry are a focus on a defined or target population and a responsibility for providing a comprehensive and integrated network of services for that population. In practice, the population is usually geographically defined by certain administrative or natural boundaries. The ideal 'community' within an urban setting ranges from 150,000 to 250,000. This lends itself to the provision of a relatively comprehensive network of services, while maintaining responsiveness to local needs. The service characteristics and the objective focus of community psychiatry are summarised in Figure 2.

To achieve these aims, community psychiatry must work closely with families' social networks in the creation of a favourable therapeutic environment and liaise with other service providers, all of whom are seen as an important part of the network of services for the mentally ill.

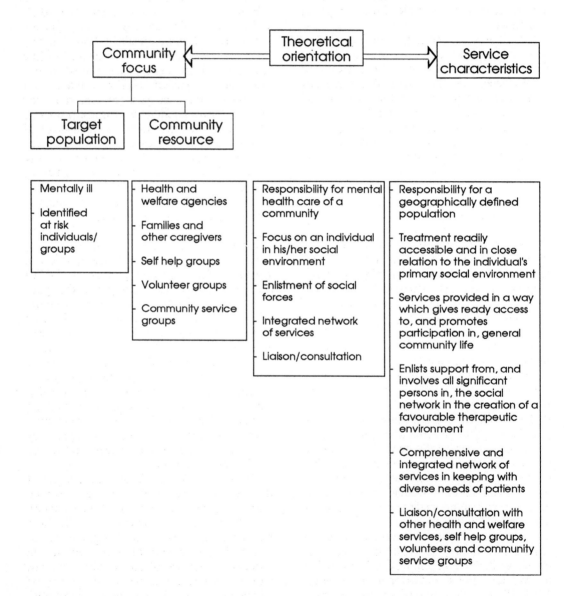

Figure 2. *Service characteristics and focus of community psychiatry.*

De-institutionalisation

In the United Kingdom, between 1954 and 1976, the mental hospital census declined from a peak of 148,000 to 83,000, a reduction of 45 per cent. In the United States, during the same period, mental hospital patient numbers fell from 558,000 to 193,000 representing a decrease of 65 per cent. Patterns in Australia and New Zealand followed a similar trend to those of the United Kingdom and America.

Over the same period, admissions more than doubled and it is clear that the decline in hospital population reflected a policy of greatly accelerated discharge. This process of decline in hospital population came to be known as 'de-institutionalisation'.

The philosophy which underlay this process has frequently been misunderstood. It was not simply the movement of patients out of psychiatric hospitals, but the shift in the focus of services from the institution to the community.

Community psychiatry

The second World War played a major role in reshaping public attitudes and policy, not least, in the care of socially, physically and mentally dependent persons. In 1946, the Curtis Committee in the United Kingdom recommended changes in the care of disadvantaged children and as a result, the Children's Act 1948 established the principle that preference be given to the care of children in private homes or small groups.

In psychiatry, the experience of psychiatrists with crisis intervention under combat conditions had a major influence on practice. It suggested that if persons received vigorous and early treatment close to home and could stay in the community, a more successful outcome could be achieved. This led to a recognition of the importance of environmental and social factors in the genesis and management of illness.

The 'community care' movement, of which psychiatry was but part had its modern origins in the United Kingdom Royal Commission on Mental Illness and Mental Deficiency, 1954–1957, which recommended a shift in emphasis from hospital to community care with the focus on support care in the family. It was the first time that the term 'community care' was used.

In 1961, Enoch Powell, Minister for Health in the United Kingdom, confidently predicted the demise of psychiatric hospitals and this was followed by the Hospital Plan (1962) and a policy document entitled 'Health and Welfare: The Development of Community Care' (1963). This latter document marked a radical departure in policy and affected all health and welfare services. On the opposite side of the Atlantic, President John Kennedy launched a similar policy direction for the mentally ill in 1963. The United States Community Mental Health Centres Act followed later that year and marked the Federal Government's entry into the provision of financial support for the development of Community Mental Health Centres. It was envisaged that these clinics would eventually replace the psychiatric hospitals by offering a full range of services to people from geographically defined populations ranging from 75,000 to 200,000 people.

In Australia, the Federal Government enacted the States Grants (Mental Institutions) Act 1955 in an effort to upgrade psychiatric hospitals. This followed a report by Stoller and Prescott, which highlighted the poor standards of facilities. With the introduction of the radical Mental Health and Related Services Act 1973, funding for capital works for hospitals was withdrawn, to be replaced by increased funding for community services. The rate of development of community psychiatric services increased dramatically. There was no single event which marked the transition from instititutional to community psychiatry. However, once embraced by government, the whole movement gained significant momentum.

There is no doubt that the introduction of the phenothiazines in 1955 was an essential part of the process of de-institutionalisation and the move to community care, but was not sufficient in itself. The changes in mental health policy should be seen within the broader framework of social policy changes which were taking place in the areas of education, criminal justice, social organisation and medicine, over this same period.

The objectives of community psychiatry

It was through the works of people like the sociologist, Irving Goffman and the psychiatrist, Russell Barton, that psychiatry began to recognise the effects of institutional care on the patients of psychiatric hospitals. This led many to believe that the picture of the deteriorated chronically mentally ill person, was the result mainly of institutional care and not of the underlying illness.

Other psychiatrists like R D Laing emphasised that mental disturbances were subject to external socio-cultural forces inherent in the community. This led to the belief amongst some community health workers that many forms of psychiatric disorder were preventable by community action or social change. However, the community psychiatry movement embraced a simpler set of objectives:

-the provision of alternative services and treatment in the community;
-the reduction of hospital admissions by community intervention;
-the maintenance of the mentally ill in the community by continuity of care.

Despite predictions that psychiatric hospitals would vanish, to be replaced by general hospital units and community based services, few have actually been closed. There are clearly many reasons for this, including the over optimistic expectations of the benefits of psychotropic medication and the failure to recognise the range and value of functions provided by psychiatric hospitals in the care of the mentally ill.

There are few mental health professionals today who would have any difficulty in accepting the broad objectives which have, to a large extent, been embraced within contemporary psychiatric practice. There are at least three fundamental assumptions underlying these objectives:

1. Community based care is more therapeutic and preferable to institutional care.
2. The community will be able and willing to provide that care.
3. Community based facilities and services can replace those previously provided by the psychiatric hospital.

The problem has been whether these assumptions are correct, particularly, for the chronically, severely mentally ill who have been managed in the psychiatric hospitals.

Evaluation of the community psychiatric movement

The level of success of the community psychiatry movement cannot be measured only by the decline in the psychiatric hospital census. Although the falls in patient population have been dramatic, ranging from 50 to 90 per cent, large numbers of dependent, mentally ill patients have ended up in community 'institutions' of one sort or another.

Many chronically ill people were discharged to private nursing homes. These homes now accommodate more psychiatric patients than the psychiatric hospitals, their quality varies and some are no better than poor quality boarding houses.

A number of Australian States established a system of licensed private hostels which attracted a State subsidy for residents. In South Australia and Western Australia, these hostels had well in excess of 600 beds, in each case. In Western Australia this was as many people as in the psychiatric hospitals.

In many Australian States, the care of the intellectually handicapped, the drug and alcohol dependent, mentally disordered offenders and psychiatrically disturbed elderly was separated from the care of the mentally ill and dealt with by newly established authorities, some of which were well funded for long term care of patients, but others were not.

Some authorities have referred to this process as the movement of patients to different care agencies, or as 'trans-institutionalisation'. Considering this, the question remains as to what extent the objectives of the community psychiatric movement have been able to be achieved.

The provision of alternative services

There has been a dramatic increase in the number and range of alternative services available for the treatment of psychiatric disorder over the past 30 years. The growth of psychiatric units attached to general hospitals had resulted, in some places, in over half of the in-patient care episodes taking place in these units. Private psychiatric hospitals have also provided a significant level of care.

Community psychiatric centres, hospital outpatient departments and private outpatient medical care account for the vast majority of psychiatric patient contacts. In many places, emergency teams provide crisis intervention in patients' homes and other community settings. Day centres, sheltered workshops and day hospitals are providing support and treatment for an increasing number of people.

Despite these developments in the pattern of patient care, there is evidence that the new forms of in-patient care have not yet substantially replaced psychiatric hospitals in caring for the severely mentally ill. Similarly, although outpatient contacts have increased dramatically, the evidence suggests that a whole new class of previously untreated patients are now using services that were unavailable to them 10–20 years ago.

Reduction of hospital admissions

The process of reduction of psychiatric hospital populations has had a differential impact upon the acute and long term care services. Although the length of stay has reduced, the admission rate has risen sharply.

Re-admissions have been particularly affected and represent over two thirds of all admissions to psychiatric hospitals. Almost one third of these are re-admissions in a single year. This pattern of brief, repeated admissions has been referred to as 'the revolving door' process.

The reduction in activity within hospitals has been in the least labour intensive, lowest cost services, namely, in the area of care for the chronically mentally ill. This, together with the demand for increased admission and higher standards of clinical care, has meant that hospital costs have not fallen as originally anticipated.

Maintenance of the mentally ill in the community

Despite some of the limitations in outcome outlined above, it would be wrong to suggest that the community psychiatry movement had not been of benefit in the care of people with mental illness. The vast majority can now be expected to be treated in public or private community services and can confidently be expected to be able to continue to lead satisfying and meaningful lives.

However, there is a group of people with severe, recurrent or chronic mental illness, who, although they may only spend relatively brief periods in hospital, are likely to have multiple admissions, in some cases many times each year. A not uncommon pattern has emerged, with many of these people remaining single and continuing to live at home with ageing parents, well into their adult lives. Poverty, unemployment, loneliness, hotel and boarding houses, continued dependency and repeated hospitalisation impair their capacity to enjoy their lives. Despite their illness 'experience', their needs are no different from their healthy peers, namely, meaningful affectional and social relationships, purposeful and fulfilling activity, economic and material security, creative use of free times, independence and a sense of self-worth.

It should be recognised that although the psychotropic medications have significantly altered the course of individual illness episodes, they have not changed the long term outcome of some of the most disabling illnesses. Almost two thirds of people with schizophrenia will experience some degree of personal and social deterioration. The time of onset of these illnesses in late adolescence or early adulthood and their extraordinary nature may significantly interfere with the fabric of adult life.

There is compelling evidence that so far, the community psychiatric movement has been geared toward the care of 'the single episode user' to the detriment of those with lifelong disorders—the very group it was designed to free from the isolating conditions of the 'asylums'. The emphasis in the developments of services has been on 'acute care' to the detriment of persons with chronic or recurrent illness who require services designed to address their disability.

Organisational models

During the past 30 years there have been a number of significant findings which are starting to influence community mental health planning. Amongst these are the following:
1. Some mental illnesses cause progressive personal and social deterioration in a significant number of sufferers. This deterioration is not simply a result of institutional care, but due to the biological process of the illnesses.
2. Long periods of hospitalisation do not necessarily confer any benefit in outcome in the long term.
3. People with these mental illness can be successfully treated in the community in most cases, although the benefits rapidly disappear if support is discontinued.
4. People with mental illness prefer to be treated in their own homes or in general hospital settings and, in most cases, this is more acceptable to their family.
5. People with schizophrenia who live in homes with high levels of tension are likely to have more frequent relapses and require more frequent hospital admission.
6. 'Good' community care is generally more expensive than mental hospital institution care.
7. Psychiatric hospitals provide a more complex array of supports for patients than was previously realised and care must be taken to *ensure* that patients find these supports through the community health and welfare services (for example, housing).

In our culture, 'community care' represents care 'in' the community rather than 'by' the community. It is recognised that care is generally divided between the State and family. However, in many cases, it is provided by the family who bear the largest burden and, are the main providers of personal and material support in the long term.

A survey conducted by the Association of Relatives and Friends of the Mentally Ill (1982) in South Australia, indicated that, in families which were caring for mentally ill members, most reported severe hardship,

financial loss, social isolation and community rejection. They identified four major requirements which they expected from psychiatric services:
1. appropriate accommodation alternatives;
2. respite care provision;
3. 24 hour crisis intervention service;
4. information from professionals.

Similar requirements have been identified by non government health and welfare agencies, which have increasingly found themselves confronted with a growing population of mentally ill people seeking companionship and shelter.

The components of a community psychiatry service, which many studies have indicated are required to care for the mentally ill in the community, are as follows:

1. Assessment and treatment services

These should provide ready access for assessment and treatment and encourage people to seek assistance before their illness has progressed to the stage where admission to hospital becomes necessary. Liaison/consultation with other relevant health and welfare professionals should be an important part of this service.

2. Crisis intervention service

A 24 hour crisis intervention service should be available to assess and treat patients in their home. Families with mentally ill members and voluntary agencies who have contact with the mentally ill, have reported immense benefit from such a service.

3. Emergency accommodation

Supervised accommodation should be available as an alternative to hospital admission. Hospital admission is frequently used to provide respite for the family, or where supervision arrangements are inadequate and this is not always necessary or desirable.

4. Support for relatives

Families have identified information as essential in assisting them to care for their mentally ill member. Since families provide the majority of aid and care for their mentally ill members, support for relatives is an essential component of community services.

5. Peer support

Sponsoring and supporting self help groups is an important role for community psychiatry. Social isolation and loss of self-esteem are common accompaniments of mental illness. Peer support groups not only assist in alleviating that isolation, but encourage patients to accept and take greater responsibility for their illness.

For the *chronically mentally ill*, certain other aspects of management are necessary. These are:

1. Case management

Patients with chronic mental illness often experience difficulty in obtaining assistance because of the social and personal deterioration associated with their illness. The use of staff members as 'case managers' to help negotiate and coordinate services between patients and agencies has proved successful in helping maintain patients in the community.

2. Accommodation

For many people with long term illness, stable, affordable accommodation is perhaps the single most important factor in the success of community care. There is a need for a network of accommodation ranging from respite accommodation to independent living units. The degree of support or supervision required for residents will determine the type of accommodation most suited to their needs.

3. Social activity programs

Drop-in-centres and social clubs can be an important adjunct to other more structured programs. This type of program has been found most suited for people who have difficulty in structured programs. Benefits include companionship, friendship, constructive use of time, increased confidence and self-esteem.

4. Living skills programs

Emphasis is on the acquisition of personal and social skills. These programs are designed to increase the patient's ability to live independently and relate to others.

5. Work related programs

Up to 87 per cent of all chronically mentally ill people are unemployed and in receipt of social security benefits. Frequent relapses in their illness and the associated social and personal handicaps interfere with their ability to hold down regular work. Programs range from teaching patients to use their time creatively to preparation for sheltered or open employment.

There are different organisational models for the delivery of these services. In practice, there are basically three systems:

1. Psychiatric or general hospitals which have progressively allocated an increasing proportion of their resources to the provision of community 'outreach' services.

2. Separate community psychiatric services which provide outpatient and community services to defined populations.

3. A system which attempts to integrate hospital and community by having administrative responsibility in a district authority which controls both hospital and community services.

All these models can lead to a community psychiatry orientation, which, it must again be stressed, is an approach to the care of the mentally ill, rather than a particular service model. Equally, each of these models can become isolated, cut off from other carers, and fail to take a community psychiatry approach.

Future challenge

The community psychiatric movement has resulted in a significant shift in the practice of psychiatry, from a focus upon people in hospitals to one of people within their social environment.

While this has proved beneficial for the majority of people with mental illness, there has been a growing awareness over the past 15–20 years amongst mental health professionals, that this shift in focus has left some of the patients behind. There is still a significant number of people with chronic mental illness for which the psychiatric hospital remains an important, if not the only, element in the service network.

One eminent British academic has said: 'The acid test of a community service lies in whether it can meet the needs of the seriously handicapped persons who used to, in the old days, become long-stay mental hospital inmates.' There would be consensus amongst many mental health professionals that the community psychiatric movement has not met this test.

The major challenge for the future is to attempt to redress this problem. It is significant, in this respect, that a number of Australian States have given policy and planning priority to services for the seriously mentally ill. There have been a number of promising studies in Australia and overseas which have clearly identified that the severely mentally ill can successfully be treated in the community providing that there is hospital backup and that support is integrated and on-going.

Further Reading

Backrach L, 'A Conceptual Approach to De-institutionalisation', *Hospital and Community Psychiatry*, Vol 29 No 9, 1978, pp 573–8.

Goldman H, 'De-institutionalisation: The Data Demythologised', *Hospital and Community Psychiatry*, Vol 34 No 2, 1983, pp 129–34.

Hoult J, Renolds I, Charbonneau-Powis M, Weeks P and Briggs J, 'Psychiatric Hospital Versus Community Treatment: The Results of a Randomised Trial', *Australian and New Zealand Journal of Psychiatry*, Vol 17, 1983, pp 160–7.

Jones D, 'Commentary: De-institutionalisation of Mental Health Services in South Australia—Out of the Frying Pan, into the Fire', *Community Health Studies*, Vol 1 No IX, 1985, pp 62–8.

Jones, K, 'Skull's Dilemma', *British Journal of Psychiatry*, Vol 141, 1982, pp 221–6.

Kosky R J, 'From Morality to Madness: A Reappraisal of the Asylum Movement in Psychiatry 1800–1940', *Australian & New Zealand Journal of Psychiatry*, Vol 20, 1986, pp 180–7.

Wing J and Olsen R, 'Community Care for the Mentally Disabled', Oxford University Press, Oxford, 1979.

Chapter 45

Aboriginal Mental Health

E M Hunter

To be concerned about Aborigines and mental health in the last decades of the twentieth century demands more than a preoccupation with the exotic, or with phenomenological comparisons. For many Aborigines, surrounded by an unremitting topography of poverty, illness, alcoholism, violence, incarceration, unemployment, inadequate housing and transgenerational welfare dependence, diagnostic categories are easy to find. Yet these provide little insight into why there have been dramatic increases in self-harmful behaviours in the last decades. These have included alcoholism, other substance abuse (kava, petrol inhalation and other street drugs), self-mutilation and suicidal behaviour, deaths due to violence and accidents, and suicide. These are clearly the most pressing 'mental health' issues for Aborigines; they demand a historically attentive social analysis. Psychiatry cannot, however, lay claim to have been in the forefront of initiatives to examine the psychological or social experience of Aboriginal Australians. It has consistently reflected the shifting visions and constructions of Aborigines prevalent in the dominant non-Aboriginal society.

Psychiatry and Aborigines

Prior to European settlement, complexity and diversity characterised Aboriginal Australia. While adaptation to colonisation varied considerably with the particular experiences of different Aboriginal groups, the consequences in terms of power over land and lives were uniform. Regardless, the experiences of Aborigines in the isolated Kimberley, with barely a century of permanent European presence, are considerably different to those of the Illawarra Aborigines south of Sydney. For the white settler the land had been 'tamed' in Eastern Australia but was still undergoing settlement and 'pacification' in the remote North-West. There is thus enormous variability between Aboriginal groups, in terms of both pre-colonial culture and their particular histories and legacies of accommodation and resistance to non-Aboriginal control. Adding an additional dimension of complexity, the last three decades have been the period of greatest socioeconomic change affecting Aborigines across the continent.

In the early decades of this century, the construction of history for the nascent nation valorised Europeans and marginalised Aborigines. Prevailing attitudes and legislation reflected tenacious stereotypes based openly on principles of social Darwinism. It was widely accepted that Aborigines were dying out and that little could, or should be done about their inevitable fate. Certain attributes were considered universal. Aborigines were childlike or, particularly if half-caste, potentially treacherous. Legislation throughout the country was openly preoccupied with recurring issues—alcohol and miscegenation (Daisy Bates' 'dreaded half caste menace') resulting in prohibition and the removal of partial descent children to institutional life. Citizenship was obtainable for a small number of Aborigines, but it was provisional, and depended on rejection of Aboriginal identity and social network. Another issue in isolated Australia was central but covert: viz cheap labour. Regardless of the various motivations across the country, the key legislative issue was control over the Aborigine, effected through isolation and 'protection'.

It was in this context that the psychoanalyst Geza Roheim conducted field work in Central Australia during 1929. Aborigines constituted a 'psycho-anthropological laboratory' in which the 'primitive' in modern man could be observed and studied. This particular orientation has continued, frequently without direct experience. Another psychoanalyst, Bruno Bettelheim, based his 1950 analysis of 'Australian rites' on the field work of Spencer and Gillen in Central Australia in the 1890s.

The policies and practices of isolation and 'protection' continued until after the second world war when the principle of assimilation of Aborigines into the prevalent white culture was advocated and guided by such figures as Sir Paul Hasluck and Professor R P Elkin. This period coincided with the growth of an Australian psychiatric profession. Through the 1960s a number of studies were published based on brief visits to discrete Aboriginal communities, in which Aborigines were observed and categorised according to the prevailing diagnostic schemas inherited from British psychiatry. This was primarily an imposed analysis concerned neither with the real internal world nor the social realities of Aborigines. It was psychopathology of the exotic laboratory.

Through the 1960s the impossibility and unacceptability of assimilation for Aborigines became evident. The economic plight of Aboriginal workers in the North was becoming a political issue and attitudes in the Australian general public were beginning to change, culminating in the 1967 referendum in which the Australian people voted to take the care of Aboriginal people out of the hands of the States and place it with the Federal Government. The ensuing era claimed to be guided by the ideals of self-determination and multi-culturalism. During this period of transition the predominant psychiatric frame was the ethno-medical/cross-cultural psychiatric orientation of John Cawte, the 'Aboriginal mental health laboratory'. This approach utilised short stay field studies and Cawte introduced for the first time a longitudinal perspective, remaining involved with particular Aboriginal groups over decades. The works of Morice, Eastwell, and Nurcombe are also characteristic of this type of psychiatric investigation. Research with Aborigines had until this period primarily concerned itself with full-descent and isolated Aborigines. This reflected an enduring preference within the wider majority culture for a conception of Aborigines that authenticated the 'traditional'. The increasing political momentum of urban Aborigines, brought effectively into the living rooms of White Australia by the 1972 'tent embassy' in Canberra, confronted entrenched stereotypes and demanded bicultural examination of post-colonial history.

A concern for the social determinants of distress was included in the work of Cawte and Nurcombe, but foregrounded in Max Kamien's studies of the town of Bourke, which placed a primary focus on non-traditional Aborigines. The intercultural realities of Aborigines confronting a non-Aboriginal dominant society became central at this level of analysis. Settings such as Bourke provided a 'social laboratory' to explore the consequences of socio-economic disparity and prejudice. It was the first step towards developing a dialogue with Aborigines and involving them in the research studies. This period saw the formation of the Aboriginal Mental Health Association in 1978.

The 1980s have been a period of Aboriginal political engagement and media presence. There has been an unprecedented interest in Aboriginal artistic creativity and its products and there have been serious attempts to address the subjectivity of Aborigines. From outside the psychiatry field there have been attempts to investigate child development, the way in which Aborigines construct their sense of self, and their social reality. There has also been a move to 'rehistoricise' Aborigines, examining their situations and experiences with greater attentiveness to questions of subjectivity. Constructions of Aboriginality in literature by Europeans and by Aborigines have been explored and a variety of Aboriginal voices have emerged through oral histories, Aboriginal literature and auto-biographies. Mental health research is only slowly following these leads, to examine Aboriginal idioms of distress in the context of their particular intercultural and intracultural experiences.

Psychiatry has, to a certain extent, been committed by political forces, particularly the Royal Commission into Aboriginal Deaths in Custody. Commissioner J H Wootten in his report into the death of Malcolm Charles Smith emphasised the critical need for a socio-historical frame, in understanding the nature of suffering for an aboriginal.

> His [Michael Charles Smith's] death is part of the abiding legacy of the appalling treatment of Aboriginals that went on well into the second half of this century in the name of protection or welfare. It is history, but history of critical importance today. It is history that few Australians know, and which our historians are only now piecing together. Without a knowledge of it we cannot hope to understand Aboriginal/White relations today, for they are deeply moulded by that history. We will not understand the ill-suppressed hatred which many Aboriginals feel towards police, and their deep distrust of officialdom generally. We will fail to appreciate how many Aboriginal men and women there are now in the community carrying deep scars from that history, scars that prejudice not only their own lives but those of their children. We will run the risk that, as happens so often, we will repeat the mistakes of the past (Wootten 1989).

Problems

Certain consequences of the upsurge of interest in Aboriginal issues need to be analysed, particularly given the popular concerns about Aboriginal people in the events surrounding the Australian Bicentennial.

In the public perception two contrasting images of Aborigines appear to have been dominant. The first is urban, educated, articulate and relatively politically empowered. This woman or man meets needs for certain sections of both Aboriginal and non-Aboriginal society. For White Australians this image of Aborigines supports a national ideology of political tolerance and humanitarian support for the underprivileged. The

second image is of a timeless traditional Aborigine, untroubled by the turmoil of change and frenzy of modernity. This stereotype appeals to paternalistic sentiments. It idealises the 'bush blackfellow' and suggests differences from this as deviance and indicative of a loss of 'Aboriginality'. The power of this view is evident in the primacy of tradition in authenticating claims under land rights legislation.

Beyond these simple typologies is another Aboriginal Australian that is neither empowered nor romantic. These are Aborigines on the fringes of the majority culture. In the 1986 census Aborigines constituted 2.45 per cent of the national population. Two-thirds lived in towns or cities.

A comprehensive analysis of the social determinants of health, and the implications for mental health of Aborigines is beyond the scope of this paper. Before touching on certain issues at this critical level of involvement for mental health professionals, I shall present several perhaps self-evident caveats.

1. There is no reason to expect that Aborigines should not be subject to a similar range of psychiatric conditions as non-Aborigines, and thus have *at least* the same needs.

2. While Aborigines generally have not had the same access to mental health services as white Australians, those sections of Aboriginal Australian in greatest need are clearly inadequately served.

3. Inter-cultural contacts for Aboriginals are often with bureaucratic agencies which tend to maintain problems rather than bring them to resolution.

4. The cultural and historical experiences of particular Aboriginal groups inform their expression of distress in a contemporary setting.

5. Institutional reactions to Aboriginal behaviour considered to be deviant or abnormal frequently minimises socio-cultural analysis in favour of certain labels—for example, alcoholism or chronic schizophrenia.

6. Such reductive diagnostic practices reduce subsequent vigilance for other conditions—such as organic disorders, depression, suicide potential and reactions to stress.

Contemporary issues

The challenge for mental health professions, indeed for an Australia that includes Aborigines, is a cooperative (ie bilateral) questioning of the asymmetries in our society and their implications for health and well-being. A telling irony lies in the fact that the major issues suggesting psychological distress of Aborigines have entered the public and professional consciousness only in the last decade, at a time when Aborigines have theoretically gained access to all the benefits of the wider society.

Contemporary issues of concern include high rates of failure to thrive, poor educational achievement, alcoholism, petrol sniffing, violence, delinquency, high rates of incarceration and recidivism, deaths in custody, and suicide. In order to examine the inter-relationship of some of these issues I shall draw from personal experience of one discrete region of Australia, the Kimberley region of North West, Western Australia, home to some 12,000 Aborigines.

The most dramatic of these contemporary issues of Aboriginal mental health has been the recent increase in suicide, brought to national attention in the late 1980s by death while in police custody and prison. Suicide among tradition-oriented populations was (and remains) rare. In mid–1989 this writer reported 24 suicides of Aborigines in or from the North-West (mean age 23 years), of which two were in custody. Twenty had occurred between 1980 and 1984, and 13 since 1985. All except two were young males; all except two (possibly one) were partial descent, and the majority occurred in an area of the Kimberley experiencing the most rapid social and economic changes. Clinical features commonly associated with these deaths were recent personal histories of disturbances in conscious state usually due to alcohol and a recent loss of someone close or a disruption in social life. Most had given warnings or had histories of previous attempts.

This emergent suicidal, phenomenon must be placed in a broader context. There has been an increase in the rate of suicide among younger age-groups in a number of European societies, including Australia, though not as dramatic as the emergent patterns of suicide among Aborigines, where suicide is almost exclusively confined to young adult males. More marked increases are reported from a number of indigenous cultures in areas of European cultural dominance, including from the Pacific Basin, Micronesians, Samoans, American Indians and Eskimos. In all of these settings it is the same group primarily involved: young adult males. Alcohol use is a consistent association.

This broader picture must also include the changes in mortality affecting Aborigines from other non-natural causes. This writer reviewed all death certificates over a 30 year period for the Kimberley, 15 years before and after full citizenship rights (and therefore alcohol use privileges) were extended to the region in 1970. For the first 15 years the proportion of deaths over one year of age from external causes (motor vehicle accidents, other accidents, homicide and suicide) was relatively constant at between 2.3 per cent and 5.3 per cent of female deaths and 4.2 per cent and 6.8 per cent of male deaths. After 1970, a linear increase in deaths from external causes occurred such that for the five year period 1982–1986 deaths in these categories increased to 15.2 per cent of female and 22.6 per cent of male deaths.

Males predominated in all categories except homicide, where females were the most common victims. Within the broader context of increasing proportions of deaths due to non-natural causes, the increase in deaths from suicide was a late event, a phenomenon of the 1980s. The five year period 1982–1986 saw an increase in male suicide at the same time that there was a plateau in male deaths from homicide and a sharp increase in female deaths from homicide. Reviewing all coroners' reports of those dying between the ages of 15 and 30 since 1980, the frequent involvement of alcohol was confirmed. Drinking males were most vulnerable to the consequences of their own reckless behaviour (motor vehicle accidents and other accidents), whereas the interpersonal environment (homicide) became particularly dangerous for females.

Much of the research on Aborigines and alcohol is now over a decade old. In a setting of such rapid change this is clearly inadequate. Old information can be misinformation. For instance, middle aged Aborigines of isolated Australia are the first generation to be legally able to purchase alcohol when they were old enough to drink. Older Aborigines were well into adult life when they were able to legally obtain alcohol. Young adult Aborigines are the first generation to have grown up with widespread parental drinking. There are no clear precedents. In a sample of Kimberley Aborigines, alcohol use was most common among 20-30 years olds (86 per cent of men and 57 per cent of women) and decreased as people became older. This was more true for women and only 17 per cent of women over 70 used alcohol. However, the issues are complicated by the pecularities of the availability of alcohol to different generations.

The effects of alcohol use in the tight social environment of camp life are, of course, extensive. In particular, it has been hard to assess the parent–child effects. In this writer's sample, 60 per cent of one or both parents aged less than 30 years were heavy alcohol users.

The patterns of alcohol use are changing in Aboriginal north-west Australia, as are the direct and indirect consequences. As mentioned earlier a number of the Kimberley suicides were reported to have experienced disorders of ideation and perception associated with alcohol. Anecdotal reports from the Kimberley indicate that alcohol hallucinosis appears to be becoming increasingly common. This is supported by data from the Northern Territory. For 1977 and 1982 the hospital admissions for most alcohol related conditions among Aborigines and non-Aborigines were roughly similar. However, for the single diagnosis of 'alcohol hallucinosis', there was a 50 per cent increase for Aboriginal males. While this may reflect a change in diagnostic practices, a real increase is suggested as the increase did not involve females or non-Aborigines. Those Aborigines given that diagnosis were also younger, the peak being in the age range 25-44, whereas for non-Aborigines this diagnosis peaked in the 45-64 age group.

The problems of suicidal behaviour and self-destruction are very great indeed. An adequate analysis must take into account not only personal problems, but also intracultural forces such as the changing inter-sex dynamics of power within Aboriginal society. Aborigines of isolated Australia in the last decade have been confronted by disruptive tradition-alien ideals promoted during the optimism of the 1970s. They too frequently lack the means (linguistic, economic, educational, etc) for negotiating and manoeuvring within the power structures of the majority culture. While clearly there are many who do not want to participate in the dominant society, the question should be rather whether in reality they have a choice. The dynamics have changed from the era of isolation and protection, but in the world of welfare dependence, Aborigines remain controlled and seemingly trapped. In a system that discourages substantial upward mobility, stifles dissonance yet prevents total collapse, Aborigines of remote Australia are suspended, immobile, powerless and contained.

It is the males who are particularly affected by the conflict of presented ideals and realisable options. For young men, often regardless of education, opportunity is extremely limited. It is thus not surprising that, as noted by Commissioner Wootten, while Aborigines comprise 1.8 per cent of the 10–17 year old population, they make up at least 25 per cent of those in prison. The high rates of pregnancy for young Aboriginal females (the fertility rate for Western Australian Aborigines aged 15–19 in 1987 was eight and a half times greater than for non-Aborigines) may be protective, both in terms of providing an avenue to economic power (maternal benefits) denied to males, and access to an ego-ideal valued by the majority culture (motherhood).

Traditionally power devolved into two broad domains—religious and economic. The power functions of the former have been radically reduced, and women have greater predictable access to the resources of a welfare economy. Indeed it has been suggested that Aboriginal women more closely approximate the 'ideal welfare recipient' than men. The tensions produced by the asymmetries accompanying this externally informed shift in power is possibly reflected in the previously mentioned homicide statistics, and also in domestic violence and sexual assault convictions, which increased ten fold for Aboriginal males in Western Australia between 1961 and 1981.

The current increase in self destructive behaviour is occurring among the generation who are the children of those who were young adults when citizenship rights were granted. These rights included industrial conditions the same as white workers, and the dependency of life in the rural missions was actively discouraged. Rural stations could no longer afford Aboriginal labour and the missions were also closed in many cases. In the Kimberley at this time, town camps grew rapidly as Aborigines were uprooted from traditional or long term homes on stations and other settlements due to the resultant economic and legislative forces that had little concern for the immediate realities of their lives. Aboriginal communities were reduced to fringe town living, often involving tense and violent proximity of groups, black and white, that would otherwise have remained far apart. Adults, were confronted by the reality of unemployment, and the unprecedented demands of budgeting (rent, electricity, rates) that were alien in the structures of dependent rural or mission life. Powerful new forces impinged on their lives—education, telephones, radio, television, videos and advertising.

In conjunction with these intrusions and upheavals came the right to drink. Aborigines were encouraged to do so not only by the ideals presented through the media and the example of heavy drinking Europeans in isolated Australia, but also by those with a profit motive for encouraging and supporting Aboriginal drinking.

Compounding the earlier mentioned impact of alcohol on parenting, heavy drinking Aborigines are at great risk (greater than non-heavy drinking Aborigines or non-Aboriginal heavy drinkers) of being arrested. This further undermines parental, particularly paternal roles. The Institute of Criminology estimated that in 1986 one in 20 Aboriginal males aged between 20 and 29 were in prison at any one time. The consequences of the rapid post-citizenship increase in the proportion of

drinkers continued to evolve in the following generation. For example, among the recently increasing number of self-mutilators in the Kimberley, a history of parental heavy drinking is common, and familial relationships seriously disturbed. It seems that the childhood environment of these individuals is a product of the above social destabilisation, being accompanied by an undermining of the traditional practices that structured the transitional periods of childhood and particularly adolescence. In addition there was a sudden withdrawal by the European agencies (mission, station and government) that had for generations imposed external controls on Aboriginal lives, including childhood.

The consequences of these social and psychological developmental issues interact with the subsequent social realities of Aboriginal powerlessness and cultural exclusion, to produce trans-generational self-reinforcing cycles impacting on the construction of the sense of identity and on self-esteem. For example, before 1960, many Aboriginal children were removed from their parents' care by Government Authorities and brought up by white foster parents or in missions and institutions. While overt European control of Aboriginal children was withdrawn from the 1960s, the proportion of young Aborigines in the Kimberley brought up by their biological parents has in fact continued to fall (just over a third of the random sample mentioned previously and aged between 20 and 30 years were raised by grandparents). While this may reflect traditional patterns of shared responsibility, it is coincident with the increase in reported of parental heavy drinking.

Thus, while social realities such as dislocation, unemployment, and welfare dependence may have structured patterns of behaviour at the time of citizenship rights nearly two decades ago (heavy drinking, increasing deaths from non-natural causes), the system in many deprived Aboriginal settings seems to have developed a self-sustaining autonomy. This cycle is reinforced by the psychological consequences of unrealised expectations and unfulfilled ideals. It is manifested by high levels of self-mutilation, suicidal behaviour, transfer of parenting responsibilities, alcoholism and violence. This is a topography of poverty and social powerlessness.

A role for mental health professionals

These issues are far from universal within Aboriginal Australia, and do not reflect the advances and achievements of Aborigines in many fields. However, it is this arena into which mental health professionals are most likely to be, indeed should be drawn. Without a theory which takes into account the reinforcing patterns of precursors and consequences, such workers are likely to be overwhelmed by the immediacy of needs. The medicalisation of social distress suggests short term medical remedies, be they clinics, psychiatrists, alcohol treatment facilities or suicide proof cells. While such measures may be helpful, they may obscure social reality and the longer term needs. If mental health professionals are to be meaningfully involved they must also work with Aborigines to confront the longer term social issues. Planning should take into account the socio-historical forces that have resulted in Aboriginal ill-health and distress. Goals can be defined socially (rates of failure to thrive, intact families, truancy, school retention, unemployment, incarceration, recidivism, alcoholism, etc) and not only in terms of resources (budgets, clinics opened, staffing numbers etc). Such planning clearly goes beyond the lifetime of a single government, and thus demands bipartisan political commitment.

Today, any discipline claiming credibility in its work with Aborigines must not only seriously consider Aboriginal views, but also stimulate and elicit Aboriginal involvement. Inter-cultural communication must thus occur not only on the level of client/patient, but between colleagues and workers. The following principles may serve as a useful guide to clinical practice in the field of Aboriginal mental health.

1. Those seeking to work among Aborigines should be conscious of inter-cultural variables, and be aware of the enormous differences between Aboriginal groups. A corollary is that stereotypes of Aborigines are invariably misleading.

2. They should develop a broad awareness of the historical, cultural and social issues affecting Aboriginal experience generally and the specifics of the regional and local groups. Much of this work will come from disciplines other than mental health.

3. Theoretical openness and integrative capacity is necessary. The corollary of this is therapeutic flexibility.

4. The work is not for those without patience, or for individuals whose work is strictly guided by schedule. For health workers it frequently entails sustained care rather than immediate cure.

5. Particularly in non-urban settings, Aborigines have been invariably exposed to a long series of transitory workers, such as health workers, teachers, advisers, anthropologists, medical researchers, sacred site recorders, welfare workers and so on. Frequently each new arrival brings values and ideals forged in a different reality. Indirectness and dishonesty are the handmaidens of paternalism and authoritarianism. Aborigines in such settings may not directly confront such attitudes, but with long experience they are keenly sensitive and will quite rightly withdraw cooperation.

6. Having accepted culture as a valid and important variable, and having developed skills relevant to one's work, mental health professionals must guard against attitudes which erode clinical vigilance by invariably considering the cultural implications. Some of these issues are discussed in Chapter 47.

Finally, health professionals should constantly be aware of the powerful position they occupy by virtue of their work. It will open doors in Aboriginal Australia that remain closed to many other Australians. However, that privileged access will only remain as long as the health professional is not entirely reliant on professional status, and gains acceptance as a caring individual.

Further Reading

Australian Institute of Criminology, 'Aboriginal Imprisonment', *Crime Digest*, 1, 1988.

Bell, D, *Of the Dreaming*, McPhee, Gribble/Gowin, Melbourne, 1983.

Broadhurst R G, 'Imprisonment of the Aborigine in Western Australia', in *Ivory Scales: Black Australia and the Law*, (ed Hazelhurst K M), New South Wales University Press, Sydney, 1987, pp 190-226.

Brody, E B, 'Cultural exclusion, character and illness', *American Journal of Psychiatry*, Vol 122 No 2, 1966, pp 852-8.

Cawte J, *Medicine is the Law*, University of Hawaii Press, Honolulu, 1974.

Hunter E M, 'Aboriginal Deaths in Custody: A view from the Kimberley, *Australian and New Zealand Journal of Psychiatry*, Vol 22, 1988, pp 273-82.

Mettingley C, *Survival in Our Own Land*, ALDAA and Hodder & Stoughton, Adelaide, 1988.

Wootten J H, *Royal Commission into Aboriginal Deaths in Custody: Report of the Inquiry into the Death of Malcolm Charles Smith*, Australian Government Publishing Service, Canberra, 1989.

Chapter 46

Remote Australia

H M Connell

Australia is slightly smaller than the United States of America (eight million square kilometres against nine million square kilometres). It is 30 times the size of the United Kingdom and 10 times the size of Japan. Currently its population is over 16 million giving an overall population density of two persons per square kilometre. In this respect it contrasts sharply with its Asian neighbours. For example the central area of Hong Kong supports nearly 200,000 persons per square kilometre.

Approximately two-thirds of the Australian population is concentrated on the coast, chiefly on the Eastern seaboard where rainfall is highest, leaving the vast interior (the Centre or outback) very sparsely populated indeed. Aside from towns associated with mining and one large centre expanded by tourism (Alice Springs) outback families live in small 'towns', often only a cluster of houses, or on large properties (called stations). The latter may be enormous; the largest owned by a single family is 7800 km^2. Those owned by companies may be much larger. In such cases the homestead is occupied by a manager and his family, sometimes by a group of families.

This chapter looks at the effects of geographical isolation on the lifestyle of families living in the outback. Queensland and Western Australia are used as examples since they offer their inhabitants the most geographically isolated conditions in the world. Together these States comprise 4,265,500 km^2 and have a population of about four million people. This area is slightly larger than the Indian sub-continent which has a population of over 900 million people.

Travel between properties is often rugged, roads (tracks) can be pot-holed, corrugated and at times obliterated by dust storms, sand drift or the occasional flood. Hazards on the road include straying stock, kangaroos and occasional emus. Remote homesteads still have no telephone, although the communications satellite, AUSSAT, has improved the situation, and brought television to many as well. The radio network associated with the Royal Flying Doctor Service, which covers the Australian continent, is of vital importance. It brings news of the outside world and provides social contacts outside the family as well as help in cases of emergency.

Typically the outback family is tough, resourceful and the survivor of many near disasters. Water is of prime importance to life. Rain brings prosperity, droughts may last for five or ten years. Fathers may be absent from home for days or weeks, working on station boundaries or hiring their services if times are lean. Mothers traditionally have been totally committed to the property: 'I have to be parent, station-hand and teacher, I never have time to do what I should'.

Aside from 'property children' whose families often have traditions derived from generations of outback existence, other groups must be considered: These are:

1. Children of railway and itinerant workers who have a far less settled environment, moving wherever their father's work takes them.

2. Children of miners—some live in extremely primitive conditions, many on the opal fields in tents or caravans for long periods of time. Others live in towns provided by large

mining companies. In keeping with the wealth derived from Australia's mineral boom, these may provide excellent physical facilities. There is less individual isolation but the towns themselves are isolated and social problems associated with a mobile population can be considerable.

3. Aboriginal children who live in communities on their tribal lands, some of which are very isolated indeed, being sited in the remote outback or in the central deserts. Their families may adopt a nomadic lifestyle and may be in and out of contact for weeks or months at a time.

The psychological effects of isolation

Most studies relating to children's psychological adjustment to their social environment have focused on life in over-crowded inner city areas. Studies of children who live in geographic isolation are few, and relate chiefly to their cognitive rather than their psychosocial development. A study of children from isolated farms in the mountains of Norway drew attention to the likelihood of emotional and social deprivation among them, often the result of their mother's investment in farm activities which left her little time to devote to children. Comparison with urban controls showed that isolated children also differed significantly in cognitive style. They acted out their feelings and ideas rather than discussing them verbally, and showed highly individual perceptions of the world. Many experienced extreme social difficulty when they went to boarding school at the age of seven years.

These findings are consistent with descriptions of isolated children in Australia whose verbal/social development lags behind that of city children. They act rather than talk, and are well known for their idiosyncratic approach to life. Some may never attend school and many do not attend until secondary level. Adults raised in the outback describe the difficulties which transition to urban life can create. 'Boarding school was the worst experience of my life' is a frequent comment.

The process of socialisation, which includes learning roles, attitudes, behaviours and perceptions from others in the environment can be regarded as a series of interpersonal interactions in progressively wider circles. Normally social interaction will be with the mother, then father, siblings, extended family, neighbourhood peers, and finally school companions. The importance of the peer group as a socialising agent as the child slowly grows to become more independent from his family, is universally recognised. The influences of school and neighbourhood on social development are of greatest importance. For the child reared in geographical isolation many of these agents are missing and the main elements in the child's lifestyle are:

1. Intense interaction with family members in the absence of outside influences. This can lead to unusually strong identification with parents. As adolescence is approached intensification of the usual rebellion against parent figures may occur as the young person strives toward individuation in the absence of support from peers.

2. Parent figures may be so involved with survival in their harsh existence that they have little time to give children intellectual stimulation and emotional support. Children may be left to their own devices. Many are expected to work on properties for long hours.

3. Lack of contact with peers may lead to difficulties in establishing an identity because there are no figures with whom to compare. At the same time individual interests and activities may be intensively pursued to the extent of producing eccentricity. The 'give and take' inherent in group membership may be inadequately learned.

4. Lack of cognitive stimulation in some areas may delay the development of certain skills. Language development is especially affected. Lack of verbal ability results in immediate action rather than premeditation when faced with a problem. General know-ledge may be lacking. A 10 year old boy, asked to describe the world's tallest building, drew a picture of the local water tower!

5. In contrast, motor development and survival skills may forge ahead. Many children of the outback show a surprising degree of self-sufficiency. One 10 year old girl drove a car 40 km over her father's land to school

daily with two younger members of her family in it.

Outback children do have advantages. The remote Australian landscape is of striking beauty. Gibber plains shimmer in the sun and mirages add to the feeling of space. Ancient mountain ranges worn by time expose rocks varying in colour from yellow to ochre to vermilion. Even in the deserts, wildlife is surprisingly abundant. Until recently, when television was unavailable over a large area, most children had a horse, among numerous pets. Their contact with the wild far surpasses that of urban children. Yet a Norwegian study drew attention to the influence space and distance have upon the behaviour of man and how too much of either may impose restrictions on the development of the child.

Air transport and radio communication have reduced considerably the 'tyranny of distance'—a phrase first used in horse and buggy days—but social isolation can still disadvantage outback children when they have to compete with others who are the products of contemporary urban society or who are judged by the mores of such a society.

Helping isolated children

Methods developed to help children living in geographical isolation will now be described. These will cover three areas: (1) Physical health (this will be touched on briefly); (2) mental health, and (3) education and psychosocial development. For the latter two, services developed in Queensland are described.

1. Ensuring physical health

Small, neglected graves in the bush give an indication of the hazards of outback life for children before the advent of the Royal Flying Doctor Service. Fifty years ago, this organisation, started by voluntary effort, began to cast its 'mantle of safety' over four-fifths of the continent. Now by means of the radio network, help can be summoned immediately in the case of accident or illness. A medicine chest with numbered bottles is supplied with each radio transceiver, and diagnosis can be made and treatment started immediately

through instructions over the air. Routine clinics are held where no school medical service could ever reach, often in outstations or even under the shade of the aircraft wing. Children can be transferred to hospital when necessary. There is also a Flying Dental Service. In Western Australia, a paediatrician (who is also a pilot) covers the State outside the metropolis and conducts emergency consultations by radio.

2. Mental health

Between 1978 and 1982 a point prevalence survey of 986 primary school children in Queensland looked at the extent of psychiatric disorder among them. This showed that the remote area children had a lower prevalence of psychiatric disorder than comparable groups from urban and metropolitan areas of Queensland. However, overall almost 10 per cent had evidence of significant psychiatric disorder. Half of these showed signs of emotional disorder and half signs of conduct disorder. Virtually none of the remote area children had access to psychiatric help although some parents described travelling over 1000 km to seek psychiatric consultation for their children.

Today, a team comprising a child psychiatrist, psychologist and paediatrician travel by plane to remote areas regularly. The furthest centre visited by the team is nearly 2000 km from Brisbane. The usual stay is 2–3 days, and peripheral areas may be visited during this time by charter plane or the Royal Flying Doctor Service. Clinics are held for assessment and treatment of any children with psychological or physical problems. Most important are discussions with professionals who supervise treatment between the team's visits. Contact is made with schools in the area to enable teachers to discuss the management of disturbed pupils. Regular consultation sessions are held on the School of the Air Radio Network. Two cases will illustrate the type of problems encountered:

1. A family travelled 200 km each way for a consultation regarding a 12 year old girl who had been sexually molested by a station hand. They had no telephone. Mother worked in a shop prior to marriage and found

315

it hard to adapt to country life. She was concerned about the child's attention seeking behaviour and her failure to achieve in schoolwork since the incident. Psychological assessment showed a minor learning disability which had gone unnoticed before. Interviews revealed that the incident had aggravated a rift between the parents and had produced intense anxiety in the mother, to which the child was reacting. There were no companions for the girl apart from a baby sibling. She spent most of her time in her mother's company.

2. A seven year old boy was brought for consultation with complaints of 'hyper-activity', difficulty in learning to read, and bed wetting. His home was 100 km from the nearest hospital. His father was away on contract work, and he had no playmates within 50 km of home. Mother lived in the city before her marriage, she reported that she often came close to maltreating her son. His early history included a difficult labour and delivery and delayed language development. This case raised problems of how the visiting team could help her.

The psychiatric unit of the State's children's hospital has also developed a program to enable rural families to gain maximum benefit from inpatient admission. The referring agency is asked to provide as much information as possible about the disturbed child in advance and to ensure that parents or someone familiar travels with the child. A two week admission is arranged (this is about the maximum time parents can leave a property), accommodation is found for the parents and they participate intensively in treatment. Aboriginal children are particularly distressed by city life and by separation from their parents. Allowances have to be made for this.

Plans for psychiatric and neurological evaluation are made before arrival. A school in the hospital grounds provides educational assessments, starts any necessary remedial work and offers explanations to the child and the parents as to why learning difficulties have developed. These can go a long way toward reversing any negative attitudes engendered by persistent failure.

Treatment involves a team effort by the ward staff. During a short admission an in-depth approach is not possible but by utilising the available time, focusing on specific problems, and working both with the family and individually with the child, an improvement in symptoms can be effected as early as the first week. If drugs are indicated, the effects of which may not be immediately apparent, it may be necessary for the parents to leave the child and return later. The value of methylphenidate can be assessed rapidly; neuroleptics and antidepressants take more time.

The essential factor in post-discharge supervision is continuing communication with a key figure from the child's environment. Family doctors, community health nurses, social workers, teachers, and the Flying Doctor Service are all important in after care and follow-up. A detailed letter explaining the treatment plans, the side effects of medication and other details is sent to the person willing to supervise. Phone contact with the parents is made whenever possible and it is equally important for someone to be easily available in the hospital should trouble arise.

3. Educational aspects

Of the 450,000 school age children in Queensland, 15,000 are scattered through outback areas. About 2000 have no access to a traditional school. Others can get to school, albeit with difficulty, but often rural schools are small, say with 10 or 12 pupils of varying ages and a single teacher. Children on 'properties' who cannot attend school but have a settled existence, often have a separate schoolroom and parents or governesses who supervise their education. Children of itinerant workers have a far more unsettled lifestyle and their school attendance can be very erratic.

Commonwealth funding has been made available to establish a Country Priority Area Program with the aim of enriching culturally, socially and intellectually, the environment of country children. Through this program library facilities are regularly upgraded and vocational guidance is supplied.

Excursions for pupils are arranged using 'mini' buses stationed at strategic centres and field studies are encouraged by the provision of a caravan and complete camping outfits. Itinerant teachers, remedial teachers and speech therapists travel from school to school by four-wheel drive vehicle or charter plane. Two trucks converted into mobile workshops visit schools for several days at a time to give pupils instruction. An itinerant music teacher pilots his own plane and visits schools regularly. There is also a 'flying' artist. Closed circuit television presenting magazine style topics is available to most schools.

For children unable to go to school the program provides itinerant teachers who visit properties and arrange for groups of four to five children to meet at the home of one of them for a mini-school. Sometimes a caravan serves as a 'mobile classroom'. During home visits emphasis is placed on teaching parents how to teach and improve attitudes to education. Parent illiteracy is a considerable problem.

In most Australian States there is a correspondence school. In Queensland this is a large organisation employing nearly 100 teachers and is subdivided into pre-school, primary and secondary school sections.

Lessons (both written and audiotaped) go out by post and are returned for correction. In recognising the need for students to identify positively with their teacher as a basis for learning, efforts are directed towards establishing the identity of the person who sends the instructions, and families are encouraged to attend a yearly camp on the coast. This gives children an opportunity to meet and take home a mental image of the teacher, as well as a taste of what life is like in a traditional classroom.

The School of the Air augments these activities. It is run in conjunction with the Flying Doctor Service, using its two-way radio network for a limited time each day.

There are Cubs, Brownies, Guides and Scouts of the Air. Every year, a Christmas party is held. At one centre for 400 students scattered over some 9000 km², Santa Claus asked about presents then listened while children sang, exchanged riddles and played musical instruments. Every day, before lessons start, a session is allowed when the children talk to each other. Sitting in on this session is fascinating.

The Distance Education Unit at Longreach, Queensland, is an example of the School of the Air Centre. It has a comprehensively equipped school yet the classrooms are often empty, only being used for 'mini-school' days. The instruction of mothers and governesses in methods of teaching is part of the program transmitted regularly over the air.

In 1985 Australia's domestic communication satellite, AUSSAT, was placed in orbit and the transponder leased for educational purposes. Expense has prevented wide usage, since each pupil has to be provided with an antenna dish, computer, printer and colour monitor for one-way video and two-way audio communication. For those who have the equipment not only can they *see* the teacher but voice communication via satellite is far superior to the radio to which they are accustomed.

Messages between pupil and teacher travel 72,000 km and take 0.27 of a second to travel between the two: this surely makes AUSSAT the largest classroom in the world.

AUSSAT is used for teacher training and by colleges of Advanced Education, universities and professional continuing education course seminars. A program for training family doctors has found that x-rays and ultrasound pictures travel well. Diagnosing the cause of an illness in a child is quite possible.

Children with learning disabilities often have problems intensified if they live in remote areas. The Queensland Isolated Children's Special Education Unit caters for them. Initially, the child and parent(s) visit a centre for assessment and a program tailored to individual needs is developed. Postal and radio supervision follows. A team of itinerant teachers visits homes regularly and gives explanations and support to parents as well as teaching the child for a few days at a time. Liaison with all the services described above is very important; in fact the education of outback children is seen as a team effort in every case.

Problems for adults

Some of the stresses to which outback life predisposes adults have been described in the foregoing section. The urban personality, pervasively influenced by social contacts, with its strong group orientation and intense striving for social prestige and financial advantage, has been well described. So far no stereotype for the dweller in remote regions of the world has reached the medical press. Although removed from many of the petty tensions of city life, those who face the harsh conditions of the outback need considerable personality strengths and a sense of mateship (helping others) in order to survive. Married couples may spend far more time in each other's company than their city counterparts. Flexible attitudes toward their relationship are essential if it is to last.

Newcomers may find adjustment hard. A husband caught up in a masculine and pioneering ethos may offer little support to his wife who may become persistently depressed as a result. Associated with the 'macho' image of the outback male comes the problem of alcoholism. Excessive drinking, aggravated by the hot, dry conditions, can result in outbursts of violence. These include wife and child abuse. Drought, with its resultant financial stresses and unemployment, may aggravate physical and emotional abuse in families, and contribute to suicide.

Social isolation and an itinerant lifestyle appeal to the individual who shrinks from contact with his fellow men. Those who migrate from cities (some with a history of a gaol sentence or psychiatric illness) to try their luck in the outback often meet disaster. An isolation syndrome is sometimes found among explorers in the wilderness and truck drivers doing long stints at night. It produces a sense of detachment, disorientation and sometimes extreme subjective experiences such as hallucinations, which are aggravated by heat and thirst.

Outback life fosters self-reliance but it also tolerates a wider pattern of eccentricity than a city lifestyle. Mental illness may reach major proportions long before help is sought and,

even then, delays occur because of the necessity for the patient to travel to a health centre or bush hospital. Symptoms such as hallucinations, delusions, paranoia and violent behaviour may be quite florid when they finally present for a medical opinion.

The extent to which the Royal Flying Doctor Service can help with such cases may depend upon the orientation and interests of the particular medical officer. Supervision of a drug regimen is possible but patients may be reluctant to be at a given place and time for a clinic visit.

Mental health problems among the Aboriginal population are only mentioned briefly here and are described further in chapter 45. Boredom, unemployment and the lack of an opportunity to hunt and enjoy 'bush tucker' can result in chronic depression. Marital disharmony can follow and alcoholism is a major problem. The latter is reflected in young people (sometimes even small children) who abuse drugs and sniff petrol. Adolescents may lack the intimate guidance of their elders when tribal structures break down. Suicide in police cells after arrest is a current and pressing problem.

Bizarre symptoms or trancelike states may develop among Aboriginal people who are stressed. Where traditional beliefs are unchallenged and malevolent supernatural forces accepted, sorcery syndromes (bone pointing) can still be found.

In summary, living in remote areas of Australia calls for a robust and flexible personality and an ability to survive and to assist others. To many it presents an incomparable way of life and city dwelling seems suffocating in contrast. Nevertheless, mental ill health may develop and can escalate among those who are unable to survive the rigours of the outback. Help for such patients may be hard to find and is often delayed despite unique and innovative approaches to the delivery of health care in remote areas of Australia.

Suggested Reading

Ashton J, *The School of the Air*, Seal Books, Rigby, Sydney, 1971.

Connell H M, Irvine L and Rodney J, 'The Prevalence of Psychiatric Disorder in Rural School Children', *Australian & New Zealand Journal of Psychiatry*, Vol 18, 1982, pp 177–80.

Haggard E A and Von Der Lippe A, 'Isolated Families in the Mountains of Norway' in *The Child and his Family*, Vol 1, (ed James Anthony E and Kaupernick C).

Rutter M, 'The City and the Child', *American Journal of Orthopsychiatry*, Vol 51 No 4, 1972, pp 610–25.

Chapter 47

Multicultural Psychiatry: General Considerations

G F Boranga

Whereas transcultural psychiatry usually refers to studies of comparisons of mental illness and health among different cultures, multicultural psychiatry specifically refers to the mental health problems which arise in a society made up of people who have different cultural backgrounds and practices. Australia and New Zealand are both pluralist societies partly made of people who have migrated from other places, or whose relatively close forebears have done so, and who have brought aspects of their original cultures with them. In addition there are other cultural characteristics of these countries.

Firstly, prior to the relatively recent waves of migration from other parts of the world, there were already present in both countries, ancient and complex native cultures. Secondly, the two countries are not simply a product of the mix and clash of cultures, but are two unique cultures themselves with laws and social practices fashioned from the experiences of the past and the efforts of legislators to create a society where people might flourish in health and well being. The social characteristics of both countries are democratic, liberal, egalitarian and humanistic.

In these respects the social principles fashioned in Australia and New Zealand were the products of rationalist views of the human condition as embodied in the Enlightenment. These principles also underpinned the establishment of the Republics of the United States of America and of France following the great revolutions in those countries. The Australian

and New Zealand societies which have developed along similar lines are by and large free of tyranny and relatively egalitarian. The Constitutions and laws of both Commonwealths embody personal freedoms and rights.

Nevertheless, the dominant cultures of each country have been criticised. In particular, it has been claimed that Australian culture is a 'hard culture', embodying 'masculine' principles which are aggressive, insensitive and competitive. A 'hard culture' is one in which religion is marginal, intellectual activity is scorned and where people are uncomfortable with differences or controversy. It has been argued that such attitudes have led to racial intolerance, antipathy towards individual excellence and resistance to change.

While such criticisms may be arguable, the xenophobic attitudes of Australian society up to fairly recent times are well documented. In the past two decades there has been a considerable shift towards acceptance of Australia's Asian geography and of migrants from Asia. The early intolerant attitudes also led, in Australia, to policies of active assimilation and integration of other cultures into the dominant anglo-celtic cultural mode. This policy led to many unfortunate consequences. Highly skilled migrants were forced to work on menial tasks for several years before they were accepted into their appropriate vocation and some never were able to work at the level of the training they had received in their country of origin.

While the Maori in New Zealand were protected to a major extent by the Treaty of

Waitangi, Australian Aborigines became the focus of active government assimilation policies. An example of these attitudes is provided in Chesson's biography of the Aboriginal poet and playwright, Jack Davis. Chesson reports that at the inaugural conference of Commonwealth and State Aboriginal Authorities in Canberra in April 1937 Mr Neville, representing the West Australian government, said that the opinion held by the State authorities was 'that the problem of the native race should be a long-range plan'. The prominent feature of this policy was the 'breeding out of colour'. 'In Western Australia' he said, 'we have the power under the Act to take any child from his mother at any stage of its life, no matter whether the mother is legally married or not.' Davis writes of his own experience of social acceptance in the small community of the country town Yarloop, Western Australia where he grew up. He describes how, when he reached adolescence, his father was reluctantly persuaded by government authorities to send him and his brother to the government Aboriginal farm training centre at Moore River. They left Yarloop excited and 'clean and spruced'. They were to discover, at the Centre, hardship, tyrannical authority, exploitation and abuse which left Davis, by nature an optimist, with a legacy of bitterness and anger for the system which allowed human beings to be treated in such a degrading fashion.

Multicultural psychiatry must take these types of social experiences into consideration with each person. To do this, those who work within its ambit must have access to and understand the social network and practices which encompass each person. The focus of multicultural psychiatry tends to challenge the ethocentricism of traditional Australasian psychiatry which has its origin and basis in British medicine and practice. Multicultural psychiatry, although concerned about interactions within families, also moves away from the narrow focus of family therapy on the internal family system to the wider, external systems of the family's culture and its relation to the society. It is a principle of multicultural psychiatry that by consideration of the relationships between a person, their

family, their cultural history and the wider present society, it is possible to begin to understand the mental health problems of many people, particularly those from minority ethnic groups.

It follows that, for mental health workers operating with these principles, it is necessary to try actively to change some of the societal attitudes which bring harm to people. These might include inappropriate assimilation policies for migrant people, inadequate language education, inappropriate or insensitive housing policies and so on. There are many examples. They need also to affirm the cultural values of others living in a pluralistic society as many people from minority backgrounds have a weak political base in their adopted country and are often overlooked or forgotten. It is also a belief among workers in the field of multicultural psychiatry that an open society, which can accept people whose culture and behaviour are different and which values this diversity because it enriches the general culture, provides, in fact, an ideal environment for promoting and defending mental health.

Language and culture

Cultural values are embodied in language and it is usually difficult to understand these values without understanding the language also. Non-English speaking people, or people who speak English poorly, can easily be misunderstood and their problems misinterpreted as symptoms of mental illness, unless they can be engaged in communication by a clinician who can speak their language and who knows, or is interested in, their cultural heritage.

The clinician who does not know a non-English speaking person's language is forced to make use of an interpreter. This practice, which is often inevitable, is not an ideal solution for a number of reasons. Firstly, the interpreter is an alien presence that can potentially interfere with the intimate nature of the relationship between the clinician and the patient. Those who try to conduct a psychiatric interview through an interpreter will discover that an already uncomfortable situation can become highly embarrassing. For example, one can understand that an elderly Southern Italian woman of great modesty cannot readily discuss intimate issues through a stranger.

Secondly, an interpreter simply decodes the verbal communications, very often putting these in their own words. However, in a clinical meeting between a psychiatrist and a patient, the verbal content is only one aspect of the communication. The inflexions, pauses, silences and other nuances of speech cannot be so easily interpreted or described in a way which makes them fully comprehensible. Witticisms, metaphors and proverbs often lose their meaning or significance if directly translated. Body language may lose its significance if the accompanying spoken language is not clear to the observer. Moreover, all these non-verbal aspects of language and communication help create the formal but friendly and stimulating atmosphere in which the person can talk freely about their doubts, fears, anguish and other problems.

In many communities a psychiatrist is perceived as an authority who can officially sanction the verdict of 'madness' which may already have been given by the social environment in which the patient lives. In other words, the psychiatrist can give scientific 'weight' to a social stigma which is attached to mental illness. Psychiatrists are also often identified with psychiatric asylums and it is from this that a fear of psychiatric internment arises.

In a situation fraught with such anxieties, the presence of an interpreter does not guarantee free and detailed communication but instead runs a distinct risk of reducing the psychiatric interview to an interrogation aimed at making the patient 'confess' his subjective disturbances so that they can be translated into the medical language of symptoms. It is difficult to produce an empathic relationship in such a context. On the contrary, there is a risk of the individual being inappropriately forced to adopt the role of a patient in a presumed illness. There is a risk of so objectifying the patient that the narrow bio-medical model gains dominance over other possible interpretations of the person's predicament, a frequent outcome of poor communication and cultural incomprehensibility on the part of the clinician.

Communication is also much more fluid, open and rich if the patient enters into intellectual and emotional harmony with the clinician and this occurs more easily when the former realises that there is a cultural affinity between them; the clinician either understands or is interested in the person's culture. Then a patient can intuitively sense that he is heard and understood. It must be remembered that a meeting with a mental health worker is always anxiety-provoking for the patient and this is even more so for ethnic patients who find themselves face to face with a clinician who may neither speak their language nor share their cultural background.

Clinicians who have the same cultural background as their patients have a great advantage, not only because they can communicate directly without intermediaries, but also because they can more accurately appreciate the patient's problems from his own perspective and understand them in the context of the patient's family. The clinicians who share common experiences of life and relationships with their patients are more naturally inclined to interpret the problems in the cultural context where they originated, distinguishing those considered normal in that context from those either partially or totally abnormal.

It is relevant here to relate the story of a 22 year old Chinese student who was diagnosed as suffering from severe depression following an attempted suicide and was subsequently unsuccessfully treated with anti-depressant medication. This young patient began showing depressive symptoms shortly after his parents joined him in Australia. He had emigrated alone four years earlier and had managed to integrate well with his Australian contemporaries, accepting some of their behavioural patterns. Masturbation was one of these, regarded in Australia as a normal practice in a young man. In his parents' culture, however, masturbation was considered to be dangerous as it was thought to lead to impotence, insanity and psychosis. Having discovered by chance that their son masturbated, the parents became alarmed and began to scold him continually. The patient progressively developed a serious depression and attempted suicide.

An interview with a psychiatrist did not discuss the masturbation problem because neither the parents nor the son mentioned it. They were too ashamed and feared they would be considered primitive. Besides, no questions were asked by the clinician about sexual behaviour. Subsequently, the parents did not accept the clinical diagnosis of endogenous depression nor the psychiatrist's medical prescriptions because they were convinced that their son's illness was caused by masturbation.

They were then referred to a Chinese social worker for help and advice and during a culturally sensitive interview, the masturbation problem came to light immediately. It proved to be the tip of the iceberg in a conflictual situation. The cause was a cultural clash between parents who were anchored in Chinese cultural traditions and a son who had adopted the Australian culture.

This case provides an example of how a system which is insensitive to cultural issues can fail to be effective in bringing help to someone in distress. It also illustrates the need for patients to have access to people who can understand relevant cultural issues.

Other cases can be provided in which, while a mental illness exists, it is still possible for a clinician without cultural knowledge to misconstrue the reported information or to miss the significant points.

For example, a young Chinese patient firmly believed that his Australian neighbour was trying to poison him by sending toxic gases into his house during the night. Objective verifications carried out by different people showed that his convictions had no real foundation. As a result the young man was diagnosed as being mentally ill, paranoid, and his beliefs about the poisoning were considered delusional. But this delusion was not entirely incomprehensible. The diagnosis did not totally invalidate him and make everything that he said false. The content of the delusion could not be ignored and considered merely an arbitrary product of a mental illness. Intolerance and racial prejudice towards Asians in Australia are not delusions but facts and it was his experiences of prejudices which were incorporated in the delusion. A closer study revealed that this Chinese patient was communicating a truth about his experiences which needed to be seriously understood.

A widowed middle-aged Italian woman, neglected by her children, lived alone in a modest house, surrounded by neighbours whose language and lifestyle were incomprehensible to her. This woman was convinced that an important person, the director of a bank, was her lover. She wrote to him, telephoned him and waited for him when he left work. The police were called and the woman was admitted to a psychiatric hospital. Her beliefs were labelled as an erotic delusion. A closer study, from a cultural perspective, revealed that this delusion symbolised a real drama involving her social isolation, her loneliness and a very human need to be loved.

By reflecting on such cases, it is not intended to suggest that the cultural problems caused the psychoses, but simply to underline the fact that psychiatric patients and the expressions of mental illness have meaning in the context of people's lives and their historical and social experiences.

If a medical diagnosis of schizophrenia is used as the sole means of defining an individual's condition, by 'homogenising' behaviours, it risks rendering the human element secondary and uninfluential. There is a particular danger of this occurring when the clinician cannot adequately communicate with the patient or is unsympathetic or ignorant of the patient's culture.

Cultural influences

Sometimes certain approaches which are normal and legitimate within a particular culture can be offensive and harmful in a different cultural context. For example, for a Southern Italian woman who has lost her husband, a period of mourning is necessary, during which attempts to engage her in occupational therapy should be avoided because they only produce diffidence, distrust and hostility towards the health workers. The pattern of her mourning should also not be seen as a symptom of depression or labelled social withdrawal. On the contrary, her desire to be alone may be a normal reaction, in perfect harmony with the values and customs of her culture. She may wish to demonstrate to herself and to convey to those around her that she is suffering for the loss of her husband by undergoing a period of mourning. This culturally consistent behaviour must be respected if the patient's trust is to be maintained by the health workers.

In dealing with families of different cultural backgrounds it is necessary to free oneself of ethnocentric attitudes, of the tendency to interpret human situations in the light of one's own personal experience and culture, making exclusive reference to the values of one's own ethnic group.

Male–female and parent–child relationships vary from society to society. Anglo-Celtic families rear their children with the aim of rendering them relatively autonomous and independent of family ties while Italian families, for example, tend to favour the maintenance of closer ties of dependence. In a traditional Italian culture, family unity is a value of primary importance. Separations and divorces have traditionally been dramatic events. Such cultural characteristics must be taken into serious consideration when one is consulted for conflictive situations within such a family. Efforts may need to be made to preserve the family unity as far as possible. Even in situations where, for example, the marital relationship is objectively oppressive, the natural inclination to press for a separation or divorce may be more harmful for the woman's immediate mental health than trying to maintain the cohesion of the family group. An Italian woman who decides to abandon her husband to go and live with another man breaks a social convention which is profoundly rooted in her culture. In fact, she is not only breaking with her husband but with her parents and children as well and they may often refuse to maintain any sort of contact with her. This decision leaves her in a situation which is just as oppressive as the previous one because she loses the affection and the respect of both her parents and her children.

However, issues of understanding of and sympathy for the cultural background of a patient are not as simple as ease with the language or knowledge of the country of origin might, at first, suggest.

The impoverishment of the spoken and written language which can be observed in many migrant communities in Australia relative to the contemporary situation in the country of origin, suggests that dislocation from the primary culture has caused the values and social conventions of the group in question to 'fossilise'. This phenomenon is particularly obvious in those migrant communities which, either for economic or geographic reasons, have little contact with their country of origin. The passage of time, accompanied by processes of linguistic and cultural adaptation to the receiving country, results in the language becoming contaminated and the original culture inflexible. In this way sub-cultural worlds are created which defend and reinforce the individual and group identity and resist the disruptive forces of assimilation with the host country's culture. Because their contact with the country of emigration is infrequent, these sub-cultural worlds are not influenced by the progressive changes occurring in the original culture.

It is, therefore, simplistic to think that the customs, social conventions and lifestyles of a certain ethnic community are identical to those in the original country. A recently arrived immigrant clinician examining patients who had entered the country a long time before, would initially have difficulty making himself understood. He may also find behavioural patterns and ways of relating that were typical of past generations but are no longer found among contemporaries in his country of origin.

In order to establish a positive relationship with these patients such a clinician would have to reflect on memories of his past, to rediscover cultural and linguistic elements that would enable understanding of the patient. It would also be necessary for this clinician to comprehend the current cultural world of patients as it is constituted in Australia, and be prepared to participate in their social lives in order to gain the experience necessary to understand the social interactions, expectations and values of the sub-culture.

Such examples above underline the complexity of multicultural psychiatry. They also should encourage psychiatrists, social workers, psychologists and others who deal with patients from different cultures to broaden the horizons of their own knowledge. This can be done by studying the languages and analysing the culture and the values of the various ethnic groups and cultivating their own intellectual curiosity for different cultures. It is this attitude which lessens the possibility of making errors in the treatment of ethnic patients and favours the realisation of an effective, open and receptive therapeutic approach which is not bound by ethnocentric assumptions.

Emigration

It is said that parting is a little like dying. Popular wisdom reminds us that leaving one's own native land, family and friends is a dramatic experience which in some ways may be similar to the experience of mourning. Emigrating is a critical event in the life of an individual and it remains constantly in one's thoughts after the event. Even for someone who appears to be well integrated into the host society, the experience of emigrating is often a memory which is loaded with agonising and distressing emotional elements.

This underlines the importance of delving into the emigration experience during the clinical interview, even with people who seem to attach little significance to the event and who declare that they have lost interest in their country of origin. Sometimes such people do not participate in the social life of their ethnic community and readily adopt the lifestyle of the host country, which may be quite different from their own cultural traditions. Where they have simply buried the migration trauma without having worked it out at an intellectual, social and emotional level, they become vulnerable to psychiatric illnesses. Such individuals may become psychologically quite dysfunctional when faced with frustrations or accidents at work, retirement, a child leaving home or even the marriage of a son or daughter. In these situations the trauma of the emigratory experience can re-emerge with intense emotional distress. The individual starts thinking about their country with excruciating nostalgia, and idealises it. They may become afraid that their life has been wasted, they may doubt their decision to emigrate, start criticising everything that is different from the original culture, feel that their roots have been lost, yet intuitively realise that it is impossible to go back because the world they have left has changed radically and they do not belong there any more. Visits home may bring disillusionment, frustration and regret.

The psychopathological symptoms manifested in such cases may lead to a diagnosis of depression which does not, however, respond to psychopharmacological treatment. It is a problem of existential despair for which treatment should start with the reactivation of the emigration trauma and provoke a critical, compassionate but rigorous reflection on the patient's life in the light of the persons' culture, choices, failures and achievements.

There are also recently emigrated individuals who experience 'cultural shock'. They are not capable of understanding the differences in values and social conventions between their culture and that of the host country. They under-rate the differences, believing they are in a cultural context which is similar to their original one. The difficulties they encounter in their social relationships and their frustrations at work are felt by them to be their own personal fault, a subjective insufficiency which is independent of the external environment. In such cases, it is necessary to clarify the different cultural characteristics of the country of origin and the country of immigration. This is often sufficient to prevent the individual losing confidence in himself. Others tend to idealise the host country, without having any in-depth knowledge of it, and have emigrated having convinced themselves that in a new environment they will be able to resolve their family conflicts. On the contrary, these conflicts are often aggravated and the divisions become wider than could have been expected—leading, for example, to separation and divorce.

It is thus important to emphasise that the clinical assessment should not be limited solely to the collection of symptoms but should attempt to identify all these elements of a cultural, social and existential nature that may be at the roots of a migrant's problems. Such an approach is crucial for the eventual choice of therapy (see also chapter 2).

The practice of multicultural psychiatry

The general approach of the clinician to the cultural aspects of mental health is not something which is widely thought about or understood in the mainstream of health disciplines. They tend to reflect the dominant Australian and New Zealand culture and perhaps their largely British origins. As with the early assimilation policies widely practised in Australia such ethnocentricity can have insensitive and destructive consequences.

In order to allow the development of a multicultural approach to mental health, as outlined above, multicultural psychiatric centres have been established in Perth and Melbourne. These centres not only provide a service orientated to the ethnic and cultural groups who live in these cities, but also help to teach others about approaches to the mental health of such groups.

The Multicultural Psychiatric Centre in Perth, Western Australia, was established in 1983 as part of the government mental health services. The Centre's permanent staff consists of an Italian psychiatric superintendent, a Bulgarian senior consultant psychiatrist, a Chinese social worker, an Italian social worker, a Polish psychologist, a Peruvian psychologist, two Italian psychiatric nurses, a Vietnamese welfare officer, a Bulgarian welfare officer, an Aboriginal welfare officer, a secretary of Italian descent and a receptionist of Yugoslav descent.

The Centre helps train psychiatrists, doctors, nurses, social workers and psychiatric nurses. The people who come to the Centre for training experience are generally chosen because of their linguistic skills or because of their manifest interest in migrants.

As well as direct work with patients, the professional activity of the Centre is characterised by visits to the patient's home, by meetings with various ethnic services, social agencies and various other resources such as general hospitals, psychiatric hospitals and health workers, including general practitioners and ethnic social workers. These meetings include informing people of the functions and policies of the Multicultural Psychiatric Centre and of the nature of multicultural psychiatry.

Members of the staff also actively participate at conferences with the aim of illustrating these ideas and experiences to as wide a public as possible.

Therapeutic groups are run on a volunteer basis at the Centre. These groups play an important part in breaking the social isolation of many patients and at the same time develop, especially for women who are isolated at home, an interest outside their home.

The languages which are spoken at the Centre include Italian, French, German, Russian, Spanish, most of the languages of the Balkan Peninsula, Mandarin, Cantonese and Vietnamese.

In a situation where a patient speaks a language which is not known by any of the staff, one of the Centre's ex-students is called in. This may be a nurse, student nurse or student social worker. Teamwork is a work practice at the Centre which arises not only from philosophy but also from objective necessity. In fact, every member of the staff has to function as an interpreter on certain occasions when the clinician does not speak the patient's language. This practice has produced very encouraging and positive results, because it has overturned the rigid roles which tend to revolve around expertise and professional function, and instead favours a permanent exchange of experiences, knowledge and information. This has broadened the staff's cultural education and created a stimulating, democratic atmosphere.

Referrals to the Centre are generally made by general practitioners, psychiatrists, general hospitals and ethnic agencies. There are also quite a few self referrals. The Multicultural Psychiatric Centre in Perth is a walk-in clinic. There are no waiting lists and in emergency situations clients are seen without having had preceding appointments.

Of the 1730 patients who have so far used the centre, Italians are the most numerous (569), followed by Yugoslavs (281), Poles (144), Vietnamese (63), and Latin Americans (63). The Centre has a particular interest in Aboriginal Mental Health and 105 Aboriginal Australians have used the Centre. This is particularly important considering that Aboriginal people rarely use conventional mental health services in Perth and it suggests that the employment and training of Aboriginal mental health workers at the Centre has been recognised and appreciated by the Aboriginal community in Perth.

In the Centre's experience the most vulnerable individuals and those most at risk of having a serious psychological breakdown are refugees, migrant women who are not sufficiently integrated into the Australian way of life, single men, adolescents affected by cultural conflicts with parents, elderly people and professional people unable to practice in their selected field because their qualifications are not recognised.

One aim of the service provided by the Centre is to prevent the patients being admitted to a psychiatric hospital. Despite all the efforts to improve them, psychiatric hospitals tend to be locked in to an unresolvable contradiction between cure and custody and mostly it is the custodial attitude which prevails over the therapeutic one. Admission to a psychiatric hospital is a sad experience for most but it is even sadder for an immigrant. He may find himself locked up against his will, often without knowing why, in an environment which he knows neither the language nor the rules, and his already precarious sense of identity can be seriously compromised. For the majority of ethnic people, mental illness is considered to be a very serious social slur and thus the admission becomes a confirmation of their social marginalisation.

Psychiatric hospitalisation and its resultant social stigma also makes reintegration into the social network difficult when the patient leaves hospital. Many ex-patients, for various reasons, are not tolerated in their community and as a result are often sent back to a psychiatric hospital for inadequate reasons and on very inconsistent pretexts.

For these reasons the Multicultural Psychiatric Centre in Perth is committed to avoiding psychiatric admissions but, where these cannot be avoided, the staff try to render them as brief as possible. At the same time they establish regular contacts with the family and the patient's social context and attempt to enlist the support of the ethnic community. This renders the admission less dramatic and makes it easier to reintroduce the individual into the community.

Conclusion

In a pluralist society, an ethnocentric approach to mental health and illness may be insensitive and lead to misinterpretation of people's problems. Multicultural psychiatry attempts to look at a person's wider socio-cultural context and to understand the influences arising from these aspects of experience. Much can be gained by clinicians who understand the language and culture of their patients or by those who are prepared to be sympathetic to cultural aspects. These are not usually taught in the health sciences in relation to mental illness but a recent development has seen the establishment of multicultural psychiatric clinics for therapeutic work and also for training mental health workers.

Further Reading

Chesson K, '*Jack Davis: A Life-story*', Dent, Melbourne, 1988.

Chrisman N J and Maretzki T W, 'Clinical Applied Anthropology, Anthropologists in Health Science Settings' from the series *Culture, Illness and Healing*, D Reidel Publishing Co, 1982.

Kleinman A, 'Patients and Healers in the Contest of Culture', *An Exploration of the Borderline between Anthropology, Medicine and Psychiatry*', University of California Press, 1980.

Littlewood R and Lipsedge M, '*Aliens and Alienists, Ethnic Minorities and Psychiatry*', Penguin, 1982.

Murphy H B M, '*Comparative Psychiatry—The International and Intercultural Distribution of Mental Illness*', Springer-Verlag, 1982.

Patience A, 'Notes for an Historical Sociology of Australian Hard Culture', *Australian Studies*, May, 1990.

Pedersen P B, Draguns J G, Lonner W J and Trimble J E, '*Counselling Across Cultures*', University of Hawaii Press, 1981.

Chapter 48

Emergencies

A T Davis

The term psychiatric emergency is used to describe a psychological disturbance that presents an immediate and substantial risk to the safety and welfare of a patient or others. In general, the disturbance is acute in onset and involves either a physical threat to others or self-damaging behaviour.

This definition is in keeping with the concept of emergency in general medicine, but excludes a number of acute psychological disorders which are commonly seen in hospital emergency departments and community settings. These include states of intense grief, marital and family crises and the emotional sequelae of accidents, assault, rape or natural disasters. These conditions are characterised by the experience of intense personal or social distress, without immediate threat to life. The concept of 'crisis' is used to delineate these conditions, which reflect a temporary disturbance in the equilibrium between the person and the environment as a result of either overwhelming external stress or impairment of coping abilities.

This chapter will outline common disturbances of behaviour that present in emergency situations and provide an approach to the assessment and management of such emergencies. Particular attention will be given to the assessment of patients with suicidal and violent behaviours. More complete descriptions of the range of psychiatric disorders mentioned in this chapter are provided in other chapters of the book.

Epidemiology

Epidemiological data concerning psychiatric emergencies is limited. Patients in need of urgent psychiatric assessment may be brought to professional attention by concerned family, friends or police officers. They may present to a variety of agencies, including general practitioners, community health centres, social services, crisis agencies (for example, Crisis Care and Lifeline) and emergency departments of general and psychiatric hospitals. In addition, psychiatric emergencies may appear in medical and surgical hospital wards, often in relation to physical illness or its treatment.

Most statistical information originates from surveys of hospital emergency departments and general wards, and refers to the presenting complaints or diagnostic assessments of patients. The most common emergencies involve suicidal and violent patients, and the most common related diagnoses are mood disorder (depression and mania), schizophrenia, drug and alcohol related disorders.

Classification

Psychiatric emergencies can be classified according to: (1) the source of referral; (2) the diagnosis; (3) the degree of disturbance of function; (4) the cause of the disorder and (5) the pattern of behaviour disturbance. For the clinician, this last approach provides the most practical means of classifying patients in emergency situations and planning management. The most common psychiatric emergencies in this system of classification are:

1. Suicidal behaviour
2. Violent behaviour
3. Disorganised behaviour
4. Paranoid behaviour
5. Stupor

Suicidal behaviour

The assessment and management of suicidal patients is one of the most challenging tasks that confronts the clinician. The nature of suicidal behaviour is fully discussed in chapter 29. In this chapter we will concentrate on the emergency aspects of suicidal behaviour. Suicidal patients make up the largest group of psychiatric emergencies and constitute a significant number of acute admissions to emergency departments and medical wards in general hospitals. A survey of admissions to the Royal Adelaide Hospital, Adelaide, South Australia between 1986 and 1988 leads to a conservative estimate of an attempted suicide rate in the Adelaide metropolitan area of 220 per 1000,00 population per annum. This rate is thought to be representative of the broader Australian population.

Between 93 and 100 per cent of suicides are associated with psychiatric illness. The most common diagnosis is depression, followed by alcohol dependence, schizophrenia and personality disorder. In patients with depression, suicide is associated with single status, living alone, older age in females, a history of suicide attempt(s) and at a clinical level, the presence of delusions, intense hopelessness and self-neglect. The risk for suicide is highest relatively early in the course of illness and during episodes of depression.

Follow-up studies show that 15 per cent of patients with primary mood disorder die by suicide, a rate which is 30 times greater than the general population. Of this group, between 30 and 50 per cent have a history of attempted suicide. In the year following a suicide attempt, between 15 and 25 per cent of subjects will repeat the act and between 1–2 per cent will die by suicide. This is 100 times the general population rate of suicide. Long term follow-up studies show that approximately 10 per cent of these patients will eventually die from suicide. A small percentage of patients will repeatedly attempt suicide. This group is characterised by a history of previous psychiatric treatment, personality disorder, drug and alcohol abuse, unemployment, low socio-economic status and criminal activity. They can present major management problems for emergency services.

Assessment

The clinician can be faced with four types of suicidal patients: (i) those who have attempted suicide; (ii) those who seek help for suicidal thoughts or impulses; (iii) those who present with various complaints and acknowledge suicidal thoughts during the course of a clinical interview and (iv) those who deny suicidal thinking but behave in a manner that indicates suicide potential. These patients are often brought to professional services by family members or friends. In all instances, a comprehensive assessment is required. Through an empathic clinical interview, the basis for a therapeutic alliance is established and the opportunity to discuss innermost thoughts and feelings is provided. The assessment interview is coupled with a mental state examination and, in some instances, a physical examination. The clinician aims to define: (i) the immediate risk of suicide and the likely subsequent risk of suicide or attempted suicide; (ii) the nature of the current crisis and the motivation of the suicidal behaviour; (iii) the type and severity of associated psychiatric disorder and (iv) the social situation and scope for intervention.

To ensure that a full psychosocial history is obtained, corroborative information should be obtained whenever possible from family or friends, the general practitioner and other health professionals involved in the patient's life. The interview with the patient should be conducted in a quiet, private room, even in the setting of a busy emergency department. If the patient has attempted suicide, the psychiatric assessment is arranged as soon as he is fit to give a reliable account of the circumstances of the attempt. This generally follows a period of hours or days in a hospital medical or surgical ward.

In the evaluation of suicidal risk, the clinician looks for the presence of suicide high-risk characteristics (see chapter 29). Careful examination of the patient's mental state is essential. In particular, the clinician looks for features of depression, namely mood disturbance, vegetative symptoms, psychomotor changes and morbid thoughts. In addition it is important to exclude psychotic illness. Signs of hallucinations, delusions, thought disorder and behaviour disturbance are sought. Further enquiry as to alcohol and drug use should follow.

In the evaluation of the patient's social situation, the clinician aims to define the patient's personality and usual coping mechanisms, the number and quality of social supports, the nature of available resources and ease of access to professional agencies and willingness to seek help.

Management

The immediate management of the emergency suicidal patient will be determined by the findings of the assessment interview. If the risk of suicide is judged to be high, hospitalisation is mandatory for the protection of the patient. In some instances, when the patient is mentally ill and is assessed as having a continuing high risk of suicide, compulsory admission under the relevant Mental Health Act may be necessary. Other indications for hospital admission include the presence of major psychiatric disorder, ongoing overwhelming stressors and lack of adequate social or other external supports.

In the hospital setting, the immediate goal is to prevent the patient from harming himself. This requires adequate staff levels, a secure environment and specific guidelines for staff concerning all aspects of observation and inpatient care. Clear communication between all staff members is critical. Appropriate physical therapy is instituted and accompanied by psychological support and education.

Subsequently, psycho-social stressors are evaluated and specific interventions arranged. This may involve individual psychotherapy, group therapy, marital or family therapy, or attention to social circumstances and supports.

When the risk of suicide or attempted suicide is thought to be low, management can be arranged through psychiatric outpatient clinics, psychiatrists in private practice, general practitioners and specialised social workers and community nurses. Specific referrals are tailored to meet individual needs, as defined by the initial assessment. When psychiatric disorder is present, standard treatments should follow. For the majority of

patients, a period of psychological support and counselling provides the opportunity to resolve the crises that underpin the suicidal behaviour (see chapters 28, 29).

Violent behaviour

The evaluation and management of violent patients is an important skill in emergency medicine. While the majority of violent behaviours in our society are not linked to physical or mental illness, patients may present with violent behaviour in diverse clinical situations, often without warning. The clinician's task is to evaluate the cause(s) of the violence and to facilitate optimal and prompt management of such patients.

The emergency assessment of a violent patient is complicated by several factors: (i) the clinician is often under pressure to 'treat' quickly or discharge the patient, which may inhibit the evaluation of the cause of the violence, (ii) the clinician may be fearful or angry, and thus lose clinical objectivity, (iii) in legal terms, the violent behaviour may have profound consequences for the patient and thus it is imperative that the clinician carefully document all findings and clinical decisions, and (iv) in practical terms, the evaluation rarely occurs in the ideal setting, with experienced staff, security and appropriate clinical resources. Nonetheless, the clinician is obliged to complete as good an assessment as the circumstances allow. Violent behaviour has multiple determinants. These include organic, psychological, social and environmental factors, which are listed in Table 1. In the evaluation of a violent patient, the relative contribution of each of these factors should be considered.

Assessment

The first step in the assessment of violent behaviour is to guarantee safety for the patient, the interviewer, the staff and others. Attention should be given to physical aspects of the environment. At the outset, objects that could be thrown or used as a weapon should be removed. Ideally, the interview should occur in a quiet room with the patient being made as comfortable as possible. The clinician

Table 1. Determinants of violent behaviour

Physical disorder

Minimal brain damage (eg perinatal hypoxia, previous head injury)

Genetic defect (eg XYY chromosome abnormality)

Central nervous system disorder (eg epilepsy, head injury, tumour)

Systemic illness (eg hypoglycaemia, infection, hypoxia)

Drug and alcohol related disorder (eg intoxication or withdrawal states)

Medication effects (adverse behavioural reactions are described with numerous prescribed medications)

Psychiatric syndromes

Psychotic illnesses (eg schizophrenia, mania, paranoid disorder)

Disorders of impulse control (eg intermittent explosive disorder)

Dissociative disorders (eg psychogenic fugue, multiple personality)

Adjustment disorders (eg with mixed disturbance of emotions and conduct)

Personality characteristics

Poor impulse control and low frustration tolerance

Propensity to put feelings of distress into aggressive actions

Poorly controlled aggressive impulses

Paranoid traits

Child and family factors

Family violence and disorganisation

Parental aggression and antisocial behaviour

Child abuse and neglect

Conduct disorder, childhood schizophrenia, mania, and temporal lobe epilepsy

Socio-cultural influences

Social deprivation (eg poverty, unemployment, discrimination)

Acceptance of violence as normative (eg movies, TV, gangs)

Cultural models of masculinity

Drug and alcohol abuse

should sit between the patient and the door and have ready access to the exit. A danger alarm should be within reach of the clinician, and attending staff should be available near the room's exit. If their assistance is required, it should be arranged promptly. The clinician should talk in a calm, nonprovocative and nonjudgemental manner, yet convey a sense of control of the situation. With open-ended questions at the outset of the interview, the clinician encourages the patient to talk freely. Appropriate concern is expressed and care offered. In the assessment interview, the clinician aims to obtain a comprehensive history of recent and past behaviour, current personal and social situation, current medical illness and use of medication, use of alcohol and drugs, past psychiatric and medical treatment, family illness, relevant developmental factors and contact with legal systems. It is often necessary to gain this history from several sources (for example, family, friends, health professionals, police).

A detailed history of the violent episode is necessary. This includes details of events preceding, precipitating and following the behaviour. As well, the patient's thoughts, feelings and physical sensations during the period of violence are sought. In addition, the social setting and behaviour of the victim and others in the immediate environment should be clarified. The degree of impulse control, premeditation and planning are questioned, as are the appropriateness of the behaviour to the setting and the consistency of the violence with past behaviours. The psycho-dynamic significance of the behaviour is explored, in particular the role of humiliation, shame or challenge to self-image which may have occurred in the setting in which the violence took place.

The mental state examination should be as thorough as possible, given the limitations of the setting. Signs of impaired consciousness or judgment, disorder of mood, thought or perception and disturbance of cognition are documented. A physical examination is indicated as early as possible in the evaluation. Direct observations of appearance, posture, gait, movement, speech, pupils, skin and respiration are helpful. Vital signs should be recorded. Attention is paid to signs of substance abuse or intoxication and other signs of CNS and systemic disorder.

Laboratory investigations may be considered, as may consultation with medical colleagues. At the completion of the evaluation, the clinician aims to provide a formulation of the patient's violent behaviour in terms of the relative contribution of physical, psychiatric, personality and socio-cultural factors. Specific management will depend on the findings of this assessment.

Management

If the patient is agitated or assaultive, particularly if suffering from an organic mental disorder or functional psychosis, verbal intervention may have little influence on behaviour. In such instances, physical means of control are necessary to protect the patient and others. Physical restraint, seclusion and neuroleptic medication are the cornerstone of immediate management. Their effective use requires the careful coordination of a team of professional staff.

Physical restraint should be performed by a large number of staff, ideally at least five in number. It is essential that the restraint technique is safe and is competently performed under the instructions of a team leader. There should be a specific plan, for example, four individuals take one limb each and one take the head of the patient and place the patient in the reclining position in a secluded area. Arm restraints may be required to secure the patient on the bed. Parenteral neuroleptic medication should be administered as soon as possible after restraint has been achieved. Restraints should be checked at frequent intervals for comfort and security, and removed as soon as effective pharmacological control is established.

The method of administration of neuroleptic medication will be determined by the degree of behaviour disturbance. If the patient is moderately agitated, oral medication can be offered. If the patient is extremely agitated or assaultive, parenteral medication is required. The drug of choice is usually haloperidol, a high potency neuroleptic with a low incidence of side-effects. An initial dose of 5-10 mg is advised, with careful titration of further doses against behaviour disturbance, sedation level and side-effects. A daily maximum dosage of 20-30 mg is generally advised.

Benzodiazepines may be used as an adjunct to haloperidol. These drugs are of low toxicity, assist with sedation and, through potentiation of the action of neuroleptic medications, reduce the total requirements of the neuroleptic drug. Diazepam and lorazepam are the most commonly used benzodiazepines in such situations.

Throughout the management of the acutely violent patient, care must be taken with observation of the patient's clinical state, particularly vital functions and neurological function. It is important that the underlying cause(s) of the violent behaviour be elucidated as quickly as possible, so that specific treatment of physical or mental disorder can proceed. The use of parenteral neuroleptics in combination with benzodiazepines in a safe, supportive environment will generally bring rapid control of the behaviour disturbance.

When a patient has been restrained or given medication against his will, the clinician must obey standing hospital regulation, and clearly document in medical files what was done and the rationale for the action. It is appropriate to authorise compulsory treatment under the relevant Mental Health Act.

Disorganised behaviour

Patients with a wide range of mental disorders may present with disorganised behaviour, ie behaviour characterised by excitement, agitation, hyperactivity or non-goal directed activity. This behaviour disturbance may be accompanied by disturbances of mood (elation, depression), perception (hallucinations, illusions), thought (delusions, incoherence), cognition and judgment. It may reflect organic or non-organic disturbance of brain function and pose a serious threat to the safety of the patient through inadvertent self-injury. Emergency situations may arise in a variety of clinical settings.

In terms of the evaluation of such patients, it is useful to consider whether the disorganised behaviour is caused by physical factors or primary psychiatric disorder. Disorganised behaviour due to physical factors may be found in: (i) alcohol intoxication or withdrawal; (ii) drug intoxication or withdrawal (for example, opiates, sedative-hypnotics, hallucinogens, stimulants, phencyclidine); (iii) delirium (non-drug causes); (iv) dementia and (v) epilepsy. Disorganised behaviour due to primary psychiatric illness may be found in: (i) acute schizophrenia; (ii) mania and (iii) psychotic depression.

The task of assessment is to establish the underlying cause of the behaviour disturbance. Management is centred on treating the basic disorder. In general terms, care must be taken to ensure the patient's safety and compliance with investigations and treatment. This is achieved through provision of a safe, low stimulus environment, close observation, clear limit-setting, attention to vital physical functions and cautious use of pharmacotherapy. In some instances of severely disruptive behaviour, when the safety of the patient and others is jeopardised, physical restraint and seclusion may be necessary. The same principles of management as outlined in the discussion of violent behaviour will apply in such cases.

Paranoid behaviour

Paranoid behaviour can present as a psychiatric emergency. A patient with persecutory hallucinations and delusions may behave dangerously, trying to kill or injure perceived persecutors and related persons. Intense fear and anger are often associated with such acute paranoid reactions.

Paranoid behaviour can occur in association with the following mental disorders: (i) organic mental disorder (including delirium, dementia and drug and alcohol-related disorders); (ii) schizophrenia; (iii) affective disorder (mania and depression) and (iv) acute paranoid (delusional) disorder.

In the assessment and management of such patients, the basic principles are the same as those guiding the management of violent (or potentially violent) patients. It is important to recognise that the predominant affects associated with paranoia are fear, anxiety and suspiciousness, and thus the appropriate clinical response is one of support and reassurance rather than confrontation or anger.

Stupor

Stupor is a term used to describe a clinical state in which the patient is immobile, mute and profoundly unresponsive to environmental stimulation or personal contact. An emergency situation arises when a state of stupor is sustained for many hours, with the potentially dangerous sequelae of dehydration and malnutrition.

In clinical practice, the most common psychiatric cause of stupor is severe depression. Less commonly it is found in catatonic schizophrenia and rarely as a manifestation of conversion disorder or mania.

A physical basis for stupor must always be considered. The most common physical causes include alcohol and drug intoxication, epilepsy (post-ictal state) and focal cerebral pathology (for example, tumour, meningitis, head injury, infarction and haemorrhage). It may also be found in association with senile or presenile dementia (late in the course of illness), endocrine disorders (for example, myxoedema, Cushing's disease, Addison's disease, hypopituitarism) and other extra-cerebral disorders (for example, uraemia, hypoglycaemia, diabetic acidosis, liver disease, electrolyte disturbance, water intoxication).

In the majority of cases of organic aetiology, there will be clinical evidence of neurological or systemic disorder. Knowledge of previous psychiatric history and context of the illness will help in determining the cause. Patients with psychiatric disorder are likely to have some ability to help with feeding and eliminative functions, and show some emotional reaction to what is said or done.

Management is based on elucidation of the cause(s) of stupor, support of vital functions and instigation of specific treatment as soon as possible.

Conclusion

Patients with psychiatric emergencies present to health professionals in diverse settings. As discussed in this chapter, the most common emergencies involve suicidal and violent behaviours which present an immediate challenge to the therapeutic skills of the clinician. In order to adequately assess patients in emergency situations it is essential that health professionals have a thorough understanding of the determinants of these complex behaviours. Optimal management is achieved through a careful analysis of the emergency situation, a confident approach to the patient's care, and the cooperative efforts of professional colleagues.

Further Reading

Hawton K and Catalan J, *Attempted Suicide. A Practical Guide To Its Nature And Management*, Oxford University Press, Oxford, 1982.

Hyman E H, *Manual of Psychiatric Emergencies*, Little, Brown and Co, Boston, 1984.

Reid W H, 'Clinical Evaluation of the Violent Patient', *The Psychiatric Clinics of North America*, Vol 11 No 4, 1988, pp 527-37.

Chapter 49

Forensic Psychiatry

J Grigor

In the traditional sense, forensic psychiatry is that area of psychiatry pertaining to courts of law. Some texts limit themselves to this area with the addition of discussion of the custodial aspects of mentally ill offenders. In this chapter we will use the term to discuss the whole interface between the law and mental health.

The criminal justice system

In democratic societies power and authority is distributed over a number of agencies to ensure the protection of individual rights. This is in contrast to totalitarian regimes where the police may have the power to arrest, charge, judge, sentence, and even execute. In Australia and New Zealand, the role of the police is more limited. Courts determine guilt or innocence and determine the punishment. A third arm of the criminal justice system, an office of corrections, prisons or parole, administers the sentence decided by the court.

The sources of law

The law derives either explicitly or implicitly from Parliament and in Australia and New Zealand it is based on English law. English common law dates back to the time of King Henry II (1133-1189) when judges were sent into the country on routes, later known as circuits, to arbitrate in various disputes. Eventually, through trial and error and attention to local customs, a *common law* was derived. In the last hundred years, the doctrine of 'judicial precedent', where decisions of

certain courts are binding on other courts, has been an important further source of law. The law is also derived from *statutes*. These began with the Magna Carta in 1225 and have increased since that time by the passage of legislation through Parliament. Queensland, Tasmania, and Western Australia have codified their criminal laws. A significant body of cases has been built up to assist in the interpretation of the Crimes Acts or Criminal Codes in order to clarify ambiguities and to provide for omissions and variations.

Criminal law

Criminal law is that branch of public law relating to offences which will be subject to criminal proceedings. A crime is an offence against the State and may be either an act of commission or omission. A criminal offence is liable to punishment. Civil wrongs are known as 'torts' and here the remedy is a common law action for compensation to an injured party in the form of damages. Some offences are both 'torts' and 'crimes'.

The essential element of a crime is that it involves guilty conduct or omissions and guilty intentions (mens rea) or a knowing mind. The broad principle is that there can be no guilty conduct unless there is an intent. The concept of mens rea or guilty intention is used to denote the accused's state of mind in regard to what he was doing at the time and the accused's awareness of the consequences of his actions.

Homicide is the killing of one human being by another human being and may be lawful or unlawful. When unlawful it is divided in most jurisdictions into murder, manslaughter and infanticide. Infanticide is defined as an unlawful homicide, where a woman, 'by wilful act or omission causes the death of her child aged under 12 months and where the balance of her mind was disturbed by reason of her not having fully recovered from the effect of giving birth to the child or by the effects of lactation'. It can be used as an offence or a defence and is limited to mental illness consequent on birth or lactation.

The legal system

The basis of our court system is the adversarial system. This is a contest between opposing parties who come before a court in an attempt to prove by argument and appropriate evidence their allegations or claims. Each side is obliged to state his case as strongly as he can and point out any flaws in the opposition's case. This contrasts with some European courts which are based on an inquisitorial system where the principal function of the court is to determine the truth by enquiry.

In an adversarial system of justice, it is up to the judge or jury to decide, on the basis of the evidence offered, whether the case has been proved 'on the balance of probabilities' in civil matters or 'beyond reasonable doubt' in criminal matters. The issues are polarised and the barrister is, in a sense, a salesperson selling a case. The judge remains an umpire and must not interfere with the trial by pointing out deficiencies in the presentation. Once experts are sought to assist the courts, they too, may become proponents of one side or the other, although they may use neutral language. Barristers put experts or other witnesses on the stand only if they will represent the interests of their clients. The rules of evidence generally are rules of exclusion and a witness is considered to belong to one side or another. Barristers are not ordinarily allowed to ask leading questions of witnesses but the barrister on the other side may cross-examine the witness. Thus, in cross-examination of a psychiatrist, the barrister may try to impugn the method of gathering information, the diagnosis, the status of the expert or the conclusions that have been drawn.

Evidence in court

Many people will give evidence in court. When they do so they swear on a Bible or make a solemn affirmation that they will tell the complete truth to the court. If this is in relation to, say, witnessing a motor vehicle accident, their status in life matters little. In such cases, direct eyewitness evidence is preferred, as this may be tested under cross-examination.

A clinician may present in court as a professional witness with expertise in matters relating to his profession by virtue of his training and experience and be required to give an *expert opinion*. Most young doctors who work in Casualty during their residency years will find themselves obliged to attend court to attest to the health or injuries of patients they have examined. They will be expected to have more knowledge than the ordinary man in the street but not necessarily to be expert in any particular area of medicine. On occasions, the court requires the assistance of experts in matters which are determined to be beyond the level of knowledge of the ordinary man in the street, that is, of the people who constitute a jury. The status of expert skills of the person is provided to the court. If such a person survives cross-examination as to his credentials, he can be regarded by the judge or jury as having the expertise claimed.

Medical reports are sought by lawyers for each side and, only when it is felt that a report is favourable to one side or the other, is that witness likely to be called. The expert witness therefore, is a witness for one side and is so regarded by the court and by the legal profession. Clinicians should take comfort in the fact that the adversarial system is designed to test, under cross-examination, any evidence given so as to arrive, ultimately, at the best and fairest result.

Fitness to plead

The law requires that a person must be mentally competent to stand trial. This issue may be raised by either party or by the presiding judge who may question whether the defendant has sufficient ability to brief his lawyer and follow court proceedings.

Generally, a defendant should be able to understand what he is charged with, how he is going to plead, understand the general nature of the proceedings of a court, be able to follow the evidence in a broad way and to brief his counsel and to provide his version of the facts. A person's mental capacity may vary over hours or days and may change during the course of a trial. It will be obvious that stress may affect mental state, that inability to speak English, deafness or other handicaps may diminish the person's fitness to plead. The courts may be alerted to these factors and are sympathetic to such issues and seek to overcome them. It is only when the person's mental illness is an issue, that a psychiatrist may be called to testify as to fitness to plead. Mental illness or intellectual disability by itself need not necessarily impair a person's capacity. It is only when the intellectual defect is so severe or the mental illness leads to a delusional misinterpretation of events, or patients are so thought disordered or demented that they are unable to follow proceedings, that they would be declared 'unfit to plead'. Consequences of such a formal finding are severe, in that a person is often kept in strict detention, either in prison or psychiatric hospital or training centre for the intellectually disabled until the Governor's Pleasure is known. If a person in these cicumstances remains unfit to plead through a continuous illness then, ultimately, the Crown will not proceed with the case and a formal *nolle prosequi* will be entered. The court will need to be satisfied on the issue of community safety. Generally such people are kept in total institutional care in hospital, training centre, or nursing home.

Disease of the mind

The concept of 'disease of the mind' is dependent on medical evidence. In legal terms, it not only embraces psychiatric illness but also dementia and intellectual disability. There is a general distinction between those conditions regarded as being due to some internal cause and altered transient mental states consequent on alcohol or drugs which are not considered as diseases of the mind.

There remain many contentious issues, the most controversial of which is hysterical dissociation or depersonalisation. These are not generally regarded, in a legal sense, as diseases of the mind but more the reaction of a sane mind to stress.

Personality disorder, not matter how severe, is not generally regarded as a disease of the mind. Amnesia, that is an inability to remember one's crime is, by itself, no excuse. However, the law does require that a person charged has the necessary criminal intent and recognises that mental malfunctions including intoxications, fits, dissociated states—either transient or permanent—may impair intent. Drunkenness is no defence unless it has led to an organic brain syndrome or in rare cases where the person becomes too drunk to form the necessary intention to kill, then a case of murder will be reduced to the crime of manslaughter.

The defence of insanity

The McNaughton Rules were formulated in 1843 and allow for a verdict of not guilty on the grounds of insanity. There must be *'a deficit of reason, from disease of the mind'* so that either the accused *'did not know the nature and quality of the act he was doing'* or *'did not know what he was doing was wrong'*. Daniel McNaughton attempted to kill Sir Robert Peel the Prime Minister of England and, instead, killed his personal private secretary. In view of the medical evidence presented, the three trial judges interrupted the trial and directed the jury to find McNaughton not guilty on the ground of insanity. He was sent directly to the Bethlem Royal Hospital to be kept in safe custody 'till Her Majesty's pleasure be known'. The public outcry which followed, and the displeasure of Queen Victoria, led to the House of Lords requesting the judges to formulate their opinions which have influenced the laws on insanity since that time. McNaughton died in the Broadmoor asylum in 1865.

A person who is acquitted on the grounds of insanity may be held in safe custody during the 'Governor's Pleasure' and as a consequence is subject to an indefinite period of incarceration. This may be in prison, where their treatment is no different from that of other prisoners, or in psychiatric hospitals if the degree of psychiatric disturbance warrants transfer. In Queensland there is provision to divert people who are mentally ill from the criminal justice system by way of a Mental Health Tribunal and place them directly into psychiatric care. In some overseas jurisdictions such persons are never sent to prison but are automatically transferred to psychiatric hospitals.

The raising of the insanity defence is often dependent on the consequences of the charge. When capital punishment was still a possible outcome for a conviction for murder, then the defence was invoked quite frequently. While indefinite sentencing 'for the term of his natural life' was still practised the insanity defence also retained a certain popularity. Now that most jurisdictions have *finite* sentences for murder and there is no capital punishment, the defence of insanity is usually only raised when it is clear that the person is floridly and chronically incapacitated and in need of continuing care and protection. It may, however, be raised in the case of minors whose imprisonment might seem inappropriate.

Some patients, acutely ill at the time of the offence, respond well to treatment. They may improve to the point where, if they were civilly committed to a psychiatric hospital, they would no longer be able to be held. The inherent conservatism of law, and the unpredictability of the course of many mental illnesses, is such that, although currently well, it is unlikely that patients who have committed serious crimes will be discharged from hospital until a very long period has elapsed.

Automatism

Automatic (ie dissociated) behaviour is a defence to a crime where it can be shown that the accused's actions were not controlled by conscious intent as, for example, in sleep walking, hypnosis, concussion or epilepsy. The laws state, if under such conditions the accused cannot be shown to have the necessary criminal intent, then the proper verdict is one of acquittal. Expert evidence is required to show that the conduct of the accused was 'involuntary' at the time of the

alleged crime as people invoking this defence claim to have no memory of the events at the relevant time. Here, psychiatric evidence by both sides will be crucial to determining guilt or acquittal.

Diminished responsibility

Many people have mental impairments which are insufficient to evoke the McNaughton defence of insanity, yet it is recognised that it would be unjust to punish them on the same basis as someone who is unimpaired. English law recognises that an 'abnormality of mind sufficient to substantially impair mental responsibility' will lead to a reduction of a murder charge to that of manslaughter. In the United Kingdom the defence of diminished responsibility has largely displaced the insanity defence. There have been difficulties in defining the breadth of circumstances which fall under this heading; these might spill over into much broader psychosocial issues such as ethnic background, emotional deprivation and so on.

In Australia, the law has generally considered that the concept of diminished responsibility is too vague to be given practical effect in criminal trials. Instead, if a person is found guilty, then his counsel may enter a 'plea in mitigation' in an attempt to lessen the severity of the expected sentence. He may produce witnesses who will attest to the person's good character or other attributes and perhaps bring forward psychiatric and psychological testimony hoping to lessen the sentence. The court itself may order a pre-sentence report seeking a more neutral assessment of the psychiatric condition of the individual. At this point, the court is no longer concerned with the person's mental state at the time of the offence, as this is no longer the issue, but is interested in questions of treatability, prognosis, recidivism and future dangerousness in order to decide the nature of the sentence within the discretion of the law.

Hospital orders

There is provision in most statutes relating to mental health, for an order to be made to transfer a person to hospital where he is found guilty of an offence and where psychiatric evidence is produced indicating that a person is mentally ill and in need of involuntary hospitalisation. In some jurisdictions, the court itself may order a brief period of hospitalisation of, say, 72 hours, in order for the court to become better informed as to the mental state of the individual. Alternatively, the court may require that a person be placed in a hospital for longer periods for a further psychiatric report to be submitted to the court before any ultimate sentence. Generally, however, where it is clear that the person is psychiatrically ill, a hospital order is made which has the effect of making a person an involuntary patient in a psychiatric hospital until such time as the illness has improved sufficiently to permit discharge.

Treatment orders

Courts have the power to order a person to seek treatment for alcoholism or other drug dependence as a condition of some other disposition. Where legally qualified practitioners certify in writing that a person is an alcoholic or a drug dependent person and suitable for treatment, then some jurisdictions have the power to commit such a person to a treatment centre for a varying period of time. In some States there is legal power to commit a person to a detention centre where there has been evidence of frequent recidivism in alcohol or drug use. There is an increasing recognition that the latter disposition is seldom successful nor fits comfortably within the ethical responsibilities of the medical profession.

The Family Court and the Children's Court

Psychiatrists may frequently be called to assist in Family Court matters in relation to divorce, custody and property settlement. The matter of custody of children and access by the non-custodial parent is a frequent cause of stress and this is recognised by Family courts who provide counselling services. In recent years there has been increasing interest in the rights of the children of a broken marriage.

Previously, in law, they had often been ignored but child psychiatrists in particular have been alert to the sensitivities and wishes of the children and the need for the children to be represented. These areas are amongst the most difficult in psychiatry.

The Children's Court setting, which deals with both juvenile delinquents and children taken into care and protection, is also an area where psychological and psychiatric intervention of high quality is required. There is a need for an accurate assessment of the child or adolescent, both from an intellectual, behavioural, and psychiatric viewpoint. Information regarding school performance, interaction with peers and parents is required in order to furnish the court with as complete a picture as possible. In addition, an accurate assessment of the parents, their coping strengths and parenting skills will be of use to the court in determining whether a child should be retained in the community within the family, fostered or, perhaps placed in institutional care.

Prediction of dangerousness

The courts are vitally interested in any evidence that may give some estimation of future likelihood of dangerousness and psychiatrists and psychologists are frequently asked to comment on this. Testimony is always given within the context of the limited predictive capacity in this area. The best predictor of future dangerousness is a past history of dangerousness. Dangerousness is at the centre of the social conflict between the issue of patients' rights and the issue of protection of the public. An enlightened society is obliged to protect the public from the risk of grave harm at the hands of dangerous mentally ill offenders by hospitalising them or by imprisoning them. This, however, exposes the offender to the risk of detention beyond that required for retribution or treatment, if there is a presumption of future dangerousness. Some social reformers believe that the public must be educated to accept the risks entailed. For them, it is necessary to recognise that the mentally ill have a right to treatment in the least restrictive settings and that punishment of offenders must be based solely on the concept of 'just deserts'. Public opinion, though, often reflects a view that the risk to innocent people should be considered paramount.

Violence is difficult to define and covers a range of behaviours, both lawful and unlawful, in a variety of settings with many different motivations. In the context of violent offending there are a range of biological, psychological and sociological theories ranging from postulated deficiencies in the central nervous system, theories based on instinct, learned responses, violence as sub-culture and violence as a consequence of economic deprivation.

The most extreme form of violence is homicide. In Australia, this is not likely to be associated with other crimes. Over three quarters of victims are either known or related to their assailant; most assailants are male and murder often occurs within the context of the family.

There are a number of possible contributing factors to the expression of violence. A majority of violent assaults are associated with alcohol and, among Aboriginal Australians there is a strong association between alcohol consumption, violence, homicide, and suicide. Hallucinogens and inhalants have been associated with aggression and homicidal behaviour. Amphetamines and cocaine can lead to increased aggressiveness and barbiturates and sedatives can have a disinhibiting effect leading to aggressive behaviour. On the other hand cannabis appears to reduce aggression, although availability through the criminal sub-culture may be associated with secondary violence.

Television violence has remained the focus of attention in many countries with the suggestion that it may lead to imitative behaviour and alter the threshold of what is acceptable behaviour. The availability of firearms is closely connected with homicide rates. Homicide studies in Australia show that firearms figure predominantly and it is reasonable to assume that restrictions on the availability of firearms may reduce homicide rates.

Mental illness and dangerousness

While most mentally ill people are not violent, there are more schizophrenic murderers than are expected by the prevalence of schizophrenia in the population. However, studies in the United States have shown that when mentally ill offenders have been released into the community or transferred to ordinary psychiatric hospitals, events of harm in the follow-up period have been about half or less than predicted.

Assessment goes beyond question of the risk of a person causing harm and must attempt to estimate under what circumstances the patient may become dangerous and then to consider how likely is it that this person will find themselves in these circumstances in the foreseeable future. Ultimately a prediction of dangerousness will reflect the experience of the clinician. However, there is a developing research interest in the clinical and statistical aspects which should improve our knowledge base in this area in the future.

Psychiatry in prisons

In contrast to the medico-legal expert witness who provides opinions for those for whom he will have no responsibility afterwards, other psychiatrists work in the correctional setting.

It is important that psychiatric services provided in prison have close links with a broader psychiatry service. A model forensic psychiatry system will have as its starting point, the view that, when people who are in prison become mentally ill and require hospitalisation, this should be provided in a hospital setting rather than in prison. The hospital should provide interaction with other hospital staff and the unit exposed to academic enquiry and therefore the unit should be part of a general teaching hospital. When the patient has improved sufficiently, he can return to prison. Prison based services can concentrate on providing psychiatric screening services for all new receptions, acute treatment and rehabilitation facilities including analogues to hostel, day-hospital, and sheltered workshops in the community.

In Australia, psychiatric evaluation for courts has traditionally been carried out within prisons while people are on remand. In other countries, there are facilities to remand patients for the purpose of psychiatric assessment, to a hospital. This allows a better assessment in which the nursing staff can play a prominent role, and where the necessary investigations can be undertaken. Assessments provided in this matter are usually of better quality and provide fuller information to assist the court.

The screening assessment of new prisoners on reception is a cornerstone of any correctional service. The act of imprisonment is stressful for all prisoners and adjustment reactions can be expected. Many prisoners charged with homicide undergo a grieving process even though it is they who have taken life. Many mentally ill people are caught up in the criminal justice system. Alcohol and drug dependent people may require treatment for withdrawal symptoms.

Recent changes to Mental Health legislation to protect patients' rights have led to either fewer admissions to psychiatric hospitals or to brief lengths of stay there. Deinstitutionalisation, described by some as trans-institutionalisation, has in some circumstances left a large number of mentally ill people inadequately cared for in the community (see chapter 44). This has put a greater stress on the criminal justice system and may have led to an increase in mentally ill people to prison. There are no accurate figures as to the incidence of mental illness in prisons but surveys have shown that at least 10 per cent of those remanded in custody may be suffering from a mental illness. In addition, the high incidence of suicide in prison has always been of concern. In the 1980s the issue of deaths of Aboriginal people in custody led to a Royal Commission and many alterations in procedures both in police cells and in prison have been recommended. Correctional staff are only in direct contact with prisoners for 8 out of every 24 hours and are unable to monitor prisoners adequately. Suicide prevention is too frequently based on incarceration in a single cell rather than assessment, increased couselling, medication and the use of extra nursing staff.

The identification of intellectually disabled people in prison is still at a distressingly poor level. Many disabled people become adroit at concealing illiteracy or their inability to tell the time and other deficits. Although they may not be obvious to custodial or therapeutic staff, intellectually disabled prisoners are readily recognisable by other prisoners and often fiercely discriminated against, assaulted and sexually abused. Recent legislation has emphasised 'normalisation' of the mentally retarded. Regrettably, the prison system cannot always protect their rights. Modern prisons usually set aside units for socially marginal prisoners to afford them greater protection and support. Psychiatric services play an important role in identifying and assisting these people and psychological and educational programs have been developed to meet their needs. The intellectually disabled offenders may also be suffering from an associated mental illness. In some States, now, intellectual disability services are creating secure units within training centres for the offender who cannot be appropriately managed within the broader prison setting.

Prisons usually provide occupational therapy, and some individual and group therapy, usually concentrating on improving social skills, assertiveness or independent living skills. There is interest in developing specific programs for particular categories of offenders. Sex offenders have to be segregated from other prisoners who regard them with contempt. In the last 20 years effective psychological therapies have been developed to enhance the social competency of sex offenders. Behavioural techniques have sometimes achieved a reduction in abnormal sex drives. These programs are frequently coupled with hormone medication. There is interest in the introduction of such programs for prisoners, particularly in the final months of sentence.

About 90-95 per cent of prisoners are male. The 5-10 per cent of female prisoners constitute a very special population and include people who are imprisoned for crimes such as prostitution. Some feminists argue that incarcerating a 'service provider' while not sanctioning the 'service user' is unjust. They also argue that women prisoners are subject to gender bias from male clinicians.

Confidentiality

Medical ethics enjoin doctors to hold confidential information which is provided to them by patients. It is accepted that in hospital situations, this information may be shared amongst other staff who form the treatment team. Beyond this circle, including the patient's family, the sharing of information requires permission from the patient. Increasingly other third parties ask for information. Government data collectors and third party insurance payers may also seek confidential medical information. The doctor is frequently in a position where disclosure is required by law. In some jurisdictions, in civil cases, unless the mental health of a patient is an issue before the court, the doctor may be protected under an Evidence Act from being compelled to disclose clinical material. However, in criminal jurisdictions the right of the court to know the truth overrides medical confidentiality.

Medical practitioners remain under a duty to act for the benefit of their patient. In forensic psychiatry the responsibility to the patient has to be balanced against the responsibility to the family of the patient and to the community as a whole. This may produce an intense conflict of interest for the psychiatrist. In prisons, psychiatrists are asked to see mentally ill prisoners on occasions for treatment, and on other occasions for administrative reasons and may be obliged to divulge information gained during the interview. It might be argued that, even when consent is given, under such circumstances the consent may have a degree of coercion derived from the prisoner being expected by the courts or legal services to comply with the psychiatric interview. It is essential, in these circumstances, that the clinician define precisely his role and responsibilities to provide reports to the courts and others.

It is recognised that common sense and professional judgment may lead to a decision to break confidentiality. Such situations might include the possibility of a patient committing a murder or suicide. Similarly a clinician may feel impelled to report a patient who has serious responsibilities as a pilot or a bus driver but who shows marked impairment of judgment. Responsibilities also rest with clinicians to report instances of child abuse which come to their attention. When clinicians who are obliged to testify, refuse to do so, they may be held to be in contempt of court and the court may impose sanctions including imprisonment. If a clinician is obliged or requested to disclose information, it is important to obtain a valid informed authorisation from the patient for the release of information. This should be in a written form and kept as a permanent record and dated. The authorisation might well also include the patient's right to inspect and copy any information that he authorises for release and also a note that the patient has the right to revoke consent at any time. The person to whom the information is to be sent should be listed and, in doubtful cases, an independent witness to the patient's signature is of use.

If a patient reveals a crime during the course of therapy the law does not generally require the clinician to report a criminal offence except in cases of child abuse. It is also true that psychiatric patients may confess to crimes that they have not committed. However, in some jurisdictions a doctor is required to report a crime if it is known to him. The treatment of people on parole conditions may require disclosure of a further offence to the parole authorities. In these circumstances it is important that the clinician make clear prior to the onset of therapy, the limitations of confidentiality in this regard.

For children under the age of 12, parental consent is required as the parents or guardian are the legal decision makers. Parents have a right to know about the course of treatment as well as the diagnosis and prognosis. Some States require the mandatory reporting of child abuse, even the suspicion of child abuse. In these circumstances the clinician is protected legally from any breach of confidentiality. When parents refuse treatment considered necessary, a request to have the child made a ward of the court may be made.

When minors in their teenage years are able to consent to treatment independently, it is generally acknowledged that they are able to control the disclosure of their personal medical information, if they are living away from the parental home and are independent, or if they are considered to be 'mature minors', that is, they are working. In many cases teenagers seek treatment for venereal disease or wish to discuss a termination of pregnancy, or gain advice and treatment for birth control. Here, there may be substantial conflicting interests between the minor's independent right to confidentiality and the parent's need to have information. There are no clear rules in these matters. It is suggested that careful judgment must be exercised by the doctor in order to include, when appropriate, the parents or guardian in the treatment decisions of a minor.

In 1966 a student at the University of California told his psychiatrist of his intention to kill a girl. The therapist took this matter seriously but the issue of breach of confidentiality was of concern to the University authorities, who vetoed the recommendation that the patient should be compulsory detained under emergency psychiatric provisions. Some two months later the patient killed the girl and her parents subsequently sued the University for negligence. The Californian Supreme Court ruled that a clinician who has reason to believe that a patient may kill or injure someone *must* notify the potential victim or their relatives or friends or the authorities. While this decision has not drastically affected medical practice, the general thrust of this ruling has been followed in other States in America although, to date, the matter has not been tested in Australia.

Informed consent

Before a doctor prescribes any treatment it is important that the patient be given a clear explanation which contains sufficient information to enable the patient to make a balanced judgment as to whether or not to participate in the treatment. In order for this to occur the patient must be given an adequate description of the benefits, discomforts, and the risks, and advised on alternative treatments, and the consequences of not participating in the recommended treatments. The particular problem for psychiatry relates to the mental capacity of the patient to understand these explanations. A depressed

and suicidal patient may be quite prepared to accept electro-convulsive therapy if he thinks that the treatment will kill him. On the other hand, a schizophrenic patient may make a delusional misinterpretation of the reasons for the prescribing of medication. Under such circumstances informed consent is impossible to obtain. In these cases, involuntary treatment must be considered. It is always wise to discuss the treatment with the next of kin. In most States now, Mental Health Acts provide for Guardianship Boards and Tribunals of Review to protect the rights of patients unable to give informed consent.

Testamentary capacity

Wills are usually attested before two witnesses but seldom is a psychiatrist present to comment on the mental state of the testator. About three per cent of wills are contested but only about a sixth of these successfully. If an individual has testamentary capacity, he has the right to make an unjust will, an unreasonable will, or even a cruel will. In order to be capable of making a will a person must have a sound mind and memory. He must know that he is executing a will, have a reasonable knowledge of the nature and extent of his property, and who would be 'the natural objects of his bounty'. These usually include the spouse and blood relatives, but may include others. The will should be freely and voluntarily executed. A failure to have knowledge of these three elements—the nature of the act, the knowledge of property, and possible heirs—constitutes, in the legal sense, lack of a sound disposing mind.

Alzheimer's disease and other dementias will often cause a challenge, but many elderly confused people can have lucid intervals or sufficient residual capacity to still be able to make a valid will. Severe infections and acute and chronic brain syndromes and severe mental deficiency may obviously interfere with testamentary capacity. Alcohol or drug intoxication, or persisting euphorias from the prolonged use of narcotics to relieve pain may interfere with testamentary capacity.

Psychiatric illness *per se* may not interfere with testamentary capacity, but delusional thinking may do so if it causes a disposition different from that which might reasonably be expected. Delusions of grandeur ('I own the world') or poverty ('I own nothing') or delusions of marital infidelity may make a will invalid. In general, society's notions of fairness usually seem to prevail in determining these matters in court. A question of undue influence may sometimes be raised. The same issues also arise in matters of contractual capacity, that is, the ability to enter into a legal contract.

Freedom of information

Freedom of Information legislation can provide patients with access to their case records, except in cases where it can be demonstrated that access may have a negative effect on the mental health of the individual. Clinicians are therefore obliged to be thoughtful in recording material and to be aware that information conveyed by third parties and written down in records, if accessible to the patient, may alter the quality of interpersonal relationships. The impact of Freedom of Information legislation has been generally to improve the quality of what is recorded. Some critics would maintain that information is now somewhat blander and less helpful in a diagnostic sense because some clinicians have refrained from recording any contentious interpersonal information. Failure to record such information may have an adverse impact on management for future admissions.

Other issues relating to the Mental Health Acts are discussed in chapter 50.

Conclusion

Forensic psychiatry has been described as the 'soft underbelly' of psychiatry, where there is a blurring between madness and badness, where issues of involuntary hospitalisation and imprisonment often seem distressingly unclear and where the body of knowledge is frequently based as much on moral preconceptions as on scientific enquiry. The discipline is a minefield of ethics, conflicting responsibilities, and confidentiality. Magistrates in courts are usually well aware of the significant psychiatric morbidity amongst people presenting before them and are equally aware of the paucity of resources available to assist the criminal justice system in assessment and diagnosis. The question of major mental illness is seldom raised except in the most severe and unusual crimes and the great majority of mentally ill people who come within the ambit of the criminal justice system can remain undiagnosed and untreated.

There is a need for improved mental health services at all points in the criminal justice system and an urgent need for further debate and enquiry into the relationships between crime and mental illness, free from judgmental and moralistic assumptions which have often characterised past debate on this subject.

Further Reading

Bates N, *Introduction to Legal Studies*, Butterworths, Sydney, 1973.
Buikhuisen W and Mednick S A, *Explaining Criminal Behaviour*, E J Brill, Leiden, 1988.
Halleck S L, *The Mentally Disordered Offender*, American Psychiatric Press Inc, Washington DC, 1987.
Power D J, *Principles of Forensic Psychiatry*, Edsall, London, 1979.
Rosner R and Harmon R B, *Correctional Psychiatry*, Plenum Press, New York, 1989.
Roth M and Bluglass R, *Psychiatry, Human Rights and the Law*, Cambridge University Press, 1985.
Simon R L, *Clinical Psychiatry and the Law*, American Psychiatric Press Inc, Washington DC, 1987.
Slovenko R, *Psychiatry and Law*, Little, Brown and Co, Boston, 1973.
West D J and Walk A, *Daniel McNaughton, His Trial and the Aftermath*, Gaskell Books, London, 1977.

Chapter 50

Mental Health Acts

J Durham

The subject of this chapter is the law governing the care of mentally ill or otherwise mentally disabled persons.

General

In New Zealand and in each of the States and Territories of Australia bodies of law have evolved independently, often in response to local concerns and historical contingencies, so that a superficial examination of the Mental Health Acts present an appearance of great variety. Even where, in response to recent currents of informed opinion, they have tended to converge, such resemblances are apt to be disguised by differences in outward form resulting from the necessity of adapting innovations to the existing, local legal and administrative machinery. Moreover, in some States a single Mental Health Act deals not only with medical, nursing and custodial aspects of care, but also with the safeguarding and administration of patients' property; in others the latter are provided for in separate legislation (for example, in New South Wales, the Disability Services and Guardianship Act and the Protected Persons' Estates Act).

These differences from one jurisdiction to another do not in themselves cause any serious inconvenience. This is not to say that one State's laws are as good as another's, but only that there is no good reason to call for the adoption of a uniform law, which would require too much in the way of harmonisation, in each separate jurisdiction, with other statutes. Moreover, the existence of nine independent centres of potential innovation should, through the opportunities it provides

for selective borrowing, be an advantage. The only kind of uniformity we need to aim for is that which results from a general prevalence of sound basic principles. The vocabulary of the law cannot be brought, in its whole extent, into unambiguous correspondence with the concepts of psychiatry; and the medical worker, while always, of course, abiding scrupulously by both the spirit and the letter of the law, will constantly meet with a necessity of interpreting it in a humane and responsible way. It is in the principles which one brings to this task that some degree of uniformity is desirable.

Because of the sheer multitude of variations in detail, a systematic comparison of all these statutes cannot be attempted here; even if it could, it would be of no practical value, because of the frequent emergence of new legislation and regulations. Exceptions will be mentioned, but for the most part, these variations of detail are of little theoretical or general interest. On the other hand, of course, the details of the current law and regulations in the particular jurisdiction within which one is working are the immediate concern of the health professional in the field, who will usually be able to obtain, from the employing authority, an up-to-date abstract of the essentials in plain, non-legal language, in which form they are quite easy to master. In this section, only the broad principles underlying the laws, and the more important and general among the practical problems, can be examined. Where the particulars of a statute are stated, it will be for the purpose of illustration or example, and should not be taken as necessarily representing the current

Scope of present statutes and directions of change

Such statutes usually begin with a lengthy section establishing the required 'machinery', designating the functionaries by and through whom various tasks are authorised and carried out, and defining the membership of supervisory boards and tribunals; and the statute or its accompanying regulations will contain provisions governing hospitals and other premises for the accommodation of patients.

The older statutes are largely hospital-oriented, and concerned mainly with custodial care and basic standards. More recent legislation takes account of the growing reliance, in public psychiatric practice, upon domiciliary treatment and other forms of non-residential care for patients suffering from major mental illness, and of the widening scope of services for the less conspicuous and disabling, but more widely-prevalent kinds of mental health problem. We may expect, in the newer legislation, some changes of emphasis, with more provisions of the 'enabling' and 'mandating' type, and an increasing attention to such matters as quality assurance, ready access to services, and the social and economic rights of psychiatrically disabled people. To this latter category belong the 'right to treatment' provisions recently incorporated in the statutes of a number of North American States.

At present, however, the essential core of the typical statute, and its historical raison d'etre, is the part which deals with the problem of the mentally ill patient, needing care and treatment, who lacks insight, and whose refusal of help is a manifestation of the very illness which makes it needful, so that there arises the question whether compulsion is justified. It is with this and with related problems that this chapter must chiefly deal.

Voluntary treatment

It should be borne in mind that the majority psychiatric admissions are voluntary, and that even when this has not been the case at the outset, most such patients elect to continue their stay voluntarily. The patient must of course, be competent to consent, but even severe mental illness does not necessarily disqualify a patient in this respect, so long as he is reasonably oriented. For some statutes, voluntary admission is 'informal' and subject to common law interpretations and presumptions of competence and consent; others require these latter to be formally attested.

Non-voluntary treatment

For the radical opponent of legally-enforced psychiatric treatment, its conventional justification in terms of concern for the patient's welfare is suspect. On this sceptical view, humanitarian motives played at best a subordinate part in the evolution of such laws, whose real, if undeclared, underlying purpose was at one level the suppression of eccentric behaviour, seen by reason merely of its eccentricity as subversive of the social order, and the segregation of persons who, without having committed any punishable offence, were simply a nuisance or a painful spectacle. At the level of the propertied classes, on the other hand, the laws served to protect family fortunes and to permit the removal from sight of socially embarrassing family members. In more recent times (so the argument runs) such laws have continued to serve purposes primarily of social control, licensing the internment of troublesome members of disadvantaged minorities, and screening from public gaze the more conspicuous or more desperate among the victims of an unjust social system. Under totalitarian regimes, when the simply arbitrary and the lawless imprisonment of disaffected persons could no longer be relied upon, the legalised 'psychiatric' detention of dissidents offered itself as a convenient alternative.

In the 1960s, the very notion of mental illness came under attack from several directions. According to some, 'mental illness' was a conventional fiction (Szasz); a valid though painful mode of perception and experience (Laing); or a cultural artefact induced by a kind of scapegoating ritual (Scheff).

As to the history of the legalised confinement of the mentally ill, the critics are on strong ground. The hardships of the solitary sufferer at large, in former times—outcast status, subjection to exploitation and casual brutality, and exposure to cold and hunger—must not be underestimated; but they may often have seemed preferable to the alternative of close confinement, of arbitrary duration, among grossly psychotic fellow inmates. Moreover, there can be no doubt that measures and institutions grounded in the best intentions regularly declined into neglect and abuse. Inadequate or scantly-observed legal process, lax supervision of attendants, venal or grasping managers, and the general harshness of the times—all of these, no doubt, were in varying degrees to blame; but many of what we would regard as the most oppressive practices were doubtless followed in good faith, in what must have seemed the want of any alternative. With the onus of absolute responsibility for the physical safety of inmates, but without the help of any specifically effective treatment, the control of violent, self-injurious, or persistently destructive patients could often be achieved only by recourse to solitary confinement or to various devices of bodily restraint. When the chronicity of the patient's condition seemed to require the prolonged use of such measures, there must have been many cases in which, by our lights, it would have been better to abandon them, follow what might; to say: 'It would be better for this man to be set at liberty, to suffer his chances, and better for the community to accept whatever hazard this may involve, than to keep him in this plight'. Until quite recently, however, such a solution would, to most people, have seemed morally indefensible.

The public was not insensitive, on the other hand, to the more obvious kinds of abuse, referred to earlier. Reforms, aimed at these, ushered in the era of the large asylum, a period roughly corresponding to the second half of the last century and the first half of this one. More rigorous standards of legal process were adopted. It may seem, however, from the great increase, during that time, in the number of asylum residents, that the new efficiency and growing capacity of the system encouraged an over-readiness to resort to committal as the easiest solution in any case of mental illness or intellectual handicap; and that once the patient had passed through its doors, the unnaturally huge size and isolated site of the standard mental hospital, with its irresistible institutional culture, favoured the severance of any remaining ties with family or community, making permanent residence the easiest option for all concerned, including the patient.

We must be wary, however, of judging the ways of our predecessors solely in the light of our own experience and moral concerns; nor should we discount the element of benevolence, misguided and excessively paternalistic though it often was, which generally actuated them. The miseries of cold and starvation were more present to their minds than they can easily be to ours; suicide was held in abhorrence of a kind and degree different from our own; and to be the victim of sexual exploitation was to suffer 'a fate worse than death'. Even in the first half of this century, institutional psychiatrists were obliged to take into account community attitudes toward mental illness, and moral priorities, markedly different from those of today. What we must learn, from the contemplation of what we now recognise as errors and abuses, is that the moral outlook of every epoch, by the lights of those that succeed it, suffers from blind spots; that we are presumably no exception; and that we must always be ready to re-examine our own attitudes and assumptions.

We need pay only brief attention to the claims of some writers to the discovery that mental illness is no such thing, and its corollary that a 'medical model' is quite out of place in any attempt to understand or deal with it. Obviously, a psychiatrist is consulted about many kinds of mental distress which are not, or do not appear to be, the products of illness in any ordinary or medical sense; and of course even when they are, as in the major psychotic disorders, the sufferer needs to be understood as an individual with a unique personal history, and a particular social setting. But the claim that illnesses like schizophrenia can be explained purely in such terms is quite untenable; and its supporters betray, in the very arguments they employ, their failure to grasp what they have undertaken to explain. It is necessary, however, for the student of psychiatry, and especially for the health worker who may be required to play some part in civil committal proceedings, to know that such doctrines have been widely influential, and that they are apt to form an element—together with a lingering mistrust of institutional psychiatry born of its sins of bygone days—in the ordinary person's attitude towards non-voluntary hospitalisation. On the other hand, it is not unusual to encounter an equally strong feeling of contrary tendency. There are still some people, impressed with an exaggerated idea of the capacity for mischief of any and every sufferer from mental illness, who feel that in any case of doubt, if the patient is not positively known to be harmless, the presumption should be in favour of confinement. The strength with which either of these views may be held, by someone involved with a psychotic patient, will often oblige the mental health worker to spend much time explaining the reasons for a decision, whether it be to recommend a committal, or not to do so.

Principles

We are now ready to consider the question: when, and upon what principles, are we justified in curtailing the liberty of an adult person who has committed no punishable offence; in subjecting the person to medical treatment without his consent; and in removing the person from the control of his affairs generally? (For the sake of simplicity, we shall henceforth use the term 'civil committal' to refer to either or both of the first two, and 'guardianship' for the third).

In the United States, it is natural for these questions to be discussed in terms of constitutional legitimacy—of State 'powers': a 'police power' to protect the basic rights of citizens from infringement by others, and a 'parens patriae' power deriving from the role of the State as guardian of last resort for those unable to care for themselves. Mention is made of these terms only because of their frequent occurrence in the American literature: for us they are not, perhaps, equally useful.

Traditionally, two classes of persons have been regarded as properly liable, though blameless, to restriction of bodily liberty: the seriously mentally ill, and those deemed likely to pass on a life-threatening infection. With the latter, of course, we are not concerned except to note—because the point has some relevance, by way of analogy, to what we shall later have to say in connection with the problem of the patient deemed to be dangerous—that personal restrictions under quarantine laws are nowadays imposed only when a gross and immediate danger can evidently be averted at the cost of a tolerably brief inconvenience to the person affected.

So far as we are concerned, then, the presence of serious mental illness in the person concerned is a necesesary condition of civil committal. Obviously, it is not a sufficient condition: the illness must be of a certain severity, and there must be other good reasons, evident in the particular case. These problems will be discussed shortly; let us first, however, be clear about why it is a necessary precondition.

When we interfere with the liberty of a mentally ill person, we usually do so—leaving out of the question, for the moment, the matter of dangerousness to others—for his own good, believing that we are for the time being better able than the patient to judge his best interests in important respects. There are, however, many varieties of folly, not involving mental illness, and of course any number of instances in which it could be persuasively argued that coercive intervention would be beneficial to the person concerned. John Stuart Mill provided, perhaps, the clearest exposition of the case against compulsion in such circumstances, arguing that coercive interference in the activities of an adult person cannot in general be justified on the sole ground that it is in his best interest. (Mill of course allowed exceptions which cover the case of mental illness or infirmity). His arguments, which are compelling, cannot be adequately summarised here; they hinge upon the questions: Who is to be appointed the judge of another's interest; and, when once we have admitted such a principle, where is it to stop?

Mill did not argue, of course, that everyone is always the best judge of his own interest, but only that any general and legally-constituted system (beyond such as might apply to persons of obvious incapacity) for revising people's choices in matters that, for better or worse, concerned them only, must rapidly lead to an absurd form of tyranny. It follows that if a course of conduct, no matter how apparently unwise, does not infringe the rights of others, we are not justified in coercive—as distinct from persuasive—intervention, unless we can say, on the basis of evidence which is, at least in a certain sense, independent of, or additional to, the particular behaviour in question, that the person's judgment is not merely at fault in this single instance, but grossly and morbidly defective over a considerable range of important concerns—in other words, that he is mentally ill in a very definite sense. (Of course, we must intervene, provisionally, even without such independent evidence, if the behaviour seems to involve imminent risk to life, and other data are for the moment lacking).

Requirements over and above the presence of mental illness

The restricted sense of the expression 'mental illness', which we should have in mind in any question of civil committal, will be discussed in more detail in connection with the problem of its definition. It is however, probably sufficiently familiar and distinct to the mind of the reader to permit us to set it on one side for the time being while we consider the other requirements referred to—special features of the illness, or particular circumstances of the case—which may be held to justify coercion. It is about these requirements that opinions are apt to vary most widely—from a theoretical viewpoint, about how exacting they should be; and, in practice, whether they have been satisfied in a particular case.

Some statutes are more explicit than others in the expression of such requirements. In Queensland, South Australia and Tasmania, it is required (the wording varies little) that the illness be of a nature and degree that warrants detention (in Tasmania, detention or a guardianship order) and such that the patient ought to be detained in the interest of his own health or safety ('welfare', in Queensland) or for the protection of others. In Western Australia it is required merely that the person suffers from 'mental disorder' and 'needs to be treated', 'in the interest of that person or of the public'. New Zealand's criteria are rather more explicit: the 'mental disorder' must pose 'a serious danger to the health or safety' of the affected person or of others, or must seriously diminish the person's ability 'to take care of himself or herself'.

In Victoria, as in some other States and in New Zealand, there are additional stipulations to the effect that treatment on a voluntary or a less restrictive basis is not an available alternative.

In the laws of other States, less is left to the discretion of the medical, judicial or tribunal authorities. In the Northern Territory an apparently mentally ill person may be taken into custody if it appears that he is in need of care *or* is 'likely, by act or neglect, to cause death or serious bodily harm to himself or another person'. Further detention, however, according to the wording of the Act, appears to require that both the foregoing criteria be satisfied—thus, that there must be risk of physical harm.

In the Australian Capital Territory, for an emergency treatment order, there must be 'mental dysfunction', together with 'an immediate and substantial risk of actual bodily harm' to the patient or to another person; but a non-emergency application may be made on the alternative ground of 'social breakdown'—meaning such gross inability to perform the functions necessary to an autonomous life as 'to cause the person to suffer severe distress or physical, material, or emotional deprivation'.

In New South Wales, under a new Act, there must be evidence that the action is necessary for the protection of the patient, or others, from 'serious physical harm' or, of the patient, from 'serious financial harm', or 'serious harm to his or her reputation'.

There are thus substantial dissimilarities among the statutes in this important respect, but also some ambiguities which, depending upon how they are interpreted, may mean fewer differences in practical result than might otherwise be expected. For example, only in the Australian Capital Territory does mental suffering, in itself, appear to be explicitly recognised among these criteria; but references in other statutes, in this connection, to the mentally ill person's 'interests', 'health', or 'welfare' might be read as admitting this consideration. Similarly, in New South Wales, 'serious damage to reputation' might seem to have a place in the Australian Capital Territory's category of 'social breakdown' or to require consideration in connection with Queensland's 'welfare'.

Concept of 'mental illness' in relation to civil committal

We must now turn to the question of what is to count, in this context of compulsory treatment, as 'mental illness'. Certainly the expression is used, in other contexts, to designate illness-like or troublesome or incapacitating mental states or conditions in general, and thus to include for example psychoneuroses and other conditions which in the opinion of most people would never justify civil committal no matter how severe the particular case. This usage is quite natural, and we cannot object to it, in these other contexts, or seek to change it—one reason being that some such conditions, in some patients, prove to be the product of ascertainable pathogenic processes, and it is likely that more will do so in the future.

Thus 'mental illness', not further defined, seems too inclusive a term for the purpose. The sense required (for reasons which will be discussed in more detail below) is a more restricted one, connoting a severe impairment of rationality and judgment which is manifested in gross and persistent misapprehension of everyday reality, or in a radical misconception of the basis of the sufferer's relations with others and/or of the meaning of their conduct toward him. This sense corresponds, of course, with the common meaning of the older terms 'mad', 'insane', 'lunatic', or 'of unsound mind'—terms too harsh in their associations to have a place in neutral official language whether medical or legal, but referring unambiguously to that set of attributes which most people have in mind, whether they are doctors, lawyers, or lay persons, when they think of 'certifiable' mental illness. It embraces, mostly, the kinds of disorders which psychiatrists range under the headings of 'psychosis' and (severe) 'dementia': but in a legal context this pair of terms would not make an appropriate substitute, for several reasons. 'Psychosis' is often used to refer to the species of illness—such as schizophrenia or bipolar affective disorder—from which the patient suffers, rather than to its characteristic mode of expression with such manifestations as those referred to above; and a person may of course suffer from an illness of this kind even in the absence of such gross manifestations. Likewise it is possible to suffer a moderately severe degree of dementia without losing insight and thus without becoming irrational.

The reasons for adhering to this restricted sense of 'mental illness', in questions of civil committal, are probably intuitively apparent to the reader, but may be briefly examined.

There is, firstly, the purely ethical one, in keeping with Mill's principle. Only the gross degree of incapacity and irresponsibility inherent in conditions answering to the description given above can justify us in substituting our judgment for that of the patient.

Secondly, it affords a defence against encroachments, in the guise of mental health ordinances, upon civil liberty. If 'mental illness' is interpreted in a very broad sense, to include psychoneuroses, personality disorders, and other kinds of maladjustment, the defining traits become difficult to distinguish from traits common, in some degree, to all humankind, and are probably distributed, not perhaps quite in accordance with the 'normal' curve (see chapter 71), but at least unimodally, so that the dividing line between 'illness' and 'non-illness' can be drawn only by an arbitrary decision. Wherever it is initially drawn, there must be, just on the further side of the line, a host of cases, excluded, but very difficult to distinguish from the adjacent ones included; there can be no firmly grounded objection to a proposal that the line be shifted so as to bring in these former, and so on. (All the pressures, in practice, would be against moving the line in the other direction).

With mental illness taken in the narrower sense, it is quite otherwise. Because of the distinctiveness of its manifestations, there is something like a 'natural', non-arbitrary dividing line, not absolute, of course, but located where there is a minimum—corresponding to the dip in a bimodal curve—of 'undecidable' cases. This is a line very difficult to ignore. (The only psychiatric condition which commonly generates 'undecidable' cases—cases in which it is impossible to obtain any large measure of agreement as to whether the patient should or should not be regarded as mentally ill in the 'committable' sense—is bipolar affective disorder, especially in the form of hypomania).

Finally, there is the clinical argument—it is only patients who are ill in this narrow sense whom we can confidently hope to help by means of treatment not voluntarily accepted in the first instance.

Definition of 'mental illness' in relation to civil committal

In Australia and abroad, most statutes supply a 'definition' of mental illness which is essentially circular or tautological, or one which confines itself to an indication of what is not to count as mental illness—such more or less obviously excluded attributes or dispositions as sexual preferences, religious or political beliefs, drug habits, or immoral behaviour.

The absence from most statutes—those of New Zealand and New South Wales being very recent exceptions—of any more positive definition of such a cardinal concept has of course attracted much criticism. The omission is not indefensible, however; the usefulness of defintions can be overestimated. Most familiar features of our daily surroundings can be recognised with high reliability without the help of a definition, and in many cases it would be very difficult to supply one which was not inadequate, trivial or circular.

The same is true of many expressions in common use, denoting abstract concepts. Such an expression, of course, often has several distinct meanings, of which the one intended, in any particular instance of its use, is usually unambiguously determined by its context. It

may be argued that 'mental illness' is such an expression, and that when it occurs in a context dealing with civil committal, everybody knows well enough what is meant; a concise definition, on the other hand, is difficult to construct and, once put to paper, may be interpreted in a manner unintended and unforeseen.

This argument is probably no longer valid. Where they occurred in the previous generation of statutes, such terms as 'insanity' and 'lunacy' were no doubt unambiguous, allowing no latitude of interpretation, and needing no definition, in that setting; and when, in the succeeding statutes, they were replaced by terms like 'mental illness', it was probably felt that the interpretation of these new terms was still sufficiently constrained by the context. Since then, however, with the emergence of changing patterns of disturbed behaviour, their interpretation has been put under considerable pressure, and a positive definition is probably called for. This seems to have been recognised in the two most recent statutes, those of New Zealand and New South Wales.

In now reviewing some of the limitations placed upon the application of the term 'mental illness', or its equivalent, in various statutes, we should not assume that actual practice varies as widely as these latter may seem to allow, and that where a particular restriction is not mentioned, it is not in practice observed.

Some States have separate statutes for the compulsory detention or treatment of persons given to the severe abuse of alcohol or other drugs. The usefulness and ethical propriety of such provisions are not matters of universal agreement, and the topic will not be further discussed here except to observe that if the principle of compulsory treatment for such problems is accepted at all, they should certainly not be regarded as forms of mental illness, but provided for in separate legislation and in separate facilities, because the processes of ascertainment, the methods of management, and the kind of residential accommodation required are completely different.

In Victoria, New South Wales, the Northern Territory, the Australian Capital Territory and

Queensland a list is given of conditions or attributes which may not count as mental illness. In general the lists comprise such obvious things as religious or political beliefs, sexual practices, and simply immoral or illegal behaviour. The first three States also exclude from consideration drug or alcohol abuse, as such, though, of course, not their neuro-psychiatric accompaniments or consequences if these amount in themselves to mental illness. The first two, and also South Australia and Western Australian, exclude developmental intellectual disability from consideration as mental illness (but institutional care can be provided, if necessary, under guardianship provisions).

The Tasmanian statute, following the dubious example of the English one of 1959, distinguishes mental illness from 'sub-normality' and 'psychopathic disorder', but recognises any of these as a valid basis for civil committal. For 'subnormality' and 'psychopathic disorder'—the latter character-ised by a persistent disposition to 'abnormally aggressive or seriously irresponsible con-duct'—there are age limits; the patient must be under 21 to be so committed, and may only exceptionally be detained past the age of 25. Moreover, the sufferer from 'psycho-pathic disorder' may be committed only if the condition 'requires or is amenable to medical treatment'—a stipulation which must in practice severely limit the use of this provision. (In most statutes, the exclusion of 'immoral conduct' can probably be taken to exclude the condition of antisocial personality disorder; in Victoria and New South Wales it is explicitly excluded).

New Zealand and New South Wales have recently opted for positive, non-tautological definitions of mental illness for the purposes of civil committal. For New Zealand (which uses the term 'mental disorder') it is 'an abnormal state of mind . . . characterised by delusions, or by disorders of mood or perception or volition or cognition . . .'. The New South Wales statute's definition, though differently worded, contains essentially the same items, except significantly, the last: there is no mention of cognitive disorder. In other words, broadly, the New Zealand definition comprises psychosis and dementia, while that of New South Wales excludes the latter, unless it is accompanied by manifestations of the former. (The omission of cognitive disorder from the New South Wales definition is discussed in the Appendix to this chapter).

The New South Wales law has another novel and unique feature: the provision for very short-term, non-voluntary care of persons, not suffering from mental illness in our sense, but exhibiting 'behaviour for the time being . . . so irrational . . .' as to justify apprehension of danger to themselves or to others. This may seem to represent an abandonment of the principle that only mental illness in the strict sense justifies civil committal. Properly regarded, however, it is only a tactical retreat, the better to hold the line. Increasingly often, nowadays, we encounter a person, not mentally ill, but in a state of angry excitement, often affected by alcohol or benzodiazepines, who has just made some suicidal gesture, or has threatened suicide or homicide in a manner which indicates that the risk will be short-lived, but that it cannot meanwhile be ignored. Often there is no alternative to brief detention in such cases even though it may be abundantly apparent that the person is not really mentally ill. Some authorities would indeed justify the measure, not simply as an expedient, but on the contention that such a state was really a brief form of mental illness. Herein lies the danger: that unless special recognition is given to this kind of problem it is likely to lead to a gradual but indefinite extension of the notion of what constitutes 'committable' mental illness, to include conditions of person-ality disorder and habitual drug abuse—conditions which, except in their emergency aspects, cannot be cared for on the same footing as mentally ill patients—and even to include, eventually, any kind of troublesome or embarrassing behaviour. Therefore, to give distinct recognition to emergencies not involving mental illness, and to provide a very short statutory maximum time for non-voluntary detention in such cases, together with a stringent limitation on repeated or consecutive use of the provision, can serve only to clarify the separate status and requirements of mental illness. Unfortunately, as enacted, the provision suffers from two blemishes: the patient can be detained for three working days, which seems too long; and a risk of 'serious financial harm' is inappropriately included as a ground for such detention.

Assessment of risk

As we have seen, some statutes may, in certain circumstances, allow consideration of the illness itself, in its own right, by reason of the suffering and desolation it brings upon the patient, as a valid ground for civil committal. Otherwise, the decision to recommend committal of a person suffering from mental illness involves the assessment of risks of one kind or another. All statutes, of course, recognise as relevant, among these, risks of grave physical harm, whether to the patient or to others; and most seem, though with less explicitness, to permit consideration of other kinds of hazard.

The New South Wales statute, however, explicitly requires risks of serious harm to the patient's reputation or finances to be taken into account. 'Reputation' here presumably refers, not to fame or renown, or even to any special standing in some local community or circle of connections, but only to that measure of respect, esteem or affection which the ordinary person enjoys among family, friends, neighbours or workmates. As a serious mental illness, untreated, can seldom fail to imperil 'reputation' in this sense, in which it is an attribute of most people, it will be seen that this provision gives the New South Wales law a very wide scope of application.

In relation to financial risks, it is necessary to distinguish two quite different forms of intervention. Under guardianship provisions of one kind or another a mentally ill person may be relieved of control of financial resources, if this would clearly be to his benefit, no matter how large or small the resources may be—even if, for example, it is merely a case of inability to husband social security payments sufficiently to obtain, regularly, the necessities of life.

The curtailment of a mentally ill person's liberty of movement, primarily in order to safeguard his property, is obviously quite another matter. In discussing its legal aspects,

some artificiality of argument is unavoidable, because the words of the statute in question imply that the necessity of safeguarding the mentally ill person's property might be the sole object and justification of the committal, whereas in most cases other considerations, such as the prospects of successful treatment, would in practice enter into the decision. With this reservation, it is evident that the relevant considerations fall mainly under the heading of urgency: the degree of the person's mobility and activity, the magnitude and liquidity of the assets in question, the proportion of them apparently at hazard, and the severity of the alternative consequences for the person and perhaps for his dependants. (Not infrequently, however, the occasion of such concerns is an episode of mild hypomania, and the difficulty lies not so much in assessing the risk as in deciding whether the person should be regarded as mentally ill in the legal sense.)

The assessment of suicide risk is dealt with elsewhere (chapter 29).

Risks arising from heedlessness of danger, or from self-neglect, generally present few difficulties of assessment. Often much more difficult are questions of a patient's dangerousness to others. It is not possible to devise, from relevant outcome statistics, a predictive instrument applicable to the individual case, and such judgments are chiefly a matter of clinical experience. In this connection, there has recently become widespread a belief that it has been shown that psychiatric predictions of dangerousness err so far on the side of over-prediction as to be quite valueless under all circumstances. In its usual form, this belief is based upon an invalid generalisation from studies conducted under very special conditions, far removed from the emergency situations in which most such judgments are required to be made.

Obviously, some acutely psychotic persons are dangerous in an immediate way which is only too obvious to anyone in their vicinity, psychiatrist or not. The long-range prediction of dangerousness is a rather different matter, concerning, in large part, mentally ill persons who have committed serious offences. All statutes make special provision for patients in this category, discussed in the chapter on Forensic Psychiatry (chapter 49). What follows, now, is to be understood not as referring to such long-term problems, but to cases in which only brief intervention may be called for.

In general, then, and with the aforementioned exceptions: if dangerousness to others is to be the sole or main justification for civil committal, the danger must be a clear and present one. In making such assessments, one must not pay undue regard to amorphous possibilities, diffusely spread as to time, place and person. A danger threatening a special individual, the subject of the patient's delusions, will generally impress as of more account than a risk which is borne, not by anyone in particular but, in an equal and infinitesimal degree, negligible to the individual, by the public at large.

One must not allow oneself to be unduly alarmed by mere braggadocio, or by threats uttered in the heat of the confrontation which has led to the patient's admission to hospital. On the other hand a patient's persistence, after any initial excitement has subsided, in menacing allusions to a particular person or other identifiable target should be regarded with caution. Mere quarrelsomeness, with a readiness to resort to fisticuffs among peers and kindred spirits in rough company does not, simply because the person concerned suffers from chronic psychosis, call for civil committal. Much must depend, in such cases, upon whether the aggressive disposition appears to be the product of psychotic illness, and upon the prospects for a lasting amelioration of the patient's condition as the result of a brief coercive intervention.

In deciding whether a perceptible but unquantifiable danger calls for coercive intervention, it is of course in many cases sufficient to rely upon a consideration of what would be the judgment of a reasonable lay person: in departing from this standard one must be prepared to adduce special reasons. Another rough yardstick can perhaps be derived from the quarantine provisions, referred to earlier, which do not attempt to anticipate every conceivable contingency at the cost of oppressive treatment of the individual.

One may sometimes hear expressions of uneasiness in the feeling that in recommending civil committal on the ground of a patient's dangerousness to others we vacate our proper role, that of ministering to the patient, and adopt instead that of the prosecutor or the agent of social control. This misgiving is unnecessary. Quite apart from the disaster to the victim, the commission of an act of homicide or arson is a disaster for the psychotic perpetrator, and if it is to be anticipated, it is our duty to protect the patient from it. The position of an external consultant giving an opinion, for example, at a review hearing about the patient of another doctor, is of course a different one, justified on other grounds.

The danger which a mentally ill parent may present to his children usually lies primarily within the province of child protection laws.

Non-custodial treatment orders

The development of community psychiatric services, with effective systems of regular treatment delivery at a distance from the hospital, has made it possible to reduce, for most patients, the duration of inpatient care, often to avoid it altogether; and it should permit even non-voluntary treatment to be administered in ways less restrictive of bodily liberty. The statutes have always made provision for non-voluntary patients to be released upon conditions. The bald references to 'conditions', however, left room for doubt as to what their scope might properly be; without well-developed community services their fulfilment was difficult to supervise; and in the case of non-compliance the only remedy provided was the abrupt, coercive readmission of the patient to hospital, which might often seem harsh and arbitrary, lacking as it usually would the visible and compelling justification of a fresh emergency. Explicit legislation has therefore been adopted in parts of the United States and of Europe and, in our part of the world, in New Zealand, Victoria, the Australian Capital Territory, and New South Wales. This permits treatment of mental illness to be given, under a certain degree of compulsion, but without detention, and the use of measures, in case of noncompliance, which may in the first instance stop short of summary readmission.

Misgivings have been expressed about this extension of coercive powers beyond the confines of the hospital, and about the possibility that it may lead to a net diminution, instead of the intended enhancement, of general liberty—that the availability of the seemingly less drastic alternative of a community treatment order may make for an increasing readiness to resort to compulsion in this form, and for a wider assumption of authority for domiciliary intrusions. Such Orwellian fears are not to be lightly dismissed. Certainly one must not assume that three or six months' compulsory pharmacotherapy is necessarily a less drastic imposition than would be a (generally much shorter) spell of hospital detention. To ensure appropriate use of such powers, two principles must be observed: firstly, that the essential criteria of justification for civil committal—mental illness in the narrower sense, and clear necessity—should be satisfied for either kind of order; and, secondly, that the community order is not to be regarded as simply a milder measure, to be applied in slight or doubtful cases, but one based upon different and specific indications. If, as with the New South Wales provisions, such orders are envisaged as generally remaining in effect (failing an appeal) for predetermined, fixed terms much longer than would ordinarily be the case for a custodial order, the indications must include a very substantial history of good response to treatment, and of repeated relapses convincingly attributable to a persistent failure to cooperate in its maintenance.

In New Zealand, the Australian Capital Terrtiory and Victoria, the criteria are essentially such as would otherwise suffice for compulsory admission, and in Victoria this is still the starting point. In the two former, however, the patient need not go to a hospital; rather, the initial presumption is reversed, and the resulting order is for management on an outpatient basis unless otherwise specified; moreover, just as with one for compulsory admission, the initial order is only provisional and short-term in effect; thus it consorts with a wider range of indications than those mentioned in the last sentence of the preceding paragraph.

In New South Wales a Community Treatment Order can be made, as in Victoria, after a patient has been compulsorily admitted to hospital; but there is also provision for what is called a Community Counselling Order (though it authorises drug therapy under some degree of compulsion). This can be made effective for six months if a magistrate is satisfied 'on the balance of probabilities' that a person who has in the past been mentally ill in such a way as to meet the requirements for civil committal (whether at that time actually committed or not) would otherwise again, within three months, become mentally ill so as again to fulfill these requirements; and is satisfied also that suitable treatment is available to prevent such an outcome. This seems to mean that the order can be made even if the person concerned is not, at the time, mentally fit at all; but in practice it is unlikely that the requisite medical testimony as to anticipated relapse within three months would be forthcoming unless some degree of illness were still unmistakably in evidence.

Procedures

For a mentally ill person's compulsory conveyance to hospital, each statute provides several alternative procedures, adapted to the various kinds of circumstances in which such a necessity may first become apparent, whether to a relative, a doctor, a police officer, or a member of the public. In New Zealand, the Australian Capital Territory, and some States there are appointed special officials (variously entitled and empowered) of appropriate training and experience, among whose tasks is the coordination of these procedures. Otherwise, authority for (if necessary, enforced) access to a mentally ill person's habitation is generally available from a magistrate.

As to further prescribed procedures, designed principally to ensure against unnecessary detention , the statutes vary very widely in detail, and to some extent in their adequacy to the purpose, but there is some agreement in certain essentials.

In general, if a medical recommendation, founded upon a quite recent personal interview, has not accompanied or preceded the patient, a psychiatric assessment must be made at the point of admission. At least one, and generally two, further concurring medical opinions (requirements as to specialist qualification vary) must follow in short course if the patient is to be detained longer than a day or two. In New Zealand two such opinions are required at the outset, prior to the patient's being admitted or required to undergo further assessment as an outpatient. In some Acts it is explicitly required that the medical opinions be arrived at independently; in any case a junior doctor must not in this matter be under any pressure, let alone instruction, from a senior.

Not all statutes require, explicitly, that a detained patient be informed of his rights; but this should be done in every case in which the patient is capable of attending to the explanation, or as soon as he is able to do so.

In New South Wales and the Australian Capital Territory, the detained patient must at this stage be brought before a magistrate. In Western Australia and the Northern Territory a magistrate is involved at an early stage but not necessarily by way of a full formal hearing. New Zealand provides an elaborate set of safeguards including the notification, within five days, of the Director of Psychiatric Services, an official visitor, the patient's regular medical attendant, a specially appointed legal official, and others; upon application by any of these, or by the patient, the case must be reviewed by a District Court judge.

In other States the patient may be detained further, on the strength of the medical documents, until the case is considered by an external Board or Tribunal. Usually such a hearing must occur within a few weeks, and again within a few months, if further detention is needed; and thereafter regularly.

Apart from the universally available remedy of habeas corpus proceedings and in addition to scheduled reviews, all statutes provide, in one way or another, for urgent appeals against detention to be lodged with some external authority.

It is an axiom of natural justice that a patient who is able to give instructions, and who wishes to be represented at such a hearing, should be accommodated in this respect. In New South Wales and South Australia, legal representation is mandatory, unless the patient refuses it. It is sometimes conducted in a robustly adversarial manner; and this may worry the testifying doctor, who may feel that the patient is likely to be embarrassed at hearing the explicit testimony demanded, that it may damage the patient–doctor relationship, or that it may turn the patient against the family or friends who have supplied information. The latter problem may call for careful handling, but seldom otherwise does there seem to be any ill-effect. Expressed tactfully, with a careful choice of words, the early review of the facts of the case, in the patient's hearing and in the presence of an impartial listener, often seems helpful rather than otherwise.

Scope of authority to administer treatment

In matters of physical custody or compulsion, guardianship provisions are usually seen as investing the responsible agent with a limited authority which, like that of the parent in the case of a minor, is enforceable only to an extent determined by the physical and mental capacities of the person in wardship. Mental health statutes, on the other hand, generally confer upon hospital personnel a rather extensive authority to administer treatment for psychiatric purposes, by force if necessary, so long as the treatment would generally be regarded as 'standard' or conventional. (The South Australian and Tasmanian mental health statutes are exceptional in that for certain purposes their guardianship provisions include such coercive functions).

For necessary non-psychiatric (for example, surgical) treatment of patients who are not competent to furnish informed consent, there exist provisions, under mental health or guardianship statutes, for others to consent on their behalf.

Statutes or regulations generally place restrictions upon certain measures, with exceptions for emergencies. The use of mechanical restraint or solitary confinement is generally made subject to stringent monitoring and reporting requirements. Electro-convulsive therapy can generally not be given to a non-consenting patient, except in a life-threatening emergency, without some special dispensation from an outside authority; and for psychosurgery this is usually required even in the case of a competent and consenting patient. It is to be anticipated that future legislation will increasingly apply more specific controls upon the use of drug treatment for non-voluntary patients. The rapid advance of knowledge means that this is best done by means of easily-up-dated regulations, rather than in the parent statute, and by way of mandatory clinical review committee, rather than by way of statutory mention of specific measures, which are difficult to define adequately in such a context.

Appendix: The New South Wales law on dementia

The omission of cognitive disorder from the New South Wales definition of legal 'mental illness', as a merely local curiosity, would merit only brief notice were it not for the illustration it affords of the problems of reconciling legal terms and categories with those of psychiatry.

In 1986, in the Supreme Court of New South Wales, a ruling was given to the effect that mental infirmity, in the sense of mere failure of intellectual powers as the result of brain changes in the senium, is not 'mental illness' as recognised in relevant extant law, the latter being characterised rather by delusions or hallucinations or other conspicuous manifestations of an exuberantly irrational nature. The ruling was apparently intended to distinguish between a state evidently envisaged as one of passive incapacity, requiring only care and assistance, on the one hand, and active psychosis, on the other other, requiring energetic treatment and sometimes coercive measures. Next, this distinction was evidently confounded with the time-honoured

psychiatric one between 'organic' and 'functional' psychoses—a distinction of long standing, which now, however, serves only as a rough-and-ready, working clinical classification. Finally, the latter of these two terms seems to have been mistaken as implying the absence of brain disease; thus cognitive disorder, as a cardinal feature of brain disease, could not count as 'mental illness'.

It is only fair to acknowledge that it has been conceded that the former does not preclude the latter, provided that psychotic manifestations are also present, and that this interpretation has been enjoined in a pro-legomenon to the statute.

The decision to enshrine the awkward Supreme Court ruling in the statute was no doubt influenced by the very proper feeling that patients suffering from dementia of Alzheimer or multi-infarct type are not best accommodated, and should not end their days, in general purpose psychiatric units; that their care is more fittingly exercised under guardianship provisions, with access, when needed, to specialised units. But of course, not all patients with dementia are elderly or suffering from irreversible brain changes; many such cases are acute or sub-acute and require urgent investigation and treatment in a hospital setting. The ordinary procedures for instituting guardianship are not well-adapted to dealing with emergencies; nor do the custodial and coercive powers normally envisaged under such arrangements seem adequte for the care of young, insightless and resistive patients. (Such powers, unlike those conferred under mental illness laws, are ordinarily regarded as limited in the same ways, and in accordance with the same kinds of contingency, as those of a parent in dealing with a minor). If the needs of elderly persons are met with suitable institutional provision, this legislative blunt instrument is superfluous; if they are not, it cannot help them.

Further Reading

Allderidge P, 'Hospitals, Madhouses and Asylums: Cycles in the Care of the Insane', *British Journal of Psychiatry*, Vol 134, 1979, pp 321-4.

Ellard J, 'The Dangerousness of Psychiatrists', *Australian & New Zealand Journal of Psychiatry*, Vol 23, 1989, pp 169-75.

Hoge S K, Appelbaum P S and Greer A, 'An Empirical Comparison of the Stone and Dangerousness criteria for Civil Commitment', *American Journal of Psychiatry*, Vol 146, 1989, pp 170-5.

Laing R, *The Divided Self*, Penguin, London, 1974.

McNeil D E and Binder R L, 'Predictive Validity of Judgments of Dangerousness in Emergency Civil Commitment', *American Journal of Psychiatry*, Vol 144, 1987, pp 197-200.

Mill J S, (ed Himmelfarb G), *On Liberty*, Penguin, London, 1974.

Roth L H, 'A Commitment Law for Patients, Doctors and Lawyers', *American Journal of Psychiatry*, Vol 136, 1979, pp 1121-7.

Roth M and Kroll J, *The Reality of Mental Illness*, Cambridge University Press, Cambridge, 1986.

Scheff T J, *Being Mentally Ill, a Sociological Theory*, 2nd ed, Aldine, New York, 1984.

Szasz T, *Insanity, The Idea and its Consequences*, Wiley, New York, 1986.

Part 7
Contemporary Issues

Chapter 51

A Feminist Perspective

Lois Achimovich

One of the most significant developments in Western society in the last one hundred years has been the movement for the emancipation of women. In the past few decades, an exciting discourse on feminism has developed, not only within academic circles, but also as a matter of public interest and debate.

Women are increasingly moving away from economic and social servitude. The difficult pursuit of equality for women, the 'feminist enterprise', is a major issue in contemporary society, although a wide socio-economic gap still exists between men and women in the work place.

Until the end of the nineteenth century, medicine was exclusively the domain of men. Women, if they were physically robust, could enter nursing, which was seen as a 'vocation' rather than an economically stable occupation. The University of Adelaide was the first in Australia to open its doors to women on equal terms with men. The University defied the Colonial Secretary and Queen Victoria in order to be able to grant degrees to women. Adelaide's first graduate, Miss Edith Dornwell, was admitted for the degree of Bachelor of Science in December 1885. Oxford and Cambridge admitted women to degrees, for the first time, in 1920 and 1948, respectively. One of the founders of the Medical School of Adelaide, Edward Stirling, supported in the South Australian House of Assembly the extension of the franchise to women and in 1896 they were the first women in Australia to exercise the vote. However, over the next few decades, the influence of women, even in a progressive University like Adelaide, was minimal and they were often

relegated to quarters separate from the men and inferior in quality. It is only in recent years that a more equitable treatment of women students has occurred at the institutions of higher education or that women have formed a significant proportion of tertiary enrolments in Health Sciences.

Feminists have been critical of medicine and other health professions, stating that they have been used as a technique to control women. In particular, they point to the high levels of sedatives prescribed to women in Australia and to the dominance of males controlling obstetrics and gynaecology services. Feminist critics have argued that pregnancy and childbirth have, in the last 150 years, been taken out of the domain of women and 'taken over' by men.

In a more general sense, the whole of the basic and social sciences have been criticised as being based on values determined by selective male attitudes. Women have rarely constituted a significant part of the scientific community, sufficient to challenge these attitudes. Some feminists argue that women are still actively excluded from science.

Just as feminist ideas have had difficulty influencing the basic gender assumptions in science and the health professions generally, so the medical and psychiatric texts have also largely failed to take into consideration the feminist criticisms. Although in recent years, issues affecting women, such as domestic violence, incest and single parenthood have become matters for discussion in the psychiatric literature, few attempts have been made to address the whole issue of sex role stereotyping and paternalistic attitudes that pervade the literature. In the eyes of some feminists, the texts are prejudiced by sexist attitudes on the part of those who are responsible for their production and for the dissemination of our psychiatric knowledge. For these critics, psychiatry represents one, albeit powerful, arm of a patriachal society in which there is a pattern of male dominance under aegis of gender.

Many health professionals are trained in hierarchies in which the position of power and influence is held most exclusively by men. Those trained in such male dominated structures are often unaware that, when they 'see' a women patient, they are likely to already have established views which are a collection of stereotypes developed by the patriachal system and which have little to do with how a women sees herself, or with an appreciation of the real social context of her 'symptomatic' behaviour.

It may be argued that psychiatrists, especially among health professionals, have always been concerned with their patients' social context. This is so, but it is equally true that the psychiatrist's professional training is informed mainly by three major conceptualisations of human behaviour, viz the biological model, the learning theory model and the psychoanalytic model. Very few psychiatrists have developed broader sociological models which would include consideration of the social role of women in which their 'illness' might be given a different significance.

Hence, it is unlikely that a woman feeling oppressed in her marital situation would be recognised as having more than a depressive illness. The likely outcome of this diagnosis is that antidepressant medication or individual psychotherapy or both, are seen as the primary 'treatment', although it would be more appropriate to see the problems as part of disturbed interpersonal relationships in which the husband's attitudes, values and behaviour are essential components.

Just as psychiatric theory and training show little evidence of the influence of feminist thought, so it is with the practice of psychiatry. General and State hospitals must deal with crises which other arms of the State are unwilling or unable to handle. If these crises are seen as episodes of mental illness which need to be treated and the patient sent home, nothing needs to be changed in the social system. If however, the psychotic, depressive or violent episode is seen as a response to an intolerable social or domestic situation, the actions of the intervening agency could and should be different.

A consideration of the life of Zelda, the wife of Scott Fitzgerald, demonstrates how vulnerable women are to the destructive effects of stereotyped values (biographies of Eugene and Carlotta O'Neill, T S and Vivienne Eliot and Janet Frame are also worth perusal). In the 1920s, Zelda was diagnosed as suffering from schizophrenia by both Eugen Bleuler and Adolf Meyer, the leading psychiatrists of their time. For many years, it was the 'received wisdom' that Scott was a great writer, but an unfortunate artist, who drank too much and who was unfortunately afflicted with a crazy wife. He used her story as the basis for one of his novels 'Tender is the Night'.

In more recent years, a different interpretation has surfaced in literary journals. Zelda wrote her own version of their story 'Save Me The Waltz' during the first six weeks of her hospitalisation for schizophrenia at the Phipps Clinic in February 1932. Scott was apparently furious that the doctors had allowed her to send the book to publishers without his seeing it. The doctors were apologetic. Judged by early critics to be of little literary merit, this book and other examples of Zelda's writing are now receiving a new reading and considerable praise from contemporary critics.

A traditional approach to the couple's problems reveals a competitive marriage in which their close friends, like Hemingway, and the professionals whom they consulted, saw the problem as emanating from the wife's jealousy of the husband's success. (Adolf Meyer, to his credit, told Scott directly that his drinking was making the situation worse). A more systemic approach might hypothesise that Zelda and Scott were at two poles of a triangle with their friends, relatives and professionals at the third. A feminist approach would recognise that, from the point of view of power, Scott held all the trump cards. He was famous, earned the money and had a symptom, alcoholism, which was socially sanctioned. Her attempts to develop her own artistic nature, through dancing, painting and writing, were seen as 'neurotic' and 'competitive'. Her early roles as 'vamp' and 'madcap' were no longer available to her, now that she was a mother and a maturing married woman. Was she meant to be happy basking in the reflected glory of her husband for the rest of her life?

A compassionate view of the couple's plight would not mean an indictment of the husband or the medical fraternity-their views were those of most Western thinkers of the time. However, an appreciation of the Fitzgeralds' predicament may lead to a richer understanding of contemporary married couples and make clinicians cautious in labelling a woman as 'mad' and thereby prejudicing the manner in which she will be treated from then on.

A woman who has multiple admissions to hospitals may be diagnosed in many ways, from inadequate personality to bipolar depressive to schizophrenic, but if nothing is done about the violence or poverty of her living situation, we simply add a diagnosis to her other problems.

Training in couple interviewing techniques and family interventions may be helpful to counteract stereotyped attitudes to gender in health professionals. Currently, such training is not a priority in tertiary courses, although there are some signs that it is becoming more acceptable, such as a Masters course in Psychotherapy at the University of New South Wales and a marital therapy program at Glenside Hospital in South Australia.

In private medical, psychological and social work practice, psychotherapy usually tends to be one to one, long term and frequent. However, individually based treatment models tend to construct psychological problems as stemming from past personal experience rather than from the social context of the patient's life. For example, a marital problem will be seen as stemming from the immaturity of one of the members of the dyad, rather than human inequity in the balance of power in the marriage. It is easy to see that individual therapy can be used to allow a woman to adapt to her oppressed situation rather than change it (although it has the potential to develop personal resources and resolve). A couple therapy approach endeavours, from the start, to engage both members in new behaviours to improve their lives *together* or, if necessary, to make a decision to divorce from a position of understanding and consideration, rather than one of mutual retribution, which is often the case. The growth of theory and practice in the group and family field has occurred concurrently with the development of awareness that women's problems may reside somewhere other than in their own 'vulnerable' feminine nature.

Largely because of the work of writers such as Kate Millett, Freud's theories of female psychology are now seen as tentative and sometimes misguided, although recently there has been an attempt, especially among French feminists, to salvage the psychoanalytic model of feminism. Nevertheless, one unfortunate consequence of Freud's decision to consider that the claims of his women patients that they had been sexually abused were mostly derived from their own forbidden, incestuous wishes, rather than descriptions of true events, was that an excuse was provided to deny the fact of child sexual abuse. How many women who reported interference by their fathers were met with interpretations of how they imagined it all because secretly they desired to have their fathers to themselves? Once again, a paternalistic attitude served to deny women their reality.

At another level of psychiatric assessment, the traditional psychiatric interview is geared to produce an individual diagnosis. The questions asked in the interview are weighted to produce this information. This can lead to absurdities, such as the failure to register significant information, for example, that a schizophrenic girl was raped when she was two years old, because 'sexual abuse doesn't cause schizophrenia'.

Family and systemic therapists have not always been free of sexism in their approach to women. Accusations of values and attitudes of sexism and sex role stereotyping have come loud and fast since the family therapy field was established. For many years the primary theorists were men. A women's conference now traditionally precedes the annual conference of family therapists. In Australia, this was a reaction to women's concerns and has provided a welcome forum for women who wanted to discuss problems amongst others who have similar theoretical values.

For women therapists, professional life is a delicate balance between giving full weight to the difficulties that women and girls face in our culture, while recognising that most patients are not looking for radical solutions to their problems. Most women want to get on better with their male friends and relatives, not to be cut off from them. In these circumstances, it is vital that clinicians do not impose their own views of the 'perfect' relationship on their patients. Therapy for the two members is possible, provided violence and threats of violence are eschewed. Most men are amenable to negotiation regarding sharing of household tasks, money and child care, although relinquishing power in any human relationship is not easy.

Women professionals also need to be informed about sexism in fields such as obstetrics where practices which favour men continue with few counterbalances. There are very few female doctors practising obstetrics. The law is another area which is decidedly sexist. European written and common law is patriachal. In Western Australia, there are no female judges in the Family Law Court and few in other areas of the judiciary in Australia.

Finally, as Dale Spender has pointed out, if women are to stop rediscovering the wheel, they need to inform themselves of the work of women who have gone before them. The singlemindedness of the nineteenth century feminists, for instance, is a great inspiration to women who feel overwhelmed by the task of their emancipation.

It will take experience of a dramatic nature to change the prevailing health professional attitudes to women. Forward thinking training programs, including at least a few sessions on sexism in the professions and even the occasional consciousness raising group, might make some sort of beginning.

Further Reading

Andrews G and Hadzi-Pavlovic D, 'The Work of Australian Psychiatrists Circa 1986', *Australian and New Zealand Journal of Psychiatry*, 1988, Vol 22, pp 153–65.

Fitzgerald Zelda, *Save Me The Waltz*, Scribner's NY, 1932 and Sollen Illinois, UP, 1976.

Goldner V, 'Feminism and Family Therapy', *Family Process*, Vol 24, 1985, pp 31–47.

Ilich Ivan, *Gender*, Marion Bryans, London, 1983.

Millet Kate, *Sexual Politics*, Doubleday and Co, New York, 1970.

Penfold P Susan and Walker Gillian A, *Women and the Psychiatric Paradox*, Open University Press, London, 1984.

Savage Wendy, *A Savage Enquiry. Who Controls Childbirth?*, Virago Press, London, 1986.

Showalter Elaine, *The Female Malady: Women, Madness and English Culture, 1830–1980*, Virago Press Ltd, London 1987.

Spender Dale (ed), *Feminist Theorists. Three Centuries of Women's Intellectual Traditions*, The Women's Press Ltd, London, 1983.

Chapter 52

Immunology and Mental Illness

D Silove

For centuries, physicians have observed that emotional stress seemed to play an important role in the causation of physical disease. However, resistence to a 'psychosomatic' view of illness is still strong amongst some Western medical practitioners and this stems partly from the philosophical tradition known as 'Cartesian Dualism'. Rene Descartes, a seventeenth century philosopher, proposed that the universe is divided into two types of reality, the spiritual and the physical. He argued that mental phenomena such as thinking and feeling are aspects of the spiritual world and are therefore the domain of religion, while the body forms part of the physical world which is accessible to scientific investigation. Most non-Western cultures do not recognise a dichotomy between body and mind, so that their traditional healers commonly use 'holistic' approaches to treatment which combine physical and spiritual interventions. In Western medicine, some doctors retain a 'dualistic' attitude and are skeptical of claims that stress (a psychological phenomenon) may be related to the onset and course of physical illness, even though the modern public increasingly seek out 'holistic' treatments for their ailments.

Immunity and stress

Earlier this century, researchers described two universal physiological responses to stress, the 'flight and fright' response to acute challenges, and the 'general adaptation response' to chronic stress. Nevertheless, it is still unclear whether persons who suffer these somatic stress reactions are at increased risk of major illnesses such as cancer or coronary artery disease. Recent developments in the field of psycho-immunology are therefore of particular interest as they may clarify some of the more *specific* psychophysiological processes whereby stress predisposes the body to illness.

The notion that stress can impair the body's resistance to disease is intuitively attractive. It is commonplace for people to blame a bout of influenza on being 'under pressure', 'run down' and having 'low resistance'. Recently, it has become clear that there are complex interactions involving the neuro-endocrine, immune and central nervous systems (CNS), indicating the presence of pathways via which emotions may influence the body's defence against disease. A number of clinical observations provide support for a link between the immune system and states of psychological disturbance. It has been noted for many years that some diseases which have a basis in altered immune functions such as systemic lupus erythematosis can have important effects on the central nervous system resulting in psychological symptoms. Certain types of depression are associated with hormonal changes such as elevations in cortisol responses which may, in turn, result in suppression of the immune response. Infections involving the CNS such as herpes simplex encephalitis, neurosyphilis, encephalitis lethargica and even influenza, may be accompanied by psychiatric symptoms and the human immunodeficiency virus (HIV) which is responsible for AIDS, causes both immunosuppression and brain disorders in which psychological disturbance is common.

Finally, studies on laboratory animals have suggested that stress can result in impairment of immune function and thereby increases the organism's vulnerability to physical disease.

The immune system serves a number of functions including the protection of the body against foreign invaders such as bacteria and viruses, the elimination of abnormal elements such as cancer cells, the rejection of foreign tissue grafts, and the mediation of allergic reactions. More detailed reviews of the immune system and its regulation are provided by O'Donnell et al, and Calabreze et al.

Immunity and psychiatric illness

1. Schizophrenia

Schizophrenia affects approximately one per cent of the population and is one of the most perplexing and disabling illnesses in psychiatry. A number of epidemiological observations have led researchers to suspect a possible infective or immunological cause for the illness. Schizophrenia-like syndromes have been observed in patients suffering from infections such as virus encephalitis and neurosyphilis as well as in auto-immune diseases such as systemic lupus erythematosis. Furthermore, patients at risk for schizophrenia are more likely to be born in the winter months when viral infections are endemic. This observation suggests that neonates born during winter may be at increased risk of viral infections which may affect the CNS, or alternatively, that foetuses conceived in winter are at greater risk of infection *in utero* because of a seasonal increase of virus infections amongst newly pregnant women. A contagious aetiology for schizophrenia is further suggested by the observation that the illness may have been rare before the nineteenth century and was apparently unknown in many parts of the world until it was putatively 'spread' by European colonisation. The pattern of variability of the condition and its onset in late adolescence and early adult life is similar to that found in some other disorders such as diabetes mellitus and thryotoxicosis which are thought to have an auto-immune pathogenesis.

For these reasons, considerable interest was generated by studies undertaken in the 1970s which reported that patients with schizophrenia exhibited increased levels of antibodies to a number of viruses such as cytomegalovirus. More recent studies, however, have failed to confirm these findings or to detect evidence of viral particles in the brains of deceased patients. Furthermore, no firm evidence of an auto-immune process has been found: for example, a recent study was unable to detect anti-brain antibodies in the cerebrospinal fluid (CSF) of patients with schizophrenia. Some recent studies have shown that certain subcategories of lymphocytes may be defective in schizophrenia, resulting in reduced secretion of cytokinese which act as messengers which regulate the immune system.

In summary, the only consistent trend in past research is that patients with schizophrenia appear to have an impairment in some measures of immunocompetence although more recently, preliminary data suggests that there may be more specific abnormalities in particular white blood cells. These deficits in immune components may be aetiologically important, especially if they represent the effects of a perinatal viral infection at a time when the immune system is vulnerable to insult. However, it should also be borne in mind that patients with schizophrenia are more likely to lead disorganised lifestyles both premorbidly and after the onset of their illness, so that they are at greater risk of poor nutrition, unsanitary living circumstances and exposure to drugs, all of which may compromise their immune functions.

It should also be noted that 'slow' viruses may infect the brain without provoking a measurable immune response, so that a CNS infection cannot yet be excluded as a cause of at least some schizophrenia-like illnesses. Specific antibodies to key brain areas resulting in alterations to the activity of neurotransmitters such as dopamine could also result in schizophrenia and these antibodies would be difficult to detect even in cerebrospinal fluid. This possibility would be compatible with the theory that schizophrenia is caused by overstimulation of neurotransmitter receptors in selective brain centres. However, while there are grounds for further investigations into a possible infective or immunological aetiology for schizophrenia, at present, the evidence supporting these causal mechanisms cannot be regarded as strong (see chapter 33).

2. Depression

For centuries, clinicians have suspected that emotional disorders such as severe depression may lead to physical illness and premature death but it is only in the last decade that research has focused on a possible immuno-logical mechanism to explain this association. While there is no evidence of reduced numbers or subtypes of white blood cells in depressed patients, recent studies have shown that depressed patients tend to exhibit a *functional* impairment of immunity reflected by a reduced proliferation of certain white blood cells when stimulated by chemical agents in the laboratory. Older depressed subjects and those with more severe emotional disturb-ances tend to show more marked impairment in immune functions, suggesting that this effect may be associated with a particular type of depressive illness.

Some investigators have suggested that depressed patients are at a greater risk of virus infections especially by the herpes simplex virus. However, exposure to viruses increases with age, and studies which have controlled for age effects have failed to confirm these early findings. It is however known that prolonged periods of lethargy and depression may follow acute illnesses caused by certain infections such as infectious mononucleosis and hepatitis, although the cause of these emotional disturbances remains unknown. Uncertainty persists therefore as to whether common virus infections which may involve the CNS are a primary cause of depression or, conversely, whether the emotional dis-turbance itself undermines immunity so increasing the host's vulnerability to new infections or to the reactivation of latent viruses.

In summary, although recent research suggests a link between depression and impairment in some immune responses, caution needs to be exercised in interpreting this association. Almost all past studies are cross-sectional in design, or have very short follow-up periods. It is unclear, therefore, whether depression is a direct cause of immunosuppression or vice versa. For example, it is possible that virus infections may cause both immunosuppression and depressed mood. Finally, questions remain as to whether the laboratory abnormalities in lymphocyte responsiveness found in depressed persons are clinically significant. Only well-designed longitudinal studies will be able to examine critically whether depressive disorders compromise the immune system to the extent that future health is substantially jeopardised (see chapter 28).

Immunity and physical illness

1. Stress

An important study undertaken in Australia in the 1970s found that men whose wives had recently died from breast cancer showed a reduction in some of their immune responses and two further studies have confirmed the association between immunosuppression and bereavement. These findings are of particular interest because they suggest a possible psychophysiological mechanism to explain the increased rates of illness and death in bereaved spouses. However, it should be noted that increased rates of illness in this group seem to be a result of cardiovascular disease and the role of immunity in this disease in unclear.

More recently, deficits in immune responses have been demonstrated in a variety of populations experiencing acute or chronic life challenges including the stress of examin-ations, loneliness, separations, poor marital relationships and unemployment. It is not only exposure to a stressor, but the person's approach to coping with the life event that appears to influence immune functions. For example, people who feel able to exert control over demanding or threatening situations are more likely to show an adequate or enhanced immune response, while suppression of the immune response is more common in those who respond to adversity in a helpless manner. It has been suggested that the context of the life event, the individual's perception of the stress, as well as the negative effects and style of coping with the challenge, are more important than the adverse event itself in influencing immunomodulation.

As in depression, it seems that it is the functional response of some immune components that is impaired by stress. More recently investigators have shown that students undergoing examinations show a reduction in those white cells which are thought to protect against cancer and invasion by viruses. In a follow-up study, students with stress-induced reductions in these white cells were at greatest risk of contracting virus infections in the months after examinations. These findings are of great interest because they suggest that stress-induced suppression of immunity may have important clinical consequences.

2. Coping and cancer

Psycho-immunologists are particularly interested in cancer because immune mechanisms are thought to be important in combating the spread of neoplastic cells in the body. There is evidence that the way people cope when they develop cancer can influence the duration of their survival. In one particular study, recently diagnosed breast cancer patients were classified according to one of four psychological response patterns, namely a determination to overcome the disease ('fighting spirit' group), an avoidance of the truth ('denial' group), a 'stiff upper lip' response ('stoic acceptors'), and a powerless, giving up attitude ('helpless–hopeless' group). Those who initially showed a 'fighting spirit' or defence of 'denial' experienced longer disease-free follow-up periods compared to those who showed an attitude of 'stoical acceptance' or 'hopeless-helplessness'.

However, there is still some uncertainty about the range of coping mechanisms which are adaptive or otherwise in cancer sufferers. For example, the use of the defence of denial appears to be beneficial for some patients, but a more extreme form of denial ('anxious denial') is associated with poor adjustment and may have adverse effects on disease outcome.

Important questions still remain concerning the definition and measurement of adaptive coping mechanisms in cancer patients. Nevertheless, recent research does suggest that the way people cope with cancer can influence the course of their illness, and that psycho-immunological mechanisms may be implicated.

Conclusion

The last decade has seen an upsurge of interest in psycho-immunology and preliminary data suggests that further examination of the relationship between emotion and immunity is warranted. Questions which need to be examined more closely include whether the immune deficits demonstrated in depression and other states of psychological distress are severe enough to impair physical health over time. Even though the implementation of longitudinal studies is difficult, such studies are crucial in order to show a clear causal link between psychological stress, immuno-suppression and the course of physical illness. As an example, an interesting question is whether styles of coping can modify the immunosuppression associated with AIDS and thereby alter patients' survival times.

Of further interest is whether the immune response can be actively manipulated by psychological interventions. Laboratory studies have demonstated that rats can be conditioned to suppress their immune responses, but uncertainty still persists as to whether the immune system of humans can be conditioned in a similar way. Speculation continues as to whether the human's immune response may be enhanced by specific psychological interventions such as meditation, relaxation training and visualisation, all of which have been used in the treatment of patients suffering from cancer. Some preliminary case-control studies involving students under stress and elderly residents of institutions have suggested that relaxation therapy can contribute to maintaining an adequate level of immune function under stress. While there is no doubt that stress-reduction techniques can improve the quality of life of patients with serious illnesses, much further work needs to be undertaken before it will be possible to claim that psychological treatments can predictably enhance immunity and thereby improve the outcome of serious illness such as cancer.

Clinical practice depends not only on scientifically verified data but also on the legacy of medical experience which has accrued over decades. While the notion that stress is an important factor in illness has stood the test of time, it is important for medical science to define the actual mechanisms which mediate these effects. In the meantime, health personnel need to maintain a critical perspective when assessing the practices of healers who claim overwhelming success in curing serious physical disease with psychological interventions. Apart from the absence of scientific data to support the efficacy of many of these treatments, patients who invest all their faith in these treatments may suffer adverse consequences. Guilt may be induced by the conviction that their previous 'faulty' lifestyles caused their illness and they may shun orthodox treatments which are vital to their chances of survival. Most seriously, they may suffer a profound sense of failure if their illnesses deteriorate despite their best efforts to adopt the positive coping styles prescribed by their healers.

It is therefore essential that psychosomatic medicine should develop into a truly scientific discipline by subjecting its hypotheses to rigorous testing, and as a new discipline within the psychosomatic tradition, psychoimmunology may help to give further direction to this endeavour. Psychiatry and immunology are both rapidly growing sciences, and in the next few decades, the combined strengths of the two disciplines may bring us closer to the goal of understanding more clearly the complex relationships involving mind, body and disease.

Further Readings

Kiecolt-Glaser J K and Glaser R, 'Psychological Influences on Immunity', *Psychosomatics*, Vol 27, 1986, pp 621–4.

King D J and Cooper S J, 'Viruses, Immunity and Mental Disorder', *British Journal of Psychiatry*, Vol 154, 1989, pp 1–7.

Levy M, VanDyke L, Temoshok L and Zegram L, *Emotions in Health and Illness: Applications to Clinical Practice*, Grune and Stratton, New York, 1983.

O'Donnell M, Silove D and Wakefield D, 'Current Perspectives on Immunology and Psychiatry', *Australian and New Zealand Journal of Psychiatry*, Vol 22, 1988, pp 366–82.

Tecoma E S and Huey L Y, 'Psychic Distress and the Immune System', *Life Sciences*, Vol 36 No 19, 1985, pp 1799–812.

Chapter 53

AIDS 1: In Children and Adolescents

B G H Waters and J B Ziegler

AIDS

Acquired Immunodeficiency Syndrome (AIDS) is caused by the human immunodeficiency virus (HIV). It is estimated that there are currently 5-10 million people in the world who are HIV seropositive, and that by 1991, 0.5-1.5 million people will have died from, or will be suffering from AIDS.

Fortunately, HIV is not highly infectious. It is very fragile outside the human body and is difficult to transmit from person to person. However, when introduced into the body it can eventually have devastating effects. HIV appears to be able to only infect cells which have a protein on their surface called CD4. This is found in greatest quantity on a class of white blood cell called T helper lymphocytes (T cells) which are essential to the development of immune function. Antibody production can only occur with the 'help' of T cells. HIV infection of T cells can lead to their destruction. HIV also infects other blood cells which bear the CD4 molecule on their surface (such as monocytes and macrophages) but it does not destroy them.

When immunodeficiency ensues following infection, susceptibility to viral, fungal and protozoan infections and certain cancers develops. These diseases are referred to as opportunistic, since they are rarely encountered in individuals who have an intact immune system which serves as an effective defence. Very characteristic is a protozoan or single celled organism known as *Pneumocystis Carinii* which causes a severe pneumonia. Kaposi's sarcoma, a cancer-like disorder originating in blood vessels of the skin, has been encountered in homosexual men with AIDS much more frequently than those in other risk groups. When a person with HIV infection has an opportunistic infection or cancer, the term AIDS may be applied. Some of the problems of severe HIV infection appear to result directly from the effects of HIV itself, though the best recognised are certainly consequences of immune dysfunction. The nervous system is often affected, especially the brain. Many people suffer an acute viral meningitis or encephalitis shortly after being infected; later a progressive from of brain damage may ensue. Some studies have indicated some degree of brain damage in almost all HIV infected people by the time AIDS develops.

Features of HIV infection including AIDS in children

Babies infected with HIV *in utero* may have small head size. Lymph node enlargement may be noted at birth or at any time subsequently. An acute viral syndrome characterised by fever, sore throat, rash and diarrhoea may occur in about half of adults at the time of seroconversion, but is rarely seen in young children. In children, developmental delay may occur; characteristically intellectual and motor development will be arrested in the second year of life.

Opportunistic infection with organisms otherwise rarely associated with serious illness is the hallmark of advanced HIV infection in older teenagers and adults. In children, failure-to-thrive, chronic diarrhoea, and frequent bacterial respiratoray infections with slow response to appropriate therapy are characteristic. Lymphoid proliferation may be striking in children. Lymph gland, liver and spleen enlargement may occur and is reflected in the elevation of immunoglobulin (antibody protein) levels in blood, though paradoxically antibody function is poor. A bleeding tendency due to reduced numbers of blood platelets may also be a manifestation of the hyperimmuno-globulinaemic state.

Diagnosis is difficult in infants of HIV-infected mothers, since these babies will be born with HIV antibodies passively acquired transplacentally, whether or not HIV infection has occurred. Perhaps two thirds of such infants will turn out to have escaped infection. Diagnosis of HIV infection can be made if: (i) HIV antibodies persist well into the second year of life (by which time, passively acquired maternal antibody will have disappeared); (ii) HIV antigen can be detected; (iii) virus culture is positive; (iv) immunodeficiency develops; or (v) characteristic clinical features develop. Improved diagnosis using molecular bioloigcal techniques to identify viral genes is currently in development.

Management of symptomatic HIV infection

Early diagnosis of HIV related infection will allow appropriate management. Once immunodeficiency is recognised, prophylaxis for bacterial and viral infections with intravenous gammaglobulin may be recommended. Lung infection with *Pneumocystis Carinii* is considered inevitable once profound immunodeficiency develops. Long term prophylaxis with co-trimoxazole is used to prevent this.

The only antiviral drug in use which is directly active against HIV is zidovudine (AZT). This drug can delay the appearance of opportunistic infection and produce prolongation of survival with improved quality of life. Its toxicity, particularly haematological, has limited its use. Some children quickly gain up to 20 per cent body weight and return to school with AZT. The financial cost however, can run to several thousand dollars per year per patient.

Intellectual function has been reported to improve and this has been attributed to control by the drug of the neurological HIV infection.

Prevention remains the most important measure to control the HIV problem. As a vaccine is not available, control of risk behaviour and associated transmission co-factors (for example, genital ulceration) is critical. Prevention of HIV in children is now dependent on the control of heterosexual spread of the virus and modification of IV needle sharing practices. Introduction of testing of donated blood in third world countries is also of paramount importance.

Transmission of HIV virus

The methods by which HIV can be spread from person to person are as follows:

1. Sexual intercourse with a person who is infected with HIV

AIDS is a sexually transmitted (venereal) disease. Semen and vaginal secretions can transmit HIV. Although sexual transmission of HIV has been more common among homosexual men than among heterosexuals in Western countries, the cases of HIV transmission occurring between heterosexuals during sexual intercourse are gradually increasing. There is a higher risk of transmission during anal intercourse than during vaginal intercourse. As in the case of other sexually transmissible diseases, the proper use of condoms reduces the risk of transmission but they are not 100 per cent effective. Adolescents may not like using condoms.

2. Sharing drug needles with an infected person

Sharing an IV (intravenous) drug needle with an infected person can inject the virus directly into the user's bloodstream. The incidence of HIV infection among IV drug users has risen several fold in the past two years. Needle use transmission is not limited to drug addicts. Occasional or 'recreational' use of intravenous drugs is more common than is generally supposed, and can be the basis for needle transmission of HIV.

3. Injection of contaminated blood products, such as in blood transfusions

This method of transmission is now extremely rare in most Western countries because of blood-screening programs put into place in 1985. No one has ever contracted AIDS through donating blood.

4. A woman infected with HIV who becomes pregnant or breast feeds can pass the virus to the baby

Such a woman may have no symptoms of AIDS, and may only become aware of her infection because of her baby's condition. This is becoming an increasing problem in the families of IV drug users, where the mother or her sexual partner may be the drug user.

5. Transmission to children and adolescents

Children and adolescents have been infected by intravenous injection of contaminated blood or blood products, from mother to infant or from unprotected sexual activity with an HIV positive partner. In Australia, exposure to contaminated blood occurred between 1980 and April 1985, mainly when potentially infected multiple transfusions or blood products were unwittingly administered to children and adolescents who fell into the following groups: ill premature infants, and children and adolescents suffering from chronic blood disorders (leukaemia, haemo-globinopathies, haemophilia) and other chronic illnesses. The proportion of trans-fusion related HIV infection has been several times higher in Australia than in the United States.

Infants have been infected either by trans-mission from an infected mother with adult risk factors (IV drug abuse, heterosexual contact or transfusion) or via an infected transfusion. More than three-quarters of infants with AIDS in the United States have acquired the virus from their mother, whereas in Australia, the predominant route of transmission has been via blood transfusions. However, a predominant pattern of maternal transmission will develop here as HIV infects more women of child-bearing age (particularly IV drug users).

Pre-school and older children have usually been infected from contaminated blood products, but sexual assault by an HIV sero-positive perpetrator would also convey risk, particularly since trauma to the ano-genital region is likely and provides a more ready avenue for infection.

While about 10–30 per cent of adults infected with HIV develop full-blown AIDS within five years, symptomatic infection or full-blown AIDS appears to occur more frequently in young infected children. Teenagers are also vulnerable to unprotected sex with an HIV positive partner or IV use of HIV contaminated needles. In fact, about three quarters of older adolescents in Australia (17–19 years) who are seropositive are either homosexual or IV drug users.

Neuropsychiatric disorders in young patients

Neurological complications are frequent in AIDS, so brain disorders affecting behaviour, emotions, intellect and perception can be anticipated. They may be evident in earlier stages of illness by the presence of subtle memory, intellectual and perceptual changes. Most CNS disorders such as encephalitis, meningitis, and progressive encephalopathy which lead to dementia, movement disorders and paralysis, herald a terminal course and are extremely disabling diseases. However, early memory and perceptual changes can be expected to occur in some otherwise well children who are attending school. There, they may represent a significant new handicap. Regular intellectual and perceptual testing may be necessary to identify early brain disorder and to enable appropriate educational support to be initiated. The HIV may also influence parts of the brain which moderate mood and affect, leading to neurologically based disorders of these emotions which amplify the problems arising from the numerous social stresses faced by these young people and their families. In fact it is well known that children with generalised neurological disorders are at increased risk of most psychiatric disorders, and this is known to be greater if there are concurrent psychosocial stresses.

Coping with HIV infection

HIV infection is a chronic illness which often occurs against a back-drop of pre-existing adversity. There is an extensive literature on the psychosocial consequences of chronic illness in childhood and adolescence. While some families are severely stressed by chronic illness, many cope well even with ultimately fatal disorders. Factors which predict adequate coping are family cohesion, the capacity of the family to adapt satisfactorily to change, and the presence of an adequate family support network.

Many HIV seropositive children and adolescents are already at psychosocial risk before being infected with HIV—some through pre-existing illness and some through pre-existing psychosocial adversity. Those who were infected by transfusion, usually suffered from prematurity or a chronic or severe medical disorder. Transmission from the mother confers additional vulnerability due to the stresses of having a chronically ill mother or a mother who is or was drug addicted and/or working as a prostitute. Adolescents who acquired HIV sexually or by IV drug abuse are likely to be socially disadvantaged and estranged from their family. Homosexual adolescents often have a very supportive gay network to fall back on, but IV drug users usually do not have an adequate support network.

Children at different developmental stages can be expected to be sensitive to different aspects of psychosocial adversity. Pre-school children know little about AIDS but may be influenced indirectly by the changes in family life and family cohesion following the diagnosis. School-aged children are aware of AIDS but are most affected by exclusion from peer groups, and effects on their family. Adolescents have to come to grips with family and peer relationships, as well as limitations on sexual activities imposed by the order and the possibility of discrimination and prejudice due to assumptions about how they contracted the virus. Many seropositive older adolescents are homosexual or IV drug users. A major implication of HIV infection for them is the extent to which it weakens their personal relationships and support network.

Nevertheless, many HIV patients and their families are extraordinarily resilient. This may be because they are often confronting AIDS after they have already had to cope with a severe and life threatening chronic illness. They have an established array of coping skills and support networks. Rather than being rendered more vulnerable by their earlier illness, many appear to be capable of taking the ominous implications of AIDS in their stride. On the other hand, those families where a parent was a drug addict or working as a prostitute, have coped poorly. In addition, the well publicised experiences of some HIV infected adults and problems with school placement and community discrimination experienced by some HIV infected children indicate the considerable psychosocial risks associated with HIV infection. As a result of the anticipated psychosocial and neuropsychiatric risks, a psychiatric assessment should be routine for all children and their families who are HIV seropositive.

Counselling needs

HIV patients and their families, where relevant, should be considered as possibly needing some counselling. Many simply require clarification of issues in a confidential atmosphere. Others will require ongoing support and for a few, more intensive counselling involving individual counselling or family sessions will be necessary. In principle, the treating doctor should be prepared to provide a range of counselling through all stages of HIV infection—from diagnosis, during symptomatic stages and during terminal stages.

At initial counselling sessions, awareness about AIDS should be established. This includes the nature of the illness, its modes of transmission and its prevention, fears about contagion, and the social consequences of wide disclosure. Correct information should be supplied where necessary. Sources of stress unique to the family (for example, material disadvantages, marital discord etc) should be identified as should the family's strengths and coping skills. Many young HIV patients and their families require a range of psychosocial interventions. Basic fact finding and education is usually required to deal with irrational sources of anxiety. The family must be guaranteed confidentiality within the medical network and advised about the appropriate level of confidentiality for their family in their community. Counselling of children, teenagers and family members should deal with depression over the uncertain future or ostracism. Some infected teenagers are so enraged that they may wish to deliberately spread the virus sexually, and angry parents of a transfusion victim may blame the medical establishment. Individual and group counselling can assist teenagers to realise they are not alone, and help build up a support network to reduce their strong sense of isolation. Marital and family counselling often has to deal with pre-existing conflicts which have been heightened by the current crisis. Information and advocacy for appropriate medical and social welfare support services is usually necessary. Finally, with the death of the child or parent, there is a need for grief counselling.

Ethical issues with HIV positive children

The complex psychosocial issues contribute to a formidable dilemma for the doctor and other carers who must help to find a balance between the rights of the pre-school or school aged child (to access to education, protection from discrimination and victimisation, and confidentiality), the rights of their family (to privacy), and the rights of peers and school staff or workmates (to protection from HIV infection).

Health, welfare and educational bodies have attempted to strike a balance between the remote possibility of HIV transmission in the school environment, and protection of HIV infected children from discrimination by formulating policy statements on school attendance. The Australian College of Paediatrics has recommended that HIV infected children will usually be able to attend pre-school or school and that a limited number of selected staff should be informed of the circumstances. Although HIV is present in saliva, tears, urine and bowel motions, no transmission via them has been proven.

Transmission via contact with blood from cuts etc or from bite wounds is also feared, and is a potential risk. Rules about school attendance must be geared to protect both healthy children and the immune deficient HIV seropositive child. In the case of school children, in order to not breach confidence, the carers should be aware whom on the staff has been informed of the diagnosis and to whom they can transmit information. While questions of school attendance are usually settled between the parents and the school with appropriate medical advice from the physician, it is important to remember that parents are not obliged to inform the school that their child is HIV seropositive. However, if the child has open exuding skin lesions or is biting other children, then the physician may have no choice but to consider informing the school principal, despite the parents' wishes.

HIV positive adolescents can also pose considerable ethical dilemmas such as: should their parents be advised of the diagnosis if the teenager has not done so and he is living at home? Should the sexual partner or either family be advised, particularly if the teenager or partner is aged under 16 years?

AIDS education

Although awareness about AIDS has increased dramatically in the last five years, there are many in the community who remain uninformed, misinformed and confused. Ignorance and misconceptions are held by teenagers in particular. The risk-related behaviours of some teenagers puts them directly in the path of the AIDS epidemic. Indeed, certain subgroups form bridges from those currently infected to a larger subgroup of young people. In New York city, heterosexual transmission is more widespread among teenagers (15 per cent) than among adults (6 per cent). Moreover, sexually active teenagers generally have a higher prevalence of sexually transmitted diseases than do adults. As the risk of HIV transmission by vaginal intercourse increases in Australia, then, the increase may well be most striking among sexually active youth.

Education is also needed to reduce prejudice and discrimination directed towards

HIV seropositive persons and AIDS patients. Providing accurate information about HIV and AIDS, and establishing a safe lifestyle prior to teenagers becoming sexually active, should enable them to carry these values into adult health and sexuality behaviours, and will reduce HIV transmission by, and to, them.

At least half of boys and a third of girls in the final years of high school have had intercourse, and may have had multiple partners. Anal intercourse may be more prevalent than generally believed. For example, 15 per cent of Canadian 18-19 year olds in the Canada Youth and AIDS Study had experienced anal intercourse. Many teenagers do not protect themselves against pregnancy or sexually transmissible diseases. In the United States, one in seven teenagers contracts a sexually transmissible disease annually, only one third of sexually active teenagers use contraception regularly, and less than one quarter of those who use contraception, use condoms. It is likely that the behaviour of Australian teenagers is closely comparable.

As many as 5 per cent of teenagers may be homosexual or bisexual. About 4000 Australian teenagers run away from home each year and many of these become involved in drug use, prostitution and drug trafficking. While intravenous drug use has been uncommon among Australian teenagers, the rate of HIV infection among those who use IV drugs is now increasing rapidly.

Teenagers who use IV drugs, or are gay or bisexual, or are homeless, or are involved in prostitution, should all be considered target groups for special efforts that will help them develop safer sexual and drug use behaviours. The urgency may be greatest in the inner city areas of larger cities.

Despite government education programs, many teenagers lack basic thorough knowledge about the transmission of, and protection against, HIV infection. Most Australian youth AIDS education programs have focused on young people attending secondary school. Other Australian programs have targeted young IV drug users and those regarded to be at risk through IV drug use. Only about one third of Australian youth have received the school-based programs, and few

of the widely distributed information pamphlets produced by national and State bodies are seen by youth as relevant to them. Very few of the programs or materials have been carefully evaluated to measure their effectiveness.

In most industrialised nations, awareness of AIDS by teenagers is very high (90-95 per cent), but many factual misconceptions still abound, and there is little evidence so far of major shifts in target behaviour among most heterosexual youth. This is in marked contrast to homosexual youth and some heterosexual youth living in high risk HIV prevalence areas who seem to have got the message.

Content of education program

HIV infection and AIDS are social and health problems. Simply providing young people with the facts is not sufficient. They need the opportunity to clarify their values, practise decision making and communication skills and learn to resist peer pressures to be sexually active and to use drugs. There is a need to establish a new peer group norm which emphasises harm reduction and endorses self-protective and safe sexual behaviour. However it is a misguided task to make sex itself unpopular, especially for adolescents.

There are three steps in effective AIDS prevention education for adolescents. Each step has sub-goals. Strategies to achieve each goal differ between risk groups (high/low risk) and between subgroups of youth (for example, rural/urban, employed/unemployed).

To be effective and achieve its goals, the program content must be relevant to the target group, the strategy must engage them, and linked components of the campaign must be introduced in an integrated way. Unfortunately however, youth have rarely been consulted, so materials of little credibility among youth have been introduced in ways which are not congruent with their lifestyles.

A shared responsibility

A number of surveys indicate that young people do see adults as important sources of AIDS information, and they wish to share responsibility for AIDS prevention with adults—parents, educators, churches, community agencies, youth-serving agencies, health services, and the private sector. Youths' responsibility includes participation in the consultation process which will yield materials and strategies about AIDS which are relevant to their values and lifestyles. Peer education and peer support groups are also valuable strategies, especially among high risk teenagers. A key responsibility of adults is to coordinate planning and implementation of programs at a national and regional level through organisations such as AIDS Councils. At a local level they must actively promote youth AIDS education, and ensure that it takes place in their community, from primary school onwards. This applies particularly to parents of young people at school, many of whom erroneously believe that their children are not sexually active or using drugs. They are well placed to contribute to the development of materials, and also to lobby schools and educational authorities to ensure that AIDS education programs are implemented in their children's schools. Community support and participation was the key difference in a United States teenage pregnancy prevention program that actually worked!

Agencies which offer a range of community services and are concerned with the overall well-being of youth, are ideally positioned to integrate AIDS education into their programs. Often they are the only consistent adult contacts for youth at highest risk. The same is true of youth health care providers. They should offer education and counselling on AIDS to their clients who are, or may soon be, sexually active. All young clients seeking contraceptive advice should be counselled about the risk of HIV infection and each individual client's risk of sexually transmitted diseases and HIV infection should be assessed. Health delivery services should also coordinate the distribution of condoms, water-based lubricants, bleach, and sterile needles and syringes.

Further Reading

American Academy of Paediatrics: Committee of School Health, Committee on Infectious Diseases, 'School Attendance of Children and Adolescents with Human T Lymphotropic Virus III/lymphadenopathy Associated Virus Infection', *Pediatrics*, Vol 77, 1986, pp 430-2.
Barbour, S D, 'Acquired Immunodeficiency Syndrome of Childhood', *Pediatric Clinics of North America*, Vol 34, 1987, pp 247-68.
Belman A L, Ultman M H, Horoupian D, Novic B, Spiro A J, Rubenstein A, Kurtzber D and Cone-Wesson B, 'Neurological Complications in Infants and Children with Acquired Immune Deficiency Syndrome', *Annals of Neurology*, Vol 18, 1985, pp 560-6.
Waters B, Ziegler J B, Hampson R and McPherson A H, 'The Psychosocial Consequences of Childhood Infection with Human Immunodeficiency Virus', *Medical Journal of Australia*, Vol 149, 1988, pp 198-202.

Chapter 54

AIDS 2: In Adults

F K Judd and B A Biggs

Since 1981, over 150,000 cases of AIDS have been reported world wide (Table 1). It is likely that many cases remain unreported. Transmission of HIV in Australia has occurred primarily by genital sexual contact (particularly anal intercourse) and through parenteral exposure to blood especially by needle sharing amongst intravenous drug users. Transmission by transfusion of blood or blood products and perinatal transmission from mother to child have also been documented. There is no evidence of casual household or vector-borne transmission. The virology of HIV is described in another section (see chapter 53).

Table 1. AIDS cases reported to WHO as of 30 April 1989 (WHO 1989)

Americas	105,612
Africa	23,262
Europe	21,136
Oceania	1,411
Asia	369
World total	151,790

Clinical features

AIDS was originally defined as 'the presence of reliably diagnosed disease suggestive of underlying cellular immune deficiency (Kaposi's sarcoma in patients under 60 years old; *pneumocystis carinii* or other opportunistic infections) in the absence of known causes of immunodeficiency such as immunosuppressive therapy or previous malignancy'. This clinical description predated knowledge

and identification of the causative agent HIV. In mid-1986 The Centre for Disease Control (CDC) issued a new classification of AIDS and its related conditions, based on HIV culture or seropositivity and detailed clinical description of the later stages of the illness. This classification of HIV infection is shown in Table 2. The common manifestations of AIDS are shown in Table 3.

Table 2. Modification of the CDC surveillance case definition for AIDS (CDC 1986)

Stage	Description
I	*Acute infection*
II	*Asymptomatic infection*
III	*Persistent generalised lymphadenopathy*
IV	*Other diseases*
A	Constitutional disease: fever, diarrhoea > 1 month weight loss > 10% body weight
B	Neurological disease
C	Secondary infectious disease
D	Secondary cancers: (eg Kaposi's sarcoma, lymphoma)
E	Other conditions (eg chronic lymphoid interstitial pneumonitis)

Neurological manifestations

Up to 50 per cent of AIDS patients have neurological symptoms at some time during their illness and at least 80 per cent show morphological abnormalities of the nervous

Table 3. Common clinical manifestations in AIDS

Opportunistic infections	Usual symptoms and signs
Pneumocystis carinii	dry cough, fever, shortness of breath, tachypnoea, cyanosis
Cerebral toxoplasmosis	seizures, focal neuro-logical signs, meningeal symptoms, confusions, coma, psychosis
Candida albicans	mucocutaneous infection of oropharynx, oesophagus, vagina
Cryptoccus neoformans	headache, fever, meningeal symptoms
Mycobacterium avium complex	non specific symptoms—fever, anorexia, weight loss, malaise, abdominal pain, diarrhoea
Cytomegalovirus	retinitis, gastrointestinal disease, pneumonitis, encephalitis
Malignancies	
Kaposi's sarcoma	multiple purplish plaque-like and nodular lesions, less commonly gastro-intestinal and other organ involvement
Non-Hodgkin's lymphoma	primary CNS lymphoma—confusion, memory loss, focal neurological signs advanced extralymphatic disease

system. Most frequently cerebral involvement is due to opportunistic infection, but primary lymphoma, secondary spread from systemic lymphoma or kaposi's sarcoma and a variety of other pathological lesions may be detected (Table 4).Direct infection of the nervous system by HIV predominately involves the hemisphere white matter. This appears as either a diffuse leucoencephalopathy with severe loss of myelin or more circumscribed, often necrotic, areas of demyelination. Central nervous system (CNS) involvement by HIV

may occur at various stages of the illness:

1. *Early symptomatic infection* (CDC stage I and II) appears to be uncommon, but when it occurs, clinical features include headache, encephalitis, aseptic meningitis, ataxia and myelopathy. Symptoms are usually indistinguishable from other acute viral illnesses and resolve in a few weeks.

2. *Early asymptomatic infection* is apparently common. Virus, viral antigens, inflammatory cell response and local synthesis of HIV-I antibody, have all been detected in the CNS of asymptomatic patients.

3. *Aseptic meningitis* may occur in CDC Stage I illness, or later, usually in CDC Stage III or IV infection.

4. *Organic mental disorders* may occur at varying times in the course of the illness. The incidence of organic mental disorders is presumed to be high. They include:

(a) *Delerium* is the most common. Multiple factors may be implicated in the causation of delerium including primary cerebral pathology (for example, infection, neoplastic, vascular), secondary cerebral effects of systemic illness (for example, hypoxia, metabolic factors, systemic infection) or iatrogenic factors particularly drug induced delerium and sensory deprivation (see chapter 41).

(b) *AIDS dementia complex* (ADC) generally occurs in stage IV infection. The incidence is uncertain. Available studies suggest ADC occurs in approximately $1/3$ of patients with neurological complications and $2/3$ of autopsied patients with AIDS. Clinical features result from impairment of cognitive, motor and behavioural function (Table 5). The onset of dementia is usually insidious and the rate of progression is variable (2–7 months). Death from aspiration pneumonia or systemic opportunistic infection usually follows severe dementia. Neuropsychological testing reveals a 'subcortical pattern' of dementia. Computerised tomography (CT) scan may show variable degree of cortical atrophy accompanied by ventricular dilatation and magnetic resonance imaging (MRI) may be useful for detection of white matter lesions. Positron Emission Tomography has demonstrated consistently abnormal patterns of regional cerebral glucose metabolism in patients with ADC.

Coping with AIDS

Many factors make coping with HIV infection difficult. It has an unpredictable clinical course, but overall a uniformly poor prognosis. It is not only debilitating, but also disfiguring. Negative interpersonal and societal reactions to news of the diagnosis are common, resulting in both loss of support and discrimination. There is no definitive treatment.

Nevertheless, the difficulties of coping with HIV infection have been likened to those of patients with other fatal illnesses. Nichols has suggested that the coping process can be conveniently divided into four stages: initial crisis, transitional state, acceptance and preparation for death. The initial crisis is characterised by alternating periods of denial and anxiety and, unless denial is excessive, is generally an adaptive response to the crisis. The transitional state whose usual features are anger, guilt, self pity and anxiety may be particularly distressing to both the patient and his family. The acceptance phase leads to changes in lifestyle and acknowledgment of the restrictions imposed by the illness. Final adjustment requires preparation for death.

AIDS organisations providing voluntary care have developed in Australia and overseas to address the various needs of people infected with HIV. Volunteer care may be provided through informal networks of family, lovers and friends, or by voluntary organisations or by a combination of these. In Australia soon after the first cases of AIDS were diagnosed, support groups were formed by members of the homosexual community to provide financial assistance and care for those affected by AIDS. Subsequently a number of community based AIDS organisations have been established. The services provided by these organisations vary but include practical home care and support for people with AIDS, for

Table 4. CNS complications of HIV infection

Meningitis	• HIV infection • Opportunistic infection—crytococcal, tuberculosis • Neoplastic–lymphoma
Diffuse brain disease	• Encephalitis—HIV • Herpes simplex, toxoplasmosis, cytomegalovirus • Metabolic encephalopathy • AIDS dementia complex
Focal brain disease	• Infection—toxoplasmosis, cryptococcus, tuberculosis • Herpes simplex • Cerebral lymphoma • Progressive multifocal leucoencephalopathy • Vascular disorders
Myelopathies	
Peripheral neuropathy	

Table 5. Clinical features of AIDS dementia complex

	Cognitive	*Behavioural*	*Motor*
Early	Forgetfulness Loss of concentration Mental slowness	Apathy Social withdrawal Irritability Emotional lability	Loss of balance Leg weakness Poor coordination
Late	Severe global dysfunction Confabulation Distractibility	Psychomotor retardation Akinetic state/mutism Agitation Socially inappropriate behaviour	Ataxia Hypertonia Urinary & faecal incontinence Myoclonus Tremor Seizures Frontal release signs

example, shopping, cleaning, gardening, cooking etc, emotional support and financial assistance.

AIDS and psychiatric illness

1. Adjustment disorder

Adjustment disorder is the most common psychiatric diagnosis amongst individuals with HIV infection who are referred for psychiatric assessment. The majority of patients with an adjustment disorder are depressed, but other common symptoms include anxiety, disturbance of conduct and hypochondriacal preoccupation.

2. Depressive illness

Depressed mood has been reported in up to 80 per cent of patients with AIDS, however only approximately 20 per cent suffer from a depressive illness. Suicidal ideation appears to be common amongst patients with AIDS. Suicide attempts were initially thought to be uncommon, however, it is suggested that they are increasingly more frequent (see chapters 25, 28 and 29).

3. Mania

Episodes of mania have been reported in patients with HIV infection, both with and without cognitive dysfunction. In both instances it is likely that hypomanic symptoms are due to the neurotropic effects of HIV. In addition, mania has been reported in AIDS patients with cryptococcal meningitis and in those receiving zidovudine (AZT) treatment (see chapter 28).

4. Schizophrenia-like psychoses

Paranoid psychoses, whose clinical features are indistinguishable from schizophrenia, have also been reported in AIDS patients (see chapter 33).

Excessive and unrealistic fear of AIDS may be found as a feature of a variety of psychiatric disorders, including obsessive–compulsive and affective disorders, monosymptomatic hypochondriacal delusional states and schizophrenia. In all of these cases it is not AIDS, but the hypochondriacal concerns of the patient which cause the pathology. Thus, terms such as 'AIDS panic', 'AIDophobia', 'The worried well' and 'pseudo AIDS' should be avoided.

Psychological treatment

1. Psychotherapy

Psychotherapeutic treatment generally focuses on themes such as uncertainty regarding the aetiology, course and treatment of the illness, and the required modifications in lifestyle. Specific difficulties coping with the illness, often resulting in anger, depression, fear or acting out must be addressed. Additional distress may result from rejection by or lack of support from friends and family. Conflicts regarding sexual orientation and lifestyle may occur and the illness may be seen as retribution for these. As the disease progresses, increasing losses such as employment, financial difficulties and loss of relationships with others need to be addressed.

Patients require information regarding the nature of the disease, available treatment, and sources of support. Education is required regarding 'safe sex', avoidance of transmission of the illness by intravenous drug use and precautions to prevent transmission of infection to family and household members. Patients require an opportunity to ventilate their feelings and assistance to avoid acting out angry or guilty feelings in self destructive ways. An opportunity to discuss terminal care and death should be available. Intervention with the patient's partner or family and contact with self help groups are often helpful (see chapter 58).

2. Psychotropic medication

Patients with HIV infection who have a depressive illness of moderate or greater severity will require antidepressant medication. Generally, these patients respond to lower than usual doses of medication and also develop side effects with low doses. Anticholinergic effects of antidepressants may exacerbate disorientation or memory impairment, while drying of mucus membranes may increase susceptibility to local infection. At present, tricyclic antidepressants with low anticholinergic activity are recommended. Monoamine oxidase inhibitors should be used with caution as these patients are often taking a variety of other medications. Psychostimulants have also been recommended for depression in this group of patients. Antipsychotic medication is indicated for the treatment of acute psychotic illness or severe behavioural disturbance, but as with antidepressants, should be used with caution. When required, anxiolytics with intermediate half life to avoid drug accumulation should be used (see chapter 56).

Education

The infectious nature of AIDS, its association with sexual and drug taking behaviour and its poor prognosis make prevention of infection a high priority. Suggested measures to minimise infection include education, counselling to prevent infection or further transmission, compulsory treatment, legal sanctions against knowingly transmitting the virus and quarantining infected people. In Australia, most efforts have been directed towards education with emphasis being placed on measures to avoid sexual transmission, transmission through sharing needles and syringes and perinatal transmission.

The promotion of safe sex practices has been fundamental to the general community education program, with emphasis being placed on sexual activity not involving intercourse and the proper use of condoms during intercourse. Strategies to minimise transmission among IV drug users include needle distribution and disposal programs; programs encouraging cleaning used injection equipment, including the use of bleach; improving the accessibility of general health services to IV drug users; and drug substitution programs. Reducing the number of drug users in the community is a long term goal.

Education is also of importance in the support of individuals infected with HIV. Education for infected individuals must address safe sex or safe drug use, general health issues, treatment options, symptom management, life planning, and practical problem solving. Community education needs to address the community's ideas of actual and perceived risks of transmission from domestic, social and occupational contact with HIV infected individuals. Misconceptions, prejudice and fears need to be addressed and corrected, allowing the development of positive and appropriate responses (see chapter 53).

In the 1986-1987 financial year, education programs, together with advertising and public relations accounted for 30 per cent of total government expenditure associated with HIV infection in Australia.

Special issues

The particular features of HIV infection have resulted in debate regarding a variety of ethical and legal issues. The diagnosis of AIDS may have widespread interpersonal, social and occupational deleterious effects. Thus, patients with AIDS are particularly sensitive to issues of confidentiality. Conflicts regarding confidentiality may arise when patients fail to inform or refuse permission for their doctor to inform others (for example, sexual partner, other medical practitioner, dentist) who may be put at risk of acquiring the infection. Following widespread debate many, but not all, professional groups have agreed that all efforts should be made to persuade patients to inform appropriate others, but when this does not occur, it may be ethical for the physician to notify the person whom he believes is in danger of contracting the virus. The groups include the General Medical Council (UK) in 1985 and the American Psychiatric Association in 1987.

The other major ethical debate has been with respect to antibody testing without informed consent. Given the implications of the test result, it has generally been agreed that HIV antibody testing cannot be regarded as 'routine' and testing should not be done without the patient's explicit consent. In some states of Australia, for example, Victoria, this is a legal requirement (Health, General Amendment Act 1988).

Health professionals treating individuals with HIV infection face numerous stresses. These include:

1. Fear of infection. AIDS is a fatal blood borne disease. Medical staff may become

infected following exposure to infected blood, for example, needle stick injuries, cuts to fingers during surgery. Transmission via mucus membrane exposure is far less likely.

2. Issues in sexuality. Heterosexual health care workers many be fearful of homosexual patients, may feel uncomfortable caring for homosexual patients, or may reveal previously concealed anxieties and prejudices regarding homosexuality. Homosexual health care workers may over-identify with or become over-involved with homosexual patients. In addition they may fear stigma or prejudice.

3. Death and dying. Patients with AIDS are generally young, usually have recurrent and lengthy hospitalisations and eventually die despite optimal care. Thus, staff may readily identify with and often develop strong therapeutic relationships with patients. The high death rate may result in repeated grief reactions for staff which, if not adequately dealt with, may lead to depression, feelings of hopelessness and frequent staff changes.

4. Stigma. Health care workers caring for HIV infected patients may experience personal or professional isolation as a result of their wish to care for AIDS patients.

5. Exposure to 'alternative lifestyles'. Working with AIDS patients may expose health care professionals to a variety of unfamiliar situations, ethical and moral dilemmas.

Strategies to deal with these stresses include:

1. education regarding medical, psychosocial, legal and ethical aspects of HIV infection;

2. staff support groups to allow ventilation of feelings and provide reassurance and strategies to deal with distressing emotions;

3. multidisciplinary team meetings are useful for providing feedback to individual team members and allowing an opportunity for effective communication and peer support.

Conclusion

AIDS is a devastating physical illness, with both disfiguring (wasting, skin lesions) and disabling (systemic and cerebral infections and malignancies) symptoms. The syndrome is regarded as having a uniformly poor prognosis and as yet there is no definitive treatment. Initial localisation of the infection to 'high risk groups' such as homosexual men and intravenous drug users has been associated with stigma and prejudice. Psychosocial morbidity may be a reaction to features of the syndrome or may be a direct consequence of cerebral pathology. Psychological intervention with the patient, the patient's family and staff must take a high priority in the treatment of the syndrome.

Further Reading

Centres for Disease Control, 'Classification System for Human T Lymphotropic Virus Type III/Lymphadenopathy Associated Virus Infection', *Morbidity and Mortality Weekly Report*, Vol 35, 1986, pp 334-9.

Gray F, Gherardi R and Scaravilli F, 'The Neuropathology of the Acquired Immune Deficiency Syndrome (AIDS)', *Brain*, Vol III, 1988, pp 245-66.

Judd F K, Biggs B A and Burrows G D, 'Ethical Issues and Acquired Immune Deficiency Syndrome (AIDS)', *Australian and New Zealand Journal of Psychiatry*, Vol 23, 1989, pp 523-8.

Levy R M, Bredesen D E and Rosenblum M L, 'Neurological Manifestations of the Acquired Immune Deficiency Syndrome (AIDS), Experience at UCSF and Review of the Literature', *Journal of Neurosurgery*, Vol 62, 1985, pp 475-95.

Navia B A, Jordan B D and Price R W, 'The AIDS-Dementia Complex: Clinical Features', *Annals of Neurology*, Vol 19, 1986, pp 517-24.

Nichols S E, 'Psychosocial Reactions of Persons with Acquired Immune Deficiency Syndrome', *Annals of Internal Medicine*, Vol 103, 1985, pp 765-7.

Perry S W and Tross S, 'Psychiatric Problems of AIDS Inpatients at the New York Hospital: Preliminary Report', *Public Health Reporter*, Vol 99, 1984, pp 200-5.

Chapter 55

A Parent's Loss:
The Sudden Infant Death Syndrome

S Beal

Sudden infant death syndrome (SIDS), otherwise known as cot death or crib death, is defined as the sudden death of any infant or young child, which is unexpected by history, and in which a thorough post-mortem examination fails to demonstrate an adequate cause of death. In Australia this examination would include full bacteriological and viral studies.

SIDS may be a single disorder or a group of related or unrelated disorders. It could be caused by an inherent problem in the infant, by adverse environmental factors, or by an inherent vulnerability to a combination of environmental conditions.

Sudden unexpected unexplained death can occur at any age but the majority of infants who die are aged between one and six months of age. In the past 17 years in South Australia, two children aged two years could have been classified as SIDS. In the same time 31 one year olds died from SIDS, while 727 infants under 12 months of age died from SIDS. In the age group one month to one year, SIDS is now responsible for more than half the infant deaths that occur. This means that the majority of infant deaths after the first month of life occur at home.

The incidence in most Western countries is about 2 per 1000 live births. Some countries (for example, Sweden) have an incidence of less than 1 per 1000 live births, and some much higher (for example, the South Island of New Zealand greater than 5.0 per 1000 live births).

Australian Aboriginal infants have a higher incidence of SIDS than Caucasian infants living in Australia, as do Negroes in America and Maoris in New Zealand. The incidence in Hispanic infants in California differs with the place of birth of the mother. Hispanic infants whose mothers were born in Mexico have only half the incidence of SIDS when compared with Hispanic infants whose mothers were born in California.

About 10 per cent of infants found unexpectedly dead will have a cause identified by careful history and thorough autopsy. These children will not be classified as SIDS.

Several factors have been found to be associated with SIDS, for example, winter, low socio-economic class and low birth weight. No factor associated with SIDS is found in all SIDS infants and many infants who die from SIDS have none of the factors usually associated with the syndrome.

SIDS is more common in winter than in summer. This is reflected in the incidence in Australia, the highest incidence being in Tasmania, followed by the Australian Capital Territory and the lowest in the Northern Territory and Queensland. An exception to this is in Sweden, where the incidence in spring and autumn is proportionally higher than in Australia. In Sweden 27 per cent of SIDS deaths occur in the three winter months compared with 43 per cent of SIDS deaths occurring in the winter in South Australia.

Other environmental factors which have been identified as associated with SIDS are weekends, early hours of the morning, and paternal tobacco smoking. Although in South

Australia the incidence is the same in city and country infants, in Western Australia country infants have a higher incidence than city and suburban infants.

Maternal factors associated with SIDS have been: age under 25 years, two or more pregnancies, multiple births and tobacco smoking. Infant factors have been low birth weight, bottle feeding and prone sleeping position.

Management of SIDS

How the family react

The family is shattered. The parents are shocked, devastated and frightened. Above all is the fear that they have done something wrong. There is an agonised moment of disbelief and then they are plummeted into a grief for which there has been no preparation. In most cases the parents' closest association with death will have been an elderly grandparent, for whom death has been both expected and accepted as the ultimate end of a long and fruitful life. Sometimes they will have known the death of a sick parent or sibling, when there has been some preliminary grieving and preparing for death.

Most families in Australia have heard about SIDS, but few believe it can happen to them. Until it does, most families believe there must have been something those parents did wrong. Their infant, whose well being has been completely dependent on their care, is dead. It is not surprising that the parents are often engulfed by guilt as they question their own ability to care for a child: 'if only I had . . .' or 'if only I hadn't . . .' statements are produced as they mix their guilt with their wish for what they know is impossible—to have their baby back again.

What do the parents need?

Parents need information about the following:

1. SIDS. They need information about SIDS: that although the cause is not known, it is a well recognised, well documented disorder with characteristic patterns, that it is not a new disorder, and that much research is being done to try and find the cause. They need to be advised how to critically read articles in newspapers and magazines about the cause of SIDS and who to approach for the true story behind the article. Written information about SIDS and about grief can be helpful for the parents, and for their friends and relatives.

2. Grief. Parents need to know that although they may feel guilty, there is no basis for this guilt. The parents need to express their fears and have accurate explanations for example, if they say 'If only I had gone in to check the baby when I woke at six o'clock'. In fact they would have found the baby asleep in which case they would have left, or found the baby already dead. The possibility that they would have checked in the few minutes in which the baby was in trouble and would have been able to resuscitate the child, is remote.

Parents have been brought up differently, and show their grief differently. Open discussion between the parents, often easier at first through an experienced counsellor, is the best way to solve these problems. Expression of anger, guilt and fear leads to resolution, while suppression often leads to panic, violence depression and despair. 'Give sorrow words: the grief that does not speak whispers the o'er-frought heart, and bids it break'.

Each parent needs time alone, time with only their spouse and time to be comforted by all their family and friends. The amount of time differs from person to person, but all need recognition by the attending nurses and medical staff.

3. Their other children. Children even under three years of age will be aware of the family upheaval and distress, they need to feel secure and not shut out from their parents. When the mother's friends and relatives arrive and put their arms around the mother, the father should be watching the small child, as in mother's arms has been the child's place (often carefully nurtured to prevent jealousy of the new baby). The father should be ready to talk to, or cuddle the young child at this time. The reverse obviously applies if the father's friends and family arrive. Helpful friends and relatives are likely to offer to take the other children. Mostly this is a time when the immediate family need to be together, especially to sleep, as the baby went to sleep and died.

Older children need to know the truth, simply expressed in words they can understand. They need to know the baby has died, and won't be back. They need to know that the parents are sad and upset and miss the baby. The need to know that although small babies die like this it does not happen to big children like them, nor to mothers and fathers, but only to very little babies or very old people. Children under seven years will have little understanding of the permanence of death, and will often continue to ask their parents to get the baby back—finally they will give up and ask the parents to get another baby— this is a normal reaction in a child who has loved this special baby. Children often believe in magic and may have wished at times the baby wasn't there, and they now feel guilty that in some way it is their fault. These children need to know that no wishing can kill the baby, and no wishing can bring the baby back.

4. The autopsy. The parents need to know what autopsy examination entails. In Australia, autopsy is mandatory. A death certificate cannot be signed unless a diagnosis is made, and SIDS cannot be diagnosed without an autopsy. The parents need to be told that the autopsy is an operation, performed by a doctor, on their infant, that small pieces of tissue will be examined under a microscope, that all bacteria and viruses will be looked for, and that certain other samples may be collected, for example some blood, and be kept for research. They need to know that the doctor will sew the wounds neatly after the autopsy, and that they can see and touch their infant following the examination.

As soon as the autopsy is finished the parents should be notified of the interim report and informed that it is extremely unlikely that this diagnosis will be changed, but that if anything further is found later (for example, a virus identified which is thought to be responsible for death) they will be notified. The parents should be offered the opportunity of going through the autopsy report when it is complete (which may take two months) with the pathologist or another doctor, for example, their local general practitioner.

5. The funeral. The parents need to know that they should ring a funeral director who will arrange to see them and organise what they wish. He will pick up the baby from the hospital and will also ensure death certification and registration have taken place. Most funeral directors charge relatively little for the funeral of a baby. If the family have no access to funds for the funeral they can contact the Department of Community Welfare before contacting the funeral director and the Department may arrange to pay for the funeral.

6. The police and the coroner. Every death that is sudden and unexpected in Australia must be reported to the coroner. The identification and investigation by the police are essential, and almost always sensitively handled, with great sympathy and kindness shown to the parents. The parents can feel comforted to know that they have been completely cleared of any responsibility for their infant's death.

7. Support organisations. Meeting someone else who has been through what they are now going through is helpful to many parents, and all Australian States have SIDS Parents Associations that can provide such a meeting.

The greatest support should, and usually does, come from the spouse. Relatives and close friends are often helpful, but their grieving is usually shorter, and they may have difficulty coping with the ongoing grief of parents. SIDS Associations often have trained counsellors who may help the bereaved parents. Many general practitioners and psychiatrists are willing to guide parents through normal grief. A good counsellor will recognise when grief reactions become abnormal or exceptionally prolonged and arrange a psychiatric referral.

When the next baby is born the parents may have mixed feelings. Memories will be stirred and the parents' reaction to the new infant will depend on how far they have progressed through their grief. They may feel a resentment that is hard for others to understand, but which may relate to their wish to have the dead infant back and the new infant being perceived as the wrong baby. There is likely to be fear for the life of the new baby.

Although they may have been reassured that recurrence is most unlikely, many parents still feel unsure. For this reason many families choose to place future infants on a cardiac or respiratory alarm, and this brings with it its own tensions.

Conclusion

There is no way out of grief brought by sudden infant death, only a way through it. Eventual resolution of grief leads to rebuilding of self-esteem, acceptance of the sadness, which is never forgotten, and an ability to retain good memories of the child. The family who have suffered SIDS will hopefully not only learn to live again despite this tragedy, but be stronger because of this tragedy.

Further Reading

Beal S and Porter C, 'Sudden Infant Death Syndrome Related to Climate', *Acta Paediatr Scand*, 1990 (in press).

Bergman A B, Beckwith J B and Ray C G, *SIDS*, University of Washington Press, 1970.

Davies D P, 'Cot Death in Hong Kong', *Lancet*, Vol 2, 1985, pp 1346–9.

Harper R M and Hoffman J C, *Sudden Infant Death Syndrome, Basic Mechanisms*, PMA Publishing Corporation, New York, 1988.

Hilton J M N and Borhani N O, 'Post-Neonatal Sudden Unexplained Death in California: A Cohort Study', *American Journal of Epidermiol*, Vol 95, 1972, pp 95–497.

Nelson E A S, Taylor B J and Weatherall I L, 'Sleeping Position and Infant Bedding may Predispose to Hyperthermia and the Sudden Infant Death Syndrome', *Lancet*, Vol 1, 1989, pp 199–201.

Norvenius S G, 'Sudden Infant Death Syndrome in Sweden in 1973–1977 and 1979', *Acta Paediatric Scad*, 1987, Suppl 333.

Tildon J T, Roeder L M and Steinschneider A, *SIDS*, Pub Academic Press, New York, 1983.

Part 8
Treatment

Chapter 56

Medication 1:
In Children and Adolescents

Brent G H Waters

Psychotropic medications, or psycho-pharmacological treatments, are at best, a small part of broader multimodal therapeutic strategies for managing child and adolescent psychiatric disorders. The other vital components include a variety of non-drug therapies—family, individual, behavioural, counselling, remedial teaching and liaison with community agencies.

Psychotropic medications are surprisingly commonly prescribed for children and adolescents. An Australian study found that in a two week period in 1983, a relatively large number of young persons took one or more psychotropic medications. The medications covered included prescribed and over-the-counter drugs. To put these figures into perspective, the rate of psychotropic medication use among pre-schoolers was about half that among young adults. Overall, minor tranquillisers were the most frequently prescribed. Stimulants and, to a lesser extent, neuroleptics were used more frequently with boys.

The child as patient

Treatment is nearly always sought by someone other than the child (such as a parent or a teacher)—the child seldom refers himself for treatment. The surveys cited above appear to confirm this.

Children are rarely consulted about the decision to prescribe psychotropic drugs for them, so it is imperative that the prescriber ensures that the child's best interests are paramount, and that the child is both informed of, and involved in the decision and in the course of therapy to whatever extent that is possible. As well, adolescents under the age of 16 do have qualified rights of consent to treatment depending on their ability to appreciate the purpose, benefits and side effects of the medication.

Developmental issues

Children and adolescents are in an active phase of growth and maturation. Some psychotropic medications may have immediate adverse effects on growth. For example, methylphenidate, a drug used in the treatment of attentional disorders, causes temporary growth supression. Drugs may also have more delayed effects on development which are only evident by different rates of entry into, or progress through, a subsequent developmental phase. For example, puberty and breast development may be accelerated by the hormonal effects of certain tranquillisers. Drugs may also have indirect effects on one facet of development by interfering with a parallel developmental process. For example, most psychotropic drugs produce some degree of sedation. Clinical experience suggests that prolonged sedation, particularly if not marked, can exert a subtle but definite effect on socialisation by reducing social spontaneity and initiative. Over time, this may reduce social participation and affect the development of the capacity for social relationships. In addition, children metabolise or break down most drugs faster than adults so they generally tolerate higher doses.

Compliance

Young children are not usually responsible for their own medications, so problems with taking medications as prescribed (compliance) generally lie elsewhere. Non-compliance is a serious problem. It means that children and adolescents who could benefit from the medications are denied the opportunity. Non-compliance may result from parents not wishing to administer drugs which they believe are potentially toxic, habit forming or which may be causing obvious unwanted side-effects that the parents fear outweigh the expected therapeutic effect. A greater problem, though, is over-compliance and over-zealous use of sedating medications with pre-school age children, particularly when the drug was prescribed for another family member and was administered to the child on an *ad hoc* basis.

The problem of non-compliance is more acute with adolescent patients. Adolescents like to be in charge of their own lives. Those who come into psychiatric care are particularly likely to resent the coercive influence of adults, and also to resent taking a medication which affects their mental processes. For these reasons, compliance by adolescents may be even lower than that found with children.

Administration

Most psychotropic drugs have many effects. It is often difficult to be certain whether a beneficial effect is due to specific, placebo, incidental, or 'side' effects of the medication. Therapeutic and side effects must also be monitored closely during treatment. To assist this, physical, behavioural, cognitive and environmental (including family) assessments should be conducted regularly. Dosage changes should follow regular reassessments of target symptoms. Once the appropriate balance is found between therapeutic effect and unwanted side effects, the medication should be maintained for only so long as it is necessary. Sometimes this period may be quite brief. Most psychotropic medications should be withdrawn slowly because of the danger of withdrawal symptoms.

Antidepressants

Monoamine oxidase inhibitors are rarely used with children. The tricyclic antidepressants are more commonly employed. They have a variety of clinically significant chemical actions on the nervous system which may be harnessed for different conditions.

Tricyclic antidepressants are fairly well absorbed orally and are mainly broken down in the liver in a number of separate steps. Because each step in the pathway is under the control of a separate enzyme which is under independent genetic control, there is a considerable genetic variation in the rate of drug breakdown. This means that some people retain a single dose for up to five times as long as others. This is a significant problem in the treatment of both children and adults. Blood levels are often the best way of monitoring treatment effectiveness in the few cases in which their use is indicated.

Tricyclic antidepressants are commonly used in the treatment of childhood *depression*, despite the failure of carefully controlled studies to demonstrate that they are significantly better than placebo. The scanty data are not encouraging and only support their use for the depressed phase of manic depressive disorder, in which case psychiatric consultation is indicated.

Imipramine is widely used for *enuresis*. Although it and the other tricyclics are often temporarily effective as symptom suppressants, enuresis recurs after a time. Moreover relapse is almost immediate when the drug is stopped.

Recent studies suggest that clomipramine is effective for childhood and adolescent *obsessive–compulsive disorder*. It also appears to be useful in *attention deficit hyperactivity disorder (ADHD)* children, although less so than stimulants. Desipramine is reported to decrease hyperactive and impulsive behaviour as well as improving performance on cognitive and attentional tasks. These drugs may be preferable for the highly anxious

ADHD child or adolescent.

The tricyclics should not be used with profoundly *retarded* children and adolescents as they may make behaviour worse. Their popularity in the treatment of *school refusal* is based on only one positive study which has not been replicated.

Serious adverse effects such as cardiotoxicity, seizures and death have been reported with imipramine and other cyclic antidepressants. Since most sudden deaths are cardiac in origin, initial ECG assessment and ECG monitoring during treatment is essential if high doses are used. Much more common autonomic nervous system side effects include dry mouth, anorexia, weight loss, nausea, constipation, dizziness, insomnia, rashes and drowsiness. These are often transient and disappear with dose reduction; persistent dry mouth accelerates plaque formation and may promote dental caries. Allergic eczema and certain blood clotting abnormalities may occur after six months on imipramine. Rare effects on behaviour include irritability, agitation and worsening of psychosis. Some tricyclics may affect memory and other cognitive processes. Withdrawal symptoms may also occur occasionally. Accidental overdosage is a real danger for young patients and their siblings who see them taking medication. Deliberate overdosage is a significant risk among depressed, moody or impulsive adolescents.

Stimulants

These include sympathomimetic amines (amphetamine, dextroamphetamine) and related compounds (methylphenidate, magnesium pemoline). They cause CNS alerting. These drugs should not be prescribed without prior specialist consultation, preferably by a child psychiatrist.

Stimulants last only a few hours in the body. Dosage should be started at a low level and should be gradually increased until the desired clinical effect is achieved. While some children require morning and noon dose, a single morning dose is sufficient for many. Children under five years should not usually receive stimulants. Their response is more unpredictable and variable; levels of activity,

attentiveness and impulsiveness are more difficult to assess; and preschoolers respond better to parent training, behavioural management programs and other environmental treatments.

Stimulants work best for primary school-aged children with pervasive *ADHD* (evident at home and school). Despite controversy over diagnosis, studies evaluating individual symptoms and behaviours indicate that most such children (65-70 per cent) respond with significant decreases in activity, impulsivity and querulousness, and improvement in performance, efficiency and attention span. They also help some ADHD adolescents. However the stimulants do not improve the learning problems which commonly co-exist with ADHD. A calming response to stimulant medication is *not* a diagnostic test for ADHD as children with conduct disorders and aggression may also derive some positive benefit. Medications ordinarily form only a minor part of a multimodal management program.

Drug holidays are recommended which enable the child to take the medication only on school days or on days during which attention and diminished restlessness are particularly important. They are also an opportunity to establish the child's ability to behave in a controlled manner in the absence of medication, so providing a guide for when the medication should be withdrawn—usually by the time of secondary school entry.

The stimulants may worsen anxiety disorders, autism, schizophrenia, dyskinesia, tics or Tourette's disorder, and are not indicated in these conditions. The most common and important adverse effects of the stimulants include sleeplessness, loss of appetite, moodiness and tearfulness: they may occur in up to a third of children. Stomach aches, headaches, hallucinosis, dyskinesia, and facilitation of tics and Tourette's disorder are much rarer. Growth suppression is a concern, but this seldom appears unless high doses are used, and may be only a temporary effect. Stimulant medications prescribed for childhood or adolescent hyperactivity have not been found to lead to dependency so far. However, dependency or illicit sale of these medications may become a problem with the recent trend towards their use with adolescents and young adults.

Neuroleptics (antipsychotics or major tranquillisers)

Children are mostly prescribed these drugs for sedation, although during adolescence it is true that they are used more frequently for psychosis. The neuroleptics comprise of several classes of drugs: principally the phenothiazines (aliphatics such as chlorpromazine, piperidines such as thioridazine, piperazines such as trifluoperazine), the butyrophenones (such as haloperidol) and the thioxanthenes (such as flupenthixol). The neuroleptics block the receptors for certain neurotransmitters (dopamine, noradrenaline and acetylcholine). Thus, they have numerous effects on many organ systems.

Neuroleptics, particularly haloperidol, have been effective in controlling behavioural symptoms associated with *autism*. Hyperactivity and self-destructive repetitive behaviour respond to higher doses, whereas irritability, uncooperativeness, angry or labile affect, withdrawal, stereotypy, fidgetiness and abnormal interpersonal relations may respond satisfactorily to lower doses. Although they have not been completely evaluated, there is good clinical evidence that they work well with *childhood and adolescent schizophrenia* and *mania*.

Haloperidol is the preferred first line treatment of *Tourette's disorder* and *chronic tics disorder*. Although neuroleptics usually suppress tics, in view of the risks of long-term use, they should be employed only when the tics are chronic (at least of one year's duration) and socially disabling. Pimozide may be preferable since it is as effective as haloperidol but is said to have fewer adverse effects such as sedation.

Neuroleptics are widely used in the treatment of *aggressive, uncooperative behaviour by institutionalised mentally-retarded* children and adolescents. Their efficacy and superiority to other non-physical (especially behavioural) methods of calming non-psychotic disturbed children remains to be demonstrated. However, with carefully selected patients, they may have beneficial effects on hyperactivity, stereotypic, bizarre, self injurious and self stimulating behaviour. With careful drug selection and use, the deleterious effects on learning may be largely avoided.

Neuroleptics are also widely used to reduce *aggressive conduct disorder* in non-retarded inpatients. Although medications such as haloperidol may reduce aggressiveness, temper tantrums and explosiveness, this is often at a dosage which causes sedation. For this reason, lithium carbonate may be preferable in such children.

Cognitive and learning impairment are most marked with the sedating neuroleptics (such as chlorpromazine, thioridazine). Though common, they are often overlooked. However, they appear to depend on the dose and stem partly from the general slowing action of the drugs, and partly from disruption of memory and other fundamental processes. Other subtle behavioural side effects have also been described—particularly dose-related depression, moodiness, irritability and aggression.

Cardiovascular adverse effects such as hypotension, tachycardia and arrhythmias become increasingly likely with high doses, but are generally not of great importance in physically healthy children. Weight gain, menstrual irregularities and other endocrine effects also appear in high doses. Lowering of seizure threshold is an important consideration, particularly in children who are already at high risk for seizure disorders (such as autistic and retarded children).

Lithium carbonate

Dosage is regulated by periodic (at least bi-monthly) blood levels. Dosage should be increased slowly until a therapeutic level is obtained.

Lithium may be as effective as haloperidol in reducing aggressiveness, temper outbursts and explosiveness among *non-retarded under-socialised aggressive* children. However, it should only be used as part of a multimodal therapeutic approach, and is best reserved for cases in which non-pharmacological treatments have failed. Lithium may also be effective in managing severe *explosive aggressiveness in some mentally-retarded* children and adolescents.

Lithium is the mainstay of the preventive treatment of juvenile-onset *bipolar mood disorder* which may present prior to the onset of puberty, and is frequently diagnosed during adolescence.

Minor tranquillisers

The benzodiazepines are the major members of this group of selective CNS depressants.

A role for benzodiazepines in childhood and adolescent psychiatric disorders has not been established. They have been recommended for properly diagnosed *sleep-walking* and *night-terrors*, but clear scientific support is lacking. However, they may be considered if the symptoms are frequent (more than two to three times a week) and seriously disrupt the sleep patterns of the child and the family, in which case those with a short duration of action are preferable.

A particularly troublesome adverse effect is their tendency to disinhibit children and make them restless and over-excited.

Anticholinergics/antihistaminics

Central anticholinergics/antihistaminics are most widely used for *night-time sedation* of children, particularly pre-schoolers for example trimeprazine or promethazine. Their value as hypnotics has not been demonstrated.

Carbamazepine

Carbamazepine is best known as an anti-convulsant. It has recently been used for a variety of psychiatric disorders of adulthood including affective disorders, psychoses, episodic dyscontrol and behavioural disorders. There are no evaluations of its usefulness in childhood and adolescent affective disorder, but it may be a useful alternative prophylactic to lithium carbonate in unresponsive *bipolar disorder*. Common side effects include nausea, drowsiness, vertigo, ataxia, blurred vision and diplopia. Serious blood disturbances had been a concern, but they are rare. Nevertheless, periodic blood counts are usually recommended.

Clonidine

Clonidine is used primarily in the treatment of hypertension (high blood pressure). It may be a useful alternative to the neuroleptics in *Tourette's disorder* if the patient is responding incompletely or is experiencing intolerable side effects. Severe tics tend to respond less satisfactorily to clonidine than to neuroleptics, but compulsive and aggressive behaviours as well as attentional problems may respond well. Recent studies also suggest clonidine may be useful with *ADHD* children. Sedation is a frequent but usually tolerable side effect. Abrupt withdrawal may lead to hypertensive crisis.

Exclusion diets

The use of exclusion diets is based on the belief that the behaviour disturbances, particularly *ADHD* and *aggressive, defiant behaviour*, in a small group of children are due to an intolerance of certain chemical or foods. True intolerance is associated with the problem behaviour worsening when the implicated substance is eaten. The intolerance may take the form of food allergy in the narrow sense (associated with an abnormal immunological reaction to food) or food intolerance. Feingold attributed hyperactivity to 'allergy' to food additives (artificial colours and flavours). Numerous trials have assessed his claims. Generally, additive exclusion diets are associated with a high placebo response. However the few double blind trials suggest that a very small minority of children show a predictable behavioural response to challenge with additives. A recent study suggests that allergic children may show an adverse behavioural response to challenge by some foods (uncontaminated by additives). In this instance, the curative diet is 'oligoantigenic'—and includes foods such as pears. Taken together, the evidence for adverse behavioural responses to either food additives or antigenic foods is scanty.

Discussion

This review indicates that very few disorders of childhood and adolescence are predictably responsive to pharmacological treatments. The exceptions include ADHD, Tourette's disorder, bipolar manic depressive disorder and schizophrenia. Few prescribers are experienced in psychiatric diagnosis in children and adolescents, nor are they sufficiently aware of the scientific literature on the effectiveness and numerous side effects of these agents. Because of the need for skill in psychiatric diagnosis, and specialised knowledge in pharmacology, safety and efficacy, it is difficult to defend the prescription of any psychotropic drugs in children or adolescents without specialist consultation—preferably by a child psychiatrist.

The parent who seeks psychopharmacological solutions from their doctor, or who capriciously administers their own medications to the child may be setting the scene for the child to reach for psychopharmacology to change their mood or behaviour, and in the long term to sow the seeds of addictive drug use. Parents and health educators should work together to instil appropriate values in respect of all medication use (see chapter 57).

Further Reading

Aman M A and Singh N N, *Psychopharmacology of the Developmentally Disabled*, Springer Verlag, New York, 1988.

Campbell M, Green W H and Deutsch S I, *Child and Adolescent Psychopharmacology*, Sage Publications, Beverley Hills, 1985.

Campbell M and Spencer E K, 'Psychopharmacology in Child and Adolescent Psychiatry: A Review of the Past Five Years', *Journal of the American Academy of Child and Adolescent Psychiatry*, Vol 27, 1988, pp 269–79.

Gilman A G, Goodman L S, Rall T W and Murad F, *The Pharmacological Basis of Therapeutics*, Macmillan Publishing Co, New York, 1985.

Taylor E, 'Drug Treatment', In *Child and Adolescent Psychiatry: Modern Approaches*, 2nd edn (ed Rutter M and Hersov L), Blackwell Scientific Publications, London, 1985.

Varley C K, 'Diet and the Behaviour of Children with Attention Deficit Disorder', *Journal of the American Academy of Child Psychiatry*, Vol 23, 1984, pp 182–5.

Werry J S, 'An Overview of Paediatric Psychopharmacology', *Journal of the American Academy of Child Psychiatry*, Vol 21, 1982, pp 3–9.

Werry J S, 'Drugs, Learning and Cognitive Function in Children: An Update', *Journal of Child Psychology and Psychiatry*, Vol 29, 1988, pp 129–41.

Chapter 57

Medication 2: In Adults

T J Stedman and H A Whiteford

Drug therapy has been used for thousands of years to prevent or control symptoms of psychiatric illness. Although drug treatments are increasingly specific and more is understood about prevention of troublesome and occasionally dangerous adverse or 'side' effects, no 'cure' for any of the major psychiatric disorders exists. Drug treatments, while crucial to the management of many patients, form part of a plan that integrates a wide range of interventions.

Table 1 outlines the major agents used in psychiatric practice and the average dose range recommended by experts in the field (see chapter 56).

Antipsychotic drugs (neuroleptics)

The discovery of chlorpromazine in 1952 revolutionised the treatment of psychosis and led to large numbers of patients with psychotic illnesses being managed outside hospitals. The major indications for this group of drugs are the schizophrenic illnesses. However, mania and organic psychoses (including drug induced psychoses) also respond to these compounds. Antipsychotic drugs have proven useful in both acute management and longer term therapy of psychotic disorders.

The two major types of antipsychotic drugs are the phenothiazines and butyrophenones. No individual drug from these classes has proved to be a more effective antipsychotic agent but they differ in their side effect profile. The antipsychotic drugs are usually given orally, tend to break down slowly in the body (half lives are often greater than 24 hours) and may take days to weeks to substantially

reduce psychotic symptoms. Some, especially the butyrophenones, can be given by injection and this is useful for the control of acute psychosis in a very disturbed patient. A more recent development has been injectable long acting preparations which are particularly useful in ensuring continuous administration of treatment. For example, intramuscular injections of depot fluphenazine can be effective for a month or more.

The common pharmacological action of all antipsychotic drugs which parallels their antipsychotic effect, is their ability to block brain receptors for the chemical transmitter, *dopamine*.

These drugs may cause adverse effects, the most common being sedation. One group of side effects results from blocking receptors for the brain chemical, acetylcholine. These effects consist of symptoms such as dry mouth, blurred vision, constipation and difficulty initiating urination. These symptoms are more common with chlorpromazine and thioridazine and can usually be managed by reducing the dose or changing the drug. A second group of symptoms results from blocking receptors to dopamine in one of the brain systems for controlling movements. These include muscle spasms (dystonic reactions), a feeling of restlessness (akathisia), and a syndrome similar to Parkinson's Disease consisting of stiffening of muscles, difficulty starting voluntary movements and tremor (usually of the hands). Reduction in dose, or using drugs such as benztropine or orphenadrine can usually control these symptoms.

With long term use of any of these drugs,

Table 1. Major agents and recommended average dose range

Generic name	Common proprietary name	Commonly used total daily dosage* for adults
ANTIDEPRESSANT DRUGS		
Tricyclics		
Amitriptyline	Laroxyl, Tryptanol	50–150 mg
Imipramine	Tofranil	50–150 mg
Nortriptyline	Allegron, Nortab	50–150 mg
Clomipramine	Anafranil	50–150 mg
Desipramine	Pertofran	25–150 mg
Trimipramine	Surmontil	50–150 mg
Doxepin	Sinequan	50–200 mg
Dothiepin	Prothiaden	50–200 mg
Monoamine Oxidase Inhibitors		
Phenelzine	Nardil	15–60 mg
Tranylcypromine	Parnate	10–30 mg
Others		
Mianserin	Tolvon	30–120 mg
MOOD STABILISERS		
Lithium carbonate	Lithicarb	0.5–1.5 gm
Carbamazepine	Tegretol	100–800 mg
MINOR TRANQUILLISERS		
Antianxiety drugs		
Benzodiazepines		
Diazepam	Valium, Ducene	5–40 mg
Chlordizepoxide	Librium	20–60 mg
Oxazepam	Serepax	45–90 mg
Lorazepam	Ativan	1–3 mg
Buspirone	Buspar	40–60 mg
Alprazolam	Xanax	0.5–4 mg
Clobazam	Frisium	10–30 mg
Bromazepam	Lexotan	3–12 mg
Clorazepate	Tranxene	5–60 mg
Hypnotic drugs		
Benzodiazepines		
Nitrazepam	Mogadon	5–10 mg at night
Temazepam	Normison, Euhypnos	10–40 mg at night
Flurazepam	Dalmane	15–60 mg at night
Flunitrazepam	Rohypnol	0.5–4 mg at night
Other		
Chloral hydrate	Noctec	500 mg–1 gm at night
ANTIPSYCHOTIC DRUGS		
Phenothiazines		
Chlorpromazine	Largactil	75–800 mg
Thioridazine	Melleril	75–600 mg
Trifluoperazine	Stelazine	2–10 mg
Fluphenazine (oral)	Anatensol	2.5–20 mg
Fluphenazine (depot)	Modecate	12.5–50 mg fortnightly to monthly
Pericyazine	Neulactil	15–10 mg
Butyrophenones		
Haloperidol	Serenace	5–40 mg
Droperidol	Droleptan	5–25 mg
Other		
Thiothixene	Navane	10–40 mg
Pimozide	Orap	2–20 mg

* These are average doses. Individual patients may require higher doses in the acute phases of their illness and certain patients (eg the elderly) may require lower doses.

involuntary movements usually of the mouth, tongue and face (tardive dyskinesia) can appear. Unfortunately, they do not always remit even if drug treatment is ceased. Some drugs have important individual side effects. For example, chlorpromazine can cause patients to be easily sunburnt, while thioridazine in high doses for long periods can result in impaired vision.

Mood stabilisers

Lithium carbonate

The therapeutic effect of lithium in psychiatric patients was originally reported in 1949, by John Cade, an Australian psychiatrist. Lithium is effective in the treatment of acute mania and in reducing the frequency and severity of recurrences of both mania and depression in bipolar affective disorder (also known as manic depressive illness). It has also been recommended in some depressive disorders and schizophrenia, but its place in these conditions remains to be firmly established.

The mechanism of the therapeutic action of lithium is unknown. It is rapidly absorbed and is excreted by the kidneys. Treatment is introduced slowly to achieve a serum level between 0.5 and 1.0 mM/L. The rate of elimination of lithium varies greatly between individuals but its half life averages about 13 hours.

At the start of treatment, nausea, abdominal discomfort and fatigue may occur but usually disappear within two weeks. Mild tremor is common. Lithium interferes with thyroid function in many patients and occasionally this results in thyroid enlargement or hypothyroidism. Up to one third of patients taking lithium show a reversible decrease in their ability to concentrate urine, resulting in frequent urination and the passing of large volumes of dilute urine. Patients whose lithium levels are maintained in the therapeutic range rarely develop serious kidney problems. Thyroid and renal function tests are recommended before initiating lithium therapy and at yearly intervals thereafter.

Toxicity occurs when lithium levels are too high (usually above 1.3 mM/L). Early manifestations include gastrointestinal symptoms (for example, loss of appetite, nausea, vomiting, diarrhoea), while nervous system effects (for example, headache, drowsiness, uncoordinated movements, shaking, and speech difficulties), may become apparent in severe cases. Patients need to be advised that situations which produce fluid depletion such as prolonged vomiting or diarrhoea, hot weather, excessive physical exertion or childbirth predispose to toxicity. Toxicity may also develop due to drug interactions such as with certain diuretics.

In recent times, other drugs such as carbamazepine have also been found useful in the treatment of some patients with bipolar disorder who are not responsive to or cannot tolerate lithium (either alone, or in conjunction with lithium Co_3.)

Antidepressants

Tricyclic antidepressants

Following the discovery of chlorpromazine for psychosis, investigation of compounds with similar structures led to studies of a substance called imipramine. These suggested that this drug had little effect on psychotic symptoms but resulted in improvement in the mood of depressed patients. Today, the main use of tricyclic antidepressants is in the treatment of depressive symptoms. In depressed patients with the typical symptoms of melancholia, over three-quarters can be expected to improve. Other uses for tricyclic antidepressants include panic disorder/ agoraphobia, childhood enuresis, attention deficit disorder, chronic pain syndromes, obsessive compulsive disorder and bulimia.

A common feature of these drugs, which may be relevant to their therapeutic effect, is their ability to block the synaptic reuptake of serotonin (5-hydroxytryptamine) and noradrenaline. The drugs are rapidly absorbed and have long half lives (for example 40 hours for amitriptyline). Large individual differences in metabolism can result in up to 40-fold variations in blood concentrations between individuals receiving the same dose. Unequivocal differences of efficacy between tricyclic drugs have not been demonstrated but differences in side effect profiles do exist.

As with most drugs, it is advisable to start patients with a low dose. Once tolerated, usually after two to three days, this dose can be increased every few days. Full therapeutic effect is not usually observed for two to six weeks. It is advisable to continue treatment, at the lowest effective dose, until there has been a complete absence of depressive symptoms for six months.

Anticholinergic side effects are common and often troublesome. They include dry mouth, difficulty with close vision, hesitancy in passing urine and constipation. The most common cardiovascular side effect is low blood pressure and dizziness on standing. Blood pressure should be checked regularly, especially early in treatment. Tricyclic antidepressants can affect cardiac function and should be prescribed with caution in patients with pre-existing heart disease. Sedation is a common side effect especially early in treatment and may be more pronounced with amitriptyline and less pronounced with imipramine. This side effect can be useful if agitation or insomnia is prominent. Overdose with these drugs is serious and can result in delirium, convulsions, distrubance of temperature regulation, hypotension, cardiac arrhythmias and, in the most serious cases, coma and death.

Newer antidepressants such as mianserin appear to have less anticholinergic and cardiotoxic side effects.

Monoamine oxidase inhibitors

These agents were discovered when a drug for treating tuberculosis was noted to produce euphoria. The introduction of the relatively more effective tricyclic antidepressants and reports of serious adverse reactions with monoamine oxidase inhibitors have limited their use. In the last 15 years knowledge about the conditions for their safe use has led to their gradual reintroduction into clinical practice. Monoamine oxidase inhibitors are used mainly as a second line treatment in depressive disorders which have not responded to other treatment, and in panic disorder.

The inhibition of monoamine oxidase leads to increased synaptic levels of serotonin and noradrenaline. This may be the mechanism of the antidepressant effect as well as the stimulant and hypertensive side effects. These drugs should be started in low doses with the last dose in the afternoon (stimulant effects may cause insomnia). After two weeks higher doses can be tried for about six weeks if side effects and the patient's condition allow.

Side effects most commonly found include postural hypotension, drowsiness, sleeplessness, weight gain, anticholinergic and stimulant effects. Interactions with certain food and drugs can cause a severe rise in blood pressure. These foods include some cheeses, wines, seasoned meats and yeast extracts. Similar reactions occur with a range of prescribed or 'over the counter' medications including cold medicines, nose drops, opiates (especially pethidine), and general anaesthetic agents. Patients should be asked to seek advice before commencing any medication and to advise their doctor should they need surgery or dental procedures.

Minor tranquillisers

Benzodiazepines were first synthesised in the 1950s and came into wide use in the 1960s. Because they are relatively safe and have few side effects, they have now largely replaced the barbiturates in the treatment of anxiety and insomnia.

Benzodiazepines are most widely used to relieve psychological manifestation of anxiety (antianxiety actions) and to induce sleep (hypnotic actions). There are many types of benzodiazepines available in Australia and they differ primarily in speed of onset and duration of action. Drugs such as diazepam, which have active metabolites, display a more rapid onset and a longer duration of action (half life approximately 48 hours), than drugs such as temazepam (half life 8 hours) which has no active metabolites. All benzodiazepines suppress activity in the central nervous system probably by potentiating the inhibitory brain chemical *gamma amino butyric acid* and this accounts for their clinical uses ranging from sedation to anaesthesia. Benzodiazepines can have important side effects. Oversedation is common if high doses are used and this can affect coordination.

Tolerance and physical dependence can occur, and if the drug is stopped abruptly after long term use, withdrawal symptoms including seizures are possible. Benzodiazepines can also potentiate the effects of other sedative drugs including alcohol.

Some general issues with drug use

With the use of drugs in the treatment of mental illness, several important issues arise. The first of these is that the drugs used are potent and can have disabling side effects. Therefore, patients and, where appropriate, relatives and/or friends, must be provided with adequate information, instruction and access to advice about drug treatments. Ensuring this, in the presence of psychiatric impairments, is vital to successful drug treatment. The second issue is ensuring adherence to the specifics of a regimen of medication (compliance). Non compliance has been estimated to be present in up to 60 per cent of patients treated for chronic illness and even about 20 per cent of psychiatric patients in hospital. Enhancement of compliance is best achieved by education about medication and the conditions for which it is used, by designing the simplest and cheapest effective regimens, and by establishing a relationship with the patient in which concerns about illness and the problems of treatment can be easily raised. Occasionally psychiatric disorders severely affect a patient's judgment. In circumstances where patients refuse treatment and/or compliance cannot be ensured and the consequences of mental illness are very serious, legal mechanisms exist to provide drug treatment without the patient's consent. Most often compulsory treatment is used when the patient's illness is of a nature sufficiently severe to place them or others at significant risk of harm.

It is clear that in the management of psychiatric illness drug treatment is often indicated. However, it is virtually always part of an approach which integrates drug therapy with psychological treatments and social interventions.

Further Reading

Berger P A and Hollister L E, 'Psychopharmacology' in *American Psychiatric Association Annual Review*, (ed Hales R E and Frances A J), American Psychiatric Association, Washington, Vol 6, 1987, pp 698–817.

Hollister L E, *Clinical Pharmacology of Psychotherapeutic Drugs*, 2nd ed, Churchill Livingstone, New York, 1983.

Tyrer P J, *Drugs in Psychiatric Practice,* Butterworths, London, 1982.

Whaley L F, 'Neuropharmacology and Neuroendocrinology', in *Companion to Psychiatric Studies*, 4th edn, (ed Kendell R E and Zealley A K), Churchill Livingstone, Edinburgh, 1988, pp 1098–36.

Chapter 58

Psychotherapy

V Carr

The term psychotherapy refers to the application of psychological principles and methods to the treatment of interpersonal problems. The treatment is conducted by means of verbal and nonverbal interactions between therapist and patient with or without participation by relevant members of the patient's social (for example, family) network. There are many different theoretical models (for example, psychoanalytic, behavioural, etc) and types (for example, individual group, family, etc) of psychotherapy. The choice of which form may be applicable in a given case depends on the nature of the problem presented, and the personal characteristics of the patient. In part, it also depends on the background and training of the therapist.

There are several elements that are common to all forms of psychotherapy. One of these is the development of a relationship with the therapist to which the patient is emotionally committed. Secondly, a rationale or explanatory framework which makes the patient's problems understandable needs to be accepted by both parties in the therapeutic alliance; it is provided by the therapist and shared with the patient. Thirdly, a sense of hopefulness needs to be instilled, a conviction that help is being provided and that, as a result, resolution of the problem is likely to occur. There is also usually a requirement that some degree of emotional arousal occurs with appropriately modulated emotional release. This needs to be accompanied at some stage by a 'corrective' cognitive, attitudinal or behavioural change in the direction of more successful adaptation.

The question, 'Does psychotherapy work?' is about as meaningless as the question, 'Is medication useful?'. In evaluating the effectiveness of medication one needs to address such questions as which drug, for which condition, with what aims, under what circumstances, at what dose and for how long? Likewise, the efficacy of psychotherapy cannot be addressed unless a number of specific variables are taken into account. These include the nature and severity of the problems; the individual characteristics of the patient; the number, variety and appropriateness of goals identified, and their suitability to the type of treatment being employed; the theoretical framework of the therapy; the pscyhotherapeutic techniques employed and their compatibility with the theoretical framework; the skill of the therapist, and the time required to reach the therapeutic goals. It is only if these variables have been specified that one can begin to discuss the efficacy of psychotherapy.

Psychoanalytic model

The psychoanalytic model of psychotherapy is based on a model of mental functioning developed within the various schools of psychoanalysis (see chapter 2). There are several concepts that are central to psychoanalytic psychotherapy.

1. The first of these is the topographic division of the mind into conscious and unconscious mental domains. The conscious domain is that which is in the current awareness. Mental contents that are not conscious but are readily accessible to consciousness (for example, memories) are said to be within the preconscious. The focus of attention governs the contents of

consciousness at any one time. For practical purposes, the conscious and preconscious are considered as one as they both tend to operate along similar lines. The unconscious is that part of the mind which is not accessible to consciousness, except in disguised form (for example, dreams, slips of the tongue, certain psychiatric symptoms). Behaviour is said to be determined by both conscious and unconscious mental processes. The conscious mind operates according to 'secondary process thinking'. This is governed by the principles of everyday (ie external) reality which entail postponement of gratification of needs. It is logical and rational in its operation. In contrast, the unconscious mind uses 'primary process thinking'. This is governed by the principles of subjective (ie internal) reality which entails immediate gratification of needs (the 'pleasure principle'). It is not logical or rational, contradictions are permitted to coexist and it employs the non-verbal operations of condensation and symbolism.

Drives are the forces which are said to energise the psyche and impel us to action. Two kinds of drive were originally described, sex and aggression. In psychoanalytic terms the sex drive is interpreted very broadly and is not confined to genital activity but includes general affiliative needs.

2. The second set of concepts is *ontogenetic* and refers to the unfolding stages of psychosexual maturation. The 'oral' phase is followed by the anal phase (1–3 years) in which drive gratification and expression occur in terms of sphincter control. In the 'phallic' phase (age 3–6 years) the drive focus is on the genitalia. This is the stage of the classical 'Oedipal conflict' in which the previously dyadic pattern of parent–child interaction becomes triangular to incorporate a key figure other than the primary caregiver. The 'latency' phase (age 7–11 years) is then entered and is followed by puberty, a phase marking the beginnings of more mature drive expression. The first three developmental phases are regarded by psychoanalytic theorists as highly important in relation to mental illness in later life. Each of these phases is said to be marked by particular conflicts, developmental challenges which require mastery and types of ego defence. If there is some difficulty in

negotiating the challenges presented by a particular developmental phase, then the individual may become 'fixated' at that point. This means that in the face of some external stress or internal conflict later in life, a 'regression' to that earlier phase of development (the 'fixation point') may occur. The term 'regression' means a return to a developmentally earlier pattern of thinking, feeling and behaving that is inappropriate to the person's chronological age.

3. The *structural* concept of mental functioning proposes a tripartite division of the mind. Of these three structures, the 'id' is regarded as the psychic representation of the drives. It is wholly unconscious. The 'ego', which is partly conscious and partly unconscious, is that component of the mental apparatus whose functions are concerned with the individual's relationship to the environment. Its functions include the control or regulation of the drives, governance of the individual's relations with external reality, interpersonal relationships, defence mechanisms and the so-called primary autonomous functions. The latter are those functions said to be independent of conflict with the id (for example, cognition). Defence mechanisms are very important in understanding personality and certain forms of mental illness. They are involuntary, unconscious, mental operations that serve to reduce the anxiety generated by unconscious conflict. Immature and 'neurotic' defence mechanisms are said to be characteristics of the early phases of psychosexual development. Mature defences are characteristic more of normal adolescence and adulthood. The third structural component is unconscious and is referred to as the 'superego'. This is the internal representation of external (social) prohibitions against the expression of needs and wishes (the drives). It is concerned with moral precepts or conscience. A related structure, the 'ego-ideal', is the representation of one's ideal aspirations.

4. The *dynamic* aspect of the psycho-analytically based model involves the concept of interaction or 'dynamic tension' between the structures of the mental apparatus. This is the notion of unconscious conflict, the so-called 'neurotic process' which is thought to

have a causal role in the production of certain forms of mental illness. Basically there arises, for various reasons, conflict between the id (ie drives that are pressing for discharge) and the superego (ie internal prohibitions against the expression of those drives) or the id and external constraints. This conflict generates a particular kind of anxiety referred to as 'signal anxiety'. Ego defence mechanisms are then brought to bear in order to reduce or contain the emergence of this anxiety . The external manifestations of these defence mechanisms are responsible for the form that neurotic symptoms take (for example, undoing compulsive hand-washing).

A psychoanalytic explanation of mental illness thus demands an account of the condition in topographic, energic (ie drive), developmental, structural and dynamic terms. It also must take into account the adaptive aspects of the processes involved in maintaining psychological equilibrium in relation to the external environment.

5. Therapies based on this model involve the concept of *transference*. This is the unconscious process whereby infantile conflicts previously experienced in relation to important figures in childhood, together with their associated feelings, thoughts and behaviours, are re-experienced in the relationship with the therapist. The therapist, also, is affected by a similar process. This is called *counter transference*. It involves the therapist's emotional attitude towards the patient and may be a disturbing influence in the therapy. Another important concept is *interpretation*. The therapist makes interpretations of psychological phenomena to the patient, the existence or significance of which the patient is unaware. Interpretations can be made within the framework of the transference and in terms of conflict, defence and the historical development of the patient's problem. The patient's task is one of working through and resolving psychological problem in these terms.

Cognitive learning model

Cognitive learning refers to the processes whereby knowledge is acquired, organised and put to use. In information processing terms, one refers to the sequence of input, storage and output of information. The first part of this sequence involves the phenomenon of perception; that is, the organisation and interpretation of sensory inputs. Fundamental to this is the concept of attention, the process by which certain sensory inputs are selected for further processing while others are not. The very earliest step in perceptual information processing is sometimes referred to as the preattentive stage in which individual stimuli are coded automatically, in parallel, and without the effort or active control demanded in conscious attention. This process, which is not subject to interference, ends with a preliminary grouping of stimuli which sets the scene for the subsequent processing stage. The latter requires focus of attention and information is processed sequentially in a limited capacity 'channel'. In contrast to preattentive processing, this requires effort, can be interfered with, and is related to level of arousal. The allocation of processing capacity in this stage can be consciously controlled and leads to the discrimination of detail in the stimulus field. Information thus registered consciously then enters short-term memory. This is of limited storage capacity. Information in this store decays very quickly unless attention is focused upon it. At this level, information that is attended then enters long-term memory which has unlimited storage capacity and from which information can be selected and produced as behavioural 'output'.

Over time, individuals develop their own unique patterns of selectively attending to these experiences and giving meaning or responding to them. These habitual patterns of processing information are referred to as cognitive strategies; for the individual they become the familiar, repetitive and predictable ways of understanding one's self and the external world. Cognitive strategies help to determine how a person will respond to certain events. For example, a person who repeatedly experiences failure, may develop a cognitive strategy characterised by a low estimation of their own capabilities and an expectation of defeat, leading to ready capitulation in the face of minimal challenge (see also chapters 61, 63).

Social learning

In human interactions individuals tend to imitate those for whom they have affection or whose qualities they admire. The person whose characteristics are acquired in this way is referred to as a model and the process is often referred to as modelling. Psychoanalytically oriented theorists refer to a similar process as 'identification'. The imitation may be intentional and conscious or may occur without the individual's awareness. If the characteristics thus acquired are reinforced by, for example, approval and praise being given by others or success in mastering certain situations, then they are likely to be maintained and become integrated with other characteristics previously acquired by the individual.

Learning theory and the therapeutic interventions based on it are described in chapter 61.

Psychoanalytic therapies

Psychoanalytic therapy can be divided into two broad groups, long-term and brief psychotherapies.

1. Long-term psychotherapy

Psychoanalysis. This is a particularly intensive form of treatment in which regression is fostered by the setting and the techniques employed. Sessions occur frequently, three to five times weekly, and it usually extends over two or more years. The patient reclines on a couch and the psychoanalyst sits in a position out of the patient's view. In contemporary practice, the analyst may sit adjacent to the patient. 'Free association' is encouraged. This is a process in which the patient talks freely about their thoughts and feelings. The analyst is relatively passive in this process and interventions are made for clarification and to interpret unconscious material, particularly as it relates to the transference. The patient's tendency to avoid certain emotionally charged topics is referred to as resistance and is also dealt with by interpretation. The development of transference and its interpretation is the therapeutic

cornerstone of psychoanalysis. Unconscious conflicts originating in early childhood are reactivated in the transference context. It is their interpretation within that framework and the subsequent working through process that leads to insight and hence therapeutic benefit.

This form of treatment is suitable for reasonably intelligent people. It can be useful for anxiety disorders, depression, some personality disorders and other conditions in which the aetiological role of unconscious conflict is thought to be paramount. Patients must have the capacity to work within the guidelines of psychoanalysis and to maintain a working alliance with the analyst. Patients with major problems of impulse control and an inability to tolerate frustration are not suitable.

Psychoanalytically-oriented psychotherapy. This is also referred to as long-term 'insight-oriented' or 'dynamic' psychotherapy. It is guided by the same principles as psychoanalysis but regression is held in check by constant referral to day to day reality. Also, the role of the transference and interpretation based on the transference, while very important, is less prominent than in psychoanalysis. Therapy occurs in a face-to-face setting without the psychoanalytic couch. Interpretations remain the major therapeutic technique and are aimed at helping the patient to acquire insight into the thoughts, feelings and behaviours that underly their current problems. This form of treatment can be used for a broad range of neurotic conditions and some personality problems. Techniques tend to be modified to suit the particular strengths and limitations of the individual patient.

2. Brief psychotherapy

This is a form of psychodynamic or psychoanalytic psychotherapy that is narrowly focused on a specific problem or circumscribed area of psychological difficulty. Hence, it is often referred to as a focal psychotherapy. It is based on psychoanalytic theories but the therapist is very much more active in the treatment than in long-term psychotherapy and there is greater flexibility in technique. Regression is not encouraged. Usually the problem is conceptualised in terms of a particular unconscious conflict, the 'nuclear' conflict, and this is taken as the focus for therapy. Good rapport must be achieved very early and transference development is actively fostered.

Transference interpretations are linked to patients' experiences of their relationships with parents and other important figure in their lives. Anxiety-provoking questions may be used in certain forms of treatment within this framework and the more maladaptive ego defences interpreted as they emerge in this context. Other techniques include the development of identification with the therapist, the acquisition of insight, encouragement of new problem-solving skills, confronting the patient with his maladaptive behaviour patterns, emotional release, support for patients' struggles to master or resolve their conflicts and therapeutic working through of termination prior to cessation of therapy.

This form of treatment often takes only six and rarely more than 20 sessions. Several varieties of brief dynamic therapy have been evaluated and each has been shown to achieve good results. A wide variety of patients and psychological problems are capable of responding to this form of treatment or suitable modifications of it. It is well suited to well-motivated people with difficulties in interpersonal relationships, provided that severe personality disorder is not present.

Supportive psychotherapy

This form of psychotherapy is sometimes called relationship psychotherapy as it is concerned with the healing qualities of the interpersonal relationship. It is useful as a form of maintenance therapy in the long-term for people with disabling or recurrent psychiatric illnesses. It is also useful as a therapy for people in crisis or with transient stress reactions.

Empathic listening is the first principle of this form of psychotherapy. The therapist must give the patient his full attention and encourage self-disclosure and emotional expression. The latter alone may provide considerable relief of inner tension provided that the intensity of feeling generated is not so great as to overwhelm the patient and

trigger regression. The aim of self-disclosure is not to gain insight into the unconscious determinants of the patient's problems but rather to provide subjective relief and clear the way for a more objective examination of the problems and how they may be solved.

The provision of reassurance is a useful technique of supportive therapy, provided it is consistent with a realistic evaluation of the situation. Reassurance helps to restore the patient's sense of well-being, self-worth and confidence. The success of this technique depends on acceptance of the therapist's authority and so one must be careful not to allow the use of reassurance to foster unrealistic expectations.

Also dependent on acceptance of the therapist's authority is the use of advice, suggestion and persuasion. These techniques should be targeted at objectives that are within the patient's capabilities to ensure successful experiences since failure to master a problem following expert advice damages the patient's self-esteem.

Additional techniques of supportive psychotherapy include explanation: the sharing of information necessary to solve the problems faced by the patient. Information should be given in clear, uncomplicated terms.

The relationship with the therapist provides opportunities for identification (modelling). A warm, friendly, accepting relationship can help to dilute the adverse influences of earlier relationships with parents and other authority figures in the patient's life who may have been hostile, violent or rejecting. At the same time, the therapist must be careful not to foster excessive dependency but to encourage the patient to exercise his own strengths and build on previously existing personal resources.

Supportive psychotherapy can be used for a wide range of psychological problems in diverse individuals. Often it is accompanied by other forms of treatment such as medication and rehabilitation.

Crisis intervention

A crisis occurs in response to intense stress. It consists initially of mounting anxiety and high arousal followed by attempts to solve or cope with the problem presented by the stressor. If this fails, further distress and behavioural disorganisation or exhaustion may ensue. In attempting to deal with the stressor and its effects an individual may use a variety of coping techniques of which the most adaptive is problem-solving. Alternatively, if the individual is especially vulnerable to the given stressor or if the stressor overwhelms the individual's psychological resources, regression may occur. A successful resolution of the crisis may not only restore equilibrium but lead to the acquisition of a level of adjustment superior to that which existed before the crisis. An unsuccessful resolution, on the other hand, may lead to long-standing psychological ill-health.

Crisis intervention is a form of psychotherapy applied in these circumstances. This therapy is largely supportive in type. Emotional distress and arousal needs to be reduced to a manageable level. Reassurance, explanation and an opportunity to express feelings (catharsis) to an empathic listener are of first importance in this regard. The person may need to be relieved of their usual responsibilities because all of their psychological resources may have to be brought to bear in dealing with the crisis. Special arrangements may need to be made (for example child-care) if this is the case and a range of supports—social, welfare, financial and accommodation— may have to be organised. Assistance in breaking down the crisis into a manageable set of problems and the identification of methods for solving them effectively can then take place in the therapy. This can help to undermine maladaptive behaviours which the patient may be inclined to employ. Examination of the sequences of events that led to the crisis may be helpful as well. Advice and education regarding the steps involved in adaptive problem-solving in the context of the crisis may help the patient to learn new ways of dealing with or avoiding stress that can be called upon in the future.

Crisis intervention may need to involve the participation of family members, hospitalisation and, occasionally, medication. Usually, only two to three outpatient sessions are required but occasionally regular visits over two to three months may be necessary.

Cognitive psychotherapy

Maladaptive cognitive strategies result in repeated, systematic 'errors' or distortions in perceiving, organising one's experiences and responding to the world. These maladaptive strategies persist in spite of objective evidence to the contrary and they lead to repeated failure to cope with ordinary stressors.

Cognitive therapy has been most highly developed in relation to depression. It has been proposed that the depressed individual adopts a negative (ie gloomy) evaluation of the self, one's current life experiences and of the future. This 'cognitive triad' forms the basis for depression. Psychotherapy of depression based on this model involves the identification of the negative cognitions and their effects on feeling or mood (affect), and pitting them against reality. This is accompanied by active attempts to help the patient develop and apply different cognitive strategies to real problems. Techniques in this form of therapy include explanation of the conceptual framework of cognitive therapy to the patient and then eliciting and challenging the negative cognitions. Behavioural techniques are usually combined with this approach and include keeping a daily diary, maintaining a daily schedule, assignment of certain tasks to the patient, cognitive rehearsal, role playing and so on. With increasing experiences of success in mastering the ordinary challenges of everyday life the patients become increasingly aware of the inaccuracies of their earlier cognitions and develop different, healthier cognitive strategies. Depressive symptoms usually subside over several weeks as the treatment progresses.

Modifications of this psychotherapeutic approach can also be applied to other conditions such as anxiety disorders, obsessive-compulsive disorder, and hypohchondriasis (see chapter 61).

Group psychotherapy

Small groups of around six to ten individuals meeting on a regular basis with a skilled group therapist can be an effective form of treatment for a range of psychological problems, especially if they involve interpersonal difficulties.

The interactions between the group members, under the guidance of the therapist, provide the means of bringing about personal change and relief from psychiatric symptoms.

There are many theoretical models for conducting group therapy. Some are based on psychoanalytic principles. Others have used a variety of interactional models focusing on the patterns of transaction between group members in the 'here–and–now'. Still others operate on learning theory lines while some, designated experimental, involve particularly intense encounters between members, including physical contact. Finally, many therapeutic groups are basically supportive in nature and use the methods of individual supportive psychotherapy but in a group setting.

Transference can also occur in various forms in the group setting. For instance, transference can be evoked between individual group members and the therapist, between one member and another or between one person and the group as a whole. The development of transference in these forms can be subject to interpretation by the therapist or other group members. The insight that is acquired by this method can then be used in the service of behaviour change.

Other therapeutic influences acting in groups include cohesiveness, the sense of belonging and willingness to work together as a whole in maintaining the integrity of the group. The realisation that one is not alone but that others share similar problems to oneself is another therapeutic influence. Emotional release, sometimes in relation to a psychological problem or conflict of which a patient was previously unaware, can also be very useful provided the group responds in a supportive way. Learning from the experiences of others is also helpful as is identification with other group members (ie imitation of modelling). The operation of group pressure can be a powerful force in inducing group members to alter their behaviour which can then be reinforced by displays of approval or greater acceptance by the group. The sense of being valued by others to the degree that they are willing to assist the individual in solving his problems can help to instil a sense of hopefulness, an important ingredient in all forms of psychotherapy. Education, the provision of information about psychological ill-health, its origins and methods of dealing with it, is another important therapeutic factor. It provides an intellectual framework within which treatment takes place.

Group therapy has been employed for numerous psychiatric illnesses and other psychological problems. Groups that operate with a confrontational, emotionally arousing style are counter-productive for schizophrenic patients. Groups that are insufficiently confrontational are generally ineffective for individuals with antisocial characteristics. The decision to refer a patient for group therapy must involve an attempt to select the type of therapeutic approach that is suited to both the type of problem presented by the patient and the personal characteristics of that patient.

An important form of group therapy that has not been discussed is that of the self-help groups. Examples include Alcoholics Anonymous, Narcotics Anonymous and Gamblers Anonymous. These groups are formed by people who all suffer the same affliction and basically operate along supportive and educational lines.

Conclusion

Finally, in considering the role of psychotherapy, it cannot be over-emphasised that the quality of the patient–therapist relationship is probably the single most important element. Two factors seem to be central in this relationship. One is the quality of empathy which needs to be conveyed to patients so that they become aware that the therapist regards them with warmth and understanding. The other is the formation of a working alliance in which patient and therapist form a partnership, a collaboration arrangement in which the task is to work on solving the patient's problems together.

Further Reading

Beck A T, *Cognitive Therapy and Emotional Disorders*, International Universities Press, New York, 1976.
Bloch S, *An Introduction to the Psychotherapies*, 2nd ed, Oxford University Press, Oxford, 1986.
Frank J D, *Persuasion and Healing*, John Hopkins Press, Baltimore, 1967.
Malan D H, *The Frontier of Brief Psychotherapy*, Plenum, New York, 1976.
Yalom I, *The Theory and Practice of Group Psychotherapy* 3rd ed, Basic Books, New York, 1985.

Chapter 59

Family Therapy 1: General Considerations

P Hazell

Family therapy is a form of psychological treatment that focuses on the interaction of family members as a means of understanding a symptom and effecting change. It is a problem oriented rather than diagnosis oriented treatment.

Family therapy has grown from the clinical observation that emotional or behavioural problems in an individual often impinge upon others with whom they live. In addition, the patterns of relationships within the family may, in turn, modify the problems. A misconception about family therapy is that it implies families cause psychiatric illness. Most family therapists do not view the family unit as necessarily dysfunctional, but rather see the family as a forum in which to solve a problem.

A wide range of health professionals use family therapy techniques. It has been particularly popular amongst social workers, but is also practised by psychiatrists, psychologists, general practitioners, clergy and other counsellors. Family therapy is both an exciting and demanding form of therapy that requires the therapist to be able to listen to and observe often quite complex communication amongst family members, while at the same time being able to formulate the problem and implement management strategies.

In some clinical settings, the family may be the initial point of contact, as in child and family clinics, whereas in other settings the decision to assess and work with the family may result from previous assessment of an individual, the so-called 'identified' patient. Commonly when a decision has been made to work with a family, all individuals living in the same household as the identified patient are invited to attend an appointment. Sometimes other significant family members such as grandparents may also be asked to come along. Some therapists refuse to proceed unless all family members are in attendance, while others will see whoever elects to come. In child psychiatry settings it is often difficult for the mother of a child to persuade the father of the importance of taking leave from work to attend the clinic. A helpful strategy under these circumstances is to offer to contact the father personally, or even telephone him during a session to seek his advice or help on a particular problem facing the family.

The family therapist may work alone, but it is also common for two family therapists to work together with a family as 'co-therapists'. Sometimes a therapist will work with the assistance of a 'team'. The team consists of one or more co-therapists who do not actively participate in the sessions, but who observe the interactions of the family members with each other and with the therapist and may provide advice or feedback to the family through the therapist. Commonly, the team will observe the session through a one way screen or on a video monitor or both.

A common feature of family therapy is to make few appointments relatively infrequently, allowing the family time between appointments to work on specific tasks defined in the sessions. Infrequent (for example, once a fortnight) appointments also protect the therapist from becoming overwhelmed by the volume of data that can often be obtained from a family.

Family therapy has been applied particularly to problems presenting in child and adolescent mental health. One reason for this is that children and adolescents are usually accompanied by at least one parent when they attend clinics, so that a transition to a family focus often occurs quite naturally. Family therapy is also used in the setting of chronic psychiatric and physical illness, where a heavy burden falls on the family to cope with the effects of the illness and to provide effective care.

Various writers attribute different origins to family therapy, but it is likely that groups of therapists in different locations developed their own forms of family therapy more or less concurrently. Of undeniable theoretical importance is the contribution of systems theory to the development of family therapy principles. Systems theory is derived from the basic biological and physical sciences and is concerned with describing and predicting the behaviour of complex systems on the basis of the interaction of the parts. An example is the interaction between a mother and her infant. The mother's behaviour exerts an influence on the behaviour of the infant, but the behaviour and responsiveness of the infant also shapes the maternal behaviour. The important principles underpinning systems theory are:

1. The notion of homeostasis, or a dynamic steady state, which is sustained by monitoring shifts of parts of the system away from the balance and correction of these shifts (negative feedback).

2. The notion that the steady state of an organism may shift from time to time through a process of 'deviation amplification' or positive feedback. This shift in steady state is conceptualised as essential for the adaptation of the organism.

The credibility of family therapy was harmed in its early stages by claims of very high success rates in people with psychosomatic conditions, such as anorexia nervosa. These claims were based on descriptive studies with no control group and a short follow-up period. A number of units practising family therapy are attempting to address the problem of a lack of systematic outcome research. A difficulty in conducting research on family therapy has been the lack of satisfactory ways of describing and measuring family interaction. This problem has been partially redressed by the McMaster group in Canada, who have devised a self report rating scale of family function called the Family Assessment Device. This instrument has seven scales: problem solving, communication, roles, affective responsiveness, affective involvement, behaviour control and general functioning.

Similarly, a group at the Hospital for Sick Children in London, England has devised the Family Interaction Summary Format, a clinician rated instrument that has the following items: atmosphere, communication, affective status, boundaries, family operations, alliances, parental functioning and relations to the environment. Other methodological difficulties will need to be overcome, however, before there is any convincing outcome research, in particular the problem of controlling the many variables that may impinge on family function.

One area that has been studied more rigorously is family intervention in the management of schizophrenia. In the 1950s it was demonstrated that schizophrenic patients were more likely to relapse if their family environments were emotionally charged. A concept of 'expressed emotion' was developed that encompassed hostility, criticism and over-involvement. An approach to the families of schizophrenic patients was then developed which combined education with attempts to reduce expressed emotion within the family. This was found to be effective in reducing the frequency of relapse of the schizophrenic patients, although the precise mechanism of action is still unknown. It may be a direct psychological effect, or the intervention may have worked indirectly by, for example, improving patient compliance with medication.

Although there are a number of competing schools of family therapy which have different theoretical orientations, there are several techniques used so widely in family therapy that they warrant brief description. *Reframing* is restating of a problem or a behaviour in a different (usually more positive) way. An example would be the reframing of a child's disruptive behaviour in the context of marital disturbance as a caring and concerning activity designed to distract the parents from their conflict with one another. *Circular questioning* is a technique that is used to elicit difference in relationships the family have experienced before and after a problem began. An example of circular questioning would be to ask the elder sibling of a child with anorexia nervosa whether mother and father had talked more with each other or less with each other since the patient began to diet. *Metaphor* is employed by many therapists as a means of illustrating a problem, or assisting the family in distancing themselves from a problem so that they can look at it more objectively. The scope of metaphor is limited only by the extent of the therapist's imagination. An example would be to liken arguments between a mother and daughter over the issue of responsibility versus freedom to a strange tennis match in which the object seems to be to hit the ball as far out of the court as possible. Each increasingly extreme behaviour manifested by the daughter is matched by and even more extreme punishment or restriction imposed by the mother, thus inviting further extreme behaviour from the daughter. The therapist uses this metaphor to clarify his role thus: 'I can help you to get along better by coaching you to hit the ball in the court rather than out of court, but I cannot be the umpire. It would be unhelpful for me to adjudicate on how far out of court each ball was.'

Paradox is a technique that stimulates the family to resolve a problem through the mechanism of deviation amplification. Instead of offering strategies that might reduce the intensity of a problem, the therapist actually suggests a counter strategy that intensifies difficulties in the short term. An example would be to suggest to the parents of an encopretic boy that they actually praise him each time they find soiled underwear, and tell him how proud they are of his achievements. *Genogram* work involves asking the family to construct their own family tree, discussing the attributes of as many family members as possible. It is possible to discover patterns of behaviour that may not have been acknowledged by family members before. An example would be to discover that all highly successful members within a family may have made career changes before they settled on their final vocations. This may be very reassuring to a family concerned about a capable but anxious student who has made several course changes during one year.

The form of an introductory family interview varies with the orientation and style of the therapist, but the following elements are usually seen: the initial contact is often by telephone and allows the therapist to obtain some preliminary information about the presenting problem and to prepare the family for the first appointment. The therapist will then develop hypotheses based on the referral data which will be tested during initial sessions. The appointment begins with an introductory phase, in which the therapist orients the family to the room, especially if a microphone, camera or one-way screen is being used. The therapist attempts to make some form of social contact with each family member present. Early involvement of young children in the session is a common way of putting families at ease. Problem-identification follows, with the therapist asking each family member to describe their own ideas of the problem. The therapist will also be observing family relationship patterns. One technique that flows naturally from problem-identification is to ask the family how they have gone about attempting to solve the problem so far. The therapist will then ask the family to define goals for treatment. Implicit in this task is the need to determine the family's expectations of therapy. A common example would be to ask a family: 'How will you know that the problem has got better?' This is particularly useful when the presenting problem is a series of vague complaints about the behaviour of a child. The therapist then makes arrangements for future appointments. The family may be set some 'homework' tasks, for example, asking a disengaged father to keep a record of the number of time his son has missed school.

Following the session the therapist will

revise the initial hypotheses. Some therapists write a brief letter to the family summarising the content of the session and restating the homework tasks. The referring agent is contacted, where applicable, to discuss the outcome of the first assessment. Sometimes the therapist will also have to contact other sources to obtain data relevant to the assessment.

In summary, family therapy is a psychological treatment that has recently evolved. It has been most widely applied in the areas of child and adolescent psychiatry where it is often the primary management and in some serious mental illnesses, where it is used as an adjunct to other treatments. There is considerable enthusiasm amongst practitioners of family therapy regarding its efficacy, but there is still a lack of systematic outcome research. Recent advances in research methods may eventually redress this problem.

Further Reading

Epstein N B, Baldwin L B and Bishop D S, 'The McMaster Family Assessment Device', *Journal of Marital and Family Therapy*, Vol 9, 1983, pp 171–80.

Loader P, Burck C, Kinston W and Bentovim A, 'A Method for Organising the Clinical Description of Family Interaction: the "Family Interaction Summary Format"', *Australian Journal of Family Therapy*, Vol 2, 1981, pp 131–41.

McDermott J J, 'Indications for Family Therapy. Question or Non-Question?' *Journal of the American Academy of Child Psychiatry*, Vol 20, 1981, pp 409–19.

Robinson M, 'Systems Theory for the Beginning Therapist', *Australian Journal of Family Therapy*, Vol 1, 1980, pp 183–94.

Smyrnios K X and Kirkby R J, 'A Review of Brief, Child Oriented Family Therapy Outcome Research. Descriptive Reports and Single Group Studies', *Australian and New Zealand Journal of Family Therapy*, Vol 10, 1989, pp 151–9.

Weber T, McKeever J E and McDaniell S H, 'A Beginner's Guide to the Problem Oriented First Family Interview', *Family Process*, Vol 24, 1985, pp 357–64.

Chapter 60

Family Therapy 2: Clinical Aspects

C Quadrio

In family therapy, a symptomatic individual is usually regarded as the one who signals distress within the family system. For example, a child complaining of abdominal pain may have appendicitis or may be reacting with symptoms of physical pain to intrafamilial stress. A 'diagnosis' may be only a beginning to identifying complex family dysfunction.

Key words enter such descriptions—of family 'systems' and 'context'—both words that are central to the family therapy approach. Humans are social creatures, they have strong *affiliative* needs and their optimal functioning usually requires a network of interpersonal relationships. For a child, this context is the 'family of origin', the family into which a child is born or reared until he is ready to become a separate individual. This process of separation from his family moves the individual into establishing a new context, a new family, while still maintaining mutually satisfying contact with the family of origin. Further, when establishing a new family, a young couple create an interface between two pre-existing families (families of their origin). This complex system of interactions constitutes the immediate context of the new family.

It is this wider perspective of the network or system of family relationships in which symptoms are embedded and which form the essential context of a person's total functioning. For this reason, some would prefer terms such as 'systemic' or 'contextual' therapy rather than the more limited notion of 'family'.

Socio-cultural context

Added to the concept of a dynamic and essential family relationship network, there is yet another dimension which is crucial to the family therapy approach (and which underscores the inadequacy of the term 'family therapy') and that is the socio-cultural matrix in which each family exists. The family is the context in which a child is 'socialised', or taught to behave in certain ways and to incorporate values which are widely accepted in the culture. The family is an essential element in the transmission of cultural values and the parents instruct their children how to be a member of that culture. This includes values relating to masculinity and femininity. However, it should be noted that there may be little a family can do to provide a child with adequate self-esteem, if that child is one which the culture itself does not value in terms of skin colour or intellectual ability.

The complex interactions of individual–family–culture is one which concerns family therapy and obviously transcends the limited notion of 'family'. A comprehensive or systemic view of humans is represented by the biopsychosocial model which includes hierarchical series of systems, starting at the cellular level and ascending to higher levels of organisation. Alcoholism, for example, can be understood in terms of the addictive properties of a chemical substance, or the propensity of an individual to become addicted, or the immediate psychosocial stresses that provoke the drinking behaviour, or the socio-cultural mores which encourage drinking as a tension reducing mechanism, or the multinational commercial interests which promote sales of addictive substances, or all of these things acting together.

Such a perspective allows of no simple notions of linear causality. One of the most crucial and useful results of systems theory is the shift away from a linear to circular causality. Thus, the interaction of an alcoholic person with a negative spouse would be viewed as a recursive process—the more one drinks, the more the other criticises; the more one criticises, the more the other drinks. A family therapy or systemic approach is concerned with interrupting this circular process.

Family therapy is a natural corollary of a biopsychosocial perspective and can be seen as an integral part of a complete approach to psychiatric assessment and treatment. When an individual's symptomatology is difficult to understand or to treat, it is not always necessary to postulate disturbance deep within the psyche. Indeed, this approach may yield less and less in the way of perspective and understanding of the total problem. Sometimes, more information may be obtained by stepping back and observing the individual in the context of his family and the family in the context of their society.

There are many situations in psychiatry where examination of individual psycho-pathology cannot readily explain what is more clearly evident by examining the family context. Anorexia nervosa is one condition where family therapy has added much to our understanding and treatment of the problem, by considering the multi-layered interaction described above.

Clinical applications

Given the preceding introduction, we may now consider clinical applications of family therapy in mental illnesses. They cover the entire spectrum of psychiatric disorders and will vary according to the orientation and expertise of the clinician and the nature of the presenting problem. The systemic therapy purist would argue that all symptoms are manifestations of dysfunctional systems and would aim to alter the interpersonal or familial

context in every case. By contrast, a psycho-analyst would focus upon effecting change within the intrapsychic world, arguing that this would result in behavioural and interpersonal change, thereby altering the larger system. More realistic systemic therapy can encompass both views, since there is a dynamic exchange between the intrapsychic and the interpersonal worlds and change in one system will bring about changes in the other.

A systemic view would regard all psychiatric disorders as occurring in a family–social context and, given the recursive nature of systems, would regard them all as amenable to family intervention. Such an approach is still radically different from more traditional individually oriented models, even when these models incorporate an acknowledgment and understanding of the influence of the family. Particularly in child psychiatry, the influence of the family and the importance of the family structure and dynamics have long been recognised.

Psychiatry is often concerned with individual dysfunction and may invoke organic, psychodynamic or behavioural causalities for symptoms. Whilst there is recognition that individual development occurs within the individual's family and social environment, the focus of assessment and treatment is usually on the dysfunction within the individual and response to treatment is similarly assessed on the basis of individual symptomatology.

There is in fact, a continuum from the predominantly individual perspective to the systems perspective. Most psychiatry treat-ment utilises aspects from many different disciplines and very few psychiatrists maintain an exclusively individual orientation. Equally few operate entirely from a systems perspective.

Individual treatment with a family system orientation

Bowen is the foremost exponent of individual treatments which aim to modify the family system. He has developed techniques which aim at moving an individual out of the 'emotional field' of intrafamilial conflict. This process he describes as 'detriangling'. Briefly, he regards symptomatic individuals as caught in (or triangled into) a conflict between two others. Often this occurs in a family where conflict between husband and wife may be resolved or stabilised by focussing upon a child who is then said to be 'triangulated'. Whilst these interactions begin as intrafamilial they eventually become internalised and the child accepts the sick role.

Minuchin has developed a similar model which has been of particular value in dealing with children with psychosomatic illness. Conflict resolution between parents are 'detoured' through the symptomatic behaviour of the child. This is not to imply that the symptoms are caused by family conflicts, because the symptoms and the family processes interact in a recursive manner. These situations are dealt with by treating the whole family.

A 37 year old woman had chronic depression. Since her childhood she had been very involved ('enmeshed') with her parents and with their relationship problems. She described her father as an arrogant and self-centred man who had pursued his own career to the exclusion of the needs of his wife and children. Her mother had been depressed during much of her married life and had suffered a variety of illnesses and was subject to episodes of angina. She had always confided in her daughter the details of her married life. The patient was still the confidante of her mother and she struggled continually to console and reassure her, while at the same time, chiding her father for his lack of consideration of her mother's health and happiness. The father would admonish her to concern herself with her own life and marriage.

This family situation illustrates the triangulation of a child which becomes a permanent pattern. In this case, the established pattern was one of feeling responsible for other people's problems and feeling depressed when unable to alter these problems. This adjustment had persisted into adult life and led to the woman's chronic depression and the failure of her separation from her parents.

A family oriented individual therapy or 'Bowenian' approach aimed at 'detriangling'

the woman was used. She was encouraged to decline, politely, to listen to any more of her mother's confidences and to resist subsequent escalation of demands, including frequent telephone calls and threatened angina attacks (which were to be referred to the local doctor). At the same time, the patient was encouraged to meet with her father and attempt to mend the rift between them. This was to be done by avoiding any criticism of him or his relationship with his wife. It was predicted that the mother would become more distressed and that the daughter should resist this invitation to restore the status quo.

The treatment reached a climax when the patient offered to accompany her father on a weekend trip to a rural property which he operated as a hobby farm. His wife would never accompany him on these trips because she suffered from car sickness and panic attacks when travelling out of town. The father was pleased with his daughter's interest and the two set off for the weekend together. By the following day the mother had joined them, having driven alone for the first time out of the city.

With continued encouragement like this, the daughter began to disengage from the parents and the mother diminished her efforts to involve her in the marital relationship and instead increased her participation in activities with her husband. The daughter's depression improved as she came to feel less responsible for her parents and more vigorously involved in her own life.

The system maintaining individual disorder

Often a dysfunctional individual will enter relationships which support or even encourage a pre-existing problem to the extent that the maintenance of these relationships prevent any change in the symptomatic behaviour. *Alcoholism* provides a common example. The partner of an alcoholic is often described as a 'co-dependent', emphasising the partner's need for the symptom to be maintained. Often a person who suffers from low self-esteem or a fear of being unwanted or rejected will enter into a relationship wherein he or she will become indispensable to a dysfunctional person. The co-dependant's need to be needed supports the system.

Agoraphobia provides another example. It is a syndrome of anxiety and panic occurring in situations of leaving home. Eventually a person with agoraphobia may be completely housebound and may require a constant companion, usually a spouse, mother or child. The spouse may support this process and maintain the symptoms.

A 34 year old woman with agoraphobia was seen with her husband for conjoint therapy. She was fearful, anxious and housebound, but her husband was also a socially withdrawn and sexually inactive man, supportive of his wife's symptoms to the extent of spending all his off work time doing the shopping and whatever other chores she could not manage. Here the symptom of one spouse offers 'protection' for the less obvious problems of the other. The symptoms of the wife which kept her housebound and heavily dependent upon her husband, offered him 'protection' from his social and sexual anxieties. While he was assured of a secure relationship with a housebound wife, there was no threat of a sexual rival and he was able to avoid social situations by supporting his wife's housebound adjustment.

Treatment here may be extremely difficult if the marital system is not modified. With individual treatment, improvement in the wife's condition may evoke symptoms in the husband. As she becomes more active, he may become depressed or may drink heavily. When the wife's phobic symptoms return, the husband's adjustment improves and the pathological adjustment is restored.

By modifying the marital system the husband's adjustment can improve as he and his wife confront the issues that bind them together. Once the agoraphobic adjustment of the couple is altered, children of the marriage are also freed from their roles as companions and are able to pursue their own development more fully.

Treating the system without the symptomatic individual

Sometimes members of a family may present complaining about another member who is unwilling or unable to be involved in treatment. This is very often the case with adolescents who are usually reluctant patients and who may view their parents' complaints as just that, the inevitable complaining of parents. It may be possible to deal with these situations even when the 'identified patient' is not seen, as in the following case.

A 15 year old boy was truanting and staying out overnight. His mother consulted her family doctor after the school told her that they could no longer control him. The general practitioner referred him for specialist help, but the boy refused to cooperate. Instead, the mother was willing to come.

At this point there are several options. Some practitioners will insist, by phone, the entire family agree to come—this is what Whitaker refers to as the 'battle for structure' and a battle which needs to be won in order to challenge the family system. If only part of the family attends, such practitioners would refuse to see them and the family would be advised to return and to ensure that the absent members attended.

The value of this approach is that the status of the identified patient is immediately challenged and the problem placed firmly in the family interactions.

An alternative strategy is to agree to see whichever members of the family are willing to cooperate, but to ensure that the system is challenged rather than reinforced. In the case referred to above, the parents, who were divorced, were seen without their son. It became apparent that the husband, despite the divorce, was still deeply attached to his ex-wife and had not made a separate life for himself. The ex-wife had no desires at all for reconciliation, but her plans for re-marriage and for a new life with a second husband were being systematically undermined by the son's behaviour. The ex-husband was continually called upon to deal with the rebellious son whilst the potential new husband refused to finalise plans for marriage until the boy was 'under control'. Thus, the boy's behaviour (not necessarily consciously contrived) was keeping his father involved with the family and blocking his mother's plans for a new life.

By working with the parents towards a resolution of these separation issues, it was possible for an effective working relationship to be developed between them. Once this was achieved, the father began restructuring his life, the boy's rebellious behaviour subsided and his school life returned to normal.

In this case, the 'patient' was never seen by the clinician, but by working with the family the symptomatic behaviour was resolved. Such an approach carries a significant *danger* that psychiatric illness in the identified patient may be missed, for example, the child may be suffering from a depressive illness.

Treating the marital system

The marital dyad may become the focus of treatment even though the initial presentation is of an individual 'identified patient'. As the executive unit of the family, the parents are most powerfully situated to modify the system and much useful change can be effected by working through them.

At times, the marital system is the focus of treatment from the outset and this is particularly so when a couple present complaining about relationship problems, threatened breakdown of marriage, or sexual problems. The following case illustrates treatment focussed entirely on the marital system.

A 34 year old man experienced premature ejaculation throughout his marriage and described himself as 'a failure as a man'. His early history was one of deprivation and hardship, he was sent to work at the age of 12 and felt that 'no matter how much I gave, it was never enough'. He was holding down two jobs, studying to further his career and was very devoted to his wife and children. The wife had also been raised in a deprived family and had been a surrogate mother to six younger siblings, supervised by a father whom she described as brutal, dominating and irresponsible. She resented her father and the family responsibilities that were foisted upon her as a child.

At initial assessment, this couple were viewed as having complementary needs—his

to work hard, to give ceaselessly and to feel that he could never give enough; hers to find a husband/father figure who would bear all the responsibility for the family and expect little from her in return. Her past experience had left her resentful and unwilling to meet the demands or needs of father or husband. Her resentment of her husband's sexual needs and her reluctance to meet those needs were a part of their interaction. While this complementarity continued, the system was stable.

Interventions aimed at altering the complementarity and encouraging each spouse to be more direct and assertive, led to a modification of the husband's 'selflessness' so that he was able to seek more gratification of his own needs, sexual and otherwise. At the same time, his wife's chronic and passive resentment was relieved by encouraging her to exercise choice in responding to demands, to have the right to say 'no' rather than accepting with resentment or avoiding intimacy altogether. Essentially, he acquired permission to demand, and she acquired permission to say 'no'. The relationship issues and the sexual problems were overcome with this conjoint approach.

Working with the family system

Even when an individual presents with psychiatric illness, it may be possible to effect positive changes by working with the family system.

A young man aged 19 years presented as very confused and disorganised, coping poorly, not knowing what he wanted to do with his life. He had peculiar religious ideas and preoccupations. He was dishevelled and undernourished and had been living away from home in very impoverished circumstances. His strange religious preoccupations dominated his thinking and working hours, so that he neglected the usual daily tasks of caring for himself. He was asked to return to his family (two parents and four siblings) and from the outset treatment was aimed at modifying the family system.

During the family assessment, it emerged that the paternal grandfather had exerted a powerful influence on this family. This man had been forced to leave school at age 13 to help support his family and later his ambitions to return to school were interrupted by the war. He was bitter about his lack of education and determined that his own children would succeed where he never had the opportunity. He nevertheless envied their opportunities and subtly undermined their successes. Effectively, his ambivalent feelings of ambitiousness/envy towards his children resulted in their own confused expectations. His eldest son did moderately well, but was never satisfied with his performance and perpetuated similar ambivalent messages to his children. In the context of this family pathology, the 'identified patient' had decompensated in his first year of university.

The powerful influence of the grandparent, evident in the history and the relationship between grandfather, father and son, illustrates what Bowen (1960) has called the 'three generational system', suggesting that a disorder is determined over three generations by the influence of one generation on the next. Thus, the grandfather's thwarted ambitions determined the father's ambivalent attitudes towards success and failure. In turn, this determined a confused set of expectations of success and failure for the son which he could not resolve and which were expressed in his strange behaviour.

Of course there was another side to this system. The young man's mother was a puritanical woman who demanded piety and industry from her children, just as her own mother had expected of her. Her son's shabby appearance and strange religious ideas mocked her values.

This case illustrates both the three generational system and the triangulation of identified patient between the parents. The aim of family therapy is to block the triangulation between the parents and the identified patient by focusing on unresolved issues between husband and wife and between each parent and his or her own family of origin.

This is achieved by challenging the communication pattern of the family so that the parents confront issues openly and directly between them rather than by talking through, or about, the patient. The parents challenge relationships within their families of origin, to free themselves from what Bowen calls the 'undifferentiated ego mass' of the family and as the parents differentiate more from their own family systems, so their son is freed to pursue his own development.

Conclusion

In the case histories presented above, a range of approaches has been demonstrated, all relating in some way to the family system.

The way in which a clinician decides to implement family therapy will vary enormously according to the orientation of the clinician and the nature of the presenting problem. It is evident from this overview that the range of applications is extremely wide. At the same time, there is no one therapy, technique or approach which automatically suits every situation, family or individual. Different people require different treatments at different times. Some situations are better dealt with by using individual therapy. It is certainly not true that family therapy is inappropriate for very disturbed individuals, but medication and other treatment modalities need to be used, if indicated.

Whether the individual is treated; with the family system in mind or whether the whole family is present in the treatment room, the clinician will be well advised to have a thorough understanding of systems theory and family dynamics.

Further Reading

Bertalanffy L V, *General Systems Theory*, Braziller, New York, 1977.

Bowen M, 'A Family Concept of Schizophrenia', in *The Aetiology of Schizophrenia*, (ed Jackson D), Basic Books, New York, 1960.

Bowen M, 'The Use of Family Theory in Clinical Practice', *Comprehensive Psychiatry*, Vol 7, 1966, pp 345-74.

Engel G L, 'The Need for a New Medical Model: A Challenge for Biomedicine', *Science*, Vol 196, 4286, 1968, pp 129–36.

Hafner J R, 'The Husbands of Agoraphobic Women and Their Influence on Treatment Outcome', *British Journal of Psychiatry*, Vol 131, 1977, pp 289–94.

Haley J, 'Marriage Therapy', *Archives of General Psychiatry*, Vol 8, 1963, pp 213–34.

Holmes J, 'Phobia and Counterphobia: Family Aspects of Agoraphobia, *Journal of Family Therapy*, Vol 4, 1982, pp 133–52.

Keith D and Whitaker C, 'Play Therapy: A Paradigm for Work with Families', *Journal of Marital and Family Therapy*, Vol 7 No 3, 1981, pp 243–54.

Minuchin S, *Psychosomatic Families: Anorexia Nervosa in Context*, Harvard University Press, Cambridge, 1978.

Quadrio C, 'Rapunzel and the Pumpkin Eater: Marital Systems of Agoraphobic Women', *Australian Journal of Family Therapy*, Vol 4 No 2, 1983, pp 81–5.

Quadrio C, 'Families of Agoraphobic Women', *Australian and New Zealand Journal of Psychiatry*, Vol 18, 1984, pp 164–70.

Chapter 61

Behaviour Therapy

A Gannoni

Behaviour therapy has become one of the most rapidly growing areas of therapy in psychology and related professions with ongoing developments in theories, models, techniques and empirical evaluation of its effectiveness.

Models of behaviour therapy

Classical conditioning

According to Kazdin (1978), the behaviourist movement emerged from work in Russia on conditioning and reflexology. Sechenov, a physiologist developed the theory that all behaviour is reflexive, with humans learning, through associations, the complex reflexes which make up their behaviour. Pavlov extended this theory to study the development of conditioned reflexes by linking stimuli to naturally occurring reflexes by substituting an experimental or 'conditioned' stimulus for the natural, or 'unconditioned' stimulus. This was referred to as Pavlovian, respondent or classical conditioning.

Another influence in the early twentieth century was the work of J B Watson, an American psychologist, who used the classical conditioning paradigm in the study of animal behaviour to transfer learning processes to humans. He stressed that learning determined abnormal behaviour and advocated the use of objective methods to study behaviour.

The classical conditioning model is an approach to learning based on the connection between stimulus and response. It is used to explain many types of emotional disorders, including neurotic and phobic behaviours.

Operant conditioning

Probably the best known and most influential model in behaviour therapy is operant, or instrumental or Skinnerian conditioning. In this approach an individual actively produces behaviour which stimulates a response from the environment. Thus, the individual is able to choose the response, providing the behaviour is in the individual's repertoire. When it is not, an individual, for example a parent or teacher, selects a similar, already established, behaviour and shapes it to the desired response. The focus in operant conditioning is on the choice of stimuli preceding the behaviour, as well as on the consequences of the behaviour. It is the response which reinforces the behaviour and determines the probability that the behaviour will occur again in similar circumstances.

Cognitive behaviour therapy

Cognitive behaviour therapies essentially focus on internal processes and their influence on behaviour. The assumption of cognitive behaviour therapy is that an individual's emotional and behavioural reactions are the result of their interpretations of events. Thus, treatment aims at modifying these interpretations. An example is Ellis' Rational Emotive Therapy, which conceptualises an ABC model of human functioning. In this paradigm, an activating event in the environment (A) triggers an individual's relevant cognitive set of beliefs (negative) (B). The individual's emotional and behavioural consequences (C) result directly from these beliefs. Thus in Ellis' model, emotional and behavioural problems are maintained by specific cognitive sets which individuals make about themselves, events or situations (see chapters 58, 63).

Social learning theory

Social learning theory (Bandura, 1969, 1977) is essentially an incorporation of the principles of classical and operant conditioning and cognitive behaviour therapy into a comprehensive explanation of human behaviour. It emphasises the importance of cognitive and environmental influences and their reciprocal interaction. In this framework it is recognised that individuals play an active role in relating to their environment (see chapter 58).

Techniques of behaviour therapy

Techniques based on models of behaviour therapy are presented and related to their clinical use and efficacy.

Classical conditioning techniques

Systematic desensitisation and implosion therapy (or 'flooding') are conditioning methods applied to the treatment of some emotional states (for example, phobias). Systematic desensitisation was developed by Wolpe (Wolpe, 1958) and involves having the individual imagine scenes related to the phobia while in a state of deep relaxation. Often achieving this state, the subject is required to imagine the anxiety provoking scenes in an hierarchical order, beginning with the scene which is least anxiety provoking. The subject, maintaining the relaxation state, moves through the hierarchy progressing to the next level, provided the degree of anxiety at each item is manageable. Exposure to the hierarchy can be imaginal or in actual circumstances (for example, in an aeroplane). Implosion therapy (or 'flooding') involves rapid exposure and intensive contact with the feared object or situation whilst being supported and reassured by the therapist. It may be of value when treating phobic reactions. The rationale behind implosive therapy is that if the individual can be induced to remain in the phobic situation despite very high levels of anxiety, extinction of the anxiety will result. It is generally used in treating adult phobic reactions, however, implosion therapy can be used with school phobics provided the therapist is sensitive, and school staff and parents are firm, understanding, and consistent (Lask and Fosson, 1989).

Operant conditioning

The basic principle of the operant conditioning approach is that behaviour is a function of its consequences. Techniques based on this approach are specifically directed to the manipulation of reinforcement and punishment as a consequence of the behaviour. Operant techniques are widely used in clinical settings, for example, parent management programs, and inpatient care. In fact, the most comprehensive application of operant principles is the token economy which is sometimes used in residential and inpatient settings and classrooms. Operant techniques are applied to a wide range of behaviours including self-mutilating behaviour and tantrums. Some operant techniques include:

Reinforcement which involves the immediate provision of attention, praise, or tokens for desired, appropriate behaviour. It is necessary that rewards be individualised with social rewards, such as praise or smiles, coupled with tangible rewards such as food. If the desired behaviour does not occur, rewards should not be provided. After the behaviour is well established, intermittent rewards (ie partial scheduling) are more effective than consistent reinforcement (ie continuous scheduling).

Shaping, which is the procedure whereby a complex response is taught by rewarding successful approximations to that response. Rewards can be given for partially successful responses, with rewards withheld until the individual emits closer approximations of the desired behaviour. The individual is rewarded for responses at least as good as that displayed on previous occasions.

Chaining, which involves the sequencing and reinforcing of simple responses to achieve desired, complex behaviour. The individual is reinforced for successful completion of each simple response and upon proficiency at one level; reinforcement is available only after successful completion of the next level in the chain. Shaping and chaining are used in a variety of settings and are especially applicable to teaching self-help skills to mentally retarded and autistic children.

Extinction, which is the withdrawal of positive reinforcement for undesired behaviour and it generally involves ignoring or withdrawing attention. Initially an increase in the undesired behaviour can be anticipated and it is vital that the extinction process be maintained, as intermittent reinforcement can strongly encourage the persistence of the undesired behaviour.

Punishment, which refers to the application of aversive conditioning to inappropriate behaviour. In this method, undesirable behaviour is subject to punishment or withdrawal from a previously reinforcing event. Forms of punishment include: (i) the techniques of response cost, that is, the withdrawal of previously acquired rewards; (ii) time-out, that is, removal of the opportunity to obtain rewards or removal of the individual to a less reinforcing situation; and (iii) overcorrection, which refers to the repeated practice of positive behaviours contingent upon negative behaviours. For example, a child suffering from encopresis must wash his soiled underwear.

An example of physical punishment is the use of electrical aversion in which a mild, but painful, electric shock serves as an aversive stimulus. The appropriateness of electrical aversion therapy for individuals must be determined through the careful evaluation of psychological and medical status.

In the main, reinforcement and punishment techniques establish relatively rapid control over behaviour. Although they can produce dramatic results, treatment gains are often lost when the program is terminated or the individual leaves the setting. Further research is required to consider techniques to produce long term maintenance and generalisation effects.

Social learning theory

Modelling refers to the exposure of the individual to the desired behaviour, for example, during modelling the subject witnesses others in contact with feared stimuli, and these individuals demonstrate ways to manipulate the stimuli with positive outcomes. There is some evidence that a coping model (that is someone who is initially afraid but who manages the situation) may be more effective than a model displaying mastery. Modelling is hypothesised to be effective because of vicarious extinction of fear responses and the acquisition of new behaviour. Modelling has been effectively used in reducing compulsive behaviour, in treating fears and phobias, and in teaching social skills.

Cognitive behaviour therapy

These techniques aim at modifying the thinking patterns of individuals and involve procedures such as consideration of irrational beliefs and statements, generation of alternative solutions to problem situations and self instruction techniques. Another example focuses on training convert cognitive processes in children and adolescents presenting with social skills problems. Specifically, subjects are taught to identify interpersonal problems, generate alternative strategies to handle the problems, evaluate solutions by considering their consequences, and finally plan and execute the action of choice. However, cognitive problem solving programs which do not include direct training in behavioural skills do not consistently produce positive outcomes in terms of social adjustment in the natural environment. Treatment programs combining cognitive behaviour therapies and behavioural approaches have been shown to be most effective.

Behaviour therapy has a wide diversity of techniques and conceptual ideas. This chapter has briefly described the models of behaviour therapy and provided a limited representation of therapeutic techniques.

Further Reading

Bandura A, *Principles of Behaviour Modification*, Holt, Rinehart & Winston, New York, 1969.

Bandura A, *Social Learning Theory*, Prentice-Hall, Inglewood Cliffs, 1977.

Ellis A, *Reason and Emotion in Psychotherapy*, Lyle Stuart, New York, 1962.

Hersen M and Van Hasselt V B, *Behaviour Therapy With Children and Adolescents*, Wiley, New York, 1987.

Kanfer F H and Phillips J S, *Learning Foundations of Behaviour therapy*, Wiley, New York, 1970.

Kazdin A E, *History of Behaviour Modification*, University Park Press, Baltimore, 1978.

Lask B and Fosson A, *Childhood Illness: The Psychosomatic Approach*, Wiley, London, 1989.

Ollendick T H, 'Behaviour Therapy with Children and Adolescents', in *Handbook of Psychotherapy and Behaviour Change*, 3rd edn, (ed Garfield S L and Bergin A E), Wiley, New York, 1986, pp 525-64.

Turner S M, Calhoun K S and Adams H E, *Handbook of Clinical and Behaviour Therapy*, Wiley, New York, 1981.

Werry J S and Wollersheim J P, 'Behaviour Therapy with Children and Adolescents: A Twenty-Year Overview', *Journal of the American Academy of Child and Adolescent Psychiatry*, Vol 28 No 1, 1989, pp 1-18.

Wolpe J, *Psychotherapy by Reciprocal Inhibition*, Stanford University Press, Stanford, 1958.

Chapter 62

Hypnosis

F K Judd and G D Burrows

Definition of hypnosis

The National Health and Medical Research Council define hypnosis as a temporary condition of altered attention in the subject which may be induced by another person and in which a variety of phenomena may appear spontaneously or in response to verbal or other stimuli. These phenomena include alterations in consciousness and memory, increased susceptibility to suggestion, and the production in the subject, of responses and ideas unfamiliar to him in his normal state of mind. Further, phenomena such as anaesthesia, paralysis and the rigidity of muscles, and vasomotor changes can be produced and removed in the hypnotic state.

Theories of hypnosis

Many competing theories to explain the nature of hypnosis exist. These can be broadly divided into physiological and psychological.

1. Physiological

Physiological changes associated with hypnotic trance are well documented, but it is argued that these may be due to hypnosis itself, or to emotions arising from the suggestion of altered perception.
(a) Hypnosis as sleep
Research, including electroencephalograph (EEG) studies, suggests that hypnosis and sleep are not the same, although they share some of the same phenomena.
(b) Hypnosis as cerebral inhibition
Pavlov suggested hypnosis is a state of partial cortical inhibition with persistence of areas of cortical excitation to explain the persisting communication between subject and therapist. Validation of such concepts requires more specialised measurement of cerebral functioning than those currently available.
(c) Pathology
A pathological state of the central nervous system is a theory which has not been pursued by contemporary research. The suggested pathological process, 'dissociation', fails to account for all the phenomena of hypnosis. Nevertheless, the similarity between hypnosis and hysterical phenomena should not be forgotten and further understanding of hypnosis may facilitate an appreciation of the aetiology of neurotic symptoms.

2. Psychological

Psychological theories are currently the most favoured explanation of hypnosis.
(a) Conditioned response
It is suggested that trance induction is a conditioned stimulus and the phenomena of hypnosis the conditioned response. Post hypnotic suggestion can be seen as analogous to a conditioned response. However, it is unlikely that hypnosis is solely a conditioned response. Many individuals are hypnotised under different conditions using various techniques which have not been associated by previous conditioning with the idea of hypnotic trance.
(b) Suggestion
Behaviourists contend that there is no

specific distinguishing feature between suggestibility in the wakeful state and the hypnotic state. They are quantitatively rather than qualitatively different. Subsequent developments have emphasised the role of learning and directed goal-oriented striving in hypnosis.

(c) Role playing

Proponents of this theory suggest hypnosis is a particular form of sociopsychological behaviour and that the hypnotic state is not intrinsically different from ordinary waking consciousness. Those who oppose this view emphasise that some phenomena produced under hypnosis are not ordinarily within the normal range of voluntary response, for example, hypnotic anaesthesia.

(d) Psychoanalytic theories

In psychoanalysis, hypnosis is viewed primarily as a regressive experience, in which transference phenomena are emphasised. Under hypnosis, normal mechanisms such as role playing and identification are thought to assume a more primitive form. As with the conditioned reflex theory, these theories fail to explain hypnosis by metronomes, rotating discs, etc where no interpersonal relationship is involved.

The phenomena of hypnosis

The phenomena of hypnosis can be separated into two distinct categories—the physical and the psychological. They may be difficult to separate, as during hypnosis alterations in bodily function may occur as a result of changes in the psychological state. Alteration may affect voluntary and involuntary muscles, the sense organs, the memory, mental activity and the emotions (Table 1).

1. Alterations in voluntary muscles include relaxation, paralysis of muscle groups (following the subject's own idea of how a paralysed person would behave), rigidity, increased muscle performance (mainly due to inability to feel fatigue) and automatic movements.

2. Alterations in involuntary muscles, organs and glands may be induced by direct suggestion—these include change of heart rate, vasoconstriction and vasodilatation, alteration of blood pressure, changes in the rate and depth of respiration excursion, and variations in gastric secretion, peristalsis, perspiration, salivation and metabolism.

3. Alterations in the sense organs may also be influenced by suggestion and the subject's perception of any of the special senses may be altered. Vision and hearing may be accentuated or diminished. Sense of smell and touch may be similarly affected. The perception of pain may be altered and in deep trance pain sensation may be totally abolished, enabling surgery to be performed with no other form of anaesthetic.

4. Illusions and hallucinations may be elicited in a deep trance. Positive hallucinations (inducing perceptions in the absence of stimuli) of taste and touch are more readily produced than hallucinations of the other special senses. Negative hallucinations (abolishing a sensory perception when a stimulus is present) are possible only in the deepest trance state.

5. Alterations of memory include age regression and post hypnotic amnesia. In age regression an adult can be told that he is going back in time and will be able to relive experiences that he underwent at the previous age chosen. This may enable the discovery of unconscious material and emotional conflicts and be a valuable technique in analytical psychotherapy. Post hypnotic amnesia is frequently seen following medium or deep trances but is complete only with the deepest trance states.

Trance induction

Preparation for hypnosis is an essential first step in the hypnotherapeutic relationship. This includes assessment of the patient's motivation (it is impossible to hypnotise a person against his will), removal of doubts, fears and misconceptions, and explanation of what will occur during the hypnotic session.

The hypnotic state is produced by fixing and narrowing of attention, usually achieved by the constant repetition of a series of monotonous, rhythmical, sensory stimuli.

Table 1. Phenomena of hypnosis

Stage	Phenomena
Light trance	Muscle relaxation
	Slow deep breathing
Medium trance	Automatic movements
	Partial anaesthesia
	Partial amnesia
	Positive hallucinations
	Imagery
Deep trance	Complete anaesthesia
	Posthypnotic analgesia/
	anaesthesia
	Posthypnotic suggestion
	Age regression
	Positive & negative
	hallucinations

Observable responses should be linked with desired responses, using where possible normal physiological responses, for example, tiredness of the eyes, blinking, muscular fatigue. As each suggestion is accepted and activated the suggestibility of the subject is increased. Suggestions should be simple, clear, unambiguous and permissive, and limited to the purpose intended.

Commonly used induction techniques include progressive relaxation with/without eye-fixation, eye fixation with/without distraction, hand levitation and confusion techniques.

Deepening the trance state

After successful induction, when the subject has entered a light trance state, many techniques may be used to gradually deepen the trance state. Various phenomena of hypnosis, which are of specific therapeutic value, can only be elicited in the deep trance state.

Methods of deepening the trance include direct suggestion, by the relating of depth to performance, by counting and breathing techniques, imagery (for example, descending staircase/lift) and non verbal techniques (for example, music).

Assessment of hypnotic responsiveness

Ninety per cent of the population can enter the hypnotic state, but only 20 per cent can achieve the deep trance state. Various standardised scales to measure depth of hypnosis have been developed. These provide quantified ratings for specified hypnotic responses. Examples include the Stanford Hypnotic Clinical Scale (SHCS) and the Hypnotic Induction Profile (HIP).

Indications for hypnosis

Hypnosis may be a valuable form of therapy for a wide range of disorders, both physical and psychological. As for all other therapies, important prerequisites of treatment include adequate assessment and diagnosis. Assessment must include evaluation of the patient's motivation for and expectations of treatment, an understanding of the patient's personality and accurate diagnosis of the cause of the symptoms which the patient describes. Alternative or additional forms of therapy must also be considered. Common indications for hypnosis include:

1. Relaxation therapy: Trance induction with direct suggestion or imagery maybe a useful form of relaxation therapy.

2. Anxiety relief: Hypnosis maybe usefully employed to reduce anxiety accompanying various medical and dental procedures or occurring as a result of physical illness. Where anxiety contributes to the production of physical symptoms, for example, somatoform disorders or other disorders such as sexual dysfunction, hypnosis maybe of benefit. Hypnosis may be a valuable treatment, alone or in combination with other therapies in the management of panic and phobic disorders, generalised anxiety disorder, obsessive—compulsive disorder and post traumatic stress disorder.

3. The phenomena of hypnosis: Specific phenomena of hypnosis may be of value in the treatment of a variety of conditions. Examples include: the use of vasoconstriction to aid dental extractions or the treatment of various dermatological problems; vaso-

dilation to aid the treatment of Raynaud's phenomena; analgesia for childbirth, various surgical procedures, dressing of wounds and treatment of chronic pain disorder; imagery for imaginal desensitisation in the treatment of phobic disorders, for example, aeroplane phobia; positive hallucination of taste for the treatment of nail biting or smoking.

4. Hypnosis in psychotherapy: Hypnosis is often used as an adjunct to psychotherapy. It may lead to more rapid discovery of unconscious conflicts. This may be achieved by a variety of techniques including age regression, the use of imagery or fantasy techniques.

Precautions and contra indications for hypnosis

There are few contra indictions for the use of hypnosis but it is important to recognise the potential dangers of this form of therapy.

1. Psychotherapy: all psychotherapeutic interventions, including hypnosis, can be harmful. Presenting symptoms may be exacerbated or new symptoms, for example, anxiety, depression or acting out may develop. Problems are generally attributed to inappropriate patient election, inadequate therapist training, the therapist's poor personal insight, transference and countertransference factors or therapeutic technique and style. With hypnosis, particular problems may arise as a result of more rapid development of insight, more intense transference feelings including wish fulfilling fantasies and the development of excessive dependency.

2. Psychiatric illness: Patients with severe depression should not be treated with hypnosis. Hypnosis is not effective in the treatment of severe depression, and relief of anxiety without relief of depression may give the patient sufficient energy to act on suicidal impulses. The use of hypnosis in the treatment of patients suffering from a psychotic illness may be hazardous. Hypnosis may precipitate or intensify a psychotic illness, hypnotic suggestion may give credence to delusions of control, and hypnosis is not effective treatment for these disorders. For neurotic disorders, one must understand the aetiology of the presenting symptom and only effect its removal by hypnosis if alternative means of anxiety management and support of the patient are not available.

3. Physical illness: Hypnosis is a valuable adjunct in the treatment of many physical illnesses. Dangers in this situation arise not as a result of hypnosis per se, but because of failure to appreciate the effects of hypnosis on the physical condition being treated. For example, difficulties may arise when the distress of asthma is reduced and reduction of bronchoconstriction is achieved with the effect of hypnosis on the autonomic nervous system, without altering mucosal swelling and secretion, or when analgesia is induced during childbirth, but failure to adequately monitor the labour leads to late recognition of complications such as obstructed labour.

Further Reading

Burrows G D and Dennerstein L, *Handbook of Hypnosis and Psychosomatic Medicine*, Elsevier/North-Holland, Amsterdam, 1980.

Hilgard E R and Hilgard J R, *Hypnosis in the Relief of Pain*, William Kaufmann Inc, California, 1975.

Judd F K, Burrows G D and Dennerstein L, 'The Dangers of Hypnosis. A Review', *Australian Journal of Clinical & Experimental Hypnosis*, Vol 13, 1985, pp 1-15.

Meares A, *A System of Medical Hypnosis*, WB Saunders, Philadelphia, 1960.

Spiegel H and Spiegel D, *Trance and Treatment: Clinical Uses of Hypnosis*, Basic Books, New York, 1978.

Chapter 63

Nursing for Mental Health

M Clinton

Many people with mental health problems face enormous challenges in managing their everyday lives. Those with worries and problems in getting along with others have no respite from self-doubt and intense anxiety. Those who hear voices and experience their innermost thoughts as alien, find it impossible to feel and express emotions spontaneously. Those with major difficulties in forming relationships experience high levels of frustration, may act aggressively and be convinced that most of their problems arise because of the actions of other people. Many such people are treated in hospital. Some live in hostels or other community facilities. Most stay with relatives or friends while receiving treatment from general practitioners or as psychiatric outpatients. Psychiatric nurses work with such people in all these settings. They fulfil several roles and use a wide range of therapeutic practices to promote and enhance mental health. The purpose of this chapter is to consider the roles of psychiatric nurses and to describe two of their most widely used interventions. First some trends influencing the practice of psychiatric nursing will be described.

Trends influencing contemporary psychiatric nursing

The past three decades have seen major changes in the education of nurses in Australasia. The rapid development of nursing as a discipline has gathered pace throughout the world and paved the way for nursing education to make the transition from hospital based schools of nursing to universities and other tertiary education institutions. In Australasia, the transition began in New Zealand some 15 years ago. The trend is continuing in Australia as new nursing programs are set up in established centres of higher education and universities. The new programs enable students to study nursing in courses which include the physical sciences, social sciences and the humanities. Such programs enable students to develop insight into their potential to practise as clinical nurses in any setting, including the mental health field. There is scope to develop the practice of psychiatric nurses through more and even better nursing education. As more practitioners complete pre and post-registration diploma and degree level programs, the number of effective role models will increase and create a pool of expertise which should improve the overall therapeutic impact of psychiatric nurses.

Changes in nurse education have taken place during a period when there have been major changes in social policies affecting mental health. World-wide there has been a massive reduction in the number of people cared for in large mental hospitals. Hospitals which had between 1500 and 2000 beds in 1969, now have between 400 and 800 beds. However, the number of psychiatric beds available in specially designed units in general hospitals has increased.

Community facilities have also increased during the same period. Many local and health authorities now have a wide range of accommodation for ex-hospital patients. However, progress has been uneven, and some parts of Australia and New Zealand are still

427

poorly served in this regard.

The discharge of patients from mental hospitals and shorter periods of admission to psychiatric units has changed the nature of psychiatric nursing. The larger mental hospitals are left with people whose problems are long standing and who are relatively unhelped by medical treatment. There is an increasing number of elderly patients, many of whom have simply grown old while in hospital. The shorter periods of hospital stay for those with acute problems have posed challenges for nurses who now have to cope with the rapid turnover of people admitted with major disorders of thinking and mood. Caring for people with mental health problems in the community has required nurses to develop new skills to maintain treatment, manage periods of crisis, support relatives and cope with community indifference or hostility.

An equally significant trend is the growing awareness among policy makers and health professionals of the characteristics of the people most likely to require mental health services. In general, the less people are educated, the lower their income, and the less they are able to remain in employment and the more likely they are to be admitted to a mental hospital. Once admitted, they are less likely to be discharged to adequate follow-up care.

Analysis of inpatient figures in both Australia and New Zealand shows that Aboriginal and Maori people are more likely to receive short and long term inpatient treatment. The explanation for this may lie in the greater readiness of health care professionals to diagnose mental illness in disadvantaged groups, due to the inability of health care systems to compensate for poor education, poor nutrition, bad housing and other social disadvantages.

In the past decade in New Zealand, there has been an increase in awareness of the plight of Maori people in the mental health system. This has accompanied general concern about the rights of the Maori as the indigenous people of New Zealand, enshrined in the Treaty of Waitangi, the founding document of the New Zealand nation. Similar concern has been expressed in Australia as a result of land claims by Aborigines and more recently the soul searching which accompanied the Australian Bicentennial celebrations of 1988. These trends require psychiatric nurses to work with people with mental health problems in many settings and to be sensitive to the need for 'culturally safe' care when nursing members of other cultures.

Cultural sensitivity is particularly important when nursing members of indigenous cultures, whose status and relationship to the land requires special recognition on the part of the nurse (see also chapters 45 and 47).

Nursing roles

The roles of the psychiatric nurse are expressed in the activities of caring, advocacy, team membership, planning, counselling and other therapies.

The fundamental role of the psychiatric nurse is to care about, and care for people with mental health problems. *Caring about people* requires the nurse to make every effort to ensure that mentally ill people receive services appropriate to their needs, continuing support from their family and loved ones, and interventions which are in their best interests.

Caring for people with mental health problems requires a wide range of skills, from accepting responsibility for the physical care and overall well-being of elderly people with severe confusion, to caring for people in the community who require little more than support and encouragement. Caring for the elderly can involve assisting patients with their personal hygiene, helping them to eat and using a wide range of activities to maintain their physical well-being and promote awareness of their present surroundings. A high level of total health care is also required for people with acute mental health problems, especially severely depressed people, those experiencing altered states of consciousness due to the abuse of alcohol or other drugs and those who are in despair or suicidal.

Most psychiatric nurses seek to involve their patients in improving self-care, however profound their mental health problems may be. The concept of self-care has been extremely influential in shaping contemporary psychiatric nursing. Many nurses use a method called the nursing process to plan, organise and evaluate the care they provide. The nursing process is a problem solving cycle applied to nursing. The nurse first assesses the patient's needs, then plans nursing interventions with the patient. Care is given to meet specifically identified objectives. The nurse completes the cycle by continually evaluating the effect of the care provided and by re-assessing the patient's needs.

Advocate

The nurse serves as an advocate when acting on behalf of the patient to protect or advance his interests. Advocacy can involve nurses in discussing side effects of medication with psychiatrists. This may lead to a reduction in dosage or to the administration of additional drugs to counteract unpleasant side effects. Nurses fulfil the advocacy role when they discuss the admission or discharge of patients to or from hospital. The advocacy role involves assessing the ethics of decisions made by other health care workers and speaking out on the patient's behalf.

An increasing amount of advocacy takes place in the community, where nurses are involved in preparing communities for the setting up of hostels, halfway houses and community homes for ex-psychiatric patients. A great deal of skill, tactfulness and determination is required to overcome community resistance to such developments. Advocacy extends to persuading health and local authorities to provide facilities such as respite care and day centres.

Team member

Many psychiatric nurses work without supervision in the community. Most belong to therapeutic teams; although the extent to which groups of health professionals function as teams differs according to the services and personalities involved. A typical therapeutic team consists of psychiatrists, psychiatric nurses, social workers, psychologists, occupational therapists and may include administrators and lay members.

Teams are often led by psychiatrists, who have legal responsibility for care of the patient. However, team responsibilities are changing as an increasing number of teams are finding ways of sharing leadership and authority. The strength of such teams is the expertise which can be pooled to assist members to design, implement and evaluate individualised treatment programs for patients. To be effective team members, psychiatric nurses must be secure in their identity as nurses and be prepared to present points of view from a nursing perspective. The nurse's role is not to take over the functions of other team members, nor to seek to impose preferred solutions to problems facing patients, but to give the clearest possible nursing advice and represent the interests of each patient. Above all, the nurse must be able to articulate clearly the nursing contribution to the patient's overall treatment and rehabilitation.

Planner

Effective psychiatric nursing requires the care of each patient to be planned systematically by the nurse. Progress has been made in individualised care, but there is scope for further development. The preparation of care plans for individual patients is the most important, but not the only planning function undertaken by psychiatric nurses. Changes in the structure of mental health services, particularly the discharge of large numbers of ex-psychiatric patients to the community, have required major planning activities. Each patient has been assessed, and services in the community planned on the basis of the information provided.

The planning role of the psychiatric nurse has three elements. First, the forward planning of existing services to ensure that they will be appropriate to the patients of the future. Secondly, the planning of future community services to take the place of services currently based in hospitals. Finally, the planning of future hospital services to meet the needs of the patients who cannot be discharged due to their frailness, chronicity or their unmanageable behaviour. The planning role includes forecasting the need for services, calculating the number and grades of nursing staff required, and the design of quality programs to ensure efficiency and to monitor effectiveness.

The planning process involves the preparation of budgets and plans for future buildings, transport and equipment. In the past service planning has been the province of health administrators and specialist nurses. It is essential that clinical nurses become more involved in planning in the future. Their involvement will allow services to be more appropriate and responsive to the needs of patients.

Counsellor

Many psychiatric nurses fulfil the role of counsellor, providing support for people with mental health problems. Much counselling is informal and intended to support patients as they think through issues and behaviours which are causing them distress, and which need to be overcome if they are to be more effective in their personal relationships. Nurses use active listening, open questioning, suggestion and reassurance to provide a high level of personal support for patients. Some are extremely experienced counsellors, using non-directive techniques to enable patients to clarify their feelings and behaviours to prepare for situations they find challenging. Role playing and family therapy are often used by skilled nurses to encourage insight and provide patients with opportunities to rehearse behaviours in a safe environment. Role playing also allows patients to receive immediate feedback from staff and family members.

The techniques used are selected carefully to assist the patient in specific ways, but they do not rely on in-depth interpretations by the nurse. Although some psychiatric nurses are trained as psychotherapists, a larger number limit themselves to supportive counselling because this is more compatible with their nursing role, as they can rely on nursing perspectives and frameworks to orient their practice. Counselling is effective for patients experiencing problems in daily living, those facing crises and those who wish to overcome lack of confidence or problems in personal relationships, especially with family members and colleagues at work.

Some psychiatric nurses receive additional training in other forms of psychotherapy.

Their potential use in helping a wide range of people, especially on an outpatient or 'at home' basis, is vast.

Milieu therapy

Milieu therapy is the conscious structuring of the environment in which the patient lives in order to promote personal growth and the ability to cope with the pressures of everyday life. Milieu therapy is used most effectively in residential care settings, but a modified form can be achieved in day centres and community based programs. To be effective in a therapeutic milieu, the nurse must recognise that every aspect of the environment in which patients live, particularly their relationships with other patients and the nursing staff, can contribute to their health and the development of coping strategies which promote self-esteem and personal effectiveness.

Residential care offers opportunities for time away from the ordinary pressures of life. It creates a breathing space in which the patient can re-assess characteristic responses to the challenges faced in life. With the support of nurses and fellow patients, the patient is encouraged to break established behaviourial patterns and to experiment with more effective ways of dealing with the stressors of life. Milieu therapy provides for the acquisition of new coping behaviours. Patients are helped to avoid distortions in their understanding of what other people say to them. They are encouraged to take responsibility for themselves. They are helped to make choices and to accept the consequences of the decisions they make. They are challenged to see how their behaviour affects others. All these are achieved through individual programs of care, by reinforcement of positive attempts at personal responsibility and self-care and through the experience of caring and sharing relationships.

The nurse acts as a role model, demonstrating effective ways of dealing with strong feelings, anxiety, frustration and occasionally, anger. Patients are encouraged to model behaviours on those of the nurse. The nurse also fulfils the roles of helper and teacher. He explains treatments, provides information on the patient's condition and medication, and supports the patient in negotiating personal objectives to be achieved with the help of the therapeutic team. The nurse participates in activities involving patients from recreation to work experience, continually striving to take part on an egalitarian basis, accepting neither too much nor too little responsibility. The nurse reviews progress with patients and solicits and reinforces strategies for their personal growth. He assists patients to value their new behaviours and supports them while they try them out in situations which provide increasingly threatening challenges. Milieu therapy is often used as a background to other forms of treatment, including cognitive therapy (see chapters 58 and 61).

Cognitive therapy relies on the capacity people have to use their imagination and experience to overcome mental health problems arising from stress. The strategies used are indispensable to nurses as both part of a set of therapeutic interventions which can be used with a wide range of patients, and as a resource for personal growth and effectiveness in all personal relationships.

Cognitive therapy is an extremely powerful personal resource in psychiatric nursing. If nurses are to be effective therapists when leading groups or managing the milieu of care, it is essential that they do not misperceive their relationships with patients and colleagues. Therapeutic effectiveness requires techniques for handling distorted perceptions.

The most important step in meeting this requirement is to accept that we are all capable of distorted interpretations, and that we can control this distortion by paying attention to how we hear and respond to others. We need to guard against perceiving with tunnel vision by failing to attend to the totality of the communications we hear, by picking out only what we want or expect to be said. We are equally likely to dichotomise what we hear into good and bad categories, seeing everything in terms of black or white, right or wrong, when we need to be comfortable with perceptions of shades of grey. We need to avoid over-generalisations about people, places and events, and to curb our tendency to think that we know what other people are thinking when they speak. Equally we need to remind ourselves that everything which is said is not intended to refer to us. We must be careful not to personalise communication to ourselves.

Finally, we must be careful not to seek to control other people, particularly patients, or to feel that the system in which we work or study controls us. To be successful in psychiatric nursing we have to be aware of our own thoughts and feelings before we can be of assistance to others. Helping patients to combat disordered thinking is an important component of cognitive therapy. It is also an indispensable skill for the psychiatric nurse.

Future responsibilities

In the future an increasing number of psychiatric nurses will utilise the treatment methods which have been described to translate their philosophies of nursing and frameworks for practice into actions which will be effective in helping people to protect and enhance their mental health. Growth in research into psychiatric nursing will help nurses identify effective therapeutic strategies and enable a wider range of treatment methods to be used. More roles for psychiatric nurses will emerge as new and more innovative educational programs are developed, many leading to postgraduate academic qualifications in this important nursing specialty.

It is probable that more psychiatric nurses in the future will work as independent nurse practitioners. Others will develop new models of community care and help with the resettlement and rehabilitation of ex-psychiatric patients. Psychiatric nurses with advanced education may be contracted by commercial and government organisations to advise on health policies in the workplace, and to assist with the design, implementation and monitoring of policies on absenteeism, fitness for work, alcohol and drug abuse and broader health education programs. As we move into the 1990s, more attention will be given to mental health and nurses will develop their roles as health educators, counsellors and therapists. They will face the challenge of providing culturally sensitive services and seek opportunities for increased autonomy. The rewards will be intrinsic satisfaction and

a career path which recognises the need for personal development as a prerequisite for assisting others with mental health problems.

Further Reading

Altschul A T, *Psychiatric Nursing: Recent Advances in Nursing*, Churchill Livingstone, Edinburgh, 1985.

Irving S, *Basic Psychiatric Nursing*, 3rd ed, W B Saunders Co, Philadelphia, Pennsylvania, 1983.

Johnson B S, *Psychiatric Mental Health Nursing: Adaptation and Growth*, J B Lippincott Co, Philadelphia, Pennsylvania, 1986.

McKay M, Davis M, and Fanning P, *Thoughts and Feelings: The Art of Cognitive Stress Intervention*, New Harbinger Publications, Oakland, California, 1981.

Meleis A, *Theoretical Nursing: Developments and Progress*, J B Lippincott Co, Philadelphia, Pennsylvania, 1985.

Peplau H, *Interpersonal Relations in Nursing*, 2nd ed, Macmillan Education Ltd, Basingstoke, Hamphire, 1988.

Chapter 64

Social Work

R Bland

Social work in psychiatry is concerned with the social context within which mental illness occurs and the social consequences of such illness. Expertise in these areas is the basis of the unique contribution of social work to the services provided by multidisciplinary teams in hospital and community psychiatry settings. Methods of practice include casework with individuals and families, group work, community work, and the formulation of social policy.

In many settings, social workers provide specialised therapies, such as psychodynamic psychotherapy or strategic family therapy, but competence in such areas require intensive instruction beyond the social work training. This chapter will outline the broad parameters of the social work role in hospital and community settings, in working with families, and in case management services. The discussion will focus on work in primary treatment and rehabilitation settings, and on social work with the seriously mentally ill and disabled. It should be remembered however, that social workers encounter such patients in the full range of health and welfare settings, such as social security and legal aid services. Many people with less severe forms of anxiety, depression or personality problems can be managed by social workers in general health setting. This chapter is a description of 'mainstream' social work in psychiatry.

Primary treatment and rehabilitation settings

In psychiatric hospitals social workers are involved in most areas of assessment and treatment planning. While considerable role overlap is now common in the multidisciplinary team, social workers are most likely to assess the *social background* of the patient and so take a social history from the patient and family. In doing so, they cover such areas as ethnicity, personal supports, family functioning, employment history, and socioeconomic issues. The basis of such assessment is to provide information about the social factors involved in the person's illness. Such basic questions as 'what work does the person do?', 'who lives at home with the person?', and 'what income does the person have?' provide an understanding of the patient as a person in their social context.

Family assessment is a central social work task in understanding the person's social context. The social worker will probably interview key family members early in the person's admission. Such areas as family roles and relationships, supports and stresses would be explored as part of the assessment process. The social worker will frequently act as the contact person between the treatment team and the family.

Mrs B, a middle aged single mother, was admitted to an acute treatment unit with an exacerbation of chronic schizophrenia. The social worker made immediate contact with the woman's family and learned that Mrs B was living with her three teenage children. The eldest child, her son, was working, while the two girls were still in High School. Her daughters were experiencing some adolescent adjustment problems, and had been in some conflict with their mother in the months prior to admission.

Her son appeared very supportive and understanding of his mother. It was discovered that Mrs B's mother who lived nearby was a source of much support, emotionally and practically, particularly when Mrs B was showing signs of relapse. This early contact with the family provided important information about the family understanding of the illness, the stresses and supports for the person, and formed a basis for treatment planning for the team.

The issue of the *consequences of admission* is the second area of social work concern. The illness itself and treatment in hospital inevitably disrupt daily routines for patient and family. Concerns about the ability to pay the rent, keep a job, or get a sickness benefit, may be very worrying for the patient, and may be considered by the patient to be of more immediate concern than controlling symptoms. In some cases, the patient's admission to hospital precipitates other family crises. For example, a depressed sole parent requiring hospitalisation needs to organise emergency care of dependent children. Dealing with the consequences of admission may involve the social worker contacting landlords, family, friends, and employers. The social worker would assess the impact of the hospitalisation on other family members. The hospitalisation may necessitate liaison with a range of other services such as social security and welfare housing.

During the treatment, and the planning for discharge, the social worker will help the person to make the transition back to life in the community. While most patients will return to family or independent living, some patients need help to find suitable accommodation, or to make links with sheltered employment or support groups.

In setting *goals for discharge*, social workers have to work sensitively to ensure plans are realistic both in terms of the person's abilities, and in relation to the reality of community resources. For example, the young person recovering from a schizophrenic episode may need to make many decisions about accommodation, work, and relationships. The social worker needs to encourage the person to make choices which allow a period of low stress recovery. In this planning, an understanding of the stressors leading to the present admission is essential. The patient may have to defer highly desirable yet stressful goals, such as resuming an apprenticeship or getting a flat, in favour of more modest short term goals, such as getting part-time or voluntary work, until a clearer picture of the extent of recovery is achieved in time.

Another social work task in this process is that of *'social manipulation'*. Where existing community resources are inadequate to meet the needs of patients, social workers may modify or initiate resources. For example, isolated psychiatrically disabled people may be assisted by the establishment of a local social club, to provide a pleasant, low stress meeting place for recreation. Setting up such a project would be an appropriate task for a community based social worker. This community work approach combines skills in building and sustaining a supportive relationship with the patient, while applying practical skills such as organising community resources.

Social work with families

In recent years a clearer understanding of the impact of severe mental illness on the family of the patient has emerged. This is a result of the increasing strength of the self help movement, and influential research showing that the family care of patients with psychiatric illness imposes considerable stress on family caregivers. It is clear that schizophrenic patients recovering from illness do best in a living situation which is supportive, understanding, and low in stress.

Social work with the family is directed at helping the family to understand the illness and its effect on the patient and other family members. Families are helped to recognise the patient's bizarre behaviour as symptoms of an illness and to develop skills in coping with such difficulties as patient withdrawal and lack of motivation.

A second aspect of the social work role involves providing understanding and emotional support for the family members in dealing with the stress of the patient's illness—

the family's sense of grief, loss and power-lessness. The social worker may help family members to make plans for the future, based on the long term welfare of patient and family. Should the patient continue to live at home? What alternatives are available? These important issues of the context and social consequences of major mental illness are the central focus of social work role with the patient's family (see chapters 59, 60).

Case management role

Social work in community settings includes, as well as the treatment role outlined above, a case management function for psychiatrically disabled patients. This service is based around the disabling impact of long term illness, principally its effect on the person's ability to work, tolerate stress, form and sustain relationships with others. *Case management* is based on a long term supportive relationship with the patient, and includes the five functions of assessment, planning, linking, monitoring, and advocacy.

The assessment and planning roles are similar to those outlined previously. Monitoring involves a close attention to the patient's level of symptoms, side effects of medication, and potential stressors. Such monitoring may avoid exacerbation of symptoms and hospitalisation through early intervention.

Liaison with the person's treatment team may be necessary from time to time. Effective monitoring, however, relies essentially on the quality of the supportive relationship developed over time with the patient.

'Linking' involves ensuring access by the patient to the full range of health and welfare services required. An advocacy role is based on prevention of discrimination and exploitation of the patient. For example, some psychiatrically disabled people have been physically or sexually abused by landlords, have had money stolen, or have been denied basic civil rights such as access to mail or privacy in telephone calls. The social worker seeks to overcome the relative powerlessness of the patient, through taking action with the patient or on behalf of the patient to redress abuses of authority or denial of rights (see chapter 44).

The importance of welfare concepts

Within the range of tasks undertaken by the social worker in the treatment team, some activities are closely related to the management of the illness, while others can be seen as part of the wider social welfare aspects of overall patient care. For example, the psychotic patient recovering from an acute attack might have lost confidence in his ability to cope with family relationships, work or community living. A warm, supportive counselling relationship may be established with the patient to help foster coping mechanisms including problem solving capacities. Such a relationship would help to build identity and self-esteem damaged by the illness. These activities are seen as part of the more therapeutic role of the social worker.

As well as these tasks, the social worker would also be concerned with the more basic aspects of the patient's life such as housing and income security. These welfare tasks are crucial to the well-being of the patient, and give recognition to the serious social consequences of the illness on the patient's quality of life. There is a tendency for social workers themselves to underestimate the importance of the welfare aspects of their work, and to give priority to the more therapeutic roles. This is unfortunate when it is recognised that, for the patient, these welfare aspects are often considered more important than the therapeutic roles. While social workers may share counselling roles with other team members, when the chips are down, team members will rely on the social worker to provide for the patient the necessary expertise in the welfare area.

Housing has been used as a vehicle for rehabilitation in a range of mental health programs, for example, the Richmond Fellowship houses. Such programs typically use the group milieu established in the house to promote the development of interpersonal skills, and capacity for independent living, and are usually transitional in nature, preparing the resident for ordinary community living as a rehabilitation goal. Beyond these special programs, housing remains a basic human need, and many patients leaving hospital need to find accommodation on discharge. Secure housing remains, for all people, basic to the development of a sense of security and identity. For emotionally vulnerable patients, a safe home is a central part of personal security so necessary to successful community adjustment.

Social workers may be concerned with the range of accommodation alternatives available to the patient, making sure that patients exercise appropriate choice in selecting accommodation, and in liaising with the management of residential facilities to facilitate resident security.

For example, a social worker on a rehabilitation ward was concerned about the shortage of low cost accommodation for patients leaving the hospital. She organised a group of patients likely to be discharged in the near future and worked with them on planning for a share house to accommodate a group of four women. The women were able to anticipate many of the decisions they would need to make in the future, such as location, costs, how to find money for the bond and rent, telephone, shopping, and bill paying arrangements. The social worker assisted in the many small steps towards the setting up of the house and was able to follow-up the women on discharge. Such a project demanded a range of social work skills and methods including problem solving, group work, building motivation, and crisis counselling. The example illustrates too, the broad range of social work activities addressing both therapeutic and welfare concerns.

Income security is a second area central to patient welfare, and like housing, remains a common human need. One of the most immediate consequences of severe psychiatric illness is a restriction in earning capacity, either temporarily through the acute attack and hospitalisation, or as a long term disability of the illness. The organisation of sickness benefits or invalid pension may moderate the stress of loss of income, and also provides a starting point for planning for the future.

Tom, a 30 year old man with schizophrenia, was married with a child. He had been searching hard to find suitable work, and trying to keep his family on an income from Unemployment Benefit. He was very worried about his capacity to handle the stress of even part-time employment, and was finding the task of job seeking, and submitting forms for unemployment benefit, both frustrating and depressing. With the help of the social worker, he was encouraged to apply for the Invalid Pension and was successful in this regard. He reported that he was more relaxed and hopeful about the future without the threat of employment and employment failure.

Such a concern with ensuring income security is based not just on the therapeutic importance of reducing stress for the patient, but in addressing the patient's rights to a basic standard of living. This broader issue of the social disadvantage of psychiatrically disabled patients is of concern to social work at the level of social administration and policy development. The long term dependence on reliable but relatively low incomes generates a form of structured poverty which is in itself a form of disability. Study of the 'poverty line' concept in Australian society by the Institute of Applied Economic and Social Research suggests that adults totally dependent on the invalid pension are living at an unacceptably low level when compared with community norms. That is, mentally disabled people who are dependent on the Invalid Pension are at risk of remaining in poverty as a lifetime condition.

In summary, the social worker seeks to improve the patient's quality of life, by ensuring access to the range of accommodation, vocational, and recreational services. For example, at the community level, social workers may become involved as consultants to a voluntary organisation providing housing for psychiatrically disabled patients. They advise on patient needs, gaps in services, possible government support, models of housing, selection of tenants, and methods of evaluating the project. These broader issues of social policy are of concern to social workers in administration and planning positions.

Summary

This overview has emphasised the importance of the social context and social consequences of mental illness as the central focus of social work in psychiatry. The role includes casework, group work, and community skills, as well as the development of social policy in such areas as treatment and rehabilitation, work with families, and in case management. Welfare aspects of the social work role have been emphasised as a central area of concern.

Further Reading

Bernheim K and Lehman A, *Working with Families of the Mentally Ill*, Norton and Co, New York, 1985.

Bland R, 'Social Work with the Family of the Schizophrenic Patient', *Australian Social Work*, Vol 40 No 2, 1987 pp 25-30.

Brieland D, 'Definition, Specialisation and Domain in Social Work', *Social Work*, Vol 26 No 1, 1981, pp 79-83.

Hudson B, *Social Work with Psychiatric Patients*, Macmillan, New York, 1982.

Jordan L, *Invitation to Social Work*, Martin Robertson, Oxford, 1984.

Segal S and Baumohl J, 'Social Work Practice in Community Mental Health', *Social Work* Vol 26 No 1, 1981 pp 16-25.

Turner F, *Psychosocial Therapy—A Social Work Perspective*, Free Press, New York, 1978.

Chapter 65

Occupational Therapy

A E Passmore

Occupational therapy's values are reflected in the profession's belief in a paradigm of wellness, a belief that, as Reilly (1962) remarked:

> 'man through the use of his hands as they are energised by mind and will, can influence the state of his own health'.

The occupational therapy paradigm derived from the early twentieth century neuropathologist, Adolf Meyer, whose psychobiological approach stressed the rhythm of life attained through a critical balance of work, play and rest. Occupational therapy practice is based upon this fundamental construct. The major tenet is that engagement in life through the processes of work, play and social interaction, facilitate and contribute to greater personal satisfaction, an increase in the quality and productivity of an individual's life. Current views emphasise the utilisation of individual strength and foster the abilities that each person has to adapt to the environment and enhance their personal survival.

Occupational therapy is concerned with the individual's occupational nature, that is, the individual's inherent goal-directed use of time, energy, interest and attention in the dimensions of work, daily living tasks and play.

Work, in its broadest sense, such as homemaking, hobbies, voluntary service and paid employment, provides the individual with an opportunity to offer a product or service which is of value to the community. It enables the person to experience working as a member of a team, relate to others and plan and reach the completion of a task.

Daily living tasks include those activities to maintain self care such as hygiene and grooming, and those involved in a household with its physical and economic demands. Daily tasks also include the day to day contact with one's family and community.

Play or leisure is seen as an important aspect of a balanced life. This includes the exploratory play of children and the leisure pursuits of adolescents, adults and the aged. Play also allows the individual to be creative and to take risks (see chapter 2).

Interaction with the non-human environment is necessary to master and manipulate the environment and to allow further development of skills and independence.

Activities

In occupational therapy, purposeful activities, the major form of intervention, are prescribed in consultation with the individual in order to meet their needs. Functional evaluation determines the patient's abilities and deficits in performance. Purposeful activities may be used to prevent and moderate dysfunction, and to elicit maximum adaptation. Activities, therefore, my involve tasks, discussion, or any occupation in which there is involvement by the patient.

Activities are analysed in the following areas:

1. The physical demands on the person, such as motor control and endurance, sensory perception and cognitive demands. Activities requiring concentration, memory, reasoning and sequencing, can be used to address deficits in cognition. Motor control abilities can be

enhanced through a variety of gross and fine motor tasks.

2. Activities are also used for their potential to allow independent involvement by the person and for the expressive opportunities they provide both at the interpersonal and intrapersonal level. Activities can provide a vehicle for communication of thoughts, ideas and emotions, such as occurs in creative, artistic outlets, or through an activity which involves the sharing of ideas and active discussion within a selected group.

3. Analysis is also made of the component stages and tasks involved in each activity.

4. Activities serve many purposes. Through observation of the person's participation in activity, such aspects as relation to others, ability to organise and approach the task, frustration tolerance, and problem-solving ability can be objectively determined. People often appear to be more competent than the functional outcome of performing a task indicates.

Activities may then be graded or adapted to meet the needs of the individual. Intervention is devised to allow the progression of a person from one activity to another in order to extend skills. For example, activities can be selected and structured to ensure a successful end product and the experience of new and alternative roles or they may involve a task that is increasingly complex. Activities are most often used to provide a familiar life situation in which the individual can be assisted to discover a greater understanding of self.

Models of treatment

Occupational therapy practices have been based upon accepted psychological theories, and trends have tended to follow those reflected in the broader mental health community. These approaches have been translated by occupational therapists into practical and functional working concepts.

The model of human occupation

The model of human occupation is concerned with system organisation. The person is seen as an open system in which the external and internal environment influence the level of function on a day to day basis. This model attempts to explain how occupational behaviour is motivated, organised and performed. Assessment is concerned with the external environment, including cultural, community, social and family relationships. The internal organisation system is also considered, which includes such aspects as motivation, values, roles and habits as well as a variety of performance skills required for daily living.

Recapitulation of growth

Models of practice for occupational therapy have been proposed based upon analytical, behavioural and developmental theories. For example, the recapitulation of ontogenesis, Mosey's developmental model, addresses those aspects of development which are vital for adequate participation in many social roles. Assessment and treatment provide a growth facilitating environment and the mastery of skills to bring about change. Learned patterns of behaviour that allow the person to deal with the environment are known as adaptive skills. Six adaptive skills are identified: sensory integrative skills, cognitive skills, dyadic interaction skills, group interaction skills, and self and sexual identity skills.

The cognitive disabilities model

The cognitive disabilities model is based on the premise that some psychiatric illnesses frequently result in residual cognitive disabilities which limit the ability of a person to function at their expected level. Cognitive disability originates in the brain and produces observable limitations in task behaviour. These areas of disability can be separated into cognitive levels of a hierarchical nature which identify, firstly, the social dysfunction observed at home or at work and next the daily functions the individual can perform and the type of assistance considered necessary to compensate for this dysfunction. Standardised instruments involving routine tasks and a structured activity are used to identify the current cognitive level in schizophrenia, major depressive illness and in dementia. The focus of occupational therapy is to facilitate the individual's performance through structuring tasks for successful completion or through compensation in the environment (see chapters 58, 61, 63).

The functional group model

Groups are part of every person's experience, and usually we claim membership to a variety of groups in our daily lives. Many theorists have documented the potential benefits of groups, their development, the nature of their membership and the effects of group dynamics upon the individual. Occupational therapy has recently developed its own orientation toward group work, which acknowledges and integrates the findings undertaken by researchers in this field. The functional group model is a specific approach to group work related to occupational therapy. It acknowledges that humans tend to have many needs which are ordered in a hierarchy, and purposeful activity is closely related to the satisfaction of these needs. Learning about adaptation to obtain these needs is one of the major goals. The model may be applied to a variety of settings from a home-management group to creative expression or stress management.

Although much of occupational therapy is based on the functional group model, many experienced therapists in the clinical field also go on to incorporate additional psychotherapeutic approaches such as action methods and family therapy. For the average clinician, a skill-oriented, action-oriented 'here and now' group approach is most commonly used. People may also be treated on an individual basis if they are unsuitable for groups or if one–to–one work is considered to be more appropriate.

Intervention may occur on different levels (see Table 1). The strategies indicated are general approaches used in working with children, adolescents, adults and the psychogeriatric population. They are utilised only as appropriate to the individual involved. The way some of these modalities are incorporated into rehabilitation are briefly addressed in relation to the areas presented throughout the life-span. Work may involve the individual, the family, a group or a community.

Table 1. Occupational therapy intervention strategies

Depth of intervention	Therapy strategy	Therapy modality
Level 1	Pychoeducational and/or task-oriented therapy	Play, leisure skills Art, music, drama, movement
		Vocational tasks Work trials Life skills, self care Home-management Community skills Stress management Relaxation, biofeedback
Level 2	Social milieu therapy	Social skills training Life skills, assertion Parenting, self-esteem Directed play therapy
Level 3	Counselling Individual therapy	Creative-expressive therapies Verbal therapies Action methods Non-directive play therapy

Areas of practice

Occupational therapists practice as members of a multidisciplinary team, and may work in psychiatric hospital departments, clinics and in community settings, industrial environments or in private practice. They may operate autonomously, or through referral from other health professionals, guidance officers, solicitors or through self-referral.

The process of intervention follows the same direction with all patients, independent of approach adopted, or the person concerned. This means screening for inclusion, assessment for individual strengths and problems, defining goals and rehabilitation strategies, and providing ongoing evaluation of the individual's progress.

Child psychiatry and occupational therapy

The major concern of the therapist in child psychiatry is to facilitate normal development. The child is viewed within the context of the current environment, including family and school. The importance of the child's social milieu is acknowledged in the treatment approaches used, involving in many instances the parents, siblings and school staff.

Occupational therapy intervention depends on an understanding of human development and the importance of play in the life of a child. Observations of the child at play and in assessing the developmental capabilities are made along many parameters including the areas of perceptual-motor cognitive, intrapsychic and social-interactional skill.

Play is an occupation of children. If normal play is restricted by the environment or limited by the child's abilities of psychological dysfunction, then self-expression is also restricted. Therapeutic play is a major focus of treatment from infancy through to middle childhood, or longer, depending upon the child. Therapy is based upon the assumption that play is the child's natural medium for self-expression and learning. Therapeutic play also acknowledges that, with non-judgmental support, children will discover and learn ways of problem-solving through exploration of the tools of play and can therefore experiment, rehearse, practise and ultimately acquire a group of capacities that leads to healthy development.

Therapeutic play utilises the environment and the activity itself and the way in which they interact. Activities and the environment in which they are performed, are important for the variable effects they have on the child's responses, such as attention, distractability and performance. Sessions may be undertaken with the therapist on an individual basis or within a small group.

A directive play approach is used to achieve a specific treatment aim such as sensory-motor and perceptual training programs, or fostering age appropriate developmental play. The therapist assumes responsibility for guidance, understanding, observing and interpreting what is occurring during the play session.

A non-directive approach allows the child to play freely. The therapist provides few boundaries but fosters self-exploration and awareness through reflection and empathy with the child.

There are three major areas of play to be considered: developmental play, expressive play and social play. *Developmental play* includes exploratory play, manipulation and coordination games, perceptual games, experience in handling basic materials, and facilitation of the development of body image. Unstructured *expressive* play is essential in the development of self-esteem and providing opportunity for the release of feelings through acceptable channels. Some children may need direction and support to develop a level of comfort to be explorative and spontaneous, whereas others, who are too immersed in fantasy, need assistance to enable them to differentiate between reality and fantasy.

Social play is a more organised approach to play used with children who are currently attending, or are preparing for, school. It is useful for children who have little positive experience of relating effectively and collaboratively with peers as it facilitates greater awareness of others, their feelings and reactions. A variety of group play therapy approaches or task activities can be used, particularly with older children, where co-operative activities, sharing, abiding by rules and completing tasks are part of the expectation. Managing stress for example is also important to the anxious child and a variety of relaxation techniques have been developed in clinical work for children using progressive muscular relaxation and imagery approaches.

Julie was referred to the psychiatry unit from the cancer ward as she was becoming a management problem both at home and in hospital. She was aggressive towards her peers and non-compliant with the current treatment regime. The major emphasis in occupational therapy was to allow the expression of feelings in a socially acceptable way through expressive play and play with paints and clay modelling. Over a four week period Julie made drawings and paintings relating to her trapped and vulnerable situation. Little information regarding the progress of her illness had been discussed with her. Her parents were encouraged to attend some of the later sessions, to enable them to become aware of the areas that were important for Julie to talk with them. A home management program was also implemented based on a behavioural reward system. The final treatment sessions taught Julie some basic relaxation methods to enable her to have some control over the stresses of her ongoing illness.

Adolescents in psychiatry settings

The adolescent also needs to be seen as part of a system in the context of family, school, community and work. A central feature of the developmental tasks of adolescence is preparation for employment. The transition from school to work includes identification of educational opportunities and training to enhance the ability to earn a living, acquisition of personal autonomy, preparation for social relationships, and acquisition of skills for independent living. The process of occupational choice includes the adolescent's efforts to define a consistent pattern of behaviour, involving responsibility and the development of skills and habits necessary to achieve the occupational role. It is the successful outcome of these tasks with which occupational therapists are primarily interested. Broadly speaking, occupational therapy programs for adolescents focus upon learning about oneself, learning about work and the community, setting goals and maximising potential.

Intervention with adolescents can be on an individual basis, but as a major adolescent task is learning to participate in a variety of groups with peers, a group approach is often used. The development of the group process and intergroup relationships are major therapeutic tools. Groups operate at differing levels of interaction and with varying objectives and may be structured or unstructured in format. They may be task-oriented or work-oriented at the interpersonal or intrapersonal level, be goal-directed or process directed, have cooperative expectations or parallel individual aims. The appropriateness of a group and the 'right fit' for a young person is usually determined by the occupational therapist.

Creative or expressive arts have a valuable role in facilitating the adolescent's health. Links with therapy are based upon the belief that the ability to express oneself creatively and spontaneously is essential in every person. This may occur through completing creative tasks. For example, there is a wide range of creative media including crafts, art work, movement and dance, music, puppetry, drama, story-telling, poetry and writing. A creative-expression group can be presented in a number of ways. It can be given structure through the use of a specific media and a theme. The theme and media can provide a means for exploration of feelings and attitudes and bringing issues into focus at a concrete level. This enables the adolescent to gain an understanding of the situation more clearly, but without having the need to express or verbalise it accurately. Alternatively creative expression may be used as a vehicle for communication both with the self and others, involving self disclosure and a heightened awareness of one's feelings and responses to the world. Adolescents can explore the techniques and qualities and nature of paint and clay, or collage, where they are free to share the outcome or retain it at a private level.

Creative drama can also provide opportunity for a person to focus on a character and to play a role other than oneself—to experience alternative roles and to explore the world through simulated experiences in a supportive environment and learn about one's ability to cope with interpersonal relationships. 'Therapy' therefore does not always have to be a serious pursuit, focusing on problems—change and learning can also arise through enjoyment.

Life skills are an important functional area to develop and to increase knowledge skills that are part of the process of growing up. Banking, cooking, budgeting, living in a flat, career exploration, using community services and leisure are part of these skills. It is important that adolescents have these basic security and survival skills. In gaining these, a sense of competence and achievement develops self-esteem. Life-skills programs can facilitate a successful transition to the community from a hospital setting by providing experiences and activities that are focused within the community.

Social skills training can assist in diminishing the difficulties adolescents may have at the interpersonal level. Deficits that influence social skills are addressed, such as decision-making and problem solving skills, learning to be appropriately assertive, developing conflict-negotiating skills and in personal organisation such as setting goals and planning time meaningfully. These skills can be developed through role-play, discussion and from modelling and observational learning.

Vocational activities such as tasks within a workshop environment, combined with specific work assessments, provide boundaries, and also provide a focus for continual assessment of the functional level of the adolescent. Evaluation of work organisation, sequencing, the ability to follow instructions, the level of impulse control, the ability to relate to authority and peers, and attention to detail can be objectively evaluated. The above are only a few of the important work related tasks that are necessary for holding a job or managing school related tasks which require initiative, attention and cooperation with others. Based upon assessment findings, referral for work trials or vocational training can be followed through.

Peter, a 15 year old high school student, was referred to occupational therapy with problems relating to school refusal. He had a history of stomach ulcers with resulting pain and described himself as tense. Being the youngest son of elderly parents, it was expected that he would follow in the footsteps of his father and older brother who were engineers. The current contact with psychiatric services was precipitated by the necessity to select subjects for the final two school years. This boy felt rejected by most of his peers, and spent his free time at school in the library or art centre.

Treatment commenced with a stress management approach, initially adopted in an attempt to demonstrate alternative methods of coping with increased physiological arousal. A passive progressive relaxation technique was first used, moving to the use of biofeedback combined with visualisation. Further sessions focused upon expressive media forms and in discussion it became clear that his interests at school lay in the humanities and art area and not with the sciences, which then provided a clear point for negotiation with parents. A graded program for return to school was initiated in conjunction with the school, therapist and parents, with roller-skating as a leisure activity reward on the weekends. He was also encouraged to join an adolescent social skills group one evening a week to explore issues of peer relationships, and through the use of role play, expressive media (music and art), and assertion techniques, develop more effective ways of relating to others.

Over a period of weeks, he reported a dramatic decrease in stomach pain and less subjective feelings of tension when in the company of peers. Defining his autonomy at home was a slower process but his parents were beginning to acknowledge him as an individual and not as an extension of themselves.

The rehabilitation of adults in psychiatry

The specific developmental life-tasks of adulthood with its particular transitions require different approaches than those previously discussed.

The nature of intervention with adults can be divided broadly into two main functional categories. Firstly, those who require *short term treatment* which is often related to the transitional phases of development. This group of people often require assistance in re-evaluating their beliefs, attitudes and coping mechanisms they have used, perhaps unsuccessfully in the past. The therapist, through a variety of group or individual sessions, acts as an agent of change by assisting the person's understanding of himself, and understanding the impact this has upon others. The major aim for this age group is to facilitate growth and, with it, the potential for change. A variety of modalities including self-expression groups, role-play, values clarification and goal-setting are used.

Those who present with *chronic and ongoing conditions* require intervention at a more practical level. Their caregivers also often require assistance both in management and education. These clients are seen in a variety of settings, from long-term hospitalisation and hostels, to community clinics. Those with chronic disorders need to be assessed in functional and practical daily life tasks and in the area of vocational skills. Work, whether in paid or sheltered employment, in a volunteer capacity or as a home-maker, offers boundaries and organises the adult into work experience. The aim is therefore to maintain or redevelop appropriate work outlets, skills and habits, wherever the person lives. Training may be needed to re-establish basic self-care habits, for instance, dressing, or it may mean retraining for a sheltered workshop position or in house-keeping tasks.

Helping people with anxiety has for many years involved the occupational therapist in coaching people in relaxation techniques. These include progressive muscle relaxation and reciprocal inhibition approaches, imagery techniques and biofeedback. However, the selection criteria for clients attending relaxation, and the specific format used must be given careful attention. With stress management a lifestyle review is important, as well as acknowledging the cognitive factors which contribute to individual stress.

Assertiveness training may be one aspect considered and explored through the use of role play techniques. Leisure is another important component in combating stress. Emphasis is placed on the need for a balanced lifestyle, and playful and creative pursuits have their place. (see chapter 2).

Peter was a young man in his late twenties who had repeated admissions to hospital with psychotic episodes. Living at home became no longer possible. He had been extremely dependent upon his mother. Intervention in occupational therapy focused on evaluating his ability to live in a minimal support hostel with a group of adults. He explored leisure alternatives and potential vocational interests for transitional employment. He had few home management and community skills required for independent living and his program was therefore structured to deal with planning, buying and preparing food, budgeting and banking, and using public transport and telephones. This was addressed through discussion, goal setting and in actual rehearsal within groups. With support, this provided him with the skills to cope with some of the practicalities of daily living. A work trial program as a ground maintenance assistant at the local community clinic was later initiated. Contact with a community support group and a local sporting organisation were facilitated by the therapist as a further step towards independent living. Weekly follow-up by the therapist continued for the first few weeks to assist with solving the problems of day to day challenges.

Rehabilitation of the elderly

Although old age brings changes in work, hobbies and the family structure, the need for role satisfaction and a lifestyle of quality still remain important. The elderly need to feel acknowledged that they can still contribute something that is worthwhile to society. Physical, cognitive and psychosocial dysfunction are closely related and the inability to carry out expected roles and responsibilities may be affected by these three inter-related aspects. The important but basic activities of the aged in which maintenance of function is essential include mobility, self-care activities such as bathing and dressing, communication, housekeeping tasks, financial management and obtaining goods and services.

The overall aim is to assist the aged person to optimise functional performance and promote quality of life whilst providing supportive services to the caregiver. This is provided through developing problem-solving, self-expression and adaptation to functional living problems. They re-learn old skills or be exposed to new options. For many, constructive intervention means well-planned modification of the environment. Sensory deprivation is a common problem with the aged. This may result from the deterioration of the senses, from an environment that provides minimal stimulation, or be due to psychological withdrawal. Findings indicate that sensory input programs involving music, touch, conversation and physical exercise lead to greater life satisfaction and should be integrated into the total daily program. Similarly the inclusion of pets in therapy has recently been found to make a positive contribution.

Activities programs aiming at physical, social and environmental stimulation have been shown to be effective in improving or at least maintaining levels of function. General recreational activities programs may be implemented by the occupational therapist.

Reality orientation is useful in terms of altering the external environment and maximising independence. This method also attempts to reduce anxiety for those with short term memory deficits.

Reminiscence or remotivation groups aim to stimulate memories from the past, increase awareness, attention and socialisation. This approach makes use of the knowledge and experiences of these people and aids in orientation and enhances dignity. Therapy aims to be developmentally age appropriate, and is graded to meet the more limited cognitive demands of the elderly.

Caregivers also require support, education and management strategies to help their elderly relatives. This includes information on functional compensation to enable the client to be independent at home for as long as possible. Community occupational therapy resources are provided to assist families maintain their family members at home. Networking to establish relevant support groups is part of the work of the community therapist.

Community work and occupational therapy

Occupational therapy's involvement in community work primarily began with the establishment of community health and mental health centres in the 1960s and 1970s. This era saw occupational therapists working together with other health professionals involved in treatment and rehabilitation programs for deinstitutionalised people with major psychiatric difficulties. After-care services such as day hospitals, day centres and community-based residential facilities were established with occupational therapists focusing on issues of quality of life in the community, and on the client acquiring skills and supports to foster independent living. The 1980s saw occupational therapy branching out into broader areas of service in order to meet the needs of the psychiatrically ill and disabled people. New areas have included an increased focus on developing functional skills and adaptive abilities through such avenues as life skills training centres, social and leisure clubs, drop-in centres, vocational and transitional employment programs, crisis intervention and health promotion programs.

Increasing evidence suggests that social supports are vital for maintaining the health and well-being of the psychiatrically ill. Occupational therapists are becoming increasingly involved as primary care workers and networkers to assist people gain and maintain access to resources and supports. This approach expands the usual individual treatment focus. It includes in its service provision for further supports such as skills training, education and provision of resources for families, volunteer helpers, neighbourhood groups and local communities.

A final area of recent expansion in the focus of community occupational therapy is a concern with health promotion and prevention of illness and disability. This 'wellness approach' includes people who may be at risk or want to improve the state of their health and quality of life, either in everyday life, residential or occupational contexts. Programs concerned with fostering 'wellness', focus on issues such as good nutrition, physical fitness, self-care, stress management, life-style planning and improving the quality of relationships (see chapters 44, 64).

Conclusion

Occupational therapy is committed to, and primarily concerned with, orienting people towards independence and health. A major concern is in the area of functional performance, which enables the person to participate in the activities of day to day living, leisure and in a chosen vocational pursuit. This is accomplished through a variety of activities, including verbal, practical, and self-expressive tasks, either at the individual or group level.

The therapeutic relationship is seen to be significant and central to treatment. Intervention derives from a knowledge base which emphasises the interaction of the biopsychosocial aspects of human performance and adaptation. The uniqueness of the individual is acknowledged and viewed from a holistic perspective.

Within the scope of psychiatry, the diagnosis and resulting symptomatology are taken into account whilst, in practice, the rehabilitation of clients is based around the assessed levels of functioning through the client's active participation in their own rehabilitation process. The holistic approach adopted by the occupational therapy profession supports the current shift in approaches to health care, through advocating mutual responsibility, by both the professional and client, in active participation in health maintenance.

Further Reading

Axline V, *Play Therapy*, Houghton Mifflin, Boston, 1947.

Banus B, *The Developmental Therapist*, Thorofare, Charles Slack Inc, New Jersey, 1979.

Black M, 'Adolescent Role Assessment', *American Journal of Occupational Therapy*, Vol 30 No 2, 1976, pp 73–9.

Brown K, 'Wellness: Past Visions/Future Roles', *Occupational Therapy in Health Care*, Vol 4 No 1, 1987, pp 155–65.

Capra F, '*The Turning Point*', William Collins & Sons, Glasgow , 1985.

Csikszentmihalyi M, 'Play and Intrinsic Rewards', *Humanistic Psychology*, Vol 15 No 3, 1979, pp 41–63.

Dulay J and Steichan M, 'Transitional Employment for the Clinically Mentally Ill', *Occupational Therapy in Mental Health*, Vol 2, No 3, 1982, pp 65–77.

Gilfoyle E, 'Transformation of a Profession', *American Journal of Occupational Therapy*, Vol 38 No 9, 1984, pp 575–84.

Gorski G and Miyake S, 'The Adolescent Life/Work Planning Group: A Prevention Model', *Occupational Therapy in Health Care*, Vol 2, No 3, 1985, pp 139–50.

Howe M and Schwartzberg S, *A Functional Approach to Group Work in Occupational Therapy*, Lippincott, Philadelphia, 1986.

Johnson J, *Wellness: A Context for Living*, Slack Inc, New Jersey, 1987.

Levy L, 'Psychosocial Intervention and Dementia', *Occupational Therapy in Mental Health*, Vol 7, No 1, 1987, pp 69–107.

Mackinnon B, 'Occupational Therapy: Life Skills Program in a Cooperative Home Study', *Canadian Journal of Occupational Therapy*, Vol 45, No 2, 1978, pp 66–70.

Mann W, 'A Quarterway House for Adult Psychiatric Patients', *American Journal of Occupational Therapy*, Vol 30, No 10, 1976, pp 646–7.

Reilly M, 'Occupational Therapy Can be One of the Great Ideas of Twentieth Century Medicine', *American Journal of Occupational Therapy*, Vol 26, 1962, p 19.

Stone J, 'The Occupational Therapist's Role in Assisting Elderly People Adjust to Retirement' *Canadian Journal of Occupational Therapy*, Vol 49, No 4, 1982, pp 129–132

Talerico C, 'The Expressive Arts and Creativity as a Form of Therapeutic Experience in the Field of Mental Health', *Journal of Creative Behaviour*, Vol 20 No 4, 1986, pp 229–48.

Acknowledgment

L Do Rozario for her contribution in the area of community practice.

Chapter 66

Speech Therapy 1: Children

K Robinson, S Hogben and K Eddy

Over the past two decades, professionals dealing with communication disorders have become increasingly involved in the fields of mental health and psychiatry. Despite this increasing awareness and participation, speech pathology remains a relative newcomer to mental health, with few speech pathologists working in this area and little Australasian research being available.

Definitions and classifications

Speech pathologists work with people experiencing communication difficulty. They deal with each of the areas which comprise communication: language, articulation, voice and fluency. Language refers to the use of meaningful units to convey messages, and to the ability to decode and understand these messages. Articulation or speech is the physical production of speech sounds which are then combined to form words. Voice refers to the production of sound, and fluency is the rhythmic production of speech.

It is important that other professionals working with young children have some knowledge of the development of normal communication. Although there is considerable variation amongst children in the age at which they acquire specific language structures, some general guidelines can be utilised. Prior to 12 months of age, children should be babbling, playing with sounds and understanding simple instructions. A child's first words generally appear between 12 and 18 months of age, and by two years of age, most children are combining two words together and have a vocabulary of over one hundred words. A three year old child should be using sentences of three words or more, and have a vocabulary of around a thousand words. Sentence length and grammatical complexity continue to develop, with most five year old children using quite complex sentences with few grammatical errors. Abstract comprehension skills continue to develop after the age of five years, as does a child's ability to use a language in more complex ways, such as in sarcasm and humour. Development of written language skills in the form of reading and writing begins in the pre-school years and continues to develop with formal learning in the education system (see chapter 11).

The acquisition of speech sounds is also a gradual process, with considerable individual variation from child to child. By age three years, a child's speech should be 75 per cent intelligible, and by five years of age should be intelligible 95-100 per cent of the time. Inaccurate production of sounds such as 'r' and 'th' are generally the only articulation errors remaining. It is not uncommon for children to have a period of poor fluency between the ages of 2-6 years. Although a normal phenomenon, this is similar to stuttering, except that the child is not aware of or, anxious about his repetitions and prolongations of words and sounds, and does not use avoidance or compensatory behaviour. Approximately 80-90 per cent of these children spontaneously recover from this normal phase.

There has been a lack of consensus on the classification systems for childhood speech and language disorders. Traditionally, speech pathologists have not used the DSM or the ICD. This has created obstacles to liaison and consultation between professionals. The most relevant DSM categories to speech pathologists are in Axis I and Axis II. In Axis I, there is stuttering, cluttering and elective mutism, and in Axis II, mental retardation, pervasive developmental disorders, developmental articulation disorder, developmental expressive language disorder, and developmental receptive language disorder (see chapter 67).

The following are some types of communication disorders seen among children and adolescents.

1. Developmental articulation disorder

This is a disturbance or delay in the production of speech sounds, resulting in speech that is considered abnormal when compared to that of peers. Examples include a five year old child who omits sounds in the middle of words (for example, 'skipping' is articulated as 'skiing'), or a four year old whose speech cannot be understood owing to numerous sound substitutions (for example, 'puttet' is said for 'bucket'). The misarticulations are not due to mental retardation, hearing loss, language impairment or the physiology of the speech mechanism.

2. Developmental expressive language disorder

This refers to a delay or disturbance in the production and use of words and sentences that is unexplained by general mental retardation, hearing impairment, neurological impairment or physical abnormalities. Examples include a six year old child whose sentences contain grammatical errors such as 'Her putted shoes on foots', or a three year old child who does not combine any words together.

3. Developmental receptive language disorder

This describes a delay or disturbance in the understanding of words, sentences and symbols that is unexplained by general mental retardation, hearing impairment, neurological

impairment or physical abnormalities. Examples include a twelve year old child who only understands the literal meaning of colloquial sayings such as 'You're pulling leg', or a five year old child who does not understand instructions such as 'Bring me the biggest red plate from the cupboard by the fridge'. Some use the term 'aphasia' to refer to developmental language disorders. However, aphasia is generally used to describe a disorder involving the loss of some or all language skills as a result of acquired brain damage.

4. Elective mutism

This refers to a refual to talk in almost all social situations, including school. There is commonly no language or articulation impairment, and no physical or intellectual problem. For example, a child who talks only to her immediate family but not to other relatives, teachers or other children would be described as being electively mute. This problem is not due to language and/or speech disorder. It is a psychiatric disorder and should be referred to a child psychiatrist.

5. Autism

This disorder is partly characterised by a pervasive lack of responsiveness to other people, serious deficits in language development, and ritualistic and compulsive behaviours. It develops before 30 months of age (see chapter 10).

6. Stuttering

This is a disruption to the flow of speech involving repetition or prolongations of words or sounds, hesitations or pauses within or between utterances. There is an awareness of the problem by the individual, often accompanied by anxiety or compensatory behaviour.

7. Cluttering

This is a disorder of speech fluency in which speech is erratically rapid and dysrhythmic, resulting in impaired speech intelligibility. It is characterised by an unawareness of the disorder by the speaker.

Prevalence of communication disorders

Recent studies report that approximately 20 per cent of the pre-school population have speech and language disorders, with approximately 15 per cent having speech disorders and 6 per cent a language disorder.

Communication disorders have a higher incidence in boys than girls, with a ratio of three to one. Fifty per cent of children with a communication difficulty also have a behavioural, emotional or social disorder. This is considerably higher than usually found in non-communication disordered children.

Among those with communication disorders, those with language disorders, in particular receptive language disorders, have the greatest likelihood of having psychiatric disorders. Conduct disorders, attention deficit disorder, avoidant disorder and adjustment disorders were some of the most frequently occurring psychiatric conditions found among these young people.

Etiology/associated factors

There are a variety of etiological factors thought to be associated with developmental articulation disorders and developmental language disorders. These include general developmental delay, deficits in oral motor skills, speech mechanism abnormalities, auditory-perceptual deficits, family history of communication or learning disorders, low birth weight, prematurity and psycho-social deprivation. The nature of the relationship between communication disorders and emotional, behavioural social problems is unclear, however, a child who has difficulty understanding language may misinterpret messages, and consequently become confused and frustrated. These feelings may lead to behavioural problems (for example, aggression or withdrawal), emotional problems (for example, low self-esteem) and/or social problems (for example, difficulty making friends). An expressive language disorder or a speech disorder may make it difficult for a child to express his feelings, ideas, fears and needs, which may in turn lead to behavioural, social and/or emotional problems.

Assessment

As children with communication difficulties are at risk of developing psychiatric disorders, it is important that all children with suspected communication problems receive appropriate assessment and treatment. Assessment of communication skills is primarily the domain of the speech pathologist and referral should be made whenever a speech or language problem is suspected. An attitude of 'wait and see' is not acceptable. Early intervention, preferably in the pre-school years, is strongly recommended.

Assessment of communication skills by a speech pathologist involves investigation of functioning in a number of areas, including receptive language, expressive language, articulation, voice, fluency, auditory perception and oral structures and co-ordination. Results are obtained through administration of standardised assessments, informal observation of a child's communication competency and information obtained from caregivers and other agencies involved. Information regarding hearing acuity, developmental history, medical history, family situation, environment, social/emotional development and education history should also be gathered. Whilst it is important that the communication problems be dealt with, it is essential that a view of the total problem be maintained. This involves close liaison and consultation between all relevant professionals, such as psychiatrists, speech pathologists, occupational therapists, physiotherapists, psychologists, social workers, nurses, teachers and family doctors.

Differential diagnosis

Language is a uniquely human quality and is intrinsically related to the development of thought, play, social skills and emotional maturity. It follows, therefore, that a disorder of language may lead to educational, social, emotional or behavioural difficulties. Recent research strongly supports this view, stating that children with delays or disorders of communication development are at risk of developing psychiatric disorders.

Children with communication disorders

frequently demonstrate behaviours that are thought to have a psychiatric basis, but which are in fact a result of the communication problem. For example, a child who is assumed to be withdrawn and oppositional because he refuses to participate in group activities may in fact have a receptive language deficit. The child's anti-social behaviour may be a result of the communication impairment in situations requiring significant linguistic skills. Children who are easily distracted and are very active, often seem not to follow instructions, and ignore what is said to them. On assessment of their language skills, it may be that a reduction in the complexity of the information being presented to them will increase their attention span.

Children with communication difficulties may perform poorly on psychological tests or in an interview owing to the reliance of these situations on language skills. The child's poor performance may be misinterpreted as a psychiatric disorder if the language problem is not known, and not taken into account.

Management

Family involvement in speech and language therapy, as in other therapies, is an important aspect of successful treatment of communication disorders. Liaison with teaching staff is also necessary, given the evidence that children with communication disorders are at risk of developing educational problems. It is important that the communication difficulty be considered along with all other aspects of the child's functioning, including the family situation and the child's behaviour. This may require a multidisciplinary approach.

The nature of speech and language therapy will vary from child to child, depending on the type and severity of the communication problem. Therapy may involve individual, family or group intervention, with a management plan established and regular review of progress conducted. The primary aim of therapy is to develop functional communication skills that generalise from the therapy setting to the 'real world'. In addition, therapy should be fun and rewarding for the child in order to maintain his interest and co-operation. Tasks are analysed and presented

to the child in steps of increasing difficulty, ensuring success.

More specifically, language therapy may involve the development of grammatical skills, training of comprehension skills and assistance in using language appropriately. Examples of therapy techniques include modelling correct grammatical structures, expansion of a child's utterance to demonstrate more complex sentence forms, reinforcement of appropriate interactions such as turn-taking and eye contact, teaching of and exposure to new concepts and the provision of opportunities to practise them. Auditory training can play an important part in both language and articulation therapy, particularly in developing a child's ability to concentrate on verbal tasks and in the area of auditory discrimination. Articulation therapy may require teaching the child how to produce a sound, how to produce this sound in words and then sentences, and finally how to practise at maintaining the sound in conversational speech. Stuttering therapy involves achieving fluency at a single word level and progressing to phrase, sentence and conversational speech level. Intervention with children who are going through a phase of normal non-fluency may involve advising parents to slow the child's speech rate down.

Outcome

Speech and language therapy, particularly in the pre-school years, can greatly assist in the elimination or reduction of a communication difficulty. Clinical evidence indicates a positive correlation between improved communication skills and improvements in emotional, behavioural and social problems. It is apparent that an ability to understand others, talk with others, and be understood by other people can have a positive impact on a child's self-esteem, ability to make friends, and ability to learn. Children with articulation disorders tend to improve more quickly and have a better outcome than do children with language difficulties. Children with receptive language problems improve at a slower rate than do children with expressive language difficulties, and are at greatest risk of developing psychiatric and educational problems.

Strategies aimed at early detection and the prevention of communication problems, such as providing information to parents and caregivers regarding the stimulation of speech and language skills, are an important adjunct to the ultimate prevention of mental health problems in children.

Conclusions

Communicatively impaired children are known to have a high incidence of emotional, social and behavioural problems. In addition, psychiatrically disordered children have a high proportion of communication disorder amongst them. It is therefore apparent that speech pathologists have an important contribution to make in the area of child psychiatry, at both assessment and treatment level. The speech pathologist should be involved in diagnosis which differentiates the communication elements of the child's problem from the behavioural, emotional and social components. This should be part of a multi-disciplinary assessment and management of a child's problem. At a treatment level, early detection and therapy of a communication problem may help to minimise or avoid the development of a psychiatric problem.

Further Reading

Baltaxe C and Simmons J, 'Communication Deficits in Preschool Children with Psychiatric Disorders', *Seminars in Speech and Language*, Vol 8, 1988, pp 81-90.

Baker L and Cantwell D, 'Psychiatric Disorder in Children with Different Types of Communication Disorders', *Journal of Communication Disorders*, Vol 15, 1982, pp 113-26.

Cantwell D P and Baker L, 'Speech and Language', in *Child and Adolescent Psychiatry: Modern Approaches* (ed Rutter M and Hersov L), Blackwell Scientific Publications, London, 1985, pp 526-44.

Cantwell D P and Baker L, *Developmental Speech and Language Disorders*, New York, Guilford Press, 1987.

Yule W and Rutter M, *Language Development and Disorders*, SIMP, London, 1987.

Chapter 67

Speech Therapy 2: Adults

J Hooper

The role of the speech pathologist in the areas of psychiatry and mental health is expanding in Australasia. However, it is true to say that the developments in this field have been achieved by a small number of clinicians, who have crossed traditional boundaries and demonstrated the need for increased awareness and involvement by speech pathologists in this important area. As with the area of child psychiatry and communication disorders the majority of research has been done in the United Kingdom and America but there have been some recent important contributions from Australia in the areas of language impairment in dementia and voice disorders. This chapter will provide a brief outline of the communication disorders that occur in adults and their interrelationship with social problems and psychiatric disorder.

Definitions and classifications

Speech pathologists are responsible for the assessment, diagnosis, and treatment of communication and swallowing disorders. Communication disorders can affect the understanding and use of spoken or written language, articulation of speech, production and quality of voice, and fluency of speech. Swallowing disorders or dysphagia can include difficulties with chewing and swallowing food and fluids safely and effectively, which may interfere with the maintenance of adequate hydration and nutrition.

The use of ICD classification is more prevalent in the area of adult communication disorders because of the use of diagnostic related groupings for the purposes of health care funding. However, they are rather general symptom codings, and do not adequately distinguish between the different communication disorders. Consequently, the same code may be used for a number of disorders described below. Additionally, there are a number of areas that cannot be easily classified into a discrete category that may be part of a constellation of problems, for example, the problems of cognition and affective disorder resulting from closed head injury. The classification and definition of communication disorders in the adult population varies in complexity and detail in different texts.

Receptive dysphasia (ICD 784.3)

Receptive aphasia is the loss of the ability to understand spoken or written language as a result of cerebral damage.

Expressive dysphasia (ICD 784.5)

Expressive dysphasia is the loss of the ability to produce spoken or written language as a result of cerebral damage.

Dyspraxia (ICD 748.69)

Dyspraxia is the impairment of the ability to perform voluntary, coordinated movements in the absence of neuromuscular weakness. Oral dyspraxia is the inability to produce gross lip and tongue movements following demonstration or on command. Verbal dyspraxia is the inability to produce and/or sequence speech sounds, syllables and words.

Dysarthria (ICD 784.5)

Dysarthria is a disorder of muscular weakness or control as a consequence of central or peripheral nervous system damage. The muscles of respiration, phonation, resonance and articulation can all be affected to varying degrees, resulting in a variety of different motor speech disorders.

Dysphagia (ICD 787.2)

Dysphagia is difficulty in swallowing, which may be neurological, mechanical or psychogenic in etiology.

Dysgraphia (ICD 784.69)

Dysgraphia is the impairment of the ability to form letters when writing, and can be a symptom of dysphasia as a consequence of cerebral damage.

Dysphonia (ICD 784.49)

Dysphonia is a change in voice quality. Changes can include hoarseness, breathiness or pitch that is inappropriate for the person's age or sex. Other symptoms often associated with dysphonia can include problems with loudness levels, vocal fatigue or any combination of these difficulties. Voice disorders can have organic, functional, or psychogenic etiology.

Stuttering (ICD 307.0)

Stuttering is a disorder of fluency that is characterised by blocks, prolongations and repetitions of syllables and words.

There are also a number of communication and/or swallowing difficulties that occur in adults as a consequence of congenital malformations of the oral cavity, trauma, or head and neck cancer. They are therefore mechanical in origin and include laryngectomy and glossectomy. These problems are treated following surgical intervention.

Prevalence

The prevalence and incidence of voice disorders in the general adult population is difficult to determine. Studies which look at the prevalence of voice disorders vary in the reported figures. One study has estimated the incidence of voice disorders that may require a specific psychological emphasis to be around 5 per cent (McFarlane and Lavarato, 1983, in Green, 1988). However, it is important to be clear about the way in which voice disorders have been defined in the literature as this will affect reported incidence figures for the different categories. One view of psychogenic disorders is that they include all disorders that have an emotional or psychological component to the problem. This definition encompasses musculoskeletal tension dysphonia, dysphonia plicae ventricularis, vocal nodules and contact ulcers in addition to the voice problems that result from a conversion reaction or those related to an hysterical personality type. Some authors would define such problems as vocal nodules and contact ulcers as organic voice disorders because of the presence of lesions in the vocal tract. Another way of defining the same problem may be to refer to the voice disorder as functional, because the problem has occurred as a result of the person using the vocal tract in such a way that a lesion has occurred. Indeed in many cases vocal nodules occur because of vocal misuse in the absence of any emotional difficulties and therefore defining the problem as functional may be appropriate. Until there is a universally agreed definition for voice disorders, any data on prevalence must be used with caution.

Etiology/Associated factors

Communication and swallowing disorders in the adult population can be:

1. congenital or developmental, such as those of the adult person with cerebral palsy, cranio-facial abnormalities, intellectual disability or congenital voice disorders

2. acquired

(a) neurological, such as those resulting from cerebral or peripheral nervous system damage (for example, following stroke, head injury, progressive neuro-muscular disease, viral infections which attack the nervous system etc)

(b) mechanical, following surgery for head and neck cancer;

(c) other physical causes (for example,

voice disorders caused by lesions of the vocal folds, local inflammation and oedema, infections or endocrine problems);

(d) psychogenic, such as certain types of fluency problems, voice disorders and swallowing difficulties;

(e) functional (for example, voice disorders as a result of incorrect vocal technique or misuse).

Communication disorders in the adult population do not usually cause psychiatric disorders, however, many adults with diagnosed psychiatric disorder have communication problems either as a feature of the disorder (schizophrenia or dementia) or co-existing with the disorder. There are also a number of conditions that are often managed in a psychiatric context that have specific speech and language characteristics (for example, Gilles de la Tourette's syndrome, Huntington's chorea etc).

These conditions are neurological in origin but the behavioural and psychological concommitants of the disorders often require a psychological emphasis in management. The adult with a communication problem, whether congenital or acquired, may experience emotional, social or behavioural problems. Anger, frustration, feelings of grief and loss, depression and family difficulties caused by the communication disorder of an individual are all reported in the literature. These aspects must be considered in the assessment, diagnosis and management of the communication impaired individual.

There is some debate in the literature concerning the occurrence of depression in relation to aphasia. It would appear that depression is common in stroke patients but is not caused by the presence of dysphasia. Depression has been found to be frequently associated with dominant hemisphere lesions and the existence of depression may affect the recovery of the person with dysphasia (Starkstein and Robinson, 1988).

The literature in the area of dysphonia or voice disorder provides many examples of the psychological and personality characteristics that consistently occur with functional or psychogenic voice disorders. However, this is an area that requires further research as

highlighted by Green (1988). She reviewed the literature on the inter-relationship between voice and personality and emphasised that 'whilst a relationship is presumed to exist, problems in research design prevent the exact nature of the relationship being determined' (p 39). However, in some patients it may be possible that the voice disorder has been the precipitating factor that produces feelings of inadequacy, anxiety and low self-worth. An excellent example of this would be a teacher presenting with dysphonia, which is interfering with the ability to maintain the voice for a full day's teaching. Many teachers express concerns about their ability as teachers, their guilt at letting their pupils and colleagues down, their anxiety about the future of their careers etc. The resulting stress may contribute to the maintenance of the problem. There are a number of occupations that require significant use of the voice and many professional voice users experience functional voice difficulties. The practical concerns about future work potential, and the effect on the self-esteem of the individual who is unable to function effectively in his chosen profession can be considerable. The presence of chemical irritants in the working environment and the use of medicinal inhalants should also be considered.

Assessment

The assessment of the adult with communication or swallowing disorders is carried out using a variety of observational, standardised and objective techniques. These may include physical, neurological, cognitive, perceptual and language areas. The choice of assessment tool and format will vary depending on a combination of factors. This incorporates the initial medical diagnosis and the hypothesis formed at the first speech pathology interview following a detailed case history and the client's report of difficulties.

The speech pathologist will analyse the person's language skills in depth. The examination of comprehension and expression of language both in the spoken and written form will include vocabulary, morphology, structural and syntactic analysis, the analysis of semantics and the examination of pragmatic skills. Pragmatics emphasises the sociolinguistic aspects of language and concentrates on the analysis of how language is used in conversation. Such problems of discourse function can occur in combination with a linguistic or cognitive deficit or in isolation.

Speech will be analysed at the phonetic and phonological levels using phonemic transcription and comparative phonology. Phonetics refers to the types of sound a person produces or is capable of producing and phonology refers to the way in which those sounds are organised in speech to convey different meanings.

In the area of communication disorders of neurological origin the speech pathologist will carry out a neurologically based, or motor assessment to determine the extent and type of dysarthria or dyspraxia. This goes beyond the simple testing of cranial nerve responses and examines the functional use of the lips, tongue and palate for communication. In addition to the observational skill and knowledge of the clinician, there are a number of standardised tests that are used for this examination.

Standardised aphasia assessment batteries are used to assess receptive and expressive language function and will also include items for the evaluation of auditory memory, certain visual skills and other cognitive operations such as problem-solving, time concepts and calculations.

It is important for the clinician to be aware of the effects of various drugs that are commonly prescribed to patients as many can affect intellectual and motor function and consequently affect test results. These include benzodiazepine derivatives, some tricyclic antidepressants, lithium carbonate, anti-convulsants and in the elderly, the mixing of a large number of medications. Careful recording of type and dose of any medication should be made at the time of an assessment in recognition that this may have implications for test–retest results. If the speech pathologist has any concerns about the patient's perform-ance that may be related to medication, this would be discussed with the referring practitioner.

Voice disorders are assessed using a com-bination of perceptual and objective measures. A detailed case history of the client's voice problem is essential, as is a report from an otorhinolaryngologist providing information on the physical state of the larynx and vocal folds. It is extremely helpful to observe vocal fold function using a fibreoptic laryngoscope, which allows the clinician to assess the way in which the client uses the vocal folds during phonation. The additional use of stroboscopy or high speed photography allows observation of the vocal folds in slow motion giving greater detail of the vibratory function of the vocal folds. This examination is usually carried out with an ENT specialist. Other objective measures are obtained with the use of a number of different instruments that measure such parameters as air-flow, pitch, amplitude and the pertubation of the voice.

In the area of transsexualism the speech pathologist is involved as part of the team that assists the person in the transition to the chosen gender. Assessment of voice and communication skills pre-operatively will be necessary for effective management of those areas of sex-related differences.

Differential diagnoses

Differential diagnosis of the nature and extent of any communication or swallowing disorder is essential for the accurate management of the problem and the prediction of prognosis. Differential diagnosis must include a full neurological assessment in the case of acquired speech, language and swallowing disorders and detailed assessment by an otorhinolaryngologist in the case of voice disorders.

It is often difficult to determine if there is primary or secondary emotional psychiatric disorder, particularly in the presence of a communication or swallowing problem. The speech pathologist will be able to assist in the process of diagnosis by careful assessment and in some cases a trial of therapy to ascertain the presence or extent of psycho-logical factors related to the communication problem. In specific diagnoses, knowledge of the precise speech and language character-istics that typify that disorder and differentiate it from other disorders is extremely important.

Adults with developmental disabilities such as autism (see chapter 10), 'intellectual disability' (see chapter 9) or 'specific learning disorder' (see chapter 11) often have significant speech and language deficits. These deficits have usually been present since childhood and may not change as result of intervention. The important aspect of differential diagnosis in such cases is to assess the extent to which the person's speech and language function differs from his non-verbal abilities and, where possible, how long any gap between these abilities has persisted. Details of any psychological testing carried out in the past and the person's educational history should be obtained and compared with his current status. It is possible that the person has had many years of speech therapy as a child and the benefits of this should be discussed with the person and/or relatives. Some adults with a developmental speech and/or language problem may be able to benefit from therapy at this late stage. The important feature of differential diagnosis in this situation would be to determine if a specific speech and/or language problem exists over and above the developmental delay related to the primary diagnosis.

The adult with a history of epilepsy since childhood and reported speech and language problems should be investigated in a similar way to the person with a developmental disorder. Previous psychometric data and educational history should be obtained to compare with current levels of speech and language functioning. There have been many studies looking at the effects of focal cognitive deficits in epilepsy, and a language related memory deficit has been found to exist in the case of left temporal lobe epilepsy. Dysarthria in a person with epilepsy may be related to phenobarbitone toxicity and if the speech pathologist is concerned, this should be discussed with the patient's neurologist. It should be remembered that the speech and language deficits of a patient with epilepsy may be related to the underlying brain damage rather than the seizure disorder.

Gilles de la Tourette's syndrome is a condition characterised by multiple involuntary motor and vocal tics. The onset is reported to be usually before the age of 21, however, there are reports in the literature of onset and diagnosis occuring in adulthood. A number of speech and voice problems are features of this disorder, the most distinctive of these being coprolalia, i.e. the irresistable urge to say obscene words. However, other problems such as palilalia, (repetition of the last syllable, word or words of a sentence), echolalia, (repeating words spoken by others), stuttering, and spasmodic dysphonia have also been reported and may occur more commonly than coprolalia. Continuous repeated throat clearing is reported as a frequently occuring initial symptom. Speech pathologists may receive referrals from otorhinolaryngologists (specialists in ear, nose and throat (ENT)) of patients with repeated throat clearing and voice difficulties and should be aware of the possibility of such a diagnosis. Case history details and observation of any other motor tics may alert the clinician to the need for further assessment. The behavioural manifestations of this syndrome has led to it being well-documented in the psychiatric literature.

Occasionally such conditions as aphasia can occur in the absence of any other obvious neurological signs; it is in this situation that the language disturbances may be mistaken as symptoms of a psychiatric disorder such as *schizophrenia* (see chapter 33). It is important to recognise the differences and similarities of language characteristics of the two disorders. A major difference between the schizophrenic patient and the dysphasic patient is the way in which they respond to their own language difficulties. The dysphasic patient will often become frustrated by his language difficulties, whereas this is not the case with the person with schizophrenia. While the person with a fluent dysphasia has considerable difficulties with comprehension, the severe schizophrenic may appear not to understand but will then demonstrate comprehension by some word or action. The content of the dysphasic's speech will contain disordered language unlike the bizarre content of the schizophrenic. The speech of the schizophrenic can include semantic and phonemic paraphasias, circumlocutions, word salad, neologisms, jargon or paragrammatism and mutism. All of these problems can be found in different types of aphasia and formal aphasia testing would be essential to make a differential diagnosis.

The differential diagnosis of the language disturbances of aphasia and dementia (see chapter 40) is an area in which speech pathologists are becoming increasingly more involved. This is not necessarily an easy task. It had been commonly thought by some authors that the cognitive impairment of the person with dementia was greater than someone with aphasia. However, some aphasic patients demonstrate cognitive impairments that are disproportionate to their language impairment. Similarly, a language deficit can be the outstanding deficit in some people with dementia. A person with fluent aphasia is most likely to be confused with someone with Alzheimer's dementia. The language characteristics of the different types of dysphasia have been compared to different types of dementia at various stages of progression. The differential diagnosis of aphasia and dementia involves using a comphrehensive battery of tests, a high level of clinical expertise and a detailed case history of language function over time.

The differential diagnosis of voice disorders must always include a full assessment by an otorhinolaryngologist. It would never be assumed that the problem is psychogenic in origin before a physical or neurological cause has been ruled out. The voice disorder occurs despite a normal larynx; often normal or partial adduction of the vocal folds can be observed during coughing or laughing. However, this is not always the case and careful case history taking and assessment of the voice should occur before diagnosis is made. Many of the patients report musculoskeletal tension with pain and discomfort in the laraynx, neck and chest. It is often possible to assist the patient to produce normal voice during the assessment using facilitating techniques and this will also aid in the differential diagnosis of the problem. Spasmodic or spastic dysphonia has been considered to be of psychogenic origin by some authors. However a recent study by Finitzo and Freeman (1989) has concluded that the condition is a supranuclear movement disorder primarily affecting the larynx. It would

therefore be essential for full neurological investigation to be an integral part of the differential diagnosis.

It is important for the clinician to be aware of the effects of affective disorder (see chapter 28) such as depression on the speech and language ability of clients. Anxiety (see chapter 27) and mental confusion can also complicate the process of differential diagnosis and any indications of these problems should be noted and discussed with the appropriate medical practitioner.

The speech pathologist does not work in isolation. The clinician is part of a multi-disciplinary team involved with the patient and the family. Team members will vary depending on the presenting problem. Differential diagnosis takes place by the collection and interpretation of the information gathered by all members of this team. In the area of psychiatry, the speech pathologist can contribute information about the patient with a presenting communication problem that may assist in the accurate diagnosis of the primary psychiatric disturbance.

Management

The management of the person with communication and/or swallowing disorders occurs within the framework of a multi-disciplinary team. Management of specific disorder will be carried out in a number of ways depending on the needs of the patient. Individual therapy, group therapy and consultation are all used in the management of communication and swallowing problems.

Where there is a psychosocial component to the communication or swallowing problem, or where intervention must take a psychosocial emphasis, the speech pathologist may choose to work in consultation with, or as a co-therapist with a psychiatrist or psychologist. Speech pathologist also have counselling skills which can be used in this context. Many have taken further postgraduate training in such areas as transactional analysis, family therapy or rational emotive therapy. It is important to recognise that with some communication problems the psychological factors are so interwoven with the communication problem itself that the two components cannot be treated separately. In the area of voice disorders, specific techniques used to rehabilitate the voice are essential to recovery and therefore the speech pathologist is the primary professional involved in treatment and needs to be able to incorporate management strategies for many underlying psychological factors.

Speech pathologists will often work in conjunction with a psychiatrist or psychologist where hypnosis is being used as a way of dealing with factors contributing to a communication disorder or as an adjunct to therapy. There have been successful accounts in the literature of the use of hypnosis with clients with problems of fluency and voice disorders.

Oates and Dacakis (1983) reviewed the speech pathology management of transsexualism and provided a number of factors that must be taken into account when gender reassignment is carried out. There is the need to take into account the anatomical and physical constraints of the person's vocal tract and ensure that the person does not develop vocal abuse in an attempt to give their voice more feminine characteristics. The transsexual may seek advice on dress, body posture, coughing, laughing, and gesture. Additionally conversational style, vocabulary usage, articulatory differences and other communication differences need to be considered and incorporated into an individualised treatment program.

Speech pathologists in Australia have only recently become more involved in the area of the specific communication disorders of dementia and schizophrenia. The speech pathologist is in a position to assess the communicative function of the person with dementia and train relatives and caregivers in the best ways to maintain and facilitate communication with that person. With the emphasis on community living for the patient with a psychiatric disorder, the ability to communicate with others effectively, using appropriate body language, pragmatic skills and verbal language can mean the difference between success and failure in the community. Speech pathologists are trained in all aspects

of communication and could assist with individual and group programs to facilitate these skills.

Outcome

The outcome of treatment for communication and/or swallowing problems in adults will obviously vary depending on the etiology of the presenting problem, the severity, and the history of the disorder.

The management of co-existing psychosocial factors will have a significant effect on the progress of some patients. Depression, lack of insight, poor cognitive functioning and impoverished social support will all have an adverse effect on prognosis.

However, the ability to communicate is a unique human skill and any person robbed of this ability will not function as effectively as he once did. It is important to treat any communication deficit promptly and as comprehensively as possible to allow the person to function with as much dignity as possible and to maintain his feelings of self-worth. The loss of the ability to communicate is devastating and cannot be underestimated as a causative factor in the manifestation of mental health problems.

Speech pathology treatment may not result in the return of normal function particularly if there is significant brain damage. However, the aim of therapy may be to use residual function in the most effective way or provide alternative methods of communication. Particularly in the area of voice disorders, treatment programs will often result in the individual being able to resume his previous occupation. The ability to function would be the desired outcome for the majority of people with communication or swallowing problems and in the majority of cases this can be achieved.

Conclusion

Speech pathologists are trained in all aspects of communication and swallowing impairment. Many adults with mental health problems have co-existing communication or swallowing difficulties.

The assessment, diagnosis and treatment of communication and/or swallowing disorders in this population are important if management of psychosocial difficulties is to occur.

Further Reading

Aronson A E, *Clinical Voice Disorders*, Thieme, New York, 1985.

Baker J, (In Press), 'The Application of Systems Theory and Principles of Family Therapy to Clinical Teaching and Supervisory Processes in Speech Pathology', *Australian and New Zealand Journal of Family Therapy*.

Bayles K A and Kaszniak A W, *Communication and Cognition in Normal Aging and Dementia*, College-Hill Press, Boston, 1987.

Finitzo T and Freeman F, 'Spasmodic Dysophonia, Whether and Where: Results of Seven Years of Research', *Journal of Speech and Hearing Research*, Vol 32, 1989, pp 541-55.

Green G, 'The Inter-relationship between Vocal and Psychological Characteristics: A Literature Review', *Australian Journal of Human Communication Disorders*, Vol 16, 1988, pp 31-44.

Groher M E and Bukatman R, 'The Prevalence of Swallowing Disorders in Two Teaching Hospitals', *Dysphagia*, 1986, Vol 1, pp 3-16.

Jankovic J, 'The Neurology of Tics', (ed Marsden C D and Fahn S) *Movement Disorders 2*, Butterworths, London, 1987.

Laguaite J K, 'The Use of Hypnosis for Communicative Disorders', *Australian Journal of Human Communication Disorders*, Vol 10, 1982, pp 37-40.

Murdoch B E, Chenery H J, Boyle R S and Wilks V, 'Functional Communicative Abilities in Dementia of the Alzheimer Type', *Australian Journal of Human Communication Disorders*, Vol 16, 1988, pp 11-22.

Oates J M and Dacakis G, 'Speech Pathology Consideration in the Management of Transsexualism', *British Journal of Disorders of Communication*, Vol 18, 1983, pp 139-52.

Rochester S and Martin J R, *Crazy Talk, a Study of the Discourse of Schizophrenic Speakers*, Plenum Press, New York, 1979.

Serradura A and Hill P, *Transitional Feeding, the Team Approach*, Julia Farr Centre, 1989.

Starkstein S E and Robinson R G, 'Aphasia and Depression', *Aphasiology*, Vol 2, 1988, pp 1-20.

Thompson I M, 'Language in Dementia', *International Journal of Geriatric Psychiatry*, Vol 2, 1987, pp 145-61.

Wahrborg P, 'Aphasia and Family Therapy', *Aphasiology*, Vol 3, 1989, pp 479-82.

Chapter 68

Prevention

R Kosky

It has been estimated by the Australian Institute of Health, that, in 1989, Australian health costs were more than $23 billion, or $1400 per person. This amounts to about eight per cent of Australia's Gross Domestic Product. Health expenditure has shown a steady increase in costs, rising 41 per cent between 1984-1985 and 1987-1988. In relation to particular disorders, it has been estimated that the direct treatment costs of new cases of schizophrenia in New South Wales in 1976 were about $25 million and, overall, if productivity losses were included, the costs may have been as high as $1 billion. Goldney has estimated that the economic impact of youth suicide in Australia may be about $200 million a year.

To these costs we could add those (as yet unestimated) resulting from alcohol abuse, motor vehicle accidents, domestic violence, child abuse and other mental health-related problems.

It is hardly surprising that health care administrators have sought ways of preventing mental illness and of improving the general level of mental health in the community. This is not a recent interest. Mental hygiene movements have a long history in public health programs. So far, the prevention of mental illness has proved an elusive goal and attempts to improve mental health have often been problematic.

The greatest difficulty confronting those who approach the issue of preventing mental illness is the absence of knowledge about the causes and mechanism involved in mental illnesses. For those who seek to improve the level of mental health in the community, the biggest handicap is the lack of certainty about what mental health is and the intricate problem of separating pathological subjective experiences from the positive and negative effects of normal living. Because of these problems, mental hygiene movements have been particularly susceptible to political enthusiasm, sometimes with tragic effects and it is wise to address these flawed examples before considering current efforts.

The problems of mental hygiene programs

In our society, roughly 10 per cent of the population is impaired by some form of mental problem. In some areas, such as inner city areas of social disadvantage, the figure may be as high as 25 per cent. Such impairments of mental health are intimately bound up with the nature of the social structure in which people live.

There have been many attempts to create societies which offer favourable circumstances for personal development. This quest is part of human civilisation and its history. For instance, the early European settlers of Australia, according to some authoritative historians, attempted to develop a community governed by social principles in which people could be free of the persecution and tyrannies which had hampered many people in Europe. Democracy, freedom of speech, equality before the law, a universal, secular, free education system and female emancipation were social principles effected in Australia and New Zealand because of efforts to develop communities where individuals might flourish in health and well-being.

Many noble aspirations for utopian communities have fallen short in practice but not usually due to intentions which can be described as evil. Yet, the public health programs undertaken by the National Socialist dictatorship in Germany between 1933 and 1945 fit this description. The Nazis, using ideas derived from eugenics, apparently attempted to improve the mental health of the German people by culling the national gene pool of those whose genetic endowment was considered by them to be degenerate. These included mentally and physically handicapped people, schizophrenics, chronic alcoholics, homosexuals and the congenitally blind and deaf. In their public hygiene programs, begun with the passage of legislation in June 1933, less than six months after Hitler had become Chancellor, 360,000 persons, or 1 per cent of the population, were sterilised, usually by castration or x-rays. By autumn of 1941, between 70,000 and 95,000 people—mainly diagnosed as schizophrenic, feeble minded or epileptic—had been deliberately killed on the principle of 'life unworthy of life'. Babies who were born handicapped were allowed to starve to death. These 'public hygiene' measures, backed by powerful legislation, were carried out by doctors, nurses and other health professionals working for the Nazi government. Such eugenic programs were not without their supporters outside Nazi Germany.

Another, less evil, but nevertheless, pernicious example of zealotry in public mental hygiene concerns the issue of 'masturbatory madness'. A century ago, it was noted that young Britons who volunteered for the Crimean and Boar Wars had poor health. It was widely believed that this was a result of chronic masturbation. Masturbation was thought to result in mental degeneration and insanity. Consequently, there was a major health drive to suppress 'self abuse'. Many thousands of young people in Britain, America and Australia between 1850 and 1930, had their lives ruined when they were subjected to sometimes ridiculous attempts to prevent them masturbating. Various mechanical contraptions were employed. Hands were put into locked leather gloves or tied to bed rails. Genitals were blistered and cauterised. As late as 1939, masturbation was included in the list of aetiological factors of mental illnesses presented in the Victorian Mental Health Department's Annual Report.

These examples should cause us to pause for thought. It is obviously necessary to maintain a clear head about public health issues, to be modest in our aspirations and sceptical of our achievements and to base them on sound ethical as well as scientific principles.

Unemployment and mental health

In considering public health issues, we cannot ignore the effects of social factors on the mental health of the community. One example is the physical and mental health consequences of unemployment. Since 1975, when rates of employment declined sharply, unemployment has been an issue for many thousands of Australians, particularly those aged between 15 and 25 years. Long term unemployed people have poorer physical health than their employed peers and they have a higher rate of psychiatric illness and symptoms. In 1981, a cross-sectional survey of unemployed youth in Canberra found that 49 per cent of the sample scored positively on a health questionnaire suggesting that they had significant psychiatric symptoms, particularly depression. This compared to less than 10 per cent for the general population. The investigators considered that most of these symptoms were a result of unemployment rather than being present before unemployment (Finlay-Jones & Eckhardt, 1981).

Stress, life 'events' and stress management

The concept of *stress* is not a simple one although it is commonly and loosely used as a target for many mental health preventive strategies. It is better to discuss a stress model rather than use the term stress without qualification. One such model, put forward by Tennant and colleagues (1985), is illustrated in Figure 1 in which social and personal factors mediate between stressor and stress response.

The stressors can include physical stimuli such as noise and pain, as well as psycho-social stimuli, such as the death of a relative or unemployment. Stressors set in train various attempts to adapt to their effects. These responses may have good or bad consequences. Earlier notions of stress suggested that it inevitably led to maladaptation. Although still widely held, this view is only part of the story, as it is apparent that stress can be successfully mastered, useful lessons learnt for the future and a qualitatively and quantitatively different level of adaptation attained. However, if stressors are perceived as unpleasant (ie have a distressing quality), they are more likely to lead to psychological maladaptation and this quality is usually more important than the event itself.

Major stressors are more likely to cause psychiatric problems than minor stressors but it is not clear whether apparently small stressors can produce a cumulative effect, nor is it clear whether there are certain forms of

stressors (for example, certain occupations) which are particularly stressful for all people.

Life event stressors which are referred to as 'exits' (for example, losses, separations, discord and deaths) are more likely to correlate with psychiatric illness than those perceived as 'entrances' (for example, births, marriages). A more complete analysis of the effects of loss and its relationship to later depression is provided in chapters 7, 25 and 28.

The immediate response to a threatening stress is arousal and fear. This includes a physiological response of rapid heart rate, raised blood pressure and increased vigilance. Under certain conditions, this response may be prolonged into a chronic state either in whole or in part; high blood pressure, anxiety, or both, may persist. Physical and psychological processes interact. Thus, an anxious response to stress may adversely affect the course of already present heart disease.

According to Tennant's model (Figure 1), mediators between the stressor and the stress effects include the individual's personality,

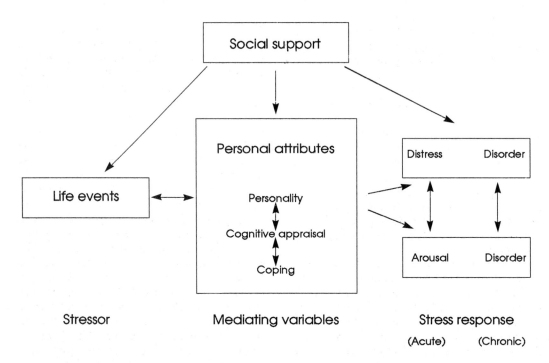

Figure 1. *A stress model (from Tennant C et al, 'The Concept of Stress', Australian & New Zealand Journal of Psychiatry, Vol 19, 1985, pp 113-18).*

and the social network available for support. Personality is itself a complex phenomenon and it is not clear whether we can define it precisely. In its widest sense it refers to the unique nature of a person. Modern ideas have stressed functional and developmental qualities such as curiosity and task resolution rather than static features such as obsessionality or intellect. Nevertheless, it is widely thought that it is possible to define character types in broad terms. One such category includes people who are aggressive, impatient, keen to work, *time-urgent* and frustrated by trivial obstacles and minor delays. In the face of stress, such individuals accentuate these characteristics and can become hostile and highly aroused. They are then considered to be vulnerable to cerebrovascular accidents and heart attacks. Others are more relaxed and easy-going and do not respond so dramatically to stress. They have been shown consistently to score less on life stress inventories than the time -urgent personalities.

Social support is also a complex notion, not easily defined for research purposes. It is a multidimensional concept. It involves the amount of actual support available and the nature of that support. The study of unemployed Canberra youth referred to earlier showed than those who could borrow a small amount of money were less likely to suffer depression than those who could not. Family, friends and co-workers may form part of the support network. Institutions such as churches, voluntary organisations or hospitals may be the key networks for others. In addition, it is not only the actual support, it is the amount of support which a person *perceives* to be available to them when they are stressed which seems important in the prevention of psychiatric disorder following a stressor.

To what extent can stress models be used to prevent mental illness and improve mental health? Common sense tells us that it should be possible to reduce the adverse effects caused by stressors by adequate preparation for stress events so that they lose some of their distressing quality. Early preparation for death seem preferable to not talking about its likelihood. Emergency drills for potential disasters may prevent panic. Techniques of time management may prevent people becoming overwhelmed by conflicting tasks. The examples are manifold and it is not surprising that stress management courses have many enthusiasts.

Programs may also be aimed at control of the physiological response to stress. Education about the effects of stress and sources of personal or work-place stressors, relaxation, exercises, yoga and mental preparation for achieving control over bodily responses, may assist some people to control the stress response.

Stress management programs have a controversial side. Some people argue that they can deflect people away from achieving social control over the stressing events. For example, some feminists have argued that stress management courses for women simply teach them to accept oppressive social relations which distress them. Instead, these critics argue, women should be prepared to get hostile and fight for social justice.

The stress model and social change

The concepts of stress/distress have also proved useful in identifying areas where social conditions can be improved with consequent improvement in mental health. One example has been in the teaching profession. A recent survey of 2000 teachers in West Australian schools found that 17 per cent had symptoms of severe psychological distress compared with 9 per cent of the general population (Finlay-Jones, 1989). The excess was associated with the teachers' exposure to a number of stressors in the teaching environment. These included lack of support from colleagues and senior staff, poor classroom design, invasion of spare time by work and a critical community attitude to teachers. The most significant factor in producing teacher stress was identified as student misbehaviour.

As a result of this study a program was instituted to help teachers develop effective management of student behaviour through means of an experimental consultancy service known as the 'Whole School Approach' whereby a team of guidance officers visit schools at weekly intervals. In the first part of the program the emphasis was on working on classroom management skills with the school's administrators and some volunteer teachers. In the second part, the approach encompassed the whole school when the goal was to review current disciplinary and pupil management procedures to ensure consistency in and support for the agreed approach.

A similar program has been developed in South Australia and is currently being evaluated on two grounds—whether it decreases the levels of distress reported by teachers and whether it improves student behaviour. Other changes relating to classroom design, conditions of service and staff development also flow from research based on this model.

Crisis intervention

Crisis intervention is based on the idea that intervention at a crucial period in a person's life could change a potential psychological or social decompensation into something which could be a positive and maturing experience for the person. The question immediately arises as to what is a critical period? In fact, crisis intervention principles have been applied to many life events such as marriage, moving house, entering school, birth, retirement and so on.

Once again, common sense might tell us that such events can be stressful for many people and that some support at these times might be useful, but few studies exist which provide scientific evidence that interventions at times of these life events can prevent mental illnesses.

However, crisis intervention principles are also used at times of unusual or unpredictable life events such as surgery, accidents, unexpected death and disaster. Studies of support given during surgery or at the time of accidents indicate that supported people do better afterwards than non-supported people. Effective support may be relatively simple—such as helping with practical issues (for example, paying house rent or ensuring pets are looked after), mobilising friends and relatives and contacting and involving social welfare agencies. It also seems clear that communicating accurate information to the patient and ensuring that they and staff have some understanding of normal responses associated with these traumatic events are aspects which improve adjustment after the event.

There have been many studies which have indicated that intervention following loss and bereavement can substantially protect against the development of symptoms of psychological distress and physical illness. Interventions which help widowed spouses, or parents who lose their children and children who lose their parents, can also be applied to health workers whose daily work brings them into contact with death and dying.

In a children's hospital in 1989, it was found that where nurses felt unsupported or busy with other priorities, or without a chance to talk to their colleagues, they were more distressed by dying patients and were more likely to 'burn out'. Such nurses were perceived by their colleagues as having become dull, insensitive, irritable, inflexible and not responding to individual patients, although they themselves did not recognise this. Simple intervention following ward deaths, such as 'debriefing' sessions or individual support from a special palliative-care nurse consultant were seen as useful in reducing levels of distress among staff and patients. These sessions consisted of those involved taking a half an hour together to go over the events, and people's reactions to them, sometimes assisted by an outside facilitator or counsellor.

Telephone counselling

There has been a rapid growth in the use of telephone counselling services which reflects a widespread belief in its preventative value. Hornblow (1986) has provided a recent comprehensive review of these services and their effectiveness. He points out that the obvious advantage is the ability to bring instantaneous counselling at the moment of personal crisis. The 'Samaritans' were established in London in 1953 with suicide prevention as their aim, and they have been widely imitated. Thirty years later there are many international branches employing over 27,000 counsellors. The counsellors are volunteers who are given some training about telephone counselling techniques.

Recent years have seen the development of many similar telephone services such as Life Line, Rape Crisis Line, Youth Line, Gay Line, AIDS hot lines and so on. In many cities, welfare agencies have developed Crisis Care Units which principally operate using telephone counselling. These developments have resulted in the mobilisation of many thousands of volunteers world-wide. The telephone counselling services are now an integral part of community mental health networks.

Despite this widespread acceptance, Hornblow points out that attempts to evaluate the preventive effectiveness of telephone counselling have usually been defeated by methodological problems. For instance, suicide rates are influenced by many social factors, some of which are by no means clear and the presence or absence of telephone counselling services are not used by those who are intending suicide. Instead, they are more likely to be used by a range of people who are ambivalent and undecided. Some have claimed that the very presence of the services may serve to suggest suicide to some members of the community. Most studies have suggested that the suicide rates remain unaffected by the presence of telephone counselling.

Most of those who call telephone services do so one or twice only and are usually found, on follow-up, to have been satisfied with the information or support given. About half comply with the advice given. The evidence to suggest that counselling via telephone can affect attitudinal or behavioural changes is controversial. Some studies have shown that high levels of emphathy and responsiveness can be achieved. This has been particularly the case for identified at-risk groups such as bereaved parents. When physicians called parents a week or so after an infant's death, these parents reported less long term problems than those who had not been called.

Legislative programs

An example of a preventive strategy arising from social action was the passing in Australia of legislation to compel occupants of motor vehicles to wear safety harnesses (seat belts). Surgeons and others concerned about the number of injuries, particularly head injuries in people involved in motor vehicle accidents, lobbied for wearing of seat belts to be made mandatory. A long public education campaign directed largely by the Royal Australasian College of Surgeons resulted in the political acceptance of seat belt legislation, despite critics who believed that such legislation was an infringement of civil liberties. Since the mandatory introduction of seat belts the number of deaths from motor vehicle accidents among young people has fallen and the number of serious head injuries has decreased. In turn, this has probably lessened the considerable burden of the neuropsychiatric sequelae of car accidents. These include intellectual impairment, depression, irritability and behaviour problems.

Other legislative measures adopted as a result of public campaigning on the part of health professionals have seen prohibitions on prescribing drugs such as amphetamines and barbiturates. Consequently, addictions, psychoses and suicide as a result of the misuse of these drugs are now rarely seen in psychiatric practice. Re-modelling of packages of antidepressant tablets and, more recently, other tablet medications, has also been aimed at preventing impulsive attempts at suicide by overdosing.

Biologically based interventions

Genetic counselling of prospective parents has proved useful in many illnesses where there are clear-cut and well understood inheritance patterns (for example, muscular dystrophy, Huntingdon's disease, some forms of mental retardation). Unfortunately the inheritance pattern and genetic contributions to the majority of most mental illnesses remain unclear.

In most cases, genetic material appears to result in a vulnerability rather than an illness per se. Yet, studies of families and of twins have shown the importance of the hereditary factor in the major psychiatric syndromes such as bipolar disorder and schizophrenia. Recent work on mapping human chromosomes has revealed marker genes for a number of conditions (for example, cystic fibrosis, Huntington's disease) and it is not unreasonable to suppose that the rapid advances in this field will soon reveal the genetic basis of the major psychiatric illnesses.

The ideal situation would be to identify people who are carriers of genes which lead to severe psychiatric disorders and to understand the laws governing their transmission from generation to generation. In this way genetic counselling about mental illnesses could be given to potential parents. This time has not yet arrived in psychiatry. At present, our best advice is that the children of a parent with bipolar disorder or with schizophrenia have a significantly increased risk (up to 20 per cent) of developing their parent's condition at some time during their life. Counselling may be important for potential parents who have these conditions.

Some preventive programs suggest biological interventions at other levels. Screening of infants for metabolic diseases such as phenylketonuria can result in early identification, and proper medical intervention preventing the development of this form of mental retardation. There has been a steady push from some psychiatrists to add thiamine (vitamin B_1) to alcoholic beverages. Many people who abuse alcohol have inadequate diets. Some develop delerium which is potentially lethal and can lead to permant memory impairment. This can be prevented by the administration of thiamine. Failure to do so may leave the patient severely incapacitated by memory loss and unable to work or care for themselves. As a result many many need permanent institutional care, or other substantial social support systems. It is argued that the addition of thiamine to beer and other alcoholic beverages would be relatively inexpensive and reasonably practical and would prevent this grave social legacy of alcohol abuse. Such a proposal seems worthy of a trial, as potential savings to the community could be enormous.

In South Australia, a major public health project has been undertaken in the Port Pirie area to reduce the levels of lead in the environment. Port Pirie is a town with a major smelting works. Blood lead levels were found to be high among the population, especially children. It was argued that this caused mild levels of lead poisoning and consequent impairment in brain functioning, manifested by lower intelligence levels and an increase in behavioural abnormalities.

The South Australian Government established a decontamination and rehabilitation program in 1984 after a community outcry over the high lead levels. From 1984 to 1987 the percentage of children above the level of concern fell from 21 per cent to 11 per cent. This compares with a 1985 study in Adelaide's western suburbs where 9.6 per cent of children had high levels of lead. The government spends about $2.5 million on the Port Pirie project each year. The program includes blood testing, community education and removing high risk factors such as contaminated soil and paint with high lead levels. Some have claimed this lead clearance program to be among the most advanced public health programs in the world.

Parents and children

There is a long history of pedagogic interest in child rearing. Many popular examples of instruction exist from all ages of recorded history (for example, the long essay, 'On Civility in Children', by Erasmus of Rotterdam, which first appeared in 1530, ran to at least 130 editions). The continuing instruction of parents about how to bring up their children has been identified as one of the 'civilising processes', by which is meant one of the mechanisms whereby society becomes progressively more structured and proficient.

In our times, much attention has been directed towards child rearing to prevent mental illness. The Child Guidance Movement was begun in the 1920s as a means of helping children enter adulthood free of neuroses. These clinics, multi-disciplinary from the start, were usually community based, free and accessible to parents and children of all social classes, ethnicity and gender. In more recent years these clinics have developed more specialised psychiatric services often associated with children's hospitals.

Attempts have been made to teach potential parents about planning families. Family planning clinics are now well established and have counselling in the forefront of their activities. Such support services are also with obstetric clinics, pregnancy termination services, in vitro fertilisation programs, adoption and fostering services, and so on. However, effectiveness of these counselling services has not been examined in any systematic way.

Much attention has also been devoted to the development of adequate early parent–child attachments. Practices surrounding child birth itself have dramatically altered in the last three decades owing to the work of child psychiatrists and others who have emphasised the importance of early emotional attachments for the later well-being of the child and the parents. Parents are now encouraged to be with the child from birth. Antenatal classes encourage active participation by mothers and fathers in the birth process. Children's hospitals encourage parents to visit and be near their children even to the extent of providing sleeping facilities for parents and siblings. In Australia, where people are often living long distances from the hospital, such practices are important as children can easily become distressed as a result of separation from family.

Aside from such sweeping changes in paediatric practice in the last few decades, more specific projects have also been aimed at disadvantaged children and at those who are seen as being vulnerable to the development of emotional disorder. Several projects, such as one in Mauritius and another in Vermont, America, have sought to identify children at risk for schizophrenia and to intervene in a preventive manner. Children identified in these projects as at-risk have included those who had excessive reactions to neurological and psycho-logical tests (Mauritius) and those who had psychotic parents, behavioural disorders or social deprivation (Vermont). In both projects, at-risk preschool children were given 'enriched' day care experiences. However, in these projects many, perhaps many thousands, of factors are uncontrolled and it has been difficult to say whether a specific intervention at one time in a person's life was able to decrease their vulnerability to later events.

The Project Headstart in the United States was a bold attempt to improve educational and social qualities for socially deprived children and to help them overcome their disadvantages as they began school. Massive funds and resources were provided for areas where people were in poverty or otherwise socially disadvantaged. It has proved impossible to quantify the effects of this program despite considerable efforts to do so and, as a result, Headstart has had severe critics. One said: 'Headstart was not working. The children were getting their teeth fixed but little else could be quantified'. On the other hand, a staunch supporter claimed that the goals had been achieved by 'pragmatic quiet actions'. The program began around 1967 and wound down after 1970 following a series of evaluation reports which failed to show measurable alterations in the cognitive abilities and educational progress of the target children.

However, on a smaller scale, the early identification of learning difficulties in school children, and their remedial correction, has been shown to advance the progress of children who, otherwise, would create difficulties in the classroom or who were at risk for developing behavioural and social disorders.

It should not be thought that all counselling and supportive interventions have positive effects, however humane they seem. One study cautions us about this. This is the Cambridge–Somerville Youth Study in which delinquent boys and so-called 'average' boys were assigned by the toss of a coin to an intervention or to a control group. There were 253 in each group. The average age of the sample was ten and a half years (range 5–13 years). Those in the intervention group were given psychiatric and medical help, counselling, tutoring and general social supports. A 30 year follow-up revealed that those in the intervention group were more likely to have committed crimes, to show signs of alcoholism, suffer serious illness and to die at a younger age. They were more likely to be in low prestige jobs and to find their work unsatisfying.

There are many problems with the conclusions from this study, not least the

467

methodological problems of conducting a 30 year follow-up. There are queries about the samples, the responses on the questionnaires and so on. There are also criticisms of the interventions themselves which seemed relatively non-specific. Despite these criticisms the results are disturbing. One possible reason for the negative results is the effect of self fulfilling prophecy and the implications, for the intervention group, of being encompassed within a highly organised welfare system.

Forms of preventive intervention

It is usual to describe preventive interventions in terms of primary, secondary and tertiary prevention. Primary interventions are aimed at preventing the occurrence of psychiatric illness (including mental retardation). Secondary interventions are aimed at preventing a disorder getting worse or reversing it in its early stages, and tertiary interventions are aimed at the rehabilitation of those with established psychiatric disorders to decrease their disabililty.

In practice such distinctions are not easy to maintain. For instance, in the crisis intervention model it is uncertain whether the person experiencing a life crisis is in the primary or secondary area for intervention. This chapter has concentrated on primary and secondary prevention.

Conclusion

Steiner, writing in 1976, after analysing the Headstart Project for the Brooking's Institute, wrote that: 'The children's policy most feasible—and most desirable—is one targeted on poor children, handicapped children and children without permanent homes. The lobbyist most needed are those urging programs targeted to those specific categories'. If we learn anything from the confusing evidence that comes from reviewing programs aimed at preventing mental illnesses or improving the mental health of communities, it is that we should identify target groups, define measurable goals, and evaluate achievements. In times of a shrinking health dollar, health professionals and administrators have a responsibility to make certain that their preventive programs, however humane their intention, have scientific credibility.

Further Reading

Caplan G, *Principles of Preventive Psychiatry*, Basic Books, New York, 1964.

Finlay-Jones, R and Eckhardt B, 'Psychiatric Disorders Among the Young Unemployed', *Australian & New Zealand Journal of Psychiatry*, Vol 15, 1981, pp 265–70.

Finlay-Jones R, 'Factors in the Teaching Environment Associated with Severe Psychological Distress among School Teachers', *Australian & New Zealand Journal of Psychiatry*, Vol 47, 1989, pp 304–13.

Hornblow A R, 'Review: Does Telephone Counselling Have Preventive Value?' *Australian & New Zealand Journal of Psychiatry*, Vol 20, 1986, pp 23–9.

McCord J, 'A Thirty-year Follow Up of Treatment Effects', *American Psychologist*, 1978, pp 284–9.

Raphael B, 'Primary Prevention: Fact or Fiction?', *Australian & New Zealand Journal of Psychiatry*, Vol 14, 1980, pp 163–74.

Tennant C, Langeluddecke P and Byrne D, 'The Concept of Stress', *Australian & New Zealand Journal of Psychiatry*, Vol 19, 1985, pp 113–18.

Weindling P, '*Health, Race and German Policies Between National Unification and Nazism 1870-1945*', Cambridge University Press, Cambridge, 1989.

Part 9
Research

Chapter 69

Epidemiology 1:
Child and Adolescent Disorders

M Sawyer and P Baghurst

The distribution of childhood psychiatric disorders refers to their frequency in terms of other factors such as age, sex or social class. For example, during the last 20 years a number of studies have shown that the prevalence of childhood disorders is much greater in impoverished inner city areas. Information like this is important for planning services and also because it suggests possible causes of childhood disorders.

In order to identify the aetiology of childhood disorders, knowledge gained in epidemiological studies is used to identify causal chains of events which appear to precede the onset of psychiatric disorders. One possible causal chain is shown in Table 1. This chain suggests that parental unemployment leads to marital disharmony, the disharmony results in inadequate management of children's behaviour and this, in turn, results in increasing antisocial behaviour by the affected children. This is, of course, only a very simple example but it is given in order to illustrate the type of information which epidemiological studies can provide about determinants of childhood disorders. As well as providing information about the aetiology of disorders, causal chains can also be used to help guide preventive programs. For example, it can be seen that steps could be taken at several different points to try and break the sequence of events shown in Table 1. If this was possible it might lead to a decrease in the number of children with antisocial behaviour.

Table 1. A possible causal chain preceding onset of psychiatric disorders

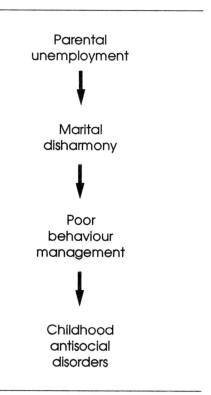

The use of information gained from epidemiological studies in order to focus preventative programs in specific areas is an important development. Epidemiological studies suggest that childhood psychiatric disorders are relatively common in the community and it will always be far too expensive to provide individualised treatment programs to help all children. The use of focused preventative programs offers a means by which the number of children with psychiatric disorders might be decreased. This could then allow treatment programs to focus on the remaining children who have established disorders.

Incidence and prevalence

Epidemiological studies generally describe findings in terms of the prevalence or incidence of disorders in specified populations (see chapter 70).

Most epidemiological studies in child psychiatry have been prevalence studies and there have been very few studies investigating the incidence of childhood psychiatric disorders. One implication of this is that much more is known about chronic psychiatric disorders of childhood than about disorders which have a short life. This is because chronic disorders, which persist over a long time period, are more likely to be identified in prevalence studies taken at a particular time.

Defining disorders to be studied

A basic problem for epidemiology in child psychiatry is how to define a disorder. Two broad approaches have been used in epidemiological studies. One approach employs the criteria identified in the DSM-III-R or ICD-9 in order to define the disorders to be studied. These diagnostic systems are widely used to define childhood disorders and were largely derived from clinical practice. It is important to notice that they are categorical in nature, that is, they assume that children can be divided into one of two categories, those having a disorder and those without a disorder. Identification of children with disorders relies on interviews with children and parents. In addition, information may also be collected from teachers. As it is too expensive to get clinicians to interview every child and family participating in broad epidemiological studies, highly structured interviews have been

developed which allow non-professionals to conduct the interviews. Results from the interviews can then be scored using computer programs in order to identify children likely to have disorders.

An alternative approach to classifying disorders relies on the use of multivariate statistical techniques in order to identify groups of symptoms which appear to cluster together (see Chapter 71). These clusters are then used to develop empirically based systems for classifying childhood psychopathology. An example is the Child Behaviour Checklist, devised by Achenbach (1985) to be filled out by parents. An important theme in this approach is that childhood psychopathology is seen as lying on a continuum. Less emphasis is placed on categorising subjects into those with and without disorders: instead the approach emphasises measurement of the frequency and severity of problems. When this approach is used, greater use tends to be made of questionnaires or checklists which can be completed independently by parents, teachers and children.

These approaches to classifying childhood disorders identify two broad groupings of disorders. The first group of disorders are called conduct disorders or externalising disorders and refer to aggressive, undercontrolled or antisocial behaviour. The second group of disorders are called emotional disorders or internalising disorders and refer to fearful, inhibited or overcontrolled behaviour.

Sources of data

An important issue for epidemiological studies investigating childhood psychiatric disorders is deciding from whom information about children should be obtained. Early studies relied heavily on information from mothers and, to a lesser extent, from teachers. More recently, it has become clear that there is only moderate agreement between parents, teachers and children reporting on the behaviour of children. In particular it is now evident that children themselves are an important source of information and should not be overlooked in epidemiological studies. A recent study conducted in New Zealand has highlighted the differences in reports which are provided by parents, teachers and children. Studies now need to give careful attention to this issue and must recognise that some children with problems may not be identified if reliance is placed on a single reporter whether that person be the mother, father or the teacher.

Strategies

Many cross-sectional studies, collecting information at only one point of time, have been conducted in child psychiatry. Two of the most well known are the Isle of Wight Study in England, and the Ontario Child Health Study (Offord, 1987). Both of these studies measured the prevalence of childhood disorders in populations of children living in a general community. As well, the studies collected large amounts of additional information about children and their families. This enabled the researchers to investigate whether childhood disorders were more frequently found in certain types of families, for example, families in which a parent had a psychiatric disorder or families where the parents reported marital problems.

Cross-sectional studies can provide a large amount of information about whether certain factors, such as marital disharmony, are associated with childhood disorders. However, one disadvantage of cross-sectional studies is that they cannot provide information about the causal relationships between factors which they find to be associated. This means that cross-sectional studies cannot be used to develop causal chains of the type discussed earlier. To take a simple example, it seems just as reasonable to suggest that children with conduct disorders might cause marital problems as it does to suggest that marital problems cause conduct disorders. To establish the cause and effect relationship between factors such as marital disharmony and conduct disorders requires that information about a population be collected at more than one point of time. There are two kinds of longitudinal studies which rely on information collected about populations at more than one point of time. The first group are called cohort studies and the second group

are called case-control studies.

Cohort studies are usually initiated before the disorder of interest has its onset. For example, if it is planned to study whether birth trauma causes autism a large number of infants will need to be identified at birth. The infants will be divided into two groups, those who suffer birth trauma and those who do not. Both groups will be followed up over several years and the proportion in each group who later developed autism will be compared. A major problem with this type of approach is that the original group of infants would have to be extremely large as autism is a very rare disorder occurring in less than 4 per 10,000 live births. Only by including an extremely large number of infants at the beginning of the study would it be possible to be sure that some children in both groups would later develop autism.

Cohort studies can provide important information about the development of children in the general community. For example, two large cohort studies have followed the development of children over a number of years in Christchurch and Dunedin, in New Zealand. These studies began with a large cohort of infants and have followed the development of the infants through their childhood and adolescence. The children are assessed at regular intervals and comprehensive information is obtained about the children and their families. This information can then be used to build up causal chains which help explain the aetiology of childhood psychiatric disorders amongst children in the community.

A major advantage of studies on children in the community is that they are free of the biases which are likely present when only children referred to psychiatric clinics are studied. For example, it is possible that children with psychiatric disorders, and their families, who attend psychiatric clinics, are different in important ways from all the children in the community with the same disorders. In light of this it is important not to assume that relationships found between factors in clinic-referred children provide an accurate picture of relationships which will be found in all children with the same disorder in the community.

In case-control studies, children who already have the disorder of interest are compared with a control or comparison group of children who do not have the disorder. For example in order to study the relationship between birth trauma and autism, a population of children who have developed autism (the 'cases') would be identified. Birth records would then be used to compare the frequency of birth trauma in this population, with the frequency in a similar population of children who are free of autism (the 'controls'). By this means it would be possible to see if birth trauma was more common amongst children who have autism. Case-control studies have two disadvantages. First, existing records often do not contain the information needed for the study or important records may be missing. Second, it is sometimes difficult to be certain that the study includes a sample representative of all children with the disorder of interest. For example, if children with disorders were identified through hospitals or clinics, those children with disorders who do not attend these services would not be represented in the study population.

A summary of current findings

There have been several studies investigating the prevalence of childhood psychiatric disorders in Australia and New Zealand. The prevalence of psychiatric disturbance in children and adolescents under the age of 20 years in Australia is approximately 10 per cent. A recent study which collected information from parents, teachers and children, reported a somewhat higher overall prevalence of 17.6 per cent in a group of 11 year old children. Of particular importance is an epidemiological study of children living in rural Queensland by Connell and colleagues which reported a prevalence of 10 per cent for psychiatric disorders amongst children living in rural settings. These results highlight the importance of epidemiological studies for planning purposes. The great size of Australia makes it very difficult to provide services to country regions but it is clear from Connell's study that psychiatric disorders are not uncommon amongst children living in remote regions.

Most studies of children report higher prevalences of disorders amongst boys, probably as a result of the higher prevalence of conduct disorders amongst boys. The prevalence of emotional disorders appears more evenly distributed amongst boys and girls.

Epidemiological studies have shown that parental criminality, parental psychiatric illness, marital disharmony, poor disciplinary methods, and the presence of a large number of siblings are all more common in the families of children with conduct disorders. Information about children with emotional disorders is less consistent.

Economically poor communities have a higher prevalence of children with psychiatric disorders than middle-class communities. The results of epidemiological studies suggest that this is due to the presence of higher prevalences in poor communities of factors which contribute to the onset of psychiatric disorders in children, such as marital disharmony and parents with psychiatric illness.

Finally, epidemiological studies in England have highlighted the very significant influence that schools can have on the development of children. What is important is that the effect of these school influences could not be accounted for by factors already present in children at the time they commenced attending the schools being studied. In addition, the size of the effects on children was large and they influenced children in a range of areas. There is a great need to further study the effect of school influences on children and the means by which they could be used to prevent the onset of psychiatric disorders in children.

Further Reading

Achenbach T M, *Assessment and Taxonomy of Child and Adolescent Psychopathology*, Sage Publications Inc, London, 1985.

Anderson J C, Williams S, McGee R and Silva P A, 'DSM-III Disorders in Preadolescent Children', *Archives of General Psychiatry*, Vol 44, 1987, pp 69-76.

Connell H M, Irvine L and Rodney J, 'The Prevalence of Psychiatric Disorder in Rural School Children', *Australian and New Zealand Journal of Psychiatry*, Vol 16, 1982, pp 43-6.

Graham P, *Epidemiological Approaches in Child Psychiatry*, Academic Press, London, 1977.

McGee R, Silva P and Williams S, 'Perinatal, Neurological, Environmental and Developmental Characteristics of Seven-year-old Children with Stable Behaviour Problems', *Journal of Child Psychology and Psychiatry*, Vol 25, 1984, pp 537-86.

Offord D R, Boyle M H, Szatmari P, et al, 'Ontario Child Health Study II, Six Month Prevalence of Disorder and Rates of Service Utilisation', *Archives of General Psychiatry*, Vol 44, 1987, pp 832-6.

Rutter M, 'Epidemiological Approaches to Developmental Psychopathology', *Archives of General Psychiatry*, Vol 45, 1983, pp 486-95.

Chapter 70

Epidemiology 2: Adult Disorders

P R Joyce and M A Oakley-Browne

Epidemiology links the clinical care of individual patients to the social, community and population context in which they live. Clinicians see only those who seek help. The epidemiologist is as much interested in those people who do not obtain treatment as those who do, and in the factors which determine who gets treated and who does not. The population orientation of epidemiology allows it to: (i) study the distribution of mental disorders in the population, and to compare rate of disorders in differing populations; (ii) decide whether certain risk factors (for example marital status) or events (for example a disaster) are associated with certain disorders; (iii) evaluate the use of health services, and whether services are providing effective interventions. This latter task of psychiatric epidemiology makes it of potential value to health administrators.

Measures and rates

The basic measures in epidemiology are those of frequency and association. These make use of the 'rate' of the disorder. A rate implies that there is a comparison between two numbers, one of these numbers (the numerator) is the number of cases, while the other number (the denominator) is the population from which the number of cases arose. There are a variety of different types of rates:

1. The *incidence* or inception rate is the number of new cases of a disorder within a certain period of time for a given population.

2. The *point prevalence* rate is the proportion of individuals in a population who have the disorder at a given point in time.

3 .The *period prevalence* rate is the proportion of individuals who have the disorder within a given period of time. Within psychiatry, common period prevalence rates are the one month or six month or one year rates. All period prevalences are affected by both the inception rate of the disorder, and by the duration of the disorder. Given that the duration of many psychiatric disorders is measured in months or years, period prevalence rates are always considerably higher than inception rates.

4. The *lifetime prevalence* or morbid risk defines the likelihood of developing a disorder in a lifetime. There is a slight difference between these terms in that the lifetime prevalence is a measure of whether a subject has had a particular disorder up to their current age, while the morbid risk makes an allowance for the fact that some individuals who have never had a disorder up to the present time may develop it in the years to come. The term morbid risk has especially been used in genetic studies, while lifetime prevalence is the more common rate reported from population surveys.

The most commonly used measures of association are *relative risk* and *attributable risk*. The relative risk is the ratio of the rate of the disorder among individuals exposed to the risk factor and those not exposed. For instance, a subject who has previously attempted suicide is 20 times more likely to kill himself by suicide than a person who has never made an attempt, ie the relative risk of completed suicide among suicide attempters is 20. The attributable risk is the rate of the disorder that can be attributed to a certain risk factor in individuals exposed to that risk factor. This measure is derived by subtracting the rate of the disorder among the nonexposed persons from the corresponding rate among exposed individuals.

Study designs

There are a variety of designs for epidemiologic studies, but a major feature which distinguishes epidemiologic studies from clinical research studies is the need for epidemiologic studies to have a defined population from which the cases are drawn. For without a reference population it is not possible to determine numbers of disorders, which are fundamental to epidemiology.

One design is a *cross sectional* descriptive study, which estimates the numbers of disorders at one point in time. Another descriptive design is a *longitudinal study* which identifies a cohort of subjects and follows them over time and observes the development of new disorders, or the recurrence of new episodes. This design can either follow a random sample of subjects over time, or can follow a group at high risk of developing a disorder (for example, the children of patients with schizophrenia (see chapter 32)).

Another design is the *case control* study (see chapter 69).

A further design is an *experimental* one in which a specific factor is altered, either by the investigators (for example, a treatment intervention for individuals, or a community intervention such as education) or by nature (for example, a natural disaster).

The development of psychiatric epidemiology

Historically, epidemiology in psychiatry first studied the severe disorders, such as schizophrenia and organic disorders (notably pellagra psychosis which was linked to a specific nutritional deficiency), in which the majority of patients were hospitalised. For a chronic disorder such as schizophrenia, this is of some value, but as soon as one is interested in major depression, anxiety disorders and personality disorders, hospital inpatient data becomes less and less relevant. For instance, over the course of one year about 250 people in 1000 will have a psychiatric disorder; of these, about 230 will attend primary medical care services; of these, psychiatric disorder will be recognised in about 140; of these only about 17 will see a psychiatrist and only about six will be hospitalised. The six psychiatric inpatients among the 250 with psychiatric disorder differ in terms of their diagnoses, the severity of their illnesses, and may differ in terms of a variety of socio-demographic variables such as age, sex and social class.

Advances in psychiatric epidemiology have been related to developments in the methods of identifying cases. Early studies thus used clinician or hospital diagnoses, and this approach may still have some value when dealing with psychotic disorders. However, as interest in non-psychotic disorders increased, it was necessary that other approaches were developed; for the last decade a common method has been to screen the population of interest with a self report screening questionnaire such as the General Health Questionnaire, and then use clinicians to interview selected subjects to have extreme scores on the screening questionnaire (see chapter 69). Commonly, with these research designs, the clinician then used the Present State Examination (PSE) as a method for determining whether a subject had a recognisable disorder or not. This approach has been used widely in Australasia. An alternative to this approach has been the development of the Diagnostic Interview Schedule (DIS), which is a structured interview which can be completed by a trained lay interviewer. The DIS was devised for epidemiologic research and is used without a screening instrument and does not require clinical expertise to administer.

In the United States, when social factors were considered to be the major risk factors for psychiatric disorder, epidemiology studies often avoided making clinical diagnoses and substituted global ratings for impairments related to psychiatric symptoms. However, this practice meant there was no common language for clinicians and epidemiologists, and the findings from epidemiology had minimal impact on clinical practice. More recently epidemiology has studied specific disorders. This has considerably increased the links between clincians and epidemiologists, and is the likely way for the future.

In recent years, several extensive psychiatric epidemiologic studies have been completed. These studies, called the Psychiatric Epidemiologic Catchment Area (ECA) studies were funded by the National Institute of Mental Health in the United States. They involved surveying five separate sites in the United States, using comparable study designs with random household sampling, and a standardised interview schedule (the DIS) which could be administered by lay interviewers. Comparable studies have been completed in Edmonton (Canada), Puerto Rico and Christchurch (New Zealand). Table 1 shows the six months prevalences for some common disorders in the various places which used comparable methodology. In general, it can be seen that rates are more often similar than different.

Future developments in psychiatric epidemiology are likely to see increasing co-operation between clinicians and epidemiologists, increasing interest in biological and genetic markers as risk factors for the development of disorders, greater use of high risk prospective cohort studies and greater interest in intervention studies. Epidemiology will also continue to have an important role in the planning and evaluation of health services.

Table 1.   The six month prevalence (%) of some common psychiatric disorders in various centres, which have completed community studies using the Diagnostic Interview Schedule

Psychiatric Disorder

	S	MD	M	Alc	Ph	Pa	OCD	ASP	Any *
Christchurch	0.2	5.3	0.1	8.3	7.5	1.1	1.0	0.9	23.4
Edmonton	0.3	3.2	0.1	5.4	5.1	0.7	1.6	1.8	17.1
New Haven	1.1	3.5	0.8	4.8	5.9	0.6	1.4	0.6	18.4
Baltimore	1.0	2.2	0.4	5.7	13.4	1.0	2.0	0.7	23.4
St Louis	0.6	3.2	0.7	4.5	5.4	0.9	1.3	1.3	16.8
Piedmont	1.3	2.0	0.2	3.8	13.7	0.7	2.2	1.0	23.1
Los Angeles (Mexican)	0.3	3.0	0.1	5.3	7.3	1.0	0.6	1.2	19.7
Los Angeles (Non Hispanic whites)	0.6	3.7	0.5	4.9	6.1	1.0	0.9	0.4	19.1
Puerto Rico	1.5	3.0	0.3	4.9	6.3	1.1	1.8	-	-

* (S=schizophrenia, MD=major depression, M=mania, Alc=alcohol abuse/dependence, Ph=phobias, Pa=panic disorder, OCD=obsessive compulsive disorder, ASP=antisocial personality disorder, Any=any diagnostic interview schedule DSM-III diagnosis covered).

Further Reading

Barrett J and Rose R M, *Mental Disorders in the Community*, The Guilford Press, New York, 1986.

Freedman D X, 'Psychiatric Epidemiology Counts', *Archives of General Psychiatry*, Vol 41, 1984, pp 931-33.

Goldberg D and Huxley P, *Mental Illness in the Community: The Pathway to Psychiatric Care*, Tavistock, London, 1980.

Henderson A S, *An Introduction to Social Psychiatry*, Oxford University Press, 1988.

Oakley-Browne M A, Joyce P R, Wells J E, Bushnell J A and Hornblow A R, 'Christchurch Psychiatric Epidemiology Study, Part II: Six Month and Other Period Prevalences of Specific Psychiatric Disorders', *Australian and New Zealand Journal of Psychiatry*, Vol 23, 1989, pp 327-40.

Robins L N, 'Psychiatric Epidemiology', *Archives of General Psychiatry*, Vol 35, 1978, pp 697-702.

Shepherd M and Wilkinson G, 'Primary Care as the Middle Ground for Psychiatric Epidemiology', *Psychological Medicine*, Vol 18, 1988, pp 263-7.

Weissman M M, 'Epidemiology Overview', in *Psychiatry Update* (ed Hales R E and Frances A J), *American Psychiatric Association Annual Review*, Vol 6, 1987, pp 574-88.

Chapter 71

Statistical Inference in Psychiatry

W Hall and K Bird

Statistics is a branch of mathematics which enables order to be discerned amid the sampling and the measurements which are essential in human sciences. This chapter will provide an overview of aspects of statistics which are of use in behavioural research and medical practice. The emphasis will be on the logic and purpose of statistical inference in psychiatric research.

Two branches of statistics are customarily distinguished: *descriptive* and *inferential*. Descriptive statistics provide a description of the main features of a set of data from a population. Inferential statistics enables inferences to be made that go beyond this sample data.

Descriptive statistics

The justification for descriptive statistics is simple: the average person is usually unable to grasp the information contained in even a small set of data.

Some types of descriptive statistics are familiar. In the case of categorical data in which subjects are assigned to one of a set of mutually exclusive categories (eg, male or female, depressed or normal) one can summarise the information by reporting the percentage of cases falling within each category.

Different types of descriptive statistics are required for measures based on *multi-item tests* which are commonly used to measure characteristics of people, such as in check lists used in epidemiological surveys. A multi-item test is one in which scores are derived by combining the answers given to a series of

items or questions. The data produced by such tests can be regarded as *continuous*, since the scores vary continuously between a maximum and a minimum value.

Scores are usually reported in numerical form (for example, 'correct' answers), or the number of ticks on a checklist. Rarely do these scores provide any useful information by themselves. In order to make sense of them (for example, 'is this patient clinically depressed?') a person's score needs to be compared with scores made by others who are depressed. Such a comparison requires the use of descriptive statistics which economically describes the main features of the group's scores, and enables an individual's performance to be compared to the group.

The first thing to be determined about an individual's score is where it lies in relation to the 'average'. One way of answering this question is to calculate where the typical score for the group lies, and how the group scores are spread around that typical score. The type of measure that summarises the typical performance of a group is a measure of *central tendency*. The most commonly used measures of central tendency are the *mean* and the *median*. The *mean* ($\overline{X}$) is the average of all the scores. It is obtained by adding up all the scores (ΣX) and dividing the sum by the number of scores (N), ie

$$\overline{X} = \frac{\Sigma X}{N}$$

The *median* is the score that falls in the middle of the set of scores. It is the score that has 50 per cent of scores above, and 50 per cent below it.

The *median* is usually regarded as a better

measure of central tendency if the scores are 'skewed' or bunched at one end, or if there is a small number of extreme scores. The mean is a widely used measure because it permits the development of more sophisticated statistical methods (t-tests, the analysis of variance.).

An individual's score can be described in relation to the mean by calculating a *deviation score*. This is the difference between an individual's score and the mean of the group $(x=X-\overline{X})$. The deviation score is only minimally informative, unless there is some indication of how typical the mean of the group of scores may be. That is, one needs to know whether the scores are widely scattered or tightly grouped around the mean.

In order to measure the spread of scores around the mean, a measure of their dispersion is required. The most widely used of these is the *standard deviation*. It is obtained by calculating the sum of the squared deviation scores (Σx^2), dividing this quantity by the number of independent pieces of information in the set (N-1), and taking the square root of the result:

$$sd = \sqrt{\frac{\Sigma x^2}{(N-1)}}$$

To see why one divides by (N-1) rather than N, consider three scores $x_1=17$, $x_2=21$, $x_3=22$. These scores provide three independent pieces of information, one of which is used in calculating their mean $[\overline{X} = (17+21+22)/3=20]$ which is a necessary step to calculating the deviation scores ($x_1=-3$, $x_2=1$, $x_3=2$). The three deviation scores contain only two pieces of information, since they must sum to zero. That is, given any two deviation scores (eg $x_1=-3$ and $x_3=2$) the third (x_2) must be equal to zero minus the sum of the other two; since all three must sum to zero.

When it comes to making statistical inferences it will be discovered that the quantity (N-1) is also known as the *degrees of freedom* for the estimate of the standard deviation, since it signifies the number of quantities that make up the estimate which are free to vary independently of one another.

By using the mean and standard deviation,

each individual's score can be described in a standardised form. This is done by calculating a z-score (or standard score) in which each subject's deviation score is divided by the group standard deviation, ie

$$z = \frac{X}{sd}$$

The z-score provides a number whose sign indicates whether the individual scored above (+) or below (-) the group mean, and its value indicates how far the individual's score is from the mean.

If assumptions are made about the shape of the distribution of scores, it is possible to use the mean and standard deviation to characterise the individual in relation to the rest of the group. An assumption that is commonly made is that the parent distribution is *normally distributed*. This means that the distribution of scores follows a normal or *Gaussian curve*, a symmetrical bell-shaped curve. This is the way many characteristics, such as height, weight, intelligence and extraversion, are distributed in the population.

The normal distribution has a number of useful statistical properties. First, a normal distribution is completely defined by its mean and standard deviation, whereas many other distributions require other measures to describe them fully, such as skew and flatness. Second, in a normal distribution, the mean and median are identical. Third, in a normal distribution there is a simple and straight-forward relationship between an individual's score and the percentage of the group that has a higher or lower score. This is provided by tables reflecting the area under a standard normal curve where two-thirds of cases will have z scores which fall within the boundaries of plus or minus 1.0 standard deviation units, and 95 per cent of z scores will fall within plus or minus 2.0 standard deviation units of the mean.

Correlation analysis

It is often useful to have an index of the strength of the relationship between different measures. The most widely used index is a correlation coefficient which quantifies the extent to which a performance on one test predicts (or covaries with) that on another test. This coefficient ranges in value from +1.0 to −1.0. A correlation of +1.0 indicates a perfect positive relationship, −1.0 indicates a perfect inverse relationship, and 0.0 indicates the complete absence of a relationship. The equation for the correlation coefficient (r) between two sets of scores x and y (also called the Pearson Product–Moment Correlation Coefficient) is given by:

$$r_{xy} = \frac{\Sigma Z_x \cdot Z_y}{N}$$

Inferential statistics

Only rarely are researchers interested in simply describing the characteristics of a sample. Usually they wish to use the sample to make inferences about the population from which the sample came. For example, a researcher may wish to use the mean score on a check list of depression symptoms from a small sample of depressed inpatients to make an inference about the mean of *all* depressed inpatients at the hospital. This is an example of statistical inference.

Inferential statistics is important in psychiatric research because of the small size of treatment effects relative to sampling and measurement errors. Suppose, for example, that a researcher randomly allocated a sample of 100 depressed inpatients to receive either an active antidepressant drug (group 1) or a placebo (group 2), and wished to evaluate the effectiveness of the drug by comparing the post-treatment mean scores of the two groups on a check list of depressive symptoms (see chapter 28). The random allocation of patients ensures that the two groups can be regarded as belonging to the same population prior to treatment. Hence, any systematic or steadily occurring differences between the means after the treatments can be attributed to differences in the effectiveness of the two treatments.

It is not a simple matter, however, to decide whether a mean difference is due to change, since differences between the means of the samples may arise because of error. Scores in the population may vary for a number of reasons (for example individual differences in intelligence, cultural differences, patient or observer bias, day to day variations in mood, etc). It is possible that chance factors may cause an unusually high proportion of high-scoring individuals to be assigned into group 2 in the example above. If this happened, group 1 might produce a lower post-treatment mean than group 2, even if the drug was no more effective than placebo. Inferential statistics is necessary to enable us to discriminate between differences that are systematic effects, and those that are chance.

In this way, inferential statistics exercises a degree of control over the tendency to mistake the peculiarities of a sample for features of a population.

The way in which inferential statistics enables us to evaluate whether observed differences may have arisen by chance is best spelt out by discussing two simple forms of statistical inference: the t-test and chi-square test of independence. The former is used to test whether the difference between means of two samples is due to chance or not, and the latter is used to test for an association between two or more categorical variables.

The t-test

The t-test, which is one of the most familiar and widely used of statistical tests, is easy to calculate and to understand, because it involves a simple comparison between two means. Suppose, that a researcher randomly allocated a sample of 100 inpatient depressed patients to either antidepressant drug treatment or a placebo. Patients' depression levels were measured six weeks later on a standardised inventory of depression symptoms. The mean and standard deviation for each group main example are shown in Table 1.

In this example, the form of treatment to which the patients have been assigned is the *independent variable*, and the score on the depression inventory is the *dependent variable*. We assume that the scores are approximately continuous, that they are normally distributed, and that in the two groups they are independent (which is ensured by the random assignment of patients).

The researcher would want to know if it

STATISTICAL INFERENCE IN PSYCHIATRY

Table 1. Depression scale experiment
Means, standard deviations and sample sizes for a hypothetical experiment in which depressed patients are randomly assigned to receive either an antidepressant drug or a placebo and assessed on a scale of depression after six weeks

	Drug	*Placebo*
$\overline{X}$	15	20
sd	10	10
N	50	50

was reasonable to infer that an observed difference between sample means (X_1 and X_2), indicated that the treatments differed in their effectiveness (that is the post-treatment population means u_1 and u_2 were different). The researcher could carry out a t-test to see whether a simpler hypothesis, that the treatments were equally effective, would be rejected. This is the *null hypothesis*. If it is true, the population means are equal, and the observed difference is likely to be due to chance.

To carry out a t-test the following ratio is calculated:

$$t = \frac{\overline{X}_1 - \overline{X}_2}{SE_{diff}}$$

that is , a ratio of (1) the difference between the two group means to (2) an estimate of the standard error of that difference (SE_{diff}), which is derived from the standard deviations within each group (sd_1 and sd_2 respectively) as follows:

$$SE_{diff} = \sqrt{\left(\frac{(N_1-1)\,sd_1{}^2 + (N_2-1)\,sd_2{}^2}{N_1 + N_2} \right) \frac{(N1 + N2)}{N_1\,N_2}}$$

The numerator in the ratio is the best estimate of the difference between the two populations means (the means of depressed inpatients who have been given an antidepressant drug and those given a placebo). The denominator is the best estimate of the standard deviation of an hypothetical distribution. This is the distribution of the values of $\overline{X}_1 - \overline{X}_2$ that would be obtained if a large number of samples of two groups of size N =50 (in our example) were taken from populations which differed in their means by

$u_1 - u_2$. Given that the two populations are normally distributed with equal variances and errors are independent, this ratio is distributed as a t-distribution.

Since the difference between the populations is not generally known, one begins by asking the question 'Is $u_1 - u_2$ different from zero or not?' This is done by testing the null hypothesis that $u_1 - u_2 = 0$ (or equivalently, that $u_1 = u_2$).

This test involves the following form of reasoning: (1) assume that the null hypothesis is true; (2) estimate the probability of the difference between the means arising if the null hypothesis is true, and (3) if this probability is sufficiently small, by convention less than 0.05, the null hypothesis is rejected; if the probability is greater than 0.05 the null hypothesis is considered true.

In our example in Table 1, calculation of the t-ratio produces the following result:

$$t = \frac{(20-15)}{2} = 2.5$$

The probability of this t-ratio arising if the null hypothesis were true is evaluated by comparing it with tables of critical values of t. These values vary with the degrees of freedom for the t-ratio, given by (N–2), where N is the total sample size. There are (N–2)=98 degrees of freedom in our example because the estimate of the standard error of the difference is based on two sets of deviation scores, 50 deviations from the mean in group 1, and 50 deviations from the mean in group 2. Since each set of deviation scores only provides 49 independent pieces of information, there are 98 degrees of freedom in all.

Comparison of the obtained value with the critical value for 98 degrees of freedom indicates that the probability is such that the null hypothesis (that the two populations have the same mean) can be rejected. That is, one can conclude that depressed inpatients who received the antidepressant drug had a lower depression score after six weeks of treatment than patients who receive a placebo.

In making this decision the probability was set at less than 0.05 and therefore the researcher accepts a risk of 5 in 100 that the decision is wrong. The error that the researcher risks making in rejecting the null hypothesis is known as a *type 1 error*. In using the t-test in this example, the researcher controls the type 1 rate (α) at 0.05.

The chi-square test

The chi-square test is the appropriate statistical test for making inferences about differences between the cases falling into various categories. Such categorical data arise when observations are classified on two or more categorical variables. An example of some cross-classified data is provided in Table 2 which displays data from a study of Finlay-Jones and Brown (1981) of the relationship between severe life events and psychiatric illness among female general practice patients.

Table 2. Psychiatric illness and the experience of a severe life event in female general practice patients

	Psychiatrically ill?		
	Yes	No	Total
Severe event	39	41	80
No severe event	6	78	84
	45	119	164

Source: Finlay-Jones and Brown, 1981.

The questions addressed, and the statistical tests used to answer it, depend upon how the data are collected. If a sample of N patients had been jointly classified as to whether or not they had a psychiatric illness *and* whether or not they had experienced a severe life event, one would perform a chi-square test of *independence*, which tests the null hypothesis that psychiatric illness and the occurrence of severe life events are independent. If fixed numbers of women who were ill, and who were well, were classified as to whether or not they had experienced a severe life event, the appropriate test would be a chi-square test of *homogeneity*, which tests the null hypothesis that the proportion of women who

have experienced a severe life event is the same among women who are well, and who are ill.

The computations are the same for whichever form of chi-square test is used. The test involves and evaluation of the goodness of fit between the *observed* frequencies (f_0), and the expected frequencies of (f_e) on the basis of a hypothesis of independence or one of homogeneity. This is given by the following formula:

$$\chi^2 = \frac{\Sigma(f_0 - f_e)^2}{f_e}$$

The pattern of data expected under either hypothesis is obtained by means of the 'product rule'. If life events and psychiatric illness are *independent*, then the expected frequency with which each of the four combinations occur will be the product of their probability of occurring separately. In the example in Table 2, this is calculated by multiplying together the two marginal totals, for example, 45 and 80, and dividing by the total number of observations, 164.

If the proportions of patients who have and have not experienced a severe life event are the same (ie homogeneous) then the number expected in each cell should be the product of the number of the psychiatrically ill, and well, and the number of those with and without severe life events multiplied by the number in the total sample.

In the example in Table 2, the data was collected on a sample of 164 patients in a general medical practice, so the appropriate chi-square test is the test of independence. Calculation of the chi-square test statistic produces a value of 35.63. The null hypothesis that psychiatric illness and the occurrence of severe life events are independent is evaluated by comparing the obtained value of χ^2 with the critical value from the chi-square distribution with the appropriate degrees of freedom. The degrees of freedom are given by the product of the number of rows minus one and the number of columns minus one, ie (R-1) (C-1). In the example, the obtained value easily exceeds the critical value ($\chi^2 = 3.84$, df=1, p<0.05). The conclusion is that there is a relationship between psychiatric illness and life events among female general practice patients. Inspection of the Table suggests that women with a severe life event are more likely to be psychiatrically ill than women who have not experienced a life event.

Statistical power

The statistical tests outlined so far control the probability of committing a false positive error (ie a type 1 error) at 0.05. That is, such tests ensure that there is only a small chance (5 in 100) that the researcher will conclude that there is a difference between the populations when no such difference actually exists.

A false positive error is not the only type of error that can be made in a statistical inference. It is also possible to make a false negative error. This occurs when one fails to reject a null hypothesis which is false. Such an error is called a *type 2 error*. Its probability of occurrence is beta (β). Ideally, one wants to minimise the chances of making false negative errors of inference. This objective is met by maximising the statistical power of a test. This is the probability of correctly rejecting the null hypothesis and its probability of occurrence is given by the complement of β (ie by $1-\beta$).

Information about the power of statistical tests is important in planning research and in interpreting the outcomes of studies. Studies should be planned to ensure that there is a reasonable chance of detecting an effect. When interpreting a failure to reject the null hypothesis, knowledge of the study's power enables one to decide whether there is no effect or whether the study had insufficient power to detect an effect. If it is known that the power of the study is adequate (for example, the chances of detecting an effect is better than 80 per cent) one can be confident that the failure to reject the null hypothesis provides good reasons for accepting it. A *power analysis* is the process of determining the sample size required to provide a high chance of detecting important differences between two treatments or a relationship between two variables.

Multiple inferences

The t-test is often used inappropriately to make statistical inferences when the research

designs are either multiple group (more than two populations are compared) or multivariate (comparisons are made on more than one measure) or both.

Assume that a researcher wished to compare two different antidepressant drugs with a single placebo and so randomly allocated 50 inpatients to each of three treatments (drug 1, drug 2 and placebo), and measured them after six weeks. The performance of multiple t-tests on this data would involve undertaking three t-tests to test the following three null hypotheses:

$$H_1: u_1 = u_2 \qquad H_2: u_2 = u_3 \qquad H_3: u_1 = u_3$$

The major problem with this approach is that it does not control the type 1 error rate for the *set* of the three decisions. The type 1 error rate for each test is 0.05 (for the reasons explained above) but the chance of making an error in *any* of the three decisions is greater than 0.05. Although one cannot be precise about what this error rate is, it cannot be greater than the number of tests multiplied by the type 1 error rate per test, ie in our example 3 x 0.05=0.15. This relationship is expressed in an inequality, which is known as the *Bonferroni inequality*, namely, the error rate for the set is $< k_{x\alpha}$ where k is the number of tests in the set and α is the type 1 error rate chosen for each test (in the example, this is 0.05).

The Bonferroni inequality provides one way of controlling the type 1 error rate for the set of decisions. If each null hypothesis is tested with a type 1 error rate of α/k, then the type 1 error rate for the set of k decisions cannot exceed α. In the example, one could test each of the three null hypotheses at a probability level of less than 0.05/3=0.0167), and thereby ensure that the error rate for the set of three tests cannot exceed 0.05.

Analysis of variance

A more commonly used method for making inferences in multiple group research designs is the analysis of variance. The analysis of variance (ANOVA) controls the type 1 error rate for tests of all possible differences between population means by testing a *joint null hypothesis*, a null hypothesis that all means are equal. In the case of the three group design outlined above (drug 1, drug 2 and placebo) the joint null hypothesis would be: $H_0 : u_1 = u_2 = u_3.$

The test of this null hypothesis is logically equivalent to a simultaneous test of all possible comparisons between pairs of means since, if all means are equal, then all possible comparisons should have a value of zero. Since ANOVA controls the type 1 error rate for the test of this joint null hypothesis, it ensures that the chances of making an error in the set of decisions cannot exceed α, the chosen type 1 error rate.

ANOVA tests the joint null hypothesis by means of an F-ratio (named in honour of R A Fisher) which is a ratio of variation *between groups* (MSB) to variation *within groups* (MSW). The former is derived from the squared deviations of each group mean from the grand mean of all observations; the latter from squared deviations of each individual's score from the mean of their group.

ANOVA assumes a model of the data in which each individual's score is composed of two components: treatment effects (if any) and error variance. Given this model, MSB estimates a composite of the squared treatment effects and error variance, while MSW estimates only error variance. When there are no treatment effects (ie all populations have the same mean) both quantities will estimate the same thing, namely, error variance. Hence their ratio should have an approximate value of 1.0.

In deciding whether an F-ratio is sufficiently large to conclude that there are treatment effects, one makes use of the same logic as was used in the t-test. The null hypothesis is assumed to be true (and thus all means are equal). One estimates how likely the obtained F-ratio would have arisen if the null hypothesis is true, by referring its value to tables of the F-distribution. If the probability of the obtained value arising is less than the conventionally accepted value (ie less than 0.05) the null hypothesis is rejected.

If the joint null hypothesis cannot be rejected, then no further testing is required to establish that the null hypothesis referring to individual comparisons cannot be rejected. If the joint null hypothesis is rejected, then it is not the case that all means are equal. Other tests are necessary in this case to identify precisely which population means differ from each other.

The analysis of multivariate data

Multivariate research designs, those in which subjects are measured on more than one dependent variable, are common in psychiatric research. If, in our example above, the researcher has measured the patient responses to each of the two antidepressant drugs and placebo by measuring depression on a number of scales (for example, on Beck, Hamilton and Zung scales) this study would be both multiple group and multivariate.

If the researcher used multiple t-tests to test three null hypotheses on each of the three outcome measures, then the type 1 error rate for the set of decisions would be less than, or equal to, 0.45 (ie 9 x 0.05). Although the Bonferroni inequality could be used to control the type 1 error rate, there are problems associated with its use. First, there is a substantial reduction in the statistical power (the probability of correctly rejecting the null hypothesis) for each individual test. Second, the *pattern* of relationships between different outcome measures is ignored. Multivariate statistical methods are required to overcome the second of these problems.

Multivariate statistical analyses take account of the pattern of relationships between the dependent variables by testing hypotheses about differences between populations on combinations of the dependent variables in which the scores on each measure are weighted positively or negatively, or given a zero weighting (linear combination). Different techniques define linear combinations in different ways. The following are the main methods.

Principal components analysis

Principal components analysis (PCA) defines linear combinations in such a way as to maximise the amount of variance 'explained' in the original variables. The first principal component (PC_1) is the linear combination of the dependent variable which has the largest variance. The second PC is the linear combination of the dependent variables with the next largest variance, subject to the constraint that it is uncorrelated with PC_1. Subsequent PCs are defined in an analogous manner. Each accounts for the maximum variance, subject to the constraint that it is uncorrelated with the previous PCs.

In general, a set of real data will require as many PCs as there are dependent variables to explain all the variance in the data. However, if the dependent variables have been chosen to measure a single construct (for example, depression in the previous example), it is often possible to summarise most of the variance in the original dependent variables by a small number of PCs. For example, a PCA of the three depression scales might indicate that the average of the three scores accounts for most of the variation in the data. If this were the case, the effect of the two drugs and the placebo on depression could be assessed by comparing the scores obtained in each group on the sum of the three depression scales.

Multivariate analysis of variance (MANOVA)

MANOVA is the multivariate analogue of ANOVA (the analysis of variance). It enables hypothesis about differences between groups to be tested on linear combinations of the dependent variables. MANOVA enables one to decide, for example, whether two groups differ on any linear combination of the measurements of the dependent variables. It does so by finding the linear combination which produces the greatest discrimination between groups. It controls the type 1 error rate at α for the test of the hypothesis that there is no difference between populations on any combination of variables. The linear combination which has the largest F-ratio is called the *discriminant function.*

If the discriminant function fails to achieve statistical significance, one concludes that the two populations do not differ on any combination of the measures. If the discriminant function is statistically significant, then one has identified a linear combination of the dependent variables on which the populations probably differ.

The coefficients of the discriminant function, when simplified, make a good starting point for an exploratory analysis to locate the combinations where the populations differ. Follow-up tests can be performed on any linear combination of a priori interest by calculating a conventional F-ratio on that particular linear combination and comparing its squared value with the critical value of the overall MANOVA test.

In multiple group multivariate research designs, the same general approach can be used. The only difference is that, in such cases, there may be more than one discriminant function to interpret. There may be up to J–1 such discriminant functions, in fact, where J is the number of groups.

Repeated measures data

Research studies which employ the same groups of subjects measured on several occasions (for example, before treatment, after treatment and at six months follow up) are called repeated measures designs. The data from such studies can be treated as a special case of multivariate data in which the repeated measures are regarded as dependent variables which are measured in the same units. Hypotheses about differences between groups in rates and degrees of change over occasions can be tested by examining linear combinations of scores over these occasions. When all hypotheses about differences between the groups and the occasions are specified independently of the data, they can be tested by means of Bonferroni-adjusted tests. When the hypotheses are defined following inspection of the data, MANOVA can be used to test the null hypothesis that the populations do not differ in the way that the mean scores change across the occasions of measurement. The advantage of MANOVA over more conventional univariate repeated measures analysis of variance is that the latter requires assumptions about the data which are often false in behavioural data which inflate type 1 error rate.

Multivariate correlational analysis

The multiple comparison problem also arises in research designs which examine the relationship between two or more variables.

For example, if one measures a cohort of inpatients on a battery of six psychological tests, and examines all possible correlations between the scores on these tests, there would be 15 t-tests of the null hypothesis that the correlation between two variables was zero. If the type 1 error rate was set at 0.05 for each individual test, the type 1 error rate for the *set* of tests could be as high as 0.75 (0.05 x 15). The Bonferroni inequality could be used to control the type 1 error rate for the set at 0.05 by testing each correlation with a type 1 error rate of 0.05/15 (ie 0.00333).

Multiple regression analysis (MRA)

A special type of multiple correlational analysis arises when a researcher wishes to use a set of variables to predict a person's score on a single outcome variable. For example, the battery of six psychological tests mentioned above may be used to predict a patient's score on a depression inventory at six month follow up. In this case, the strategy of testing all possible pairs of correlations would be an inefficient way of examining how well the test scores predict outcome. It would be more efficient to examine the possibility that linear combinations of the predictor variables do better than any of them singly. The latter type of question is best addressed by multiple regression analysis.

Two types of multiple regression analysis— simultaneous and hierarchical—can be distinguished in terms of the questions that they address. Simultaneous multiple regression analysis enables a hypothesis to be tested that there is no relationship between any combination of the predictors and the outcome variable. It searches for the linear combination of predictors which has the largest correlation coefficient with the outcome variable.

If this correlation is not statistically significant, one cannot reject the null hypothesis that there is no relationship between the set of predictors and the outcome variable. If this correlation is statistically significant one can reject the null hypothesis, and the linear combination of the predictors which leads to rejection of the null hypothesis provides the starting point for follow-up tests.

The regression coefficients (the coefficients each predictor variable receives in the *regression equation*) indicated the independent contribution of each variable, given the scores on the other variables, to the prediction of the outcome.

Hierarchical multiple regression is a technique for testing hypotheses about the incremental contribution of individual variables to prediction. It examines what each variable adds to our ability to predict the outcome. For example, one may be interested in asking: 'what does the 'locus of control' scale add to the ability of the 'neuroticism' scale to predict the severity of neurotic symptoms at six months' follow up?' In this case, the 'neuroticism' score would be entered first into the multiple regression analysis and its ability to predict neurotic symptoms examined in the standard way. Then, the 'locus of control' scale would be entered into the analysis to see if the new regression equation was better able to predict outcome than the equation which only included the neuroticism scale. This would be assessed by examining whether the increase in the squared correlation coefficient after the addition of 'locus of control' was statistically significant.

Canonical correlation analysis (CANONA)

When there are multiple predictor and outcome variables, multiple regression is no longer appropriate. For example, one may wish to use a battery of six psychological tests to predict outcome at six month follow up on four measures of depression symptoms. One could carry out four separate multiple regression analyses using the six predictors to predict each outcome variable separately, but this strategy would take no account of the correlations between the four outcome measures. An appropriate multivariate statistical method in the case is canonical correlation analysis (CANONA).

CANONA tests the overall null hypothesis that all correlations between combinations of variables in the predictor and outcome sets are zero. It does so by obtaining linear combinations of the predictor and outcome variables which produce the largest possible correlation coefficient. If this canonical correlation is not significant, one accepts the null hypothesis that there is no relationship between the predictor and outcome variable sets. If it is significant, the null hypothesis can be rejected. The coefficients of the canonical functions provide a starting point for follow-up tests to identify linear combinations of predictor and outcome variables that have meaning clinically.

Multivariate categorical data

Multivariate categorical data arise when subjects are cross-classified on more than two categorical variables. For example, a researcher may want to predict whether or not depressed patients commit suicide after treatment, using as a predictors gender (male or female), Newcastle depression diagnosis (endogenously or neurotically depressed), treatment (ECT or not) and family history of depression or not. A common way of dealing with such data is to perform multiple chi-square tests on pairs of the variables making up the multiple classification. Such a strategy is analogous to performing multiple t-tests, and it suffers from the same problem of failing to control the type 1 error rate for the set of tests. The problem in controlling the type 1 error rate for the set can be dealt with by using Bonferroni-adjusted critical values but this ignores relationships between combinations of categorical variables. Better approaches to the analysis of multivariate categorical data make use of log-linear models to test for interactions between the variables making the cross-classification.

Summary

Descriptive statistics provide a way of economically characterising the scores of a sample of patients on multi-item scales, and of comparing an individual's score with that of a reference group. Inferential statistics provide a basis for making an inference from the characteristics of a sample to the characteristics of the population from which the sample was taken.

The most commonly used form of statistical inference in psychiatry is the null hypothesis significance test which exercises a degree of control over unconstrained speculation by demanding that researchers first demonstrate that any relationships in their data cannot be attributed to chance. The logic of the null hypothesis significance test is simple: assume that the null hypothesis is true, estimate the probability of the relationship in the data occurring, reject the null hypothesis if this probability is sufficiently small (by the usual convention less than 0.05) or, otherwise, fail to reject the null hypothesis.

The most frequently used forms of tests of the null hypothesis are (i) the t-test for relationships between two continuous variables, or for differences between two populations on a continuous dependent variable, and (ii) the chi-square test for relationships between two categorical variables, or for differences between two populations in the proportion of cases falling into a particular category. More complicated forms of data require different tests. When there are multiple groups of patients being compared on a single continuous dependent variable the analysis of variance (ANOVA) is the method of choice, with appropriate follow-up tests to detect the pattern of departures from equality of means.

Multivariate statistical methods are appropriate when patients are measured on many dependent variables and the researcher is interested in either examining the relationships between these variables, or in testing hypotheses about differences between the groups on sets of dependent variables. In the case of continuous variables, relationships between measures can be examined by principal components analysis, multiple regression analysis, and canonical correlational analysis. Principal components analysis can provide useful linear combinations of multiple dependent variables based on the pattern of their inter-correlations. Multiple regression analysis can be used to identify linear combinations of a set of variables which best predict some outcome. Canonical correlational analysis (CANOVA) can be used to explore relationships between linear combinations of sets of predictor and outcome variables. Log-linear models can be used to test hypotheses about relationships between multiple categorical variables.

Multivariate analysis of variance (MANOVA) can be applied to test hypotheses about differences between populations on linear combinations of dependent variables.

Further Reading

Bird K D and Hall W, 'Statistical Power in Psychiatric Research', *Australian and New Zealand Journal of Psychiatry*, Vol 20, 1986, pp 189–200.

Cohen J and Cohen P, *Applied Multiple Regression/Correlation Analysis for the Behavioural Sciences*, Lawrence Erlbaum Hillsdale, 1975.

Finlay-Jones R and Brown G W, 'Types of Stressful Life Events and the Onset of Anxiety and Depressive Disorders', *Psychological Medicine*, Vol 11, 1981, pp 803–815.

Hall W and Bird K D, 'The Problem of Multiple Inference in Psychiatric Research', *Australian and New Zealand Journal of Psychiatry*, Vol 19, 1985, pp 265–74.

Hall W and Bird K D, 'Simultaneous Multiple Comparison Procedures in Psychiatric Research', *Australian and New Zealand Journal of Psychiatry*, Vol 20, 1986, pp 46–54.

Harris R J, *A Primer of Multivariate Statistics*, Academic Press, New York, 1985.

Lumsden J, *Elementary Statistical Method*, University of Western Australia Press, Perth, 1971.

Tabachnick B G and Fidell L S, *Using Multivariate Statistics*, Harper and Rowe, New York, 1983.

Index

AIDS (*see* **Acquired immunodeficiency syndrome**)

Aboriginal mental health *305–12*
contemporary issues *308–11*
alcoholism *308*
death in custody *308*
delinquency *308*
failure to thrive *308*
incarceration *308*
Kimberley region, in *308*
mortality *308*
petrol sniffing *308*
poor educational achievement *308*
recidivism *308*
suicide and self-destructive behaviour *308*
problems *307*
psychiatry and Aborigines *305*
role of mental health professionals *311*

Acquired immunodeficiency syndrome (AIDS) in adults *377–82* (*see also* **AIDS in children**)
AIDS cases reported to WHO (Table 1) *377*
CNS complications (Table 4) *379*
clinical features (see also *370*) *379*
dementia complex, of (Table 5) *379*
clinical manifestation (Table 3) *378*
coping with *373, 379*
definition for (Table 2) *377*
neurological manifestations *377*
psychiatric illness *372, 380–81*
adjustment disorder *380*

depressive illness *380*
mania *380*
schizophrenia-like psychosis *380*
treatment *371, 380*
education *381*
psychotherapy *380*
psychotropic medication *380, 392, 393, 396, 397, 398*
special issues *381–82*
death and dying *382*
ethical *381*
fear of infection *381*
sexuality *382*
staff *382*
stigma *382*

Acquired immunodeficiency syndrome (AIDS) in children and adolescents (*see also* **AIDS in adults**) *370–76*
coping *373, 379*
counselling needs *373*
education *374*
content *375*
a shared responsibility *375*
ethical issues *374, 381*
features of HIV infection *370, 379*
opportunistic infection *370*
neuropsychiatric disorders *372, 380–81*
behaviour problems *372*
dementia *372*
emotional problems *372*
encephalitis *372*
intellectual deficit *372*
memory deficit *372*
meningitis *372*
perceptual changes *372*
management *371*
transmission of HIV virus
children and adolescents, to *372*

infected breast feeding *372*
infected pregnancy *372*
injection of contaminated blood product *372*
sexual intercourse *371*
sharing drug needles *371*
transfusion *372*

Adolescent development *49–56*
cognitive *50*
formal operations *50*
emotional *51*
'false self' *53*
foreclosure *53*
growth of *51*
identity *51*
individuation *51*
intimate reciprocal relationships *54*
peer relations *54*
pseudomaturity *53*
relatedness *54*
social context *54*
self-image *52*
self-responsibility *52*
separation *51*
sexuality *52*
social context *54*
sub-culture *54*
physical *49*
role of parents *53*
and health professionals *53*
social and cultural context *55*
family *55*
school *55*
teachers *55*

Affective (mood) disorders *190–8*
aetiology *193*
adult social environment *193*
childhood experiences *193*
(*see also* **Death, disharmony and divorce, effects on**

491

children and **Emotional disorders in children**)
genetics *193*
neurobiological factors *194*
personality *193*
physiological factors *194*
recent life events *194*
bipolar, treatment and management of *197*
acute mania *197*
antimanic drugs *197, 392, 393, 396, 397*
continuing *198*
diagnosis *197*
outcome *198*
classification *192*
bipolar *192*
depression *192*
organic *192*
clinical features *190*
major depression *191*
mania *190*
mixed mood states *191*
other depressive states *191*
epidemiology *193*
major depression, treatment and management of *195*
outcome and long term *197*
plan *195*
physical therapies *196*
psychotropic drugs (*see also* **Medication**) *196*
recognition and diagnosis *195*

Alcohol dependence and related problems *276-86*
acute alcohol intoxication *278*
alcohol abuse *278*
alcohol amnestic syndrome (Wernicke-Korsakoff syndrome) *281*
thiamine (vitamin B₁) *281*
alcohol dependence *279*
alcohol hallucinosis *281*
alcohol withdrawal *280*
alcohol withdrawal delirium (delirium tremors) *280*
assessment *284*
causes *276*
family pattern *276*
genetic *276*
learned behaviour *276*
occupation *277*
psychiatric illness *277*
psycho-analytic theory *276*
classification *277*
definition *276*

dementia *282*
idiosyncratic intoxication *278*
management *283*
abstinence *285*
assessment, and *284*
controlled drinking *284*
minimal intervention *284*
primary prevention *283*
secondary prevention *284*
NH & MRC guidelines for responsible drinking (Table 1) *277*
polysubstance dependence *281*
psychological conditions associated with alcoholism, other *282*
anxiety disorders *283*
major depression *282*
morbid jealousy *282*
personality disorders *283*
schizophrenia *283*
responsible drinking in social situations (Table 2) *277*

Anorexia nervosa *241-4*
causes *242-4*
clinical features *241*
eating disorders (*see also* **Bulimia nervosa**) *241-6*
management *243*
prevalence *242*
prognosis *244*
psychopathology *242*

Anxiety disorders *171-9, 184-9*
aetiology *186*
anxiety *184*
disorders *184*
state *184*
symptoms *184*
trait *184*
physical causes (Table 1) *184*
symptoms of anxiety *184*
behavioural *185*
physical *185*
psychological and cognitive *185*
treatment *186*
behaviour therapy *188*
drug *187*
benzodiazepines *187, 393, 398*
beta-blockers *188*
general *186*
monoamine oxidase inhibitors *188, 398*
other drugs *188*

tricyclic antidepressants *187, 390, 397*
psychotherapy *188*

Attention deficit—hyperactivity disorder *167-70*
causes *168*
clinical features *167*
diagnosis *168*
outcome *169*
prevalence *167*
treatment *169*

Behaviour therapy *419-22*
cognitive *402, 405, 419, 421*
models *419*
operant conditioning *419*
social learning theory *403, 420*
techniques *420*
classical conditioning *420, 429*
cognitive *419, 421*
operant conditioning *420*
chaining *420*
extinction *421*
punishment *421*
reinforcement *420*
shaping *420*
social learning *420, 421*

Biological investigations *136-42*
(*see also* **Neurological investigations**)
affective symptoms (Table 4) *140* (*see also* **Affective mood disorders**)
physical causes *140*
anxiety disorders (Table 5) *141* (*see also* **Anxiety disorders**)
differential diagnosis *141*
drug abuse *141*
problems with screening *142*
psychotic patient *138*
and medical disorders (Table 2) *139*
laboratory tests for (Table 3) *140*
history *136*
neuro-endocrine tests *138*
types of laboratory tests *137*
use for laboratory tests (Table 2) *137*

Brain imaging in psychiatry *146-51*
modern technologies *146*

functional *148*
  electro-encephalogram
    (EEG) *144, 148*
  electromyography
    (EMG) *144*
  event-related potentials
    (ERPs) *148*
  magnetoencephalography
    (MEG) *149*
  positron emission
    tomography (PET) *150*
  regional cerebral blood flow
    (RCBF) *149*
  single photo emission
    computed tomography
    (SPECT) *149*
  structural (Figures 1
    and 2) *146*
  computed tomography
    (CT) *146*
  magnetic resonance imaging
    (MRI) *147*
problems and future
  direction *150*
radio-isotope (Table 1) *147*
spectrum of brain imaging
  systems employed in
  psychiatry (Table 1) *147*

Bulimia nervosa *244-6*
causes *245*
clinical features *244*
management (*see also* **Anorexia
  nervosa**) *245*
prevalence *245*
prognosis *246*

Classification *129-35*
axis I disorders *133*
axis II disorders *134*
  personality *134*
childhood and
  adolescence *132*
categorical and
  dimensional *132, 482*
DSM–III–R axis I
  disorders *133*
anxiety *133*
  separation *133*
  obsessive compulsive *133*
  phobic *134*
disruptive behaviour *133*
eating disorders *134*
  anorexia nervosa *134*
  bulimia *134, 244*
  pica *134*
  rumination *134*
elimination *134*

encopresis *134*
  enuresis *134*
gender identity *134*
  identity *134*
reactive attachments *134*
  failure to thrive *134*
speech disorders *134*
  cluttering *134*
  stuttering *134*
tics *134*
Tourette's syndrome *134*
DSM–III–R, axis II
  disorders *134*
  mental retardation *134*
  pervasive developmental *134*
    autism *134*
  specific developmental *134*
    articulation, co-ordination
      (clumsiness) *134*
    reading (dyslexia) *134*
general *129*
how to classify and
  diagnose *129*
multivariate *133, 486*
practice, in *130*
  Diagnostic and Statistical
    Manuals of Mental
    disorders (DSM) *130, 132*
  International Classifications of
    Diseases (ICD) *130, 132*
why classify? *129*

**Community
  psychiatry** *297-304*
assessment and treatment
  services *302*
  case management *303*
  chronically mentally ill *303*
  crisis intervention *302*
  emergency
    accommodation *302*
  living skills *303*
  peer support *303*
  social activities *303*
  support for relatives *302*
  work *303*
bio-psycho-social system
  (Figure 1) *297*
de-institutionalisation *299*
  evaluation of *300*
  objection of *300*
  provision of alternative
    services *300*
  maintenance of mentally ill in
    the community *301*
  organisational models *302*
  reduction of hospital
    admisssions *301*

theoretical orientation
  (Figure 2) *298*
**Death, disharmony and divorce,
  effects on children** *67-72*
death of a parent *67*
factors modifying effects on
  children *69*
  economic *70*
  institutionalisation *70*
  parenting *69*
  parents' post divorce
    contact *69*
  re-marriage *70*
  social relationship *70*
adult life *71*
  attitudes to marriage and
    pre-marital pregnancy *71*
  marriage and its quality *71*
  vulnerability to other
    stressors *71*
family disharmony and
  divorce *68*
Delirium *272-5*
aetiology *273*
clinical course *274*
clinical features *272*
definition *272*
diagnosis *274*
differential diagnosis *273*
epidemiology *273*
management *274*
prognosis *274*
risk factors *273*
Dementia *266-71*
assessment and
  diagnosis *259-68*
causes *267*
  AIDS *267*
  alcohol *267*
  Alzheimer's disease *267*
  cerebral circulation *267*
  endocrine disorders *267*
    thryoid diseases *267*
  Huntington's chorea *267*
  meningioma *267*
  multi-infarct *267*
  normal pressure
    hydrocephalus *267*
  Parkinson's disease *267*
  subdural haematoma *267*
  syphilis *267*
  vitamin deficiency *267*
clinical course and
  prognosis *269*
definition and clinical
  features *266*
differential diagnosis *268*

delirium   *268, 272, 273*
depression   *195, 268, 390, 397, 398*
focal brain lesion   *269*
mental retardation   *269*
schizophrenia (*see also* **Schizophrenia**)   *268*
epidemiology   *267*
management   *269*
availability of interventions   *269*
behavioural   *270*
aggressive patients, of   *270*
wandering patients, of   *270*
legal mechanism for intervention   *271*
psychotropic drugs   *269, 395*
residential care   *269*
risk factors   *267*

Development in children   *15*
defence mechanisms   *22-4*
denial   *23*
displacement   *23*
dissociation   *23*
identification   *23*
intellectualisation   *23*
introjection   *23*
isolation   *23*
projection   *23*
rationalisation   *23*
reaction formation   *23*
regression   *23*
repression   *23*
somatisation   *23*
sublimation   *23*
undoing   *23*
drawing   *31*
course of   *32*
use of   *32*
dreams   *32*
factors influencing development   *15*
ability and disability   *16*
birth   *15*
child rearing practices   *17*
constraint   *17*
discipline and aggression   *17*
effect of television   *18*
temper tantrum   *17*
feeding   *17*
over-protection and constraint   *17*
constitution   *15*
ethnic group   *20*
experience and environment   *16*

genes   *15*
gestation   *15*
ordinal position   *19*
preconception   *15*
social class   *19*
socio-cultural   *19*
temperament   *15*
difficult   *16*
personality, and response to stress   *16*
stability   *16*
play   *29-31*
culture, and   *29*
definition   *29*
sex, and   *29*
therapy   *31*
types of   *29*
games with rules   *31*
practice   *29*
symbolic   *30*
sleep and its disorders   *36*
hypersomnia   *37*
insomnia   *37*
nightmares   *37*
night terror   *37*
restlessness   *37*
sleep talking   *38*
sleep walking (somnambulism)   *38*
treatment   *38*
social behaviour   *27*
acute distress reaction on separation   *28*
attachment   *28*
morality   *27*
smiling   *27*
socialisation   *27*
theories of development   *20*
psychoanalytic   *20*
anal phase   *21*
latency period   *22*
oral (first year)   *20*
phallic phase   *21*
Piaget's concept of cognitive   *24*
concrete   *26-7*
pre-operational   *25*
intuitive   *25*
preconceptual   *25*
sensory motor   *24*
social learning   *20*

Development in middle and later life   *57-61*
contextual factors   *61*
developmental sequences   *59*
stages and themes   *58*

Disruptive behaviour (*see also* **Attention deficit—hyperactivity disorder**)   *161-6*
conduct disorders   *17, 18, 19, 162*
aggression   *162*
socialisation   *162*
types   *162*
group   *162*
solitary-aggressive   *162*
undifferentiated   *162*
oppositional-defiant disorder   *161*
treatment   *163-6*

Eating disorders (*see* **Anorexia nervosa; Bulimia**)   *241-6*

Emergencies   *328-34*
classification   *328*
disorganised behaviour   *332*
epidemiology   *328*
management of   *330*
suicide   *329, 330* (*see also* **Suicidal behaviour; Affective (mood) disorders**)
paranoid behaviour   *333*
suicidal behaviour   *329*
assessment   *329*
management   *330*
stupor   *333*
violent behaviour   *331*
assessment   *330*
determinant of (Table 1)   *331*
management   *332*

Emotional disorders in children   *171-9*
anxiety   *28, 31, 172, 189, 210*
DSM-III-R, and   *171*
avoidant disorders   *171*
over-anxious disorders   *171*
separation anxiety   *28, 171*
depressive   *175, 191, 192*
ICD-9, and   *171*
anxiety and fearfulness   *171*
misery and unhappiness   *171*
sensitivity, shyness and social withdrawal   *171*
prevalence   *171*
suicide (*see also* **Suicidal behaviour**)   *176*
treatment   *177*
family therapy   *177, 408-18*
group   *178*
hospitalisation   *178*
milieu   *178, 427*
physical   *177*

medication   *177, 389-99*
psychological   *178, 400, 403*
psychodynamic   *178*
social environment   *178*

Encopresis (soiling)   *98-100*
clinical picture   *98*
  aggressive   *99*
  regressive   *99*
  retention   *98*
  training   *98*
investigation   *99*
outcome   *100*
treatment   *99*

Epidemiology   *471-9*
current findings, summary
  of   *474*
defining disorders to be
  studied   *472*
incidence and prevalence   *472,
  476*
measures and rates   *476*
possible cause   *471*
prevalence (Table 1)   *478*
  life   *476*
  period   *476*
  point   *476*
psychiatric, development
  of   *477*
sources of data   *472*
strategies   *472*
study designs   *477*
  cross sectional   *477*
  longitudinal   *477*

Family therapy   *408-18*
clinical aspects   *412*
clinical application   *413*
general consideration   *408*
individual in   *413*
marital system   *416*
socio cultural context   *412*
treating the system   *415*

Feminist perspective   *361-4*

Forensic psychiatry   *335-44*
confidentiality   *342*
criminal justice system   *335*
criminal law   *335*
dangerousness   *339*
  mental illness and   *339*
  prediction of   *339*
defence of insanity   *337*
  automatism   *338*
  diminished responsibility   *338*
  hospital orders   *338*
diseases of the mind   *337*
evidence in court   *336*

Family Court and Children's
  Court   *339*
fitness to plead   *336*
freedom of information   *344*
informed consent   *343*
legal system   *336*
psychiatry in prisons   *340*
sources of law   *335*
testamentary capacity   *343*
treatment orders   *339*

Fostering and adoption   *73-8*
adoption   *74*
adoptive parents   *76*
fostering   *73*
relinquishing parents   *76*
special circumstances   *77*
special problems   *75*
telling the child   *77*
temporary adjustment
  problems   *77*

Gender identity   *251*

Genes   *15*
genetic factors   *200, 224, 247,
  276*

Genetic counselling   *465*

Gilles de la Tourette's syndrome
  (*see* **Tourette's syndrome**)

**History of mental health
  services in Australia and
  New Zealand**   *3-11*
allied health professionals   *9*
Australian States and New
  Zealand   *5-7*
early treatment methods   *6*
general hospital and community
  psychiatric services   *9*
profession of psychiatry   *7*
psychiatric nursing   *8*

Hypnosis   *423-6*
assessment of   *425*
contra-indications   *426*
definition   *423*
indications for   *425*
phenomena of (Table 1)   *424*
precautions   *426*
theories of   *423*
  physiological   *423*
  psychological   *423*
  trance induction   *424*
  deepening of   *425*

**Immunology and mental
  illness**   *365-9*
immunity and physical
  illness   *367*

coping and cancer   *368*
  stress   *367*
immunity and psychiatric
  illness   *366*
  depression   *367*
  schizophrenia   *220, 214, 366*
immunity and stress   *365*

Interviewing adults   *121-8*
general considerations   *121*
presentation of data   *127*
presentation of problem   *123*
structure of interview   *123*
  additional information   *126*
  concluding   *127*
  family and personal
    history   *123*
  formulation   *127*
  past medical and psychiatric
    history   *124*
  presenting problem   *123*
  mental status
    examination   *124*
  affect or mood   *125, 190*
  appearance   *118, 129*
  behaviour   *118, 129*
  cognition   *126*
  conversation   *129*
  insight   *126*
  intelligence   *126*
  mood (*see* affect)   *125*
  perception   *125, 220*

Interviewing children   *115-20*
background information   *115*
interview   *116*
interviewing   *117*
  the child   *117, 226*
  the family   *117*
mental state examination   *118*
  appearance   *118, 124*
  behaviour   *118, 124*
  cognitive   *119, 126*
  insight and judgment   *126,
    229*
  language   *119*
  mood or affect   *119*
  motor function   *119*
  relationship   *119*
  self-concept   *119*
  sensorium   *119*
  thoughts   *119*
physical examination   *120*

Jealousy   *282*

Joint null hypothesis   *485*

**Learning disabilities
  (LD)**   *93-7*
assessment   *93*

classification   93
  academic skills   93
    arithmetic   93
    language and speech   93
    reading   93
    writing   93
  motor skills (*see also*
    Occupational therapy)   93
  definition   93
  factors associated with   94
  PET (*see also* **Neurological
    investigations**)   94
  intervention and remedial
    education   96
  mathematical   94
    and psychiatric disorders   96
  prognosis   97
  psychiatric disorders and
    reading difficulties   95
  conduct disorder   95
  specific reading retardation   93
    and associated factors   93
    and psychiatric disorders   95
    assessment   95
    differential diagnosis   95
    medication   97
  specific spelling retardation   94

Medication   389-99
  administration   390
  anticholinergics/antihistaminics
    393
  antidepressants   390, 397
    MAOI   398
    tricyclic   397
  carbamazepine   393
  child as patient, the   389
  clonidine   393
    ADHD   169, 393
    Tourette's disorder   393
    and haloperidol   393
  compliance   390
  developmental issues   389
  discussion   393
  dosage   396
  exclusion diet   393
  lithium carbonate   392, 397
  major agents (Table 1)   396
  minor tranquillisers   393, 398
    anti-anxiety and
      hypnotics   398
  mood stabilisers   397
    lithium carbonate   397
  neuroleptics
    (antipsychotics)   395
    ADHD   169, 392
    aggressive conduct
      disorders   392

chronic tic disorder   392
  lithium   392, 397
  Tourette's disorder   392
some general issues with drug
  use   169, 291, 399
stimulants   391
  amphetamine   391
  methylphenidate   391

Mental Health Acts   345-58
  assessment of sick   353
  concept of mental illness   356
  definition of mental illness   357
  dementia
  NSW law on (Appendix)   357
  general   345
  non-custodial treatment orders
    scope of application   354
  non-voluntary treatment   346
  principles   348
  procedures   355
  requirement of presence of
    mental illness   349
  scope of authority to administer
    treatment   356
  scope of present status and
    direction of change   346
  voluntary treatment   346

Mental retardation   81-7
  causes   83-4
  clinical features   82-3
  psychiatric disorders   81-2
  sexuality   86
  syndromes   84
    affective   85
    anxiety   84
    attention deficit   84
    autism   84, 88
    conduct   85
    organic mental disorders   84
    personality   85
    schizophrenia   85, 220
  testing mentally ill   86
  treatment   86

**Multicultural
    psychiatry**   320-7
  general consideration   320
  cultural influences   19, 323
  emigration   20, 323
  language of culture   207, 321
  practice of   326

**Neglect and abuse of
    children**   62-6
  physical abuse   63
  prevention   65
  sexual abuse   64

Neurological investigations (*see
    also* **Biological
    investigations**)   143-5
  medical investigations   143
  specific neurological
    investigation   143
    computerised tomography
      scanning of the brain
      (CT scan)   144
  electroencephalography
    (EEG)   144
  lumbar puncture (CSF)   143
  magnetic resonance imaging
    (MRI)   144
  other investigations   144
    cerebral angiography   144
    electromyography   144
    evoked potentials   144
    positron emission
      tomographic scanning
      (PET)   144
    radioactive isotope
      studies   144
    radiography of the
      skull   144

Nocturnal enuresis   101-5
  aetiology   101
  clinical features   101
  definition   101
  emotional factors   102
  initial investigation   103
  medical screening   103
  physical factors   101
  psychological factors   103
  treatment   103
    conditioning   104
    medical   103
    simple behavioural
      measures   103

**Nursing for mental
    health**   427-32
  future responsibility   431
  nursing roles   428
    advocate   429
    counsellor   430
    milieu therapy   430
    planner   429
    team member   429
  trends influencing   427

Obesity   247-9
  genetic   247
  illness, and   247
  management   248

**Obsessive compulsive
    disorders**   208-12
  aetiology/causes   209, 211

clinical features *211*
  compulsion *210*
  obsession *210*
  rumination *210*
definition *208*
diagnosis *208, 211*
differential diagnosis *209*
outcome *209*
prevalence *208, 211*
treatment *209, 212*

Occupational therapy *438–46*
activities *438*
  play *438*
  work *438*
adolescents, and *442*
areas of practice *441*
child psychiatry, and *441*
community work, and *445*
models of treatment *439*
  cognitive disabilities *439*
  functional group *440*
  human occupation *439*
  intervention strategies
    (Table 1) *440*
  re-capitulation of growth *439*
rehabilitation of adults *443*
rehabilitation of the
    elderly *444*

Pain *231–5*
conversion disorders *232*
hypochondriasis *232*
management of chronic, non-
    malignant *233*
  cognitive-behaviour
    therapy *234, 419*
  general principles *233*
  marital and family
    therapy *235*
  psychopharmacological *234,
    389*
  psychotherapeutic *234, 400*
  relaxation and biofeed-
    back *234*
prognosis *235*
psychological significance
    of *233*
somatisation disorders *232*
somatoform pain disorder *233*

Personality disorders *100–12*
cluster A *107*
  paranoid *107*
  schizoid *107*
  schizotypal *107*
cluster B *108*
  antisocial *108–9*
  borderline *109*

  histrionic *109*
  narcissistic *109*
cluster C *109*
  avoidant *110*
  dependent *110*
  obsessive-compulsive *110*
  passive-agressive *110*
DSM–III–R, and *110*
  disorder of impulse
    control *110*
ICD–9, and *110*
  explosive *110*
sadistic *110*
self-defeating *110*
treatment *111*

**Pervasive developmental
    disorders (PDD)** *88–92*
autism *88*
  criteria for diagnosis *88*
  language and speeech
    disorders (Table 2) *88*
  obsessive-compulsive
    phenomena (Table 3) *89*
  other symptoms
    (Table 4) *89*
  social behaviour
    (Table 1) *88*
aetiology *89*
associated factors and
    features *89*
course and prognosis *92*
differential diagnosis *90*
  autistic-like syndromes *90*
  disintegrative psychosis *90,
    218*
  later onset autistic-like
    syndrome *90*
  other disorders *90*
    blind children *91*
    hearing defect *91*
    Leber's congenital
      amaurosis *91*
    very anxious/shy
      children *91*
  schizophrenia-like
    syndrome *90, 214, 220*
  very severe specific
    developmental language
    disorder *90, 448, 452*
treatment *91*
  education *91*

**Post traumatic stress
    disorder** *236–40*
aetiology *237*
assessment *238*
clinical features *236*

  onset *237*
  management *239*
  prevalence *237*

**Pregnancy, birth and
    parenthood** *40*
accidental crisis in
    reproduction *44*
  crisis of miscarriage *46*
  infertility and new
    reproductive
    technology *44*
  perinatal bereavement *46*
  postnatal depressive *46*
birth *43*
bonding during the critical
    period *44*
psychology of normal
    pregnancy *40*
  desire for children *40*
  developmental crisis
    (Fig 1) *41–3*
  losses and threats *41*

**Prevention of mental
    illness** *460–8*
biological *465*
  genetic counselling *465*
crisis intervention
  forms of *468*
legislative programs *465*
mental hygiene programs, the
    problem of *460*
parents and children *466*
stress, life events and stress
    management (Fig 1) *461*
stress model and social
    change *463*
telephone counselling *465*
unemployment and mental
    health *461*

Psychiatry of late life *256–65*
assessment and
    management *259*
  behavioural approaches *261*
  diversional therapy *262*
  drugs *260*
  medical tests *259*
  occupational therapy *262*
  psychological tests *259*
  psychotherapy *261*
  self-help group *263*
  social work *261*
different ethnic
    background *262*
ethical and legal issues *263*
  euthanasia *264*
  informed consent *263*

rights versus risks   263
grief   258
mental disorders   256
  alcoholism   257
  benzodiazepine abuse   257
  delirium   256
  depression   256
  paranoid   277
  personality   257
  schizophrenia (see also
     Schizophrenia)   256
  sleep   258
  suicide   258
normal experience of
     ageing   258
retirement   258
problem of morale   262
service provision   260
  community treatment and
     burden of caring   260
  institutions   260
  property management   265

Psychological testing   152–8
academic achievement   95, 155
  Neale analysis of reading
     ability   156
  wide range achievement test
     (WRAT)   156
  Woodcock-Johnson   156
adaptive behaviour and
     behaviour problems   156
  child behaviour checklist
     (Achenbach and
     Edelbrock)   156
  Vineland scales   156
background   152
classification for intelligence
     quotients (Table 1)   154
intelligence tests   153, 154
  developmental tests   153
     Bayley   153
     McCarthy   154
     Stanford-Binet   154
     Wechsler   155
       for children   155
       for adults   155
       for pre-school and
          primary   155
  nature of   152
  neuro-psychological   158
  personality   157
     Eysenck & Eysenck   157
     high school (Cattell, Cattell
        and Johns)   157
     house-tree-person   157
     Minnesota   157

Rorschach ink blot   158
  use of   152
WISC–R   155
WPPSI   155

**Psycho-sexual development and
     function problems**   250–5
gender identity   251
  during childhood   251
  transsexualism   251
homosexuality   252
paraphilias   252
  exhibitionism   252
  paedophilia   253
  sexual sadism   253
sexual arousal   263
  aetiology   254
  most common disorders   254
     dyspareunia   254
     erectile dysfunction   254
     inhibited orgasm   254
     premature ejaculation   254
     vaginismus   254
theories   250
treatment   254

**Psychosis in
     adolescents**   214–19
affective (see also **Affective
     (mood) disorders**)   190,
     216
disintegrative   90, 218
drug induced   218, 276, 278,
     280, 281, 283,
schizophrenia   214, 220
(see also **Schizophrenia**)

Psychotheraphy   400–7
cognitive   405
cognitive learning model   402,
     419, 421
crisis intervention   404
group   405
psycho-analytic model   400
psycho-analytic therapies   403
  long term   403
     psycho-analysis   403
     psycho-analytically
        orientated   403
     brief   403
social learning   403, 420
supportive   404

Remote Australia   313–19
methods to assist isolated
     children   316
  educational aspects   316
  mental health   315
  physical health   315
  problems for adults   317

psychological effects of
     isolation   314

SIDS (see **Sudden infant death
     syndrome**)

Schizophrenia   220
aetiology and
     pathogenesis   223
  mediating mechanism   225
     neurochemical   225
     psychophysiological   226
  precipitating factors   225
  predisposing factors   224
     environmental   224
     genetic   224
  perpetuating factors   225
  protective factors   225
  stress-diathesis model
     (Fig 1)   223
clinical features   221
  acute form   221
  prodromal form   221
  residual   222
diagnosis   222
  differential   222
epidemiology   220
outcome   229
rehabilitation   229
subtypes   222
treatment   226
  hospitalisation   226
  medication (see also
     Medication)   227
     antipsychotic   227
     delayed or specific
        effect   227
     immediate or non-specific
        effects   227
     long term effects   227
  electro-convulsive therapy
     (ECT)   228
  psychosocial therapy   228
     behaviour   229
     family   228
     group   228
     individual   228

School refusal   180–3
assessment   181
background   17, 180
clinical features   180
definition   180
management   181
prevalence   180
previous personality   180
prognosis   182

Social work   433–7
case management   435

primary treatment   *433*
rehabilitation   *433*
welfare concept, importance
   of   *435*

**Speech therapy in
   adults**   *452-9*
assessment   *454*
classification   *452*
   dysarthria   *453*
   dysgraphia   *453*
   dysphagia   *453*
   dysphonia   *453*
   dyspraxia   *452*
   expressive dysphasia   *452*
   receptive dysphasia   *452*
   stuttering   *453*
differential diagnosis   *455*
definition   *452*
etiology/associated factors   *453*
management   *457*
outcome   *458*
prevalence   *453*

**Speech therapy in
   children**   *447-51*
assessment   *449*
classification   *447*
   autism   *448*
   cluttering   *448*
   developmental articulation
      disorder   *448*
   developmental expressive
      language disorder   *448*
   developmental receptive
      disorder   *448*
   elective mutism   *448*
   language disorder   *448*
   stuttering   *448*
definition   *447*
differential diagnosis   *449*
etiology/associated factors   *449*
management   *450*
outcome   *450*
prevalence   *449*

Statistical inferences   *480-90*
analysis of multivariate
   data   *486*
   canonical correlational
      analysis   *488*
   correlation coefficient (r)   *481*

multiple regression
   analysis   *488*
multivariate analysis of
   variance   *486*
multivariate categorical
   data   *489*
principal component
   analysis   *486*
repeated measure data   *487*
descriptive   *480*
   central tendency   *480*
   correlation analysis   *481*
   degrees of freedom   *481*
   mean   *480*
   median   *480*
   standard deviation   *481*
   Z-score   *481*
inferential statistics   *482*
   analysis of variance   *485*
      joint null hypothesis   *485*
   Chi-square test
      (Table 2)   *483, 484*
      homogeneity   *484*
      observed frequency   *484*
      test of independence   *484*
   multiple inferences   *485*
      inequalities   *485*
      placebo   *485*
      type 2 error   *485*
   statistical power   *485*
      analysis   *485*
      type of errors   *485*
   t-test   *482*
      dependent variable   *482*
      depression scale experiment
         (Table 1)   *483*
      independent variable   *482*
      null hypothesis   *483*
      probability   *483*
      standard error   *483*
      standard error of
         difference   *483*
      standard error
         frequency   *483*
      t-ratio   *483*
      type I error   *484*

**Sudden infant death syndrome
   (SIDS)**   *383-6*
cause   *383*
incidence   *383*
management   *384*

family reaction   *384*
parents's needs, information
   about   *384*
autopsy   *384*
funeral   *385*
grief   *384*
other children's
   reaction   *384*
police and coroner   *385*
SIDS   *384*
support organisation   *385*

Suicidal behaviour   *199-207*
availability of method   *203*
causes   *200*
   biochemical   *200*
   genetic   *200*
   interpersonal   *203*
   intra-psychic   *203*
   peri-natal   *201*
   physical illness   *201*
   psychiatric illness   *201*
   social   *201*
classification   *200*
management   *204*
   assessment, and   *204*
   bereavement   *206*
   evaluation (Table 1)   *205*
   prevention   *204*
prediction   *204*
prevalence   *204*

Tourette's syndrome   *134, 456*

**Unemployment and mental
   health**   *461, 471*

Violent behaviour   *330*

Voluntary treatment   *346*

Wernicke-Korsakoff Syndrome
   (*see* **Alcohol dependence
   and related problems**)

**Wide range achievement test
   (WRAT)** (*see* **Psychological
   testing**)

WISC-R (*see* **Psychological
   testing**)

Work   *438*

Work related programs   *303*

WPPSI (*see* **Psychological
   testing**)

Writing   *93*